Comprehensive Virology 9

Comprehensive Virology

Edited by Heinz Fraenkel-Conrat
University of California at Berkeley

and Robert R. Wagner
University of Virginia

Volume 1:   *Descriptive Catalogue of Viruses* – by Heinz Fraenkel-Conrat

Reproduction

Volume 2:   *Small and Intermediate RNA Viruses* – Contributors: J.T. August,
L. Eoyang, A. Siegel, V. Hariharasubramanian, L. Levintow,
E. R. Pfefferkorn, D. Shapiro, and W. K. Joklik

Volume 3:   *DNA Animal Viruses* – Contributors: L. Philipson, U. Lindberg, J.A. Rose,
N.P. Salzman, G. Khoury, B. Moss, B. Roizman, and D. Furlong

Volume 4:   *Large RNA Viruses* – Contributors: P.W. Choppin, R.W. Compans,
R.R. Wagner, and J.P. Bader

Volume 7:   *Bacterial DNA Viruses* – Contributors: D.T. Denhardt, D.S. Ray, and
C.K. Mathews

Structure and Assembly

Volume 5:   *Virions, Pseudovirions, and Intraviral Nucleic Acids* – Contributors:
T.I. Tikchonenko, John T. Finch, Lionel V. Crawford, and H. Vasken
Aposhian

Volume 6:   *Assembly of Small RNA Viruses* – Contributors: K.E. Richards,
R.C. Williams, L. Hirth, P.P. Hung, Y. Okada, T. Ohno, and R.R. Rueckert

Volume 13: *Bacterial Virus Sequences and Assembly* – Contributors: G. Air, D.L.D. Caspar,
F. A. Eiserling, W. Fiers, R. V. Gilden, J. King, B. Seston, and W.B. Wood

Regulation and Genetics

Volume 8:   *Bacterial DNA Viruses* – Contributors: D. Rabussay, E. P. Geiduschek,
R. A. Weisberg, S. Gottesman, M. E. Gottesman, A. Campbell, R. Calendar,
J. Geisselsoder, M.G. Sunshine, E.W. Six, and B.H. Lindqvist

Volume 9:   *Genetics of Animal Viruses* – Contributors: H. S. Ginsberg, C. S. H. Young,
W. Eckhart, J. H. Subak-Sharpe, M. C. Timbury, C.R. Pringle, E.R. Pfefferkorn,
P. D. Cooper, L. K. Cross, B. N. Fields, P. K. Vogt, M. A. Bratt,
and L. E. Hightower

Volume 10: *Viral Gene Expression and Integration* – Contributors: A. J. Shatkin,
A. K. Banerjee, G. W. Both, A. S. Huang, D. Baltimore, D. H. L. Bishop,
W. Doerfler, and H. Hanafusa

Volume 11: *Plant Viruses* – Contributors: L. Van Vloten-Doting, E. M. J. Jaspars,
G. Bruening, J. G. Atabekov, H. Fraenkel-Conrat, M. Salvato, L. Hirth,
I. Takebe, T. O. Diener, and A. Hadidi

Additional Topics

Volume 12: *Newly Characterized Protist and Invertebrate Viruses* – Contributors: T. W. Tinsley,
K. A. Harrap, K. N. Saksena, P. A. Lemke, L. A. Sherman, R. M. Brown, Jr.,
T. I. Tikchonenko, and L. Mindich

Volume 14: *Newly Characterized Vertebrate Viruses* – Contributors: P.E. McAllister,
F.L. Schaffer, D.W. Verwoerd, A. Granoff, W.S. Robinson, J.A. Robb,
D.H.L. Bishop, and W.E. Rawls

Interaction of Viruses and Their Hosts (several volumes)
Effects of Physical and Chemical Agents

Comprehensive

Edited by

Heinz Fraenkel-Conrat

Department of Molecular Biology and Virus Laboratory
University of California, Berkeley, California

and

Robert R. Wagner

Department of Microbiology
University of Virginia, Charlottesville, Virginia

Virology

9

Regulation and Genetics

Genetics of Animal Viruses

PLENUM PRESS · NEW YORK AND LONDON

Library of Congress Cataloging in Publication Data

Fraenkel-Conrat, Heinz, 1910-
  Regulation and genetics, genetics of animal viruses.

  (Their Comprehensive virology; v. 9)
  Includes bibliographies and index.
  1. Viral genetics. I. Wagner, Robert R., 1923–   joint author. II. Title. III.
Title: Genetics of animal viruses. IV. Series.
QR357.F72 Vol. 9 [QH434]   576'.64'08   [576'.6484]
ISBN 0-306-35149-8   77-1176

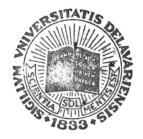

© 1977 Plenum Press, New York
A Division of Plenum Publishing Corporation
227 West 17th Street, New York, N.Y. 10011

Printed in the United States of America

Foreword

The time seems ripe for a critical compendum of that segment of the biological universe we call viruses. Virology, as a science, having passed only recently through its descriptive phase of naming and numbering, has probably reached that stage at which relatively few new—truly new—viruses will be discovered. Triggered by the intellectual probes and techniques of molecular biology, genetics, biochemical cytology, and high-resolution microscopy and spectroscopy, the field has experienced a genuine information explosion.

Few serious attempts have been made to chronicle these events. This comprehensive series, which will comprise some 6000 pages in a total of about 22 volumes, represents a commitment by a large group of active investigators to analyze, digest, and expostulate on the great mass of data relating to viruses, much of which is now amorphous and disjointed, and scattered throughout a wide literature. In this way, we hope to place the entire field in perspective, and to develop an invaluable reference and sourcebook for researchers and students at all levels.

This series is designed as a continuum that can be entered anywhere, but which also provides a logical progression of developing facts and integrated concepts.

Volume 1 contains an alphabetical catalogue of almost all viruses of vertebrates, insects, plants, and protists, describing them in general terms. Volumes 2–4 deal primarily, but not exclusively, with the processes of infection and reproduction of the major groups of viruses in their hosts. Volume 2 deals with the simple RNA viruses of bacteria, plants, and animals; the togaviruses (formerly called arboviruses), which share with these only the feature that the virion's RNA is able to act as messenger RNA in the host cell; and the reoviruses of animals and plants, which all share several structurally singular features, the most important being the double-strandedness of their multiple RNA molecules.

Volume 3 addresses itself to the reproduction of all DNA-containing viruses of vertebrates, encompassing the smallest and the largest viruses known. The reproduction of the larger and more complex RNA viruses is the subject matter of Volume 4. These viruses share the property of being enclosed in lipoprotein membranes, as do the togaviruses included in Volume 2. They share as a group, along with the reoviruses, the presence of polymerase enzymes in their virions to satisfy the need for their RNA to become transcribed before it can serve messenger functions.

Volumes 5 and 6 represent the first in a series that focuses primarily on the structure and assembly of virus particles. Volume 5 is devoted to general structural principles involving the relationship and specificity of interaction of viral capsid proteins and their nucleic acids, or host nucleic acids. It deals primarily with helical and the simpler isometric viruses, as well as with the relationship of nucleic acid to protein shell in the T-even phages. Volume 6 is concerned with the structure of the picornaviruses, and with the reconstitution of plant and bacterial RNA viruses.

Volumes 7 and 8 deal with the DNA bacteriophages. Volume 7 concludes the series of volumes on the reproduction of viruses (Volumes 2–4 and Volume 7) and deals particularly with the single- and double-stranded virulent bacteriophages.

Volume 8, the first of the series on regulation and genetics of viruses, covers the biological properties of the lysogenic and defective phages, the phage-satellite system P 2–P 4, and in-depth discussion of the regulatory principles governing the development of selected lytic phages.

The present volume provides a truly comprehensive analysis of the genetics of all animal viruses that have been extensively studied to date. Described in ten detailed chapters are genotypes and phenotypic expression of conditional, host range, and deletion mutants of three major classes of animal DNA viruses followed by seven genera of RNA viruses. Principles and methodology are presented and compared to provide insight into mechanisms of mutagenesis, selection of mutants, complementation analysis, and gene mapping with restriction endonucleases and other methods. Whenever appropriate, the genetic properties of viruses are related to nucleic acid structure and function as well as recombination, integration of viral with host genome, malignant transformation, and alteration of host cell functions.

The following volume (10) will deal with transcriptional and translational regulation of viral gene expression, defective virions, and integration of tumor virus genomes into host cell chromosomes. Later volumes will be concerned with regulation of plant virus development, covirus systems, satellitism and viroids. Two or three additional volumes will be devoted largely to structural aspects and the assembly of bacteriophages and animal viruses, as well as to special groups of newer viruses.

The complete series will endeavor to encompass all aspects of the molecular biology and the behavior of viruses. We hope to keep this series up to date at all times by prompt and rapid publication of all contributions, and by encouraging the authors to update their chapters by additions or corrections whenever a volume is reprinted.

Contents

Chapter 1

Genetics of Polyoma Virus and Simian Virus 40

Walter Eckhart

1. Introduction 1
2. Restriction Enzyme Maps of the Polyoma and SV40
   Genomes 3
3. The Lytic Growth Cycle 4
   3.1. Viral DNA Replication 4
   3.2. Transcription during Lytic Infection 5
   3.3. Virion Proteins 6
4. Mutants of Polyoma and SV40 8
   4.1. Temperature-Sensitive Mutants 8
   4.2. Host Range Mutants 12
   4.3. Defective Mutants 13
   4.4. Adenovirus–SV40 Hybrid Viruses 14
5. Viral Functions and the Early Region of the Genome 15
   5.1. Cellular DNA Synthesis 15
   5.2. T Antigen 17
   5.3. SV40 Helper Function for Adenovirus Growth 17
6. Temperature-Dependent Properties of Transformed Cells   18
7. References 22

Chapter 2

Genetics of Adenoviruses

Harold S. Ginsberg and C. S. H. Young

1. Introduction 27
   1.1. The Virion 28

xi

    1.2.   Viral Biosynthesis   34
2. Adenovirus Mutants   41
    2.1.   Types of Mutants   41
    2.2.   Mutagenic Procedures   42
    2.3.   Isolation of Mutants   44
    2.4.   Genetic Constitution of the Mutants   46
3. Characteristics of the Adenovirus Genetic System   47
    3.1.   Aims of Genetic Analysis   47
    3.2.   Complementation   47
    3.3.   Recombination and Mapping of the Adenovirus
          Genome   54
4. Phenotypes of Adenovirus Mutants   62
    4.1.   Temperature-Sensitive Mutants   62
    4.2.   Plaque Morphology and Host Range Mutants   66
5. Functional Studies Using Adenovirus Mutants   67
    5.1.   Viral DNA Replication   67
    5.2.   Transcription of the Viral Genome   68
    5.3.   Transport of the Hexon Protein   69
    5.4.   Transformation   70
    5.5.   Helper Function   73
6. Critique and Perspectives   74
7. Note Added in Proof   76
8. References   78

Chapter 3

Genetics of Herpesviruses

John H. Subak-Sharpe and Morag C. Timbury

1. Introduction   89
2. Virus Mutants   93
    2.1.   Specialized Mutants   93
    2.2.   Nonspecialized Mutants: Conditional Lethals   96
    2.3.   Temperature-Sensitive Mutants   97
3. Characterization of Mutants 105
    3.1.   Viral DNA Synthesis 107
    3.2.   Virus-Specified Enzymes 108
    3.3.   Shutoff of Host Cell DNA Synthesis 109
    3.4.   Proteins 109
    3.5.   Particles 112
    3.6.   Temperature-Shift Experiments 112

3.7.   Effect of Host Cells on *ts* Mutant Phenotype 112
3.8.   *ts* Mutants *in Vivo* 113
4.   Recombination 113
5.   Effective Genomes 115
6.   Validity of Recombination Analysis 116
7.   The Genes of HSV 117
8.   Mixed-Morphology Plaques 117
8.1.   Infectious DNA and Marker Rescue 118
8.2.   Thymidine Kinase 119
8.3.   Intertypic Complementation and Recombination .. 120
9.   Transformation 122
10.   Latency 124
11.   References 125

Chapter 4

Genetics of Picornaviruses

Peter D. Cooper

1.   Introduction 133
2.   Definition of a Picornavirus 134
3.   The Schizon 135
4.   Classification of Picornaviruses 136
5.   Genetic Methods 138
5.1.   Markers and Mutant Isolation 139
5.2.   Covariant Reversion 139
5.3.   Temperature-Shift Experiments 140
6.   Interactions of Picornavirus Genomes 141
6.1.   Genetic Recombination 141
6.2.   Genetic Complementation 145
6.3.   Genetic Reactivation 147
6.4.   Phenotypic Mixing 147
6.5.   Homologous Interference-with-Multiplication 147
6.6.   Defective Interfering (DI) Particles 148
6.7.   Homologous Interference-without-Multiplication .. 149
6.8.   Heterologous Interference 150
6.9.   Interferon 151
6.10.   Implications for Gene Function 151
7.   The Genetic Recombination Map of Picornaviruses 152
7.1.   Obtaining a Map for Poliovirus 152
7.2.   Properties of the Genetic Map of Poliovirus 153

    7.3.   Scale of the *ts* Map of Poliovirus 154
    7.4.   The Genetic Map of Aphthovirus 157
  8. Relation of Genetic Map to Gene Functions 157
    8.1.   The "Primary" Gene Functions of Poliovirus 157
    8.2.   The Secondary Gene Functions of Poliovirus 161
    8.3.   Host-Controlled Modification and Nonpermissive
          Cell Systems 166
    8.4.   Summary of Picornavirus Gene Functions 168
  9. Relation of Genetic Map to Gene Products 169
    9.1.   Mode of Production of Picornavirus Polypeptides .. 169
    9.2.   Structural Proteins 169
    9.3.   Replicase Proteins 170
    9.4.   5′-3′ Orientation 172
    9.5.   Cleavage Pathways 173
    9.6.   Information from *in Vitro* Translation 175
    9.7.   Is Picornavirus RNA Comprised of Two
          Independent Translation Units? 176
    9.8.   Cleavage Enzymes 181
 10. Sites of Action of Viral Growth Inhibitors 182
 11. The Strategy of the Picornavirus Genome 184
    11.1. Regulation Mechanisms 184
    11.2. Genome Expression 188
    11.3. The Growth Process as Indicated by Genetic and
          Other Studies 190
 12. Conclusions 195
 13. References 196

Chapter 5

Genetics of Togaviruses

Elmer R. Pfefferkorn

  1. Review of the Structure and Replication of Group A
    Togaviruses 209
  2. Types of Mutants 211
    2.1.   Plaque Morphology Mutants 211
    2.2.   Host Range Mutants 211
    2.3.   Mutants in Which the Stability of the Virion
          Is Altered 212
    2.4.   Mutants in Which the Morphology of the Virion
          Is Altered 212

2.5.   Mutants with Reduced Virulence 213
2.6.   Defective Interfering Mutants 213
2.7.   Temperature-Sensitive Mutants 214
3. Interactions of Togavirus Mutants in Mixed Infections . . 216
3.1.   Phenotypic Mixing 216
3.2.   Recombination 217
3.3.   Complementation 218
3.4.   Interference 222
4. Physiological Defects in Temperature-Sensitive Mutants . 223
4.1.   Temperature-Sensitive Mutants with Defective or
       Altered Viral RNA Synthesis 223
4.2.   Temperature-Sensitive Mutants with an Apparent
       Defect in the Assembly of Nucleocapsids 226
4.3.   Temperature-Sensitive Mutants with Defects
       in Envelope Protein 229
4.4.   Temperature-Sensitive Mutants and the Synthesis
       of Cellular Macromolecules 231
4.5.   Virulence of *ts* Mutants 232
5. References 233

Chapter 6

Genetics of Rhabdoviruses

C. R. Pringle

1. Introduction: Some Relevant Biological Features
   of Rhabdoviruses 239
2. Coding Capacity of the Genome of Rhabdoviruses 241
3. Rhabdovirus Mutants 242
3.1.   Phenotypes 242
3.2.   Spontaneous Mutants 243
3.3.   Induced Mutants 246
3.4.   Techniques for Isolation of *ts* and *hr* Mutants 247
3.5.   Isolation of *tl* Mutants 248
4. Absence of Recombination 249
5. Complementation 250
5.1.   General Characteristics 250
5.2.   Classification of *ts* Mutants into Complementation
       Groups 252
5.3.   Interstrain Complementation 253

6. Temperature-Sensitive Mutants in the Analysis of
    Genome Function 254
    6.1. Phenotype and Complementation Group 254
    6.2. Phenotypic Characterization of the VSV Indiana
          Complementation Groups 256
    6.3. Polymerase Mutants 257
    6.4. Glycoprotein Mutants 262
    6.5. A Nucleoprotein Mutant 263
    6.6. Matrix Protein Mutants 263
7. Defectiveness 265
    7.1. T Particles and *ts* Mutants 265
    7.2. Physical Mapping of the Genome 266
8. Phenotypic Mixing and Pseudotypes 268
9. Host-Controlled Modification 271
10. Virulence and Persistent Infection 272
    10.1. Role of T Particles 272
    10.2. *ts* Mutants and Neurotropism 274
    10.3. *ts* Mutants as Vaccines 277
    10.4. Pathogenesis of Rabies Virus *ts* Mutants in Mice . 277
    10.5. Mechanism of Cell Killing 278
11. Sigma Virus and Germinal Transmission 278
12. Future Prospects 280
13. References 281

Chapter 7

Genetics of Reoviruses

Rise K. Cross and Bernard N. Fields

1. Introduction: Structure and Replication of Reoviruses
    as They Relate to Genetics 291
2. Genetic Interactions 294
    2.1. Conditional Lethal Temperature-Sensitive
          Mutants 294
    2.2. Two-Factor Crosses 295
    2.3. Three-Factor Crosses 301
    2.4. Complementation 304
    2.5. Nongenetic Variables 306
    2.6. Multiplicity Reactivation 307
    2.7. Deletion Mutants 308

3. Gene Function 309
    3.1. Phenotype of Genetic Groups 309
    3.2. Transcription 310
    3.3. Replication 312
    3.4. Translation 314
    3.5. Assembly 318
    3.6. Oligonucleotides 322
    3.7. Specific Gene Lesions 324
4. Effect on Host 331
    4.1. Virus–Cell Interaction 331
    4.2. Role in Disease 334
5. References 336

Chapter 8

Genetics of RNA Tumor Viruses

Peter K. Vogt

1. Introduction 341
    1.1. Scope of This Chapter 341
    1.2. A Synopsis of RNA Tumor Virus Infection 342
2. Basic Properties of the Virus Genome 345
    2.1. The Virion Contains Cellular and Viral RNA 345
    2.2. The Molecular Weight of the 60–70 S RNA Is
          About $6–8 \times 10^6$ 346
    2.3. The 60–70 S Complex Consists of Two 35 S
          RNA Molecules 346
    2.4. The Genome of RNA Tumor Viruses Appears to
          Be Diploid 348
    2.5. The 35 S RNAs of an RNA Tumor Virus Contain
          the Same Sequences in Fixed Order 349
    2.6. The 60–70 S RNA Is an Inverted Dimer of 35 S
          RNAs Linked at the 5′ Ends 350
    2.7. Summary and Conclusions 352
3. Nonconditional Mutants and Markers 353
    3.1. Defective Viruses 354
    3.2. Host Range Variants 372
    3.3. Transformation Markers 378
4. Interactions between RNA Tumor Viruses 380
    4.1. Complementation and Phenotypic Mixing 380
    4.2. Recombination between RNA Tumor Viruses 383

5. Conditional Mutants 389
   5.1. *ts* Mutants of Avian Sarcoma Viruses 390
   5.2. Conditional Mutants of Murine Leukemia and
        Sarcoma Viruses 407
6. Biochemical Approaches to RNA Tumor Virus Genetics . 413
   6.1. RNA Tumor Virus Species: Genetic Relationships
        and Distribution among Various Hosts 413
   6.2. Occurrence and Origin of *src* Sequences 416
   6.3. The Genetic Map of Avian Sarcoma Viruses
        Probably Reads *gag-pol-env-src-C*-poly(A) 418
7. Concluding Speculations 423
   7.1. On Recombination 423
   7.2. The Product of *src* 426
   7.3. Interaction between Virus and Cell Genomes 428
   7.4. Analysis of the Viral Genome and of Integration
        Sites with DNA Restriction Enzymes 429
8. References 430

Chapter 9

Genetics and Paragenetic Phenomena of Paramyxoviruses

Michael A. Bratt and Lawrence E. Hightower

1. Introduction 457
2. Properties Relevant to Genetic Analyses 459
   2.1. Summary of Virus Structure and the Infectious
        Process 460
   2.2. Identification and Synthesis of Viral Proteins 461
   2.3. Identification and Synthesis of Viral RNA 462
   2.4. Relationships among Viral Genomes, mRNAs,
        and Proteins 465
   2.5. Properties of Virions and Infected Cells 466
3. Virus Populations 472
   3.1. Adaptation and Selection in Culture 473
   3.2. Growth of Stocks 474
   3.3. Particle Size Variation 475
   3.4. Host-Induced Modification 478
   3.5. Distinctions between Genetically Different
        Populations 480

4. Origins of Mutants and Variants 483
   4.1. Spontaneous vs. Mutagenized Isolates 483
   4.2. Mutagens 484
5. Types of Mutants and Variants 486
   5.1. Selection for Specifically Altered Properties 487
   5.2. Plaque-Type Mutants and Variants 489
6. Genetic and Paragenetic Phenomena 492
   6.1. Recombination 492
   6.2. Phenotypic Mixing 493
   6.3. Heterozygotes and Multiploid Particles 494
   6.4. Multiplicity Reactivation 497
   6.5. Defective or Incomplete Virus 499
7. Temperature-Sensitive Mutants 501
   7.1. Temperature-Sensitive Mutants of NDV 503
   7.2. Temperature-Sensitive Mutants of Sendai Virus ... 506
   7.3. Temperature-Sensitive Mutants of Measles Virus .. 508
   7.4. Summary 513
8. Persistent Infection 515
   8.1. Variants from Persistent Infection 516
   8.2. Possible Involvement of DNA 520
   8.3. Summary and Conclusions 521
9. Other Directions 522
10. References 523

Chapter 10

Genetics of Orthomyxoviruses

Lawrence E. Hightower and Michael A. Bratt

1. Introduction 535
   1.1. Scope of This Chapter 535
   1.2. Historical Perspective 537
   1.3. Organization of This Chapter 539
2. Molecular Biology of the Genome 540
   2.1. The Genome 540
   2.2. Gene Products 543
   2.3. Replication and Assembly 548
3. Virus Population 552
   3.1. Plaque-Forming and Non-Plaque-Forming
        Particles 552

3.2. Interference 554
3.3. Genetic Dimorphism 556
3.4. Phenotypic Mixing 557
3.5. Genotypic Mixing 558
4. Temperature-Sensitive Mutants 559
4.1. Genetic Interactions 559
4.2. Isolation and Characterization 564
4.3. Variants 583
5. Conclusion 586
6. References 588

Index 599

CHAPTER 1

Genetics of Polyoma Virus and Simian Virus 40

Walter Eckhart

The Salk Institute
Post Office Box 1809
San Diego, California 92112

1. INTRODUCTION*

Polyoma virus and simian virus 40 (SV40) are the smallest known tumor viruses. Their genomes are double-stranded circular DNA molecules, approximately 3.4×10^6 daltons in molecular weight, sufficient to code for the synthesis of approximately 200,000 daltons of protein. Infection of cells by polyoma and SV40 results in alterations in cell growth properties, sometimes leading to malignancy. Cells having altered growth properties are referred to as "transformed" or "neoplastic," and the process which leads to the acquisition of new growth properties is called "cell transformation." It should be emphasized that viral genes are not the only determinants of altered cell growth properties. Cellular genes and regulatory systems are major factors in the emergence of a malignant cell from a normal population.

---

* Much of the earlier work included in this chapter is described in *The Molecular Biology of Tumor Viruses* (Tooze, 1973) and a recent review (Eckhart, 1974). To avoid unnecessary references in the text, publications prior to 1973 which can be found in these volumes will generally not be cited here. The biochemistry of polyoma and SV40 infection has been described in detail by N. Salzman and G. Khoury in "Reproduction of Papovaviruses" in Volume 3 of this series. Interested readers should also consult the 1974 *Cold Spring Harbor Symposium on Tumor Viruses* (Vol. 39, 1975), which contains many pertinent articles.

Therefore, a description of cell transformation by tumor viruses necessarily requires an understanding of the interaction between viral and cellular regulatory systems.

Genetic studies of polyoma and SV40 seek to define the detailed structure of the viral genomes, and to identify the functions of each of the viral genes. Because of the limited coding capacity of these viral genomes, they provide a useful system for examining the ways in which expression of viral genetic information may influence growth regulation of infected cells. In addition, these viruses have been particularly important for studying the processes of DNA replication, transcription, and protein synthesis in mammalian cells.

The results of infection of a susceptible cell by polyoma or SV40 depend on the kind of cell that is infected. Lytic infection, which involves virus replication, production of infectious progeny, and death of the host cell, occurs after infection of mouse cells by polyoma and monkey cells by SV40. In many other cell systems, the infection is abortive: viral genetic information is expressed to a limited extent, and the infected cell survives. In a fraction of the abortively infected cells, viral genetic information is retained and passed on to the progeny of the infected cell. Cells transformed by polyoma or SV40 retain viral genetic information and express part of this information as messenger RNA (mRNA) and virus-specific protein. In some cases, cells which usually undergo lytic infection can survive the infection and become transformed. Presumably, these cells have been transformed by defective viral genomes which are unable to express all the information required for lytic infection. (These cells are not simply resistant to viral infection, because in many cases they can be superinfected with nondefective viral genomes to produce a lytic infection.)

A variety of mutants of polyoma and SV40 have been selected and used for genetic analysis. Four types of mutants have been particularly useful: (1) *temperature-sensitive* mutants, which are selected on the basis of ability to grow at a permissive temperature, usually 31–33°C, but which are unable to grow at a restrictive temperature, usually 39–41°C; (2) *host range* mutants, which have been selected for their ability to grow on one cell type, but not on another, whereas wild-type virus can grow on both cell types; (3) *defective mutants,* which contain deletions, insertions, or other rearrangements in their genomes, rendering them able to grow only poorly, or not at all, in the absence of a coinfecting helper virus; and (4) *adeno-SV40 hybrid viruses* consisting of adenovirus genomes containing limited amounts of SV40 genetic material covalently inserted into their DNA. The properties of these virus mutants will be discussed in more detail subsequently.

2. RESTRICTION ENZYME MAPS OF THE POLYOMA AND SV40 GENOMES

The availability of bacterial restriction enzymes, which cleave DNAs at defined sites, has permitted the construction of maps of the polyoma and SV40 genomes. The fragments produced by enzymatic digestion have characteristic sizes, and can be arranged in the order corresponding to their positions in the circular viral DNA molecule. The site of cleavage by the *Escherichia coli* RI restriction enzyme (*Eco·RI*), which cleaves both polyoma and SV40 at a single defined site, is used as a reference point to define the 0/1.0 map unit position. Danna *et al.* (1973) arranged the 11 fragments of SV40 produced by digestion of SV40 DNA with a restriction enzyme from *Haemophilus influenzae* (*Hin*) in the circular map shown in Fig. 1a. Griffin *et al.* (1974) arranged the eight fragments of polyoma DNA produced by digestion with a restriction enzyme from *H. parainfluenzae* (*Hpa II*) in the order shown in Fig. 1b. Maps have been constructed using other restriction enzymes, including a map of 22 fragments of polyoma produced by an enzyme from *H. aegyptius* (Summers, 1975). These will be described in more detail in a subsequent volume of this series.

Restriction enzyme analysis has been extremely useful in defining important features on the polyoma and SV40 genomes, including the origins of DNA replication, the location and direction of regions of transcription, and the sites of numerous mutations.

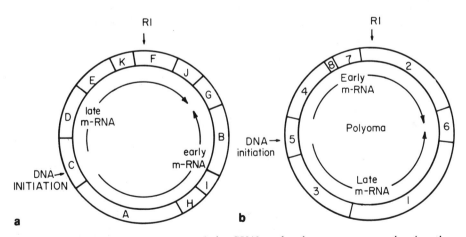

Fig. 1.   Restriction enzyme maps of the SV40 and polyoma genomes, showing the regions and directions (5′ → 3′) of transcription of stable messenger RNAs. (a) SV40: fragments produced by a restriction enzyme from *H. influenzae*. (b) Polyoma: fragments produced by a restriction enzyme from *H. parainfluenzae*.

3. THE LYTIC GROWTH CYCLE

Lytic infection of polyoma and SV40 can be divided into two stages, early and late, corresponding to the times before and after viral DNA replication, respectively. The expression of viral genetic information is different during the two stages of infection: the cytoplasmic mRNA species during the early stage of infection are derived from only half the genome, whereas during the late stage they are derived from the whole genome. The patterns of virus-specific proteins synthesized during the two stages of infection also are different. The major structural proteins of the virion are synthesized exclusively during the late stage of infection.

During the early stage of infection, a variety of changes occur in the infected cell. The synthesis of a number of cellular enzymes increases, and cellular DNA synthesis is induced in resting cells as a result of virus infection. Changes take place in the surface properties of infected cells. These surface changes include enhanced agglutinability by plant lectins, increased uptake of sugars, and the appearance of new surface antigens. A new antigen, the T antigen, appears in the cell nucleus.

3.1. Viral DNA Replication

For both polyoma and SV40 viral DNA, replication usually begins at a unique origin approximately 0.7 map unit from the RI restriction enzyme site and proceeds bidirectionally to terminate approximately 180° away from the origin on the circular DNA molecule (Fareed *et al.*, 1972; Nathans and Danna, 1972; Crawford *et al.*, 1973). The termination point is not unique because in certain defective viral DNA molecules containing multiple origins of replication the termination point is 180° from whichever origin is used for initiation of replication. Robberson *et al.* (1975) have made the interesting observation that polyoma DNA contains a second origin of replication near the RI restriction enzyme site. Replication is initiated infrequently from this origin, but proceeds unidirectionally either to the left or to the right from the RI site. Electron microscopic analysis of replicating polyoma and SV40 DNA molecules has shown that the parental DNA strands remain in a closed circular configuration for most of the time during which replication takes place, although periodic nicking and resealing are necessary to allow unwinding. Supercoiled regions are confined to the unreplicated portion of the parental DNA.

In vitro systems are very useful for studying the details of the process of polyoma and SV40 DNA replication. Systems consisting of partially purified nuclei (Winnacker *et al.*, 1972) or lysates of polyoma infected cells (Hunter and Francke, 1974*a*) have shown that synthesis proceeds at least partly in steps, beginning with the synthesis of an RNA primer, approximately ten bases long, which is extended to form a short DNA fragment, joined to the RNA primer by a link with little or no specificity (Magnusson *et al.*, 1973; Pigiet *et al.*, 1973; Francke and Hunter, 1974; Hunter and Francke, 1974*b*). When the DNA fragment reaches a size of 200–300 nucleotides, the RNA primer is removed, the gap filled, and the DNA fragment joined to the growing daughter strand. Several different enzymatic activities are required for the steps in this process, and efforts are under way to fractionate and reconstitute the systems so that the necessary factors can be isolated and characterized. A major difficulty with the *in vitro* systems used so far is that there is little or no initiation of new rounds of viral DNA replication in these systems: replicative intermediates present in the infected cell at the time the *in vitro* system is prepared are completed, but little initiation of new rounds takes place. At present, only one viral-coded protein appears to be involved in viral DNA replication, and this protein apparently is involved in the initiation of each round of replication (see below). Therefore, cellular enzymes are responsible for most or all of the steps involved in elongation of daughter viral DNA strands and termination of replication.

3.2. Transcription during Lytic Infection

The transcriptional patterns of polyoma and SV40 have been studied in detail recently, using hybridization of RNA from infected cells to restriction enzyme fragments of the viral genomes. It now seems clear that, as originally proposed by Aloni, transcription in the cell nucleus during the late stage of infection can be symmetrical; i.e., the majority of the sequences of both strands of the viral DNA are transcribed (Aloni, 1975; Kamen *et al.*, 1975; Khoury *et al.*, 1975*a,b*), although not necessarily in equal amounts. However, the stable mRNA species found in the cytoplasm of infected cells correspond to only 50% of each of the viral DNA strands, representing the early and late regions shown in Fig. 1 (Kamen *et al.*, 1975; Khoury *et al.*, 1975*b*). These results suggest that a posttranscriptional processing or transport mechanism operates to ensure that only "true" early and late mRNA species appear in the cytoplasm.

The early region of the viral DNA appears to be larger than originally estimated, covering close to 50% of the viral genome (Kamen *et al.*, 1975; Khoury *et al.*, 1975*b*). The estimates of the size and location of the SV40 early and late regions by hybridization to restriction enzyme fragments are in agreement with the results of Dhar *et al.* (1974, 1975), who have sequenced the terminal regions of SV40-specific RNA.

During the early stage of infection, only RNA sequences corresponding to the early region of the viral genome are present in the cytoplasm. The nature of the switch leading to the appearance of RNA sequences of the late region, which occurs at the time of viral DNA replication, is not clear.

The sizes of cytoplasmic viral RNA transcripts in SV40-infected cells have been estimated by Weinberg *et al.* (1972, 1974). Early RNA has a sedimentation coefficient of 19 S, whereas late RNA consists of two classes, having sedimentation coefficients of 16 S and 19 S. The 16 S and 19 S late classes appear to share common sequences, because both hybridize to "late" fragments of SV40 DNA (Weinberg *et al.*, 1974). There is evidence that suggests a precursor–product relationship between the two late classes (Aloni *et al.*, 1975). An RNA of 19 S would correspond to approximately half the viral genome.

3.3. Virion Proteins

Virion proteins, which are coded for in the late regions of polyoma and SV40 DNA, have been analyzed by polyacrylamide gel electrophoresis. A typical pattern of polyoma virion proteins is shown in Fig. 2. The major structural protein, of approximately 45,000 molecular weight, accounts for about 70% of the total protein of the virion. The band at approximately 100,000 molecular weight is a dimer of the 45,000 protein. The three candidates for virus-coded proteins have molecular weights of approximately 45,000, 30,000, and 20,000. The smaller proteins in the region of 10,000–18,000 molecular weight are cellular histones. Recent analysis of the tryptic peptide patterns of the 45,000, 30,000, and 20,000 molecular weight proteins of polyoma suggests that the 30,000 and 20,000 proteins have a large number of peptides in common, but are different from the 45,000 protein (Gibson, 1974; Fey and Hirt, 1975; Hewick *et al.*, 1975).

The candidates for virus-coded proteins in the SV40 virion have molecular weights of approximately 43,000, 32,000, and 23,000 (Crawford, 1973; Pett *et al.*, 1975). Tryptic peptide analysis of the 43,000 and

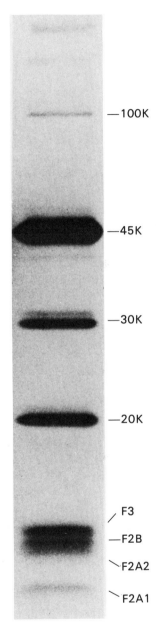

Fig. 2.   Separation of the proteins of purified polyoma virions by SDS-polyacrylamide gel electrophoresis. Courtesy of W. Gibson.

23,000 molecular weight proteins indicates that they are unrelated (Wright and diMayorca, 1975; W., Gibson, unpublished results; B. Hirt, personal communication). Cellular histones are also present in purified SV40 virions (Pett *et al.*, 1975).

Taken together, the results of the analysis of polyoma and SV40 virion proteins suggest that the viral coding capacity required to specify the virion proteins is approximately 75,000 daltons of protein. Studies of the synthesis of these proteins *in vitro* are under way in a number of laboratories, and should help to define the portions of the viral genome coding for each of the virion proteins.

4.   MUTANTS OF POLYOMA AND SV40

4.1.   Temperature-Sensitive Mutants

Temperature-sensitive mutants which affect most, if not all, of the genes of polyoma and SV40 required for lytic infection have been isolated (Tooze, 1973; Chou and Martin, 1974; Eckhart, 1974). A variety of mutagens have been used, including nitrous acid, hydroxylamine, and nitrosoguanidine. The mutants have been isolated on the basis of defects in lytic infection at the restrictive temperature: plaques picked at the permissive temperature are replated at the per- missive and the restrictive temperatures, and mutants which form plaques at the permissive but not the restrictive temperature are found at a frequency of approximately 1% in the mutagenized population. The mutants are then tested to determine the stage at which they are blocked during lytic infection at the restrictive temperature, usually by measuring induction of cellular DNA synthesis, viral DNA synthesis, and the appearance of virion antigens or virus particles. Complementa- tion analysis usually is performed by comparing the yield of pairwise mixed infections at the restrictive temperature with the yields of single infections. High ratios of the yields of mixed to single infections (10– 1000) are taken to indicate complementation. Complementation can be intercistronic or intracistronic. Intercistronic complementation results from the ability of each mutant to make a functional gene product in which the other is defective. Intracistronic complementation results from restoration of function because of the interaction of the same gene products which are altered differently in each of the two mutants.

The "leakiness" of the temperature-sensitive mutants—which reflects their ability to escape the block at the restrictive temperature— is measured by comparing the virus yields after one cycle of growth at the permissive and the restrictive temperatures. With some mutants, the degree of leakiness depends on the multiplicity of infection: leakiness is more pronounced at higher multiplicities.

The temperature-sensitive mutants analyzed so far fall into early and late classes. The early mutants are blocked at a step prior to the synthesis of viral DNA during infection at the restrictive temperature.

The late mutants synthesize viral DNA at the restrictive temperature, but do not yield infectious progeny virus.

The major class of early mutants of both polyoma and SV40 is called the *ts*A class. These mutants are defective in a viral function required for the replication of the viral DNA. This function appears to be required for the initiation of each round of viral DNA replication, but not for the elongation or maturation of the daughter strands, because in cells infected by *ts*A mutants and shifted from the permissive to the restrictive temperature, replicative intermediates are converted to mature viral DNA molecules, but little or no initiation of new rounds of replication occurs at the restrictive temperature (Tegtmeyer, 1972; Francke and Eckhart, 1973). No other classes of mutants affecting viral DNA replication directly have been found, so it appears that all of the steps of viral DNA replication except initiation of each round are carried out exclusively by cellular functions.

The late mutants of polyoma and SV40 can be arranged in groups on the basis of complementation tests (Chou and Martin, 1974; Eckhart, 1974, 1975). The significance of these groups is questionable, because much of the complementation observed in pairwise crosses seems to be intracistronic (Chou and Martin, 1974; Lai and Nathans, 1974*b*). A variety of evidence, including alterations in the tryptic peptide patterns of mutant proteins, suggests that some of the late mutants are altered in the 45,000 molecular weight major virion protein (Friedmann and Eckhart, 1975; Gibson and Eckhart, unpublished observations).

A class of SV40 mutants with unusual properties is referred to as class D (Chou and Martin, 1974). These mutants are blocked at an early stage of infection at the restrictive temperature, after adsorption and penetration, but prior to viral DNA synthesis. These mutants also fail to induce the synthesis of cellular DNA at the restrictive temperature. The mutants have two unusual properties: they fail to complement with other classes of temperature-sensitive mutants in one cycle of growth after mixed infection, and the first cycle of virus replication is not temperature sensitive when infection is carried out with purified viral DNA rather than with virions. The *ts*3 mutant of polyoma virus also displays these properties during lytic infection (Eckhart and Dulbecco, 1974). A possible explanation for these properties is that the class D mutants are altered in a protein which is associated with the viral DNA in the virion, and which must be removed or activated before viral gene expression can occur in the infected cell. In support of this idea, Chou and Martin (1975*a*) have analyzed the products of mixed infection between pairs of temperature-sensitive mutants. The class D mutants exhibit a phenomenon termed "delayed complementation," in which the virus yields after mixed infection between class D and other mutants at the restrictive temperature are low after the time required for one cycle of growth, but high after the time required for several cycles of growth. Chou and Martin propose that this phenomenon can be explained by a low level of leakiness in the first cycle of growth, followed by phenotypic mixing, which produces class D mutant genomes carrying a functional DNA-associated virion protein provided by the coinfecting mutant. These phenotypically mixed particles could then replicate normally in a second cycle of infection at the restrictive temperature. Efforts are under way to isolate and characterize DNA-associated virion proteins which may be altered in the class D mutants.

Lai and Nathans (1974b) have developed an extremely useful technique for mapping the position of mutations on the SV40 genome. This method is based on one used to map mutations in the bacteriophage ϕX174. Single-stranded circular mutant viral DNA molecules are annealed with fragments of wild-type viral DNA produced by restriction enzymes. These molecules are then used to infect cells at the restrictive temperature. If the wild-type DNA fragment corresponds to the site of the mutation, DNA replication and segregation of daughter molecules permit the formation of plaques by wild-type segregants at the restrictive temperature. This process is shown in Fig. 3. Wild-type

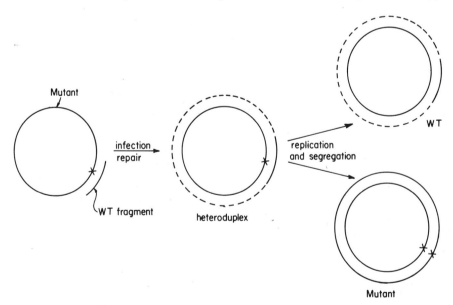

Fig. 3.   Mapping of the position of mutations on the viral genome by fragment rescue (Lai and Nathans, 1974b).

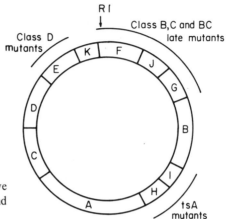

Fig. 4. Position of temperature-sensitive mutations on the SV40 genome (Lai and Nathans, 1974*b*, 1975).

fragments which do not cover the mutant site will be unable to lead to the segregation of wild-type daughter molecules.

Using the technique, Lai and Nathans (1974*b*, 1975) have located the position of a number of temperature-sensitive SV40 mutants on the circular viral DNA molecule. The results, shown in Fig. 4, have several interesting features. Seven of eight *ts*A class mutants that have been mapped occur in a small portion of the early region of the genome, in *Hin* fragment I (see Fig. 1). This fragment comprises only about 5% of the genome. Whether the clustering of *ts*A mutants reflects some special feature of the protein coded by the early region, a requirement for only part of the early region for lytic infection, or a "hot spot" for mutagenesis is not known. The late mutants in complementation classes B, C, and BC occur interspersed in a part of the late region comprising about 22% of the genome. This region is large enough to code for a protein of 45,000 molecular weight, and most likely represents the region coding for the major virion protein. The interspersed positions of class B, C, and BC mutants implies that complementation among these late mutants is intracistronic. The class D mutants map in the late region of the genome, again suggesting that they are blocked early during lytic infection because of a defect in a protein which enters the cell together with the viral DNA, rather than because of a defect in a protein which must be synthesized early during infection.

A second useful method for defining the location of mutant sites on the viral genome has been developed by Shenk *et al.* (1975*a*). This method relies on the ability of a single-strand-specific nuclease, S1, to cleave viral DNA at or near unpaired regions. Mutant and wild-type viral DNAs are converted to linear molecules using restriction enzymes that cleave the viral DNA at single defined sites. These linear DNAs are denatured and annealed together, producing heteroduplex molecules with a mispaired region at the site of the mutation. The heteroduplex molecules are then cleaved with the S1 nuclease to yield fragments whose length reflects the distance of the mutant site from the ends of the linear molecules. This method is most efficient for locating the site of deletions or insertions, where the mispaired region is larger than that for mutations involving single base changes, but it has been used to confirm the location of at least one temperature-sensitive mutant of SV40 (Shenk *et al.*, 1975*a*,*b*).

The phenotypes of the major classes of temperature-sensitive mutants are summarized in Table 1.

4.2. Host Range Mutants

Host range mutants of polyoma were originally selected by Benjamin for their ability to grow on polyoma-transformed mouse cells, but not on normal mouse cells (Tooze, 1973). It was hoped that this selection technique would pick up mutants in viral functions that are expressed in the transformed cell. In agreement with expectations, these host range mutants are unable to transform hamster or rat cells, suggesting that they are defective in viral functions required for the transformation. More recently, the mutants have been shown to be able to grow on a variety of cells in addition to polyoma-transformed mouse cells (Goldman and Benjamin, 1975), including some normal cell types.

TABLE 1

Phenotypes of the Major Classes of Temperature-Sensitive Mutants of Polyoma and SV40

	Function at the restrictive temperature[a]		
Mutant class	Induction of cellular DNA synthesis	Viral DNA synthesis	Infectious progeny
A. Mutants blocked early during lytic infection			
1. *ts*A (polyoma and SV40)	+	–	–
2. *ts*D (SV40)			
*ts*3 (polyoma)	–	–	–
B. Mutants blocked late during lytic infection			
1. *ts*B, C, and BC (SV40)			
Late mutants (polyoma)	+	+	–

[a] +, Normal; –, minus.

These results suggest that cellular factors can affect the ability of these mutants to carry out lytic infection. So far, more than a dozen host range mutants have been shown to be unable to transform hamster or rat cells (T. Benjamin, personal communication), and it will be important to define the defects in these mutants that render them unable to transform.

4.3 Defective Mutants

A variety of defective mutants of polyoma and SV40, having deletions, insertions, substitutions, or other rearrangements in their DNA, have been isolated and characterized (Brockman and Nathans, 1974; Brockman et al., 1975; Carbon et al., 1975; Davoli and Fareed, 1975; Fried, 1974; Fried et al., 1975; Lai and Nathans, 1974a, 1975; M. Martin et al., 1975; Mertz and Berg, 1974a,b; Mertz et al., 1975; Robberson and Fried, 1974; Winocour et al., 1975; Yoshiike et al., 1975). Some of these mutants arise naturally during serial passage of the virus at high multiplicity. These natural defective mutants are enabled to grow by the presence of nondefective helper virus particles in the virus stock. If the defective molecules are sufficiently different in size from the wild-type viral DNA, they can be selected on the basis of their size.

Defective mutants which occur naturally can also be selected by using restriction enzymes to cleave a population of viral DNA molecules and selecting the molecules that are resistant to cleavage. These resistant molecules have alterations in the restriction enzyme site. Generally, these mutants must be grown in the presence of a nondefective helper virus. Alterations in specific regions of the genome can be selected by using appropriate restriction enzymes, and complementing defective mutants can be isolated by using a temperature-sensitive mutant as the helper virus. The genomes carrying deletions can be separated from the helper DNA by treating the DNA population with the restriction enzyme used to select the deletion mutant. This will cleave the helper DNA but not the deleted DNA.

Deletion mutants can also be generated in a nondefective viral DNA population. This has been accomplished by cleaving the viral DNA with restriction enzymes that convert the circular molecules to linear molecules with cohesive ends. Infection with these molecules apparently results in recombinational events in the region of the cohesive ends that produce deletions of varying sizes. These deletions occur at sites dictated by the particular restriction enzyme used. A variation of this technique can be used to produce deletions at random sites in the genome: viral DNA molecules can be cleaved with DNase I in the presence of manganese to produce random breaks, and the broken molecules treated with exonuclease to create extended regions of cohesive ends. Infection by these molecules in the presence of appropriate helpers could lead to the isolation of deletions in many parts of the viral genome.

Insertion mutants also have been constructed by introducing a short stretch of poly(dA:dT) into the SV40 genome (Mertz *et al.*, 1975).

These various defective mutants are extremely useful for studying the structure and function of the polyoma and SV40 genomes. Two observations that have been made so far are especially intriguing. It seems that the region of the polyoma and SV40 DNA molecules close to the origin of replication may have unusual properties. There are deletions which occur near the origin of replication in SV40 that cause the growth of the mutant virus to be slowed, but these deletion mutants are able to grow in the absence of a helper virus, suggesting that they have been affected in a region that is not essential for replication (Mertz and Berg, 1974*b*). Likewise, for polyoma the DNA restriction enzyme fragments near the origin of replication can vary in size from one virus strain to another, suggesting that alterations in this region may not be lethal for the virus (Fried *et al.*, 1975).

Studies of highly defective SV40 DNA molecules suggest that the origin of replication is the only region which is essential to be present in *cis* configuration in order for DNA replication to occur. One variant containing as few as 150 nucleotide pairs of SV40 DNA linked to host cell DNA in tandemly repeating units is still able to replicate in the presence of helper virus, indicating that all functions required for replication, except the initiation site, can be supplied in *trans* (Brockman *et al.*, 1975). Viral DNA molecules containing repetitions of regions including the origin of replication occur very frequently in defective viral DNA populations. Presumably the presence of multiple origins of replication confers some advantage on these molecules during replication.

4.4. Adenovirus–SV40 Hybrid Viruses

Adeno-SV40 hybrid viruses are especially useful for studying the early region of SV40 DNA. These hybrid viruses consist of adenovirus genomes containing covalent insertions of SV40 genetic material. The hybrid viruses arose originally because adenoviruses are unable to repli-

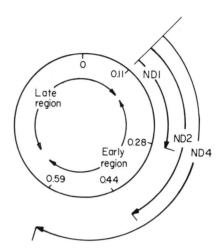

Fig. 5. Regions of the SV40 genome present in the adenovirus–SV40 hybrid viruses, ND1, ND2, and ND4.

cate efficiently in some monkey cells, but do replicate efficiently if the monkey cells are coinfected with SV40. Recombination between the adenovirus genome and the SV40 genome produces hybrids which carry the SV40 "helper function" for adenovirus growth, and therefore are nondefective in monkey cells. The structure and properties of those hybrids have been described extensively previously (Tooze, 1973) and will be mentioned only briefly here. Figure 5 shows the regions of the SV40 genome that are present in the nondefective hybrids, ND1, ND2, and ND4. Different antigens are expressed in cells infected by the various nondefective hybrids. ND1-infected cells express U antigen, ND2-infected cells express U antigen and tumor-specific transplantation antigen (TSTA), and ND4-infected cells express U, TSTA, and T antigens. The fact that the SV40 helper function for adenovirus growth can be expressed by hybrids carrying only part of the early region of SV40 DNA suggests that the early region is divided into two or more functional units. The possible nature of the SV40 helper function will be discussed later in this chapter.

5. VIRAL FUNCTIONS AND THE EARLY REGION OF THE GENOME

5.1. Cellular DNA Synthesis

Polyoma and SV40 have the ability to induce the synthesis of cellular DNA in resting cells. Several lines of evidence suggest that this induction results from the expression of an early viral gene. In particular, the ability of the virus to induce cellular DNA synthesis can be inactivated by treating the virus with ultraviolet radiation. The *ts*A mutants of both polyoma and SV40 are blocked in a function which appears to be required for initiation of viral DNA synthesis. This observation has led to the idea that initiation of cellular DNA synthesis may result from the same function that is altered in the *ts*A mutants. For example, a viral protein which might act at the initiation site in viral DNA to initiate a round of replication might recognize similar initiation sites which are present, perhaps by chance, in cellular DNA. This idea predicts that the initiation of cellular DNA synthesis after viral infection occurs by a process which affects the DNA replication machinery directly, rather than by a process which affects earlier events leading ultimately to cellular DNA synthesis, such as happens in the case of induction of cellular DNA synthesis by serum factors.

One difficulty with the hypothesis that cellular DNA induction results from the action of the protein which is altered in the *ts*A mutants is that these mutants have been reported to induce cellular DNA synthesis normally at the restrictive temperature, where the viral function is inactive as measured by the lack of viral DNA synthesis. Chou and Martin (1975*b*) have reported recently that cellular DNA induction by *ts*A mutants of SV40 is depressed when experiments are carried out at a temperature above the usual restrictive temperature. Even in these experiments, the effects on cellular DNA synthesis are much less than the effects on viral DNA synthesis, and more experiments are needed to clarify the situation.

An alternative hypothesis to explain the induction of cellular DNA synthesis by viral infection is that an early viral gene function is responsible for altering the surface or internal environment of infected cells (for example, by affecting protein synthesis) and that these alterations result in the release of resting cells from a block in the G_0 or G_1 stage of the cell cycle.

A number of changes occur in infected resting cells prior to the replication of cellular DNA (induction of cellular enzymes and changes in sugar uptake, for example); therefore, it would appear that these changes are not a consequence of altered patterns of cellular DNA synthesis. Presumably they result from expression of a different early function from that which affects viral DNA synthesis, although it is possible that a single protein coded in the early region would have pleiotropic effects. Considerable progress is being made in isolating the products of the early viral genes, and characterization of these products should help to resolve the questions about their functions.

5.2. T Antigen

Several lines of evidence indicate that the T antigens of polyoma and SV40 are coded for by the viral genome. The most direct evidence has come from experiments of Graessmann *et al.*, (1974) with SV40 and of Paulin and Cuzin (1975) with polyoma. Graessmann *et al.* injected complementary RNA made with *E. coli* RNA polymerase using SV40 DNA as template into susceptible monkey cells. They showed that cells injected with the SV40-specific RNA express T antigen. The appearance of T antigen was blocked when the cells were pretreated with interferon. T antigen was expressed in cells treated with actinomycin D to block transcription, however. Therefore, it is likely that the SV40 complementary RNA could serve as a messenger RNA for T-antigen synthesis. Paulin and Cuzin studied the properties of T antigen isolated from mouse 3T3 cells transformed by the *ts*A mutant of polyoma, and from cells transformed by wild-type polyoma. The T antigen in the *ts*A mutant transformed cells was more heat labile than the T antigen from wild-type transformed cells, when assayed both intracellularly and *in vitro* by immunoflourescence and complement fixation. This suggests that the T antigen in the *ts*A mutant transformed cells is altered because of the *ts*A mutation, rendering it more heat labile than the wild-type.

Presently, several laboratories are attempting to purify T antigen and to synthesize it *in vitro*. Although it seems clear that T antigen is coded for by the viral genome, it may have to act in association with cellular factors to carry out its function, and these cellular factors, in turn, could modify the effects of T antigen in different cells. Since some *ts*A mutants synthesize altered T antigen, it is reasonable to speculate that the T antigen may be a protein involved in initiation of viral DNA synthesis. In support of this idea, Reed *et al.* (1975) have reported that partially purified SV40 T antigen binds preferentially to the region of the SV40 DNA molecule containing the origin of replication.

5.3. SV40 Helper Function for Adenovirus Growth

As mentioned previously, human adenoviruses grow poorly in some monkey cells, and this restriction of growth can be overcome by coinfecting the cells with SV40. The restriction of growth occurs at the level of the synthesis of the adenovirus structural proteins, which are present in much lower amounts in monkey cells infected with adenovirus alone than in cells coinfected by SV40.

What is the portion of the viral genome which codes for the SV40 helper activity for adenovirus growth? From the structure of the adeno-SV40 hybrid ND 1 (see Fig. 5), it would be expected that the necessary information lies in approximately one-fifth of the early region adjacent to the early–late border opposite the origin of replication. It is not clear whether a function specified by the SV40 genome acts directly as helper, or whether it causes the synthesis of cellular functions which provide the helper activity. Host cell factors can affect the ability of monkey cells to support adenovirus growth because some monkey cell lines are permissive for adenovirus growth, and because treatment of nonpermissive cells with iododeoxyuridine causes them to become partially permissive (Jerkofsky and Rapp, 1975; Staal and Rowe, 1975). Lopez-Revilla and Walter (1973) and Grodzicker et al. (1974) have studied the proteins made in cells infected by the ND1 hybrid, and have identified a protein of molecular weight 25,000–30,000 which is present in the ND1 hybrid infected cells, but not in cells infected with adenovirus alone. Purification and characterization of this protein may help to establish whether it plays a role in the enhancement of adenovirus replication.

Several of the tsA mutants of SV40 have been shown to exhibit normal helper activity for adenovirus growth at the restrictive temperature (Jerkofsky and Rapp, 1973, and personal communication), suggesting that the product of the region altered in the tsA mutants is not involved in producing helper activity. However, Kimura (1974) has reported that an early SV40 tsA mutant is defective in helper activity at the restrictive temperature. The site on the viral genome of the mutant studied by Kimura has not been determined.

6. TEMPERATURE-DEPENDENT PROPERTIES OF TRANSFORMED CELLS

One way of studying the effects of viral gene expression on cell growth properties is to study the properties of cells transformed by temperature-sensitive mutants of polyoma and SV40. Cells grown at the permissive temperature should contain functional viral gene products, whereas cells grown at the restrictive temperature should contain a nonfunctional viral gene product specified by the temperature-sensitive mutant. The process of neoplastic transformation is a progressive one involving both cellular and viral functions, and different transformed cells display different combinations of altered growth properties compared to normal cells. A variety of altered growth properties can be used to characterize transformed cells, including altered morphology, ability to grow in medium containing low levels of serum, ability to clone on monolayers of normal cells, ability to grow to higher saturation densities than normal cells, ability to grow in soft agar, and biochemical changes such as agglutinability with plant lectins, enhanced sugar uptake, or fibrinolytic activity. In considering the relationship between viral gene expression and altered cell growth properties, it is important to keep in mind that many of the properties being studied may result from cellular gene expression, or may represent secondary changes not directly related to the function of the viral gene being examined. Although this makes the situation complicated, it is a more useful way of trying to unravel the effects of viral gene expression on cell growth properties than to treat transformation or transformed cells as though they possessed a distinct and uniform phenotype compared to normal cells.

Earlier studies of cells exhibiting temperature-dependent growth properties after transformation by temperature-sensitive mutants are summarized by Tooze (1973) and Eckhart (1974). More recently, a number of workers have characterized the properties of cells transformed by *ts*A mutants of polyoma and SV40.

Tegtmeyer (1975*b*) reported that six *ts*A mutants of SV40 are unable to induce piled-up colonies of cells after infection of mouse 3T3, rabbit kidney, or Syrian hamster embryo cells at the restrictive temperature, confirming that *ts*A mutants are defective in transformation, measured by this criterion, at the restrictive temperature. When cultures of hamster embryo cells were infected and serially passaged at the permissive temperature until the cultures showed transformed morphology, then assayed for colony-forming ability at the permissive and restrictive temperatures, five of the six *ts*A mutant infected cultures showed twenty- to fiftyfold fewer colonies at the restrictive temperature compared to the permissive temperature, although colonies that did arise at the restrictive temperature appeared transformed. Wild-type infected and late mutant infected cells showed only two- to fivefold differences. Uninfected cells, like the *ts*A mutant infected cells, showed twentyfold fewer colonies at the restrictive temperature. The *ts*A mutant-infected cells which did not divide at the restrictive temperature remained viable. When shifted to the permissive temperature, these cells were able to divide and form colonies. Mouse 3T3 cells transformed by two *ts*A mutants did not show temperature dependence of colony-forming ability. Rabbit kidney cells transformed by one *ts*A mutant did not show temperature dependence of colony-forming ability, whereas cells transformed by a second *ts*A mutant did. Tegtmeyer concluded that the SV40 *ts*A function is required to initiate stable morphological transformation of cells, but may also affect the ability of transformed cells derived from nonestablished cultures to form colonies. Because the effects observed depend on the particular *ts*A mutant and cell type used, Tegtmeyer emphasized that cellular factors are important in determining the phenotype of a transformed cell.

Osborn and Weber (1975*a,b*) studied rat embryo cells transformed by wild-type SV40 and two *ts*A mutants. Transformed cells were selected as dense, piled-up colonies with altered morphology. Cells transformed by the *ts*A mutants showed slower growth rates, lower saturation densities, and abnormal flat morphology when they were grown at the restrictive temperature, compared to the permissive temperature. Temperature-dependent morphological properties also could be demonstrated in the *ts*A-transformed cells by staining with antibody to actin. Wild-type transformed cells showed few thick, actin-containing fibers, whereas *ts*A-transformed cells at the restrictive temperature showed many long, thick fibers. The temperature dependence of morphology, growth rate, and saturation density in *ts*A-transformed rat embryo cells implicates the product of the SV40 *ts*A gene in affecting the growth properties of these cells.

Martin and Chou (1975) and R. Martin *et al.* (1975) studied the properties of secondary Chinese hamster lung cells transformed by wild-type SV40 and *ts*A mutants. Cultures infected with *ts*A mutants, and judged as transformed by their ability to grow at the permissive temperature in low-serum medium, showed poorer cloning ability at the restrictive temperature than at the permissive temperature, and failed to form piled-up colonies. Athough wild-type and late mutant transformed cultures also showed temperature-dependent growth properties, the differences were greatest with *ts*A mutant transformed cells.

Brugge and Butel (1975) and Butel *et al.* (1975) studied several mouse, hamster, and human cell cultures infected and transformed by SV40 *ts*A mutants. A variety of properties of the *ts*A mutant infected cultures were found to be temperature dependent, including morphology, saturation density, colony formation, and hexose uptake. These properties were either not temperature dependent or much less temperature dependent in corresponding wild-type infected cultures.

Kimura and Itagaki (1975) have reported that two clones of rat cells morphologically transformed by an SV40 *ts*A mutant show reduced colony-forming ability at the restrictive temperature compared to the permissive temperature. Kimura (1975) also has reported that four out of seven clones of rat cells transformed by a *ts*A mutant of polyoma show temperature-dependent growth rates in low-serum medium, again suggesting that cellular factors can influence transformed cell properties.

Previous studies had indicated that cells transformed by *ts*A mutants of polyoma and SV40 did not show temperature-dependent properties. The differences between the results described above and the earlier ones may be accounted for in a number of ways. In several of the recent studies, higher temperatures were used, and the higher temperature might inactivate a temperature-sensitive viral gene product more efficiently or might modify cellular factors involved in growth regulation. Also, several of the recent studies employed primary or secondary cell cultures, rather than established cell lines, and it is likely that established cell lines have already acquired spontaneously some of the characteristics—such as high cloning efficiency—which are attributed to transformed cells.

It seems clear that many *ts*A mutant transformed cells have growth properties different from those of wild-type transformed cells at the restrictive temperature. A variety of explanations have been proposed to account for the effects observed. One possible explanation mentioned frequently is that the product of the *ts*A gene changes the normal patterns of cellular DNA synthesis, and affects cell growth properties either directly in this way or by changing the expression of regulatory proteins whose synthesis is governed by the patterns of DNA synthesis in the cell.

A number of other kinds of cells exhibiting temperature-dependent properties have been described. These include mouse 3T3 cells transformed by wild-type SV40 (Renger and Basilico, 1972), hamster BHK cells transformed by the *ts*3 mutant of polyoma (Eckhart *et al.*, 1971), 3T3 cells transformed by the *ts*D101 mutant of SV40 (Robb, 1973, 1975), and transformed 3T3 cells not containing detectable polyoma DNA (Rudland *et al.*, 1974). This variety of cells exhibiting temperature-dependent properties, and the evidence that cellular factors are important in determining the properties of transformed cells, indicate that more needs to be understood about the viral functions themselves and the regulation of their expression before firm conclusions can be made about the effects of viral functions on cell growth properties.

The functions of the early region of the polyoma and SV40 genomes, and the changes that occur early after infection, suggest several ways that the expression of viral information could influence cell growth properties. The T antigen interacts with DNA, and could influence both replication and transcription. The SV40 helper function for adenovirus growth leads to alterations in protein synthesis. Changes in the cell surface lead to altered uptake of nutrients, new antigens, and changed physical properties. It seems likely that effects on DNA synthesis, protein synthesis, and cell surface properties all will be important in influencing cell growth properties. Therefore, the effects of viral gene expression in a transformed cell are likely to be complex rather than simple, and should continue to pose intriguing questions for some time to come.

7. REFERENCES

Aloni, Y., 1975, Biogenesis and characterization of SV40 and polyoma RNAs in productively infected cells, *Cold Spring Harbor Symp. Quant. Biol.* **39**:165.

Aloni, Y., Shani, M., and Reuveni, Y., 1975, SV40 RNA's in productively infected monkey cells: Kinetics of formation and decay in enucleate cells, *Proc. Natl. Acad. Sci. USA* **72**:2587.

Brockman, W. W., and Nathans, D., 1974, The isolation of simian virus 40 variants with specifically altered genomes, *Proc. Natl. Acad. Sci. USA* **71**:942.

Brockman, W. W., Lee, T. N. H., and Nathans, D., 1975, Characterization of cloned evolutionary variants of simian virus 40, *Cold Spring Harbor Symp. Quant. Biol.* **39**:119.

Brugge, S., and Butel, J., 1975, Role of simian virus 40 gene A function in maintenance of transformation, *J. Virol.* **15**:619.

Butel, J. S., Brugge, J. S., and Noonan, C. A., 1975, Transformation of primate and rodent cells by temperature-sensitive mutants of SV40, *Cold Spring Harbor Symp. Quant. Biol.* **39**:25.

Carbon, J., Shenk, T. E., and Berg, P., 1975, Biochemical procedure for production of small deletions in simian virus 40 DNA, *Proc. Natl. Acad. Sci. USA* **72**:1392.

Chou, J. Y., and Martin, R. G., 1974, Complementation analysis of simian virus 40 mutants, *J. Virol.* **13**:1101.

Chou, J. Y., and Martin, R. G., 1975a, Products of complementation between temperature-sensitive mutants of simian virus 40, *J. Virol.* **15**:127.

Chou, J. Y., and Martin, R. G., 1975b, DNA infectivity and the induction of host DNA synthesis with temperature-sensitive mutants of simian virus 40, *J. Virol.* **15**:145.

Crawford, L. V., 1973, Proteins of polyoma virus and SV40, *Br. Med. Bull.* **29**:253.

Crawford, L. V., Syrett, C., and Wilde, A., 1973, The replication of polyoma DNA, *J. Gen. Virol.* **21**:515.

Danna, K., Sack, G., and Nathans, D., 1973, Studies of simian virus 40 DNA. VII. A cleavage map of the SV40 genome, *J. Mol. Biol.* **78**:363.

Davoli, D., and Fareed, G. C., 1975, Formation of reiterated simian virus 40 DNA, *Cold Spring Harbor Symp. Quant. Biol.* **39**:137.

Dhar, R., Zain, S., Weissman, S. M., Pan, J., and Subramanian, K., 1974, Nucleotide sequences of RNA transcribed in infected cells by *E. coli* polymerase from a segment of simian virus 40 DNA, *Proc. Natl. Acad. Sci. USA* **71**:371.

Dhar, R., Subramanian, K., Zain, B. S., Pan, J., and Weissman, S., 1975, Nucleotide sequence about the 3′ terminus of the SV40 DNA transcript and the region where DNA synthesis starts initiation, *Cold Spring Harbor Symp. Quant. Biol.* **39**:153.

Eckhart, W., 1974, Genetics of DNA tumor viruses, *Annu. Rev. Genet.* **8**:301.

Eckhart, W., 1975, Properties of temperature-sensitive mutants of polyoma virus. *Cold Spring Harbor Symp. Quant. Biol.* **39**:37.

Eckhart, W., and Dulbecco, R., 1974, Properties of the ts3 mutant of polyoma virus during lytic infection, *Virology* **60**:359.

Eckhart, W., Dulbecco, R., and Burger, M. M., 1971 Temperature-dependent surface changes in cells infected or transformed by a thermosensitive mutant of polyoma virus, *Proc. Natl. Acad. Sci. USA* **68**:283.

Fareed, G. C., Garon, C. F., and Salzman, N. P., 1972, Origin and direction of simian virus 40 deoxyribonucleic acid replication, *J. Virol.* **10**:484.

Fey, B., and Hirt, B., 1975, Fingerprints of polyoma virus proteins and mouse histones, *Cold Spring Harbor Symp. Quant. Biol.* **39**:235.

Francke, B., and Eckhart, W., 1973, Polyoma gene function required for viral DNA synthesis, *Virology* **55**:127.

Francke, B., and Hunter, T., 1974, *In vitro* polyoma DNA synthesis: discontinuous chain growth, *J. Mol. Biol.* **83**:99.

Fried, A. M. C., Griffin, B. F., Lund, F., and Robberson, D. L. 1975, Polyoma virus— A study of wild type, mutant and defective DNA's *Cold Spring Harbor Symp. Quant. Biol.* **39**:45.

Fried, M., 1974, Isolation and partial characterization of different defective DNA molecules derived from polyoma virus, *J. Virol.* **13**:939.

Friedmann, T., and Eckhart, W., 1975, Virion proteins of temperature-sensitive mutants of polyoma virus: Late mutants. *Cold Spring Harbor Symp. Quant. Biol.* **39**:243.

Gibson, W., 1974, Polyoma virus proteins: A description of the structural proteins of the virion based on polyacrylamide gel electrophoresis and peptide analysis, *Virology* **62**:319.

Goldman, E., and Benjamin, T. L., 1975, Analysis of host range of nontransforming polyoma virus mutants, *Virology* **66**:372.

Graessmann, A., Graessmann, M., Hoffmann, H., Niebel, J., Bradner, G., and Mueller, N., 1974, Inhibition by interferon of SV40 tumor antigen formation in cells injected with SV40 cRNA transcribed *in vitro, FEBS Lett.* **39**:249.

Griffin, B. E., Fried, M., and Cowie, A., 1974, Polyoma DNA—A physical map, *Proc. Natl. Acad. Sci. USA* **71**:2077.

Grodzicker, T., Anderson, C., Sharp, P. A., and Sambrook, J., 1974, Conditional lethal mutants of adenovirus 2–simian virus 40 hybrids. I. Host range mutants of Ad2⁺ND1, *J. Virol.* **13**:1237.

Hewick, R. M., Fried, M., and Waterfield, M. D., 1975, Nonhistone virion proteins of polyoma: Characterization of the particle proteins by tryptic peptide analysis using ion-exchange columns, *Virology* **66**:408.

Hunter, T., and Francke, B., 1974*a*, *In vitro* polyoma DNA synthesis: Characterization of a system from infected 3T3 cells, *J. Virol.* **13**:125.

Hunter, T., and Francke, B., 1974*b*, *In vitro* polyoma DNA synthesis: Involvement of RNA in discontinuous chain growth, *J. Mol. Biol.* **83**:123.

Jerkofsky, M., and Rapp, F., 1973, Host cell DNA synthesis as a possible factor in the enhancement of replication of human adenoviruses in simian cells by SV40, *Virology* **51**:466.

Jerkofsky, M., and Rapp, F., 1975, Stimulation of adenovirus replication in simian cells in the absence of a helper virus by pretreatment of the cells with iododeoxyuridine, *J. Virol.* **15**:253.

Kamen, R., Lindstrom, D. M., Shure, H., and Old, R. W., 1975, Virus-specific RNA in cells productively infected or transformed by polyoma virus, *Cold Spring Harbor Symp. Quant. Biol.* **39**:187.

Khoury, G., Howley, P. M., Brown, M., and Martin M. A., 1975a, The detection and quantitation of SV40 nucleic acid sequences using single-stranded SV40 DNA probes, *Cold Spring Harbor Symp. Quant. Biol.* **39**:147.

Khoury, G., Howley, P., Nathans, D., and Martin M. 1975b, Post-transcriptional selection of simian virus 40-specific RNA, *J. Virol.* **15**:433.

Kimura, G., 1974, Genetic evidence for SV40 gene function in enhancement of replication of human adenivirus in simian cells, *Nature (London)* **248**:590.

Kimura, G., 1975, Temperature-sensitive growth of cells transformed by ts-a mutant of polyoma virus, *Nature (London)* **253**:639.

Kimura, G., and Itagaki, A., 1975, Initiation and maintenance of cell transformation by simian virus 40: A viral genetic property, *Proc. Natl. Acad. Sci. USA* **72**:673.

Lai, C. -J., and Nathans, D., 1974a, Deletion mutants of simian virus 40 generated by enzymatic excision of DNA segments from the viral genome, *J. Mol. Biol.* **89**:179.

Lai, C.-J., and Nathans, D., 1974b, Mapping temperature-sensitive mutants of simian virus 40: Rescue of mutants by fragments of viral DNA, *Virology* **60**:466.

Lai, C.-J., and Nathans, D., 1975, Mapping the genes of simian virus 40, *Cold Spring Harbor Symp. Quant. Biol.* **39**:53.

Lopez-Revilla, R., and Walter, G., 1973, Polypeptide specific for cells with adenovirus 2-SV40 hybrid Ad2$^+$ND1, *Nature (London) New Biol.* **244**:165.

Magnusson, G., Pigiet, V., Winnacker, E. L., Abrams, R., and Reichard, P., 1973, RNA linked short DNA fragments during polyoma replication, *Proc. Natl. Acad. Sci. USA* **70**:412.

Martin, M. A., Khoury, G., and Fareed, G. C., 1975, Specific reiteration of viral DNA sequences in mammalian cells, *Cold Spring Harbor Symp. Quant. Biol.* **39**:129.

Martin, R. G., and Chou, J. Y., 1975, Simian virus 40 functions required for the establishment and maintenance of malignant transformation, *J. Virol.* **15**:599.

Martin, R. G., Chou, J. Y., Avila, J., and Saral, R., 1975, The semi-autonomous replicon: A molecular model for the oncogenicity of SV40, *Cold Spring Harbor Symp. Quant. Biol.* **39**:17.

Mertz, J. E., and Berg, P., 1974a, Defective simian virus 40 genomes: Isolation and growth of individual clones, *Virology* **62**:112.

Mertz, J. E., and Berg, P., 1974b, Viable deletion mutants of simian virus 40: Selective isolation using HpaII restriction endonuclease, *Proc. Natl. Acad. Sci. USA* **71**:4879.

Mertz, J. E., Carbon, J., Herzberg, M., Davis, R. W., and Berg, P., 1975, Isolation and characterization of individual clones of simian virus 40 mutants containing deletions, duplications and insertions in their DNA, *Cold Spring Harbor Symp. Quant. Biol.* **39**:69.

Nathans, D., and Danna, K., 1972, Specific origin in SV40 DNA replication, *Nature (London) New Biol.* **236**:200.

Osborn, M., and Weber, K., 1975a, Simian virus 40 gene A function and maintenance of transformation, *J. Virol.* **15**:636.

Osborn, M., and Weber, K., 1975b, T antigen, the A function and transformation, *Cold Spring Harbor Symp. Quant. Biol.* **39**:267.

Paulin, D., and Cuzin, F., 1975, Polyoma virus T antigen. I. Synthesis of modified heat labile T antigen in cells transformed with the *ts-a* mutant, *J. Virol.* **15**:393.

Pett, D. M., Estes, M. K., and Pagano, J. S., 1975, Structural proteins of simian virus 40. I. Histone characteristics of low molecular weight polypeptides, *J. Virol.* **15**:379.

Pigiet, V., Winnacker, E. L., Eliasson, R., and Reichard, P., 1973, Discontinuous elongation of both strands of the replication forks in polyoma DNA replication, *Nature (London) New Biol.* **245**:203.

Reed, S. I., Ferguson, J., Davis, R. W., and Stark, G. R., 1975, T antigen binds to simian virus 40 DNA at the origin of replication, *Proc. Natl. Acad. Sci. USA* **72**:1605.

Renger, H. C., and Basilico, C., 1972, Mutation causing temperature sensitive expression of cell transformation by a tumor virus, *Proc. Nat. Acad. Sci. USA* **69**:109.

Robb, J. A., 1973, Simian virus 40–host cell interactions. I. Temperature-sensitive regulation of SV40 T antigen in 3T3 mouse cells transformed by the ts* 101 temperature-sensitive early mutant of SV40, *J. Virol.* **12**:1187.

Robb, J. A., 1975, Regulation of SV40 tumor antigen in transformed mouse 3T3 cells, *Cold Spring Harbor Symp. Quant. Biol.* **39**:277.

Robberson, D. L., and Fried, A.M.C., 1974, Sequence arrangements in clonal isolates of polyoma defective DNA, *Proc. Natl. Acad. Sci. USA* **71**:3497.

Robberson, D. L., Crawford, L. V., Syrett, C., and James, A. W., 1975, Unidirectional replication of a minority of polyoma virus and SV40 DNA's, *J. Gen. Virol.* **26**:59.

Rudland, P. S., Eckhart, W., Gospodarowicz, D., and Seifert, W., 1974, Action of a fibroblast growth factor on cell transformation mutants in culture: Loss of growth initiating ability at permissive temperature, *Nature (London)* **250**:337.

Shenk, T. E., Rhides, C., Rigby, P., and Berg, P., 1975a, Biochemical method for mapping mutational alterations in DNA with S1 nuclease: The location of deletions and temperature-sensitive mutations in simian virus 40, *Proc. Natl. Acad. Sci. USA* **72**:989.

Shenk, T. E., Rhodes, C., Rigby, P. W. J., and Berg, P., 1975b, Mapping of mutational alterations in DNA with S1 nuclease: The location of deletions, insertions and temperature-sensitive mutations in SV40, *Cold Spring Harbor Symp. Quant. Biol.* **39**:61.

Staal, S. P., and Rowe, W. P., 1975, Enhancement of adenovirus infection in WI-38 and AGMK cells by pretreatment of cells with 5-iododeoxyuridine, *Virology* **64**:513.

Summers, J., 1975, Physical map of polyoma viral DNA fragments produced by cleavage with a restriction enzyme from *Haemophilus aegyptius,* endonuclease R · Hae III, *J. Virol.* **15**:946.

Tegtmeyer, P., 1972, Simian virus 40 deoxyribonucleic acid synthesis: The viral replicon, *J. Virol.* **10**:591.

Tegtmeyer, P., 1975a, Altered pattern of protein synthesis in infection by SV40 mutants, *Cold Spring Harbor Symp. Quant. Biol.* **39**:9.

Tegtmeyer, P., 1975b, Function of simian virus 40 gene A in transforming infection, *J. Virol.* **15**:613.

Tooze, J. (ed.), 1973, *The Molecular Biology of Tumour Viruses,* Cold Spring Harbor Laboratory, Cold Spring Harbor, N.Y. 743 pp.

Weinberg, R. A., Warnaar, S. O., and Winocour, E., 1972, Isolation and characterization of simian virus 40 ribonucleic acid, *J. Virol.* **10**:193.

Weinberg, R. A., Ben-Ishai, Z., and Newbold, J. E., 1974, SV40 transcription in productively-infected and transformed cells, *J. Virol.* **13**:1263.

Winnacker, E. L., Magnusson, G., and Reichard, P., 1972, Replication of polyoma DNA in isolated nuclei. I. Characterization of the system from mouse fibroblast 3T6 cells, *J. Mol. Biol.* **72**:528.

Winocour, E., Frenkel, N., Lavi, S., Osenholts, M., and Rozenblatt, S., 1975, Host substitution in SV40 and polyoma DNA, *Cold Spring Harbor Symp. Quant. Biol.* **39**:101.

Wright, P., and diMayorca, G., 1975, Virion polypeptide composition of the human papovavirus, BK: Comparison with simian virus 40 and polyoma virus, *J. Virol.* **15**:828.

Yoshiike, K., Furuno, A., Watanabe, S., Uchida, S., Matsubara, K., and Takagi, K., 1975, Characterization of defective simian virus 40 DNA: Comparison between large plaque and small plaque types *Cold Spring Harbor Symp. Quant. Biol.* **39**:85.

CHAPTER 2

Genetics of Adenoviruses

Harold S. Ginsberg and C. S. H. Young

Department of Microbiology
College of Physicians and Surgeons
Columbia University
New York, New York 10032

1. INTRODUCTION

Since the initial discoveries of adenoviruses (Rowe *et al.*, 1953; Hilleman and Werner, 1954), these agents have generated intense interest because of the varied clinical and cellular responses they induce. *In vivo,* adenoviruses produce infections which range from acute, febrile diseases to latent infections and induction of malignancy in unnatural hosts. Similarly, in cell cultures the reactions vary from acute cytopathic effects to cellular transformation. This array of host responses evolves from the nuclear infection which adenoviruses establish, and thus offers the opportunity to investigate intranuclear replication and transcription of an easily identified and manipulated species of DNA in eukaryotic cells. Since mammalian cells are so complex and contain on the order of 10^7 genes, it is a most difficult task to study directly the molecular reactions regulating cellular DNA synthesis, transcription of its complex genome, modification of its mRNAs, and translation of its messengers into functional gene products. Study of the smaller adenovirus genome, which contains a maximum of 50 genes and replicates in the nucleus of an eukaryotic cell, offers a simpler model which should yield evidence germane to the molecular biology of mammalian cells as well as to viral biosynthesis. Investigations with bacteriophages, however, pointed to the problem

27

that biochemical techniques alone were insufficient to reveal the controls governing many intracellular reactions. Selected deletion and conditionally lethal mutants were essential to expose the balanced mechanisms regulating the biosynthesis and assembly of bacteriophage components.

In recognition of the critical requirement for appropriate mutants, several laboratories (see Table 1) have selected conditionally lethal temperature-sensitive mutants of adenoviruses to investigate the reactions that control adenovirus replication as well as to study the genetic mechanisms of an easily manageable DNA-containing virus. It is the objective of this chapter to review the types of mutants thus far detected, the mutagenesis and selection of adenovirus mutants, their use in formal genetic studies (which also led to a comparison of the genetic and physical maps of the adenovirus genome), their phenotypes, and their utility in functional studies to understand the regulation of adenovirus replication and cellular transformation.

Adenovirus replication has been detailed in another volume of this series (Philipson and Lindberg, 1974), and a number of reviews have described different aspects of adenovirus structure and replication (Norrby, 1968; Ginsberg, 1969; Schlesinger, 1969; Green, 1970; Philipson and Pettersson, 1973). To familiarize the nonspecialist with the data pertinent to this chapter, however, the essential evidence will be summarized.

1.1. The Virion

1.1.1. Architecture of the Virion

The viral particle is an icosahedron with a mean diameter of 70–80 nm. Contrary to the initial prediction of Crick and Watson (1956), the isometric virus is not composed of identical repeating subunits, but rather the capsid is made of three unique major multimeric proteins and several minor proteins (Maizel *et al.,* 1968*a,b*; Norrby, 1968; Ginsberg, 1969; Schlesinger, 1969; Green, 1970; Philipson and Pettersson, 1973; Philipson and Lindberg, 1974). Owing to the early demonstration that the virion can be dissociated into intact native subunits, it has been possible to describe the architecture of the virion and the topography of its components (Wilcox *et al.,* 1963; Valentine and Pereira, 1965). These studies have further shown that the capsid components are identical with the great excess (approximately tenfold) of unassembled "soluble antigens" present in infected cell extracts, and that the capsid

TABLE 1

Publications Describing Isolation of Adenovirus Mutants

Virus and mutant type	Mutagen[a]	Killing or yield depression	Frequency of mutant (ts plaques/total)	References
H2 ts	NNG	~10^{-4}	7/172	Bégin and Weber (1975)
	HNO$_2$	~10^{-3}	5/170	
H5 ts	NH$_2$OH	10^{-5}	14/146	Williams et al. (1971)
	HNO$_2$	10^{-5}	8/95	
	BrdUrd	10^{-3}	2/355	
H5 ts	NH$_2$OH	10^{-5} ⎫		Ensinger and Ginsberg (1972)
	HNO$_2$	10^{-5} ⎬ 0.01–0.10%		
	NNG	0.5 ⎭		
H5 ts	NH$_2$OH	—	8/372	Takahashi (1972)
	NNG	—	2/317	
H5 ts	BrdUrd	—	3/165	Rubenstein and Ginsberg (1974)[b]
H12 ts	NNG	0.63	10/1440	Lundholm and Doerfler (1971)
H12 ts	UV	10^{-2}–10^{-3}	45/700	Shiroki et al. (1972)
	NH$_2$OH	10^{-2}–10^{-3}	24/370	
	BrdUrd	10^{-2}–10^{-3}	2/260	
	NNG	10^{-1}–10^{-3}	17/250	
H12 ts	HNO$_2$	5×10^{-4}	5/679	Ledinko (1974)
	NNG	10^{-1}	5/550	
H31 ts	UV	10^{-1}–10^{-4}	17/506[c]	Suzuki et al. (1972)
Al ts	NH$_2$OH	8×10^{-4}	27/238[d]	Ishibashi (1971)
H12 cyt	Spontaneous UV	—	5- to 6-fold increase over spontaneous background	Takemori et al. (1968)
Ad2+ND1 host range	NH$_2$OH	10^{-4}	3/250	Grodzicker et al. (1974a)
H5 host range	NH$_2$OH	—	7/372	Takahashi (1972)
H5 heat stable	Spontaneous	—	Only one mutant isolated	Young and Williams (1975)

[a] Abbreviations: BrdUrd, bromodeoxyuridine; NNG, N-methyl-N'-nitro-N-nitrosoguanidine; UV, ultraviolet irradiation.

[b] Owing to an unfortunate error, the wild-type virus used was type 5 rather than type 12 adenovirus as reported. Hence the mutants isolated and characterized have been shown to be independently isolated type 5 ts mutants.

[c] Range varied from 1/85 for 10^{-1} survivors to 7/144 for 2×10^{-4} survivors to 3/94 for 10^{-4} survivors.

[d] Ts mutants isolated from stocks that had been inactivated to give only from 0.5 to 3.0% ts.

proteins have the unusual feature of being soluble in aqueous media while remaining in their native functional forms. The capsid consists of 252 capsomers (Fig. 1), of which the faces and edges of the 20 equilateral triangles are comprised of 240 *hexons,* so termed because each has six neighbors (Ginsberg *et al.,* 1966). At each of the 12 vertices of the icosahedron, the axis of fivefold symmetry, is a *penton* (Valentine and Pereira, 1965), which consists of a *base,* the vertex capsomer, and a *fiber.* Three minor proteins of less than 25,000 daltons (proteins VI, VIII, and IX, Fig. 1) are reported to be associated with the hexons that make up the faces of the triangles, and one minor protein (protein IIIa) is said to be adjacent to the hexons surrounding the pentons, the so-called peripentonal hexons (Maizel *et al.,* 1968*a,b*; Everitt *et al.,* 1973). These minor proteins have been isolated in relatively constant amounts and may serve to assemble and stabilize the capsid, but until chemical evidence is presented showing that each is indeed a unique protein the possibility must also be entertained that some are degradation products of one or more of the major virion proteins. Internally, there are two core proteins (proteins V and VII) (Fig. 1) closely associated with the viral DNA (Laver, 1970; Prage and Pettersson, 1971; Russell *et al.,* 1971).

1.1.2. Virion Proteins

The hexon, which induces the production of type-specific neutralizing antibodies (Wilcox and Ginsberg, 1963*a*; Kjellén and Pereira, 1968; Kasel *et al.,* 1964), as well as broad cross-reacting antibodies which immunologically identify the adenoviruses as being related (Wilcox and Ginsberg, 1961; Pereira, 1960), is composed of three identical polypeptides of 100,000–120,000 daltons each, depending on the type (Maizel *et al.,* 1968*a,b*; Franklin *et al.,* 1971; Cornick *et al.,* 1973; Stinski and Ginsberg, 1975). The fiber varies morphologically in length in different types (Wilcox *et al.,* 1963; Valentine and Pereira, 1965; Norrby, 1968, 1969) and therefore probably in molecular weights. The type 2 and type 5 fibers have molecular weights of 183,000 (Dorsett and Ginsberg, 1975) to 200,000 (Sundquist *et al.,* 1973*b*) and consist of three polypeptide chains of 60,000–65,000 each (Dorsett and Ginsberg, 1975; Sundquist *et al.,* 1973*b*). The fiber, which is glycosylated (Ishibashi and Maizel, 1974*b*) and phosphorylated (Russell *et al.,* 1972*b*), appears on the basis of biochemical evidence to be composed of either two polypeptide chains which are chemically identical and one which is unique or three chemically different chains (Dorsett and Ginsberg, 1975). Physical and transcription maps which are presently being

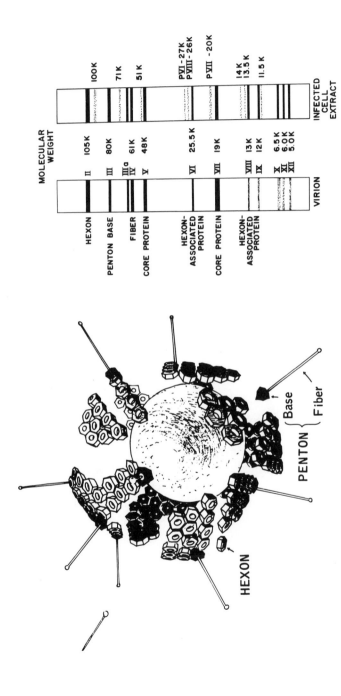

Fig. 1. Diagrammatic representation of a type 5 adenovirus particle partially disrupted to demonstrate the viral capsid and nucleoprotein core. Drawings of representative patterns of the denatured virion proteins and of infected-cell extracts, electrophoresed in SDS-polyacrylamide gels, show the relative sizes of the polypeptide chains. The nomenclature follows that of Maizel et al. (1968a) and Everitt et al. (1973). The molecular weights of the major type 5 virion polypeptide chains are presented since some are significantly different from the values given for the comparable proteins of type 2 adenovirus (Kauffman, unpublished data). In electrophoretic pattern of infected-cell extract, solid bands represent virion proteins and dotted bands represent nonstructural proteins.

constructed should furnish more precise data, however, on the proportion of the genome that codes for fiber proteins, and hence will indicate the number of unique polypeptide chains. The penton base is relatively unstable and highly sensitive to proteolytic enzymes (Pereira, 1958; Everett and Ginsberg, 1958), and it therefore has not yet been well characterized except to note that it consists of several polypeptide chains (four or five) of 70,000–80,000 molecular weight (Maizel *et al.,* 1968*a,b*). The fiber is associated with the base through noncovalent bonds which are disrupted by 2.5 M guanidine-HCl (Norrby and Skaaret, 1967), 8% pyridine (Pettersson and Höglund, 1969), or 33% formamide (Neurath *et al.,* 1968).

1.1.3. Viral DNA

The viral genome is a linear, double-stranded DNA molecule of 20–25×10^6 daltons (Green *et al.,* 1967; van der Eb *et al.,* 1969), depending on the immunological type and animal host (there are 31 human, 23 simian, 8 avian, 6 bovine, 4 porcine, 2 canine, and 1 murine types reported). It is striking that the viral DNA is neither circularly permuted nor terminally redundant, but each strand of the molecule contains an inverted terminal repetition (Garon *et al.,* 1972; Wolfson and Dressler, 1972), like the adeno-associated virus DNA (Koczot *et al.,* 1973). Hence, when the viral DNA is denatured at a limited concentration, both strands can form single-stranded circles through hydrogen bonds between the complementary ends (Garon *et al.,* 1972; Wolfson and Dressler, 1972). Concordant with an inverted terminal repetition, the $3'$ termini of both molecular ends of type 2 and 5 DNAs have been shown to have identical sequences consisting of . . . pCpC . . . pGpApTpG$^{3'}$ (Steenbergh *et al.,* 1975). However, the function of this novel DNA structure is unclear. It has also been reported that a small protein molecule associated with the viral DNA maintains the genome in a circular form when in the virion and when artificially released from it (Robinson *et al.,* 1973). A similar circular genome has not been detected, however, after intracellular uncoating of the virion (Robinson *et al.,* 1973) or during viral DNA replication (Sussenbach *et al.,* 1972; Pettersson, 1973).

Just as adenoviruses have been divided into subgroups according to biological properties, such as oncogenicity or hemagglutination (Huebner *et al.,* 1965; Rosen, 1960), the viral DNAs of different types may be similarly classified according to base composition (Piña and Green, 1965) and DNA–DNA hybridization (Green, 1970; Garon *et al.,* 1973). Thus adenoviruses have been arranged into three subgroups (A,

B, and C) according to their oncogenic potential in newborn hamsters (Huebner *et al.*, 1965). The viruses fall into similar subgroups when divided according to G + C content and nucleotide sequence homology. The G + C content of subgroup A, which consists of the most oncogenic adenoviruses (types 12, 18, and 31), is 48–49%; subgroup B, which contains weakly oncogenic viruses (e.g., types 3, 7, and 21), has a G + C content of 49–52%; and subgroup C, which consists of viruses that are essentially nononcogenic (e.g., types 1, 2, and 5), has a G + C content of 55–60% (Green, 1970; Piña and Green, 1965). It is also striking that between members of a subgroup the nucleotide sequences are up to 95% homologous, whereas DNA-DNA hybridizations between selected members of different subgroups show only about 10% homology (Green, 1970; Garon *et al.*, 1973). Electron microscopic examination of heteroduplexes formed between DNAs from different subgroup viruses reveals considerable heterology (Garon *et al.*, 1973), while DNAs from viruses belonging to the same subgroup show almost complete homology (Garon *et al.*, 1973; Bartok *et al.*, 1974) except for two discrete regions of nonhomology, one located 0.08 fractional map unit from one terminus, and the second 0.52 fractional map unit from the opposite end of the genome (Bartok *et al.*, 1974).

Study of partially denatured type 2 and 12 adenovirus DNA molecules using electron microscopic techniques has revealed regions of the genome that are particularly rich in adenine–thymine base pairs (Doerfler and Kleinschmidt, 1970; Doerfler *et al.*, 1972). It is striking that the right-hand end (according to the orientation adopted for restriction enzyme maps, Fig. 2) of the genome is particularly rich in A · T base pairs, but both ends of the DNA molecules are relatively abundant in A · T base pairs, and one or two major internal A · T-rich regions are also detectable. The unique denaturation maps also present additional evidence that the genome is nonpermuted.

The similarities and disparities in fine structure of adenovirus DNAs from different serological types have been further described using bacterial restriction enzymes which cleave the double-stranded molecule at sites containing unique palindromes. Thus the restriction endonuclease *Eco* · RI, isolated from *Escherichia coli* strain RY-13 (Yoshimori, 1971), cleaves DNA by introducing single-strand breaks between the guanine and adenine residues on each of the two DNA strands at sites containing the base sequence (Hedgpeth *et al.*, 1973).

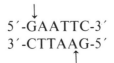

TYPE 2 ADENOVIRUS

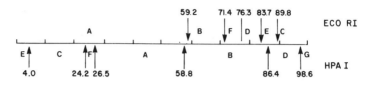

TYPE 5 ADENOVIRUS

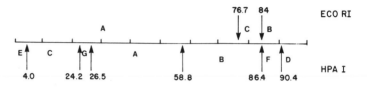

Fig. 2.   Endonuclease cleavage maps of type 2 and 5 adenovirus DNAs. The *E. coli* RI
(*Eco*·RI) and *Haemophilus parainfluenzae* I (*Hpa*I) endonucleases were used; the
DNA fragments were separated by electrophoresis on 1.4% agarose gels, and denaturation maps were developed to position each fragment on the viral genome. From Mulder
et al. (1974*a*).

The DNA fragments can be separated according to size by electrophoresis through agarose gel (Pettersson *et al.*, 1973) and ordered on
the genome by heteroduplex and denaturation loop mapping. More
than 20 different restriction enzymes have now been isolated and
characterized using a variety of DNA molecules. Representative
restriction maps of type 2 and 5 adenovirus DNAs using *Eco*·RI and
*Hpa*I (*Haemophilus parainfluenzae*), shown in Fig. 2, indicate the similarities and differences in their DNA structures which were revealed by
this relatively simple procedure (Mulder *et al.*, 1974*b*).

1.2.   Viral Biosynthesis

1.2.1.   Virion Replication

Production of infectious virions follows from an ordered series of
reactions which is initiated by association of a viral particle with a susceptible cell and culminated by the assembly of virions from its
subunits. Replication of type 2 and 5 adenoviruses has been most extensively studied because the yield is great (about 10^4 PFU/cell), and the
virion, as well as most of the components, can be easily purified and
analyzed. Accordingly, the molecular biology of adenovirus infection is
known in greatest detail with these types, and the description of

adenovirus replication that follows will summarize the investigations with type 2 and 5 viruses. A single cycle of type 5 adenovirus multiplication with the accompanying biosynthetic events is diagrammatically summarized in Fig. 3. The temporal characteristics and viral yield vary, however, with different types of adenoviruses. For example, in contrast to type 5 virus, the eclipse period for type 12 adenovirus at 36°C is 16–18 h (Gilead and Ginsberg, 1965) and biosynthesis of the viral DNA cannot be detected until 12–15 h (Piña and Green, 1969) after infection. The virion attaches to a susceptible cell's receptor sites via the fiber (Levine and Ginsberg, 1967; Philipson *et al.*, 1968), but the nature of the cell's specific receptors has not yet been identified. Attached virions enter susceptible cells by phagocytosis (Dales, 1962; Chardonnet and Dales, 1970) or direct penetration of the plasma membrane (Morgan *et al.*, 1969). Whether either entry mechanism is preferred is still unclear, but even after phagocytosis the virions must directly penetrate the membrane of the phagocytic vacuole to gain access to the cytoplasm. Once within the cytoplasm, viral uncoating (i.e., viral eclipse) is rapidly initiated, with disengagement of the pentons (Sussenbach, 1967) which is soon followed by dissociation of the capsid and release of the nucleoprotein core (Sussenbach, 1967; Lawrence and Ginsberg, 1967; Lonberg-Holm and Philipson, 1969). Neither synthesis of proteins nor replication of nucleic acids is required for these initial uncoating reactions (Lawrence and Ginsberg, 1967; Lonberg-Holm and Philipson, 1969). The partially uncoated virus appears to be transported in microtubules to nuclear pores (Chardonnet and Dales, 1970), where further dissociation of DNA from the internal proteins occurs at the nuclear membrane (Morgan *et al.*, 1969) or in

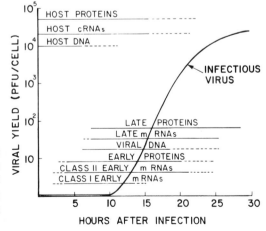

Fig. 3. Schematic representation of sequential biosynthetic events in replication of type 5 adenovirus, and the effect of viral infection on biosynthesis of host macromolecules.

the nucleus (Lonberg-Holm and Philipson, 1969). However, the extent and the mechanisms of the terminal uncoating reaction have not been determined.

The description of viral penetration and uncoating presented carries with it a caveat. The ratio of total viral particles to infectious virions (i.e., plaque-formers) varies from ten to several hundred, according to the viral species (type), and all the experiments described employed large multiplicities of infection. Consequently, the sequence of events that was observed, which was followed by biochemical analysis of isotopically labeled virus and electron microscopic observations, involved a large population of viral particles in each cell, but the virion or virions that established the infectious process may not necessarily have followed the same sequence. This unfortunate situation plagues many of the biochemical investigations of viral replication.

1.2.2. Transcription

Shortly after the viral DNA reaches the nucleus, 2–3 h after infection, transcription begins (Thomas and Green, 1969; Lucas and Ginsberg, 1971; Parsons and Green, 1971). Since protein synthesis is not required (Parsons and Green, 1971) and the virion does not contain its own RNA polymerase, transcription apparently involves a host enzyme. This has been shown to be α-amanitin sensitive and therefore probably corresponds to the DNA-dependent RNA polymerase II (Ledinko, 1971; Price and Penman, 1972). Prior to viral DNA replication, only a portion of the genome is transcribed, yielding *early mRNAs* (Thomas and Green, 1969; Parsons and Green, 1971; Lucas and Ginsberg, 1971; Tibbetts *et al.*, 1974). However, the extent of the genome copied into early transcripts is still uncertain, with reports varying from 10–20% (Thomas and Green, 1969; Lucas and Ginsberg, 1971) to 40–50% (Tibbetts *et al.*, 1974). It is particularly important to note that the genes for early transcripts are not limited to a single region but are distributed throughout the genome (Craig *et al.*, 1975). Following the initiation of DNA replication, "late" transcripts appear (Bello and Ginsberg, 1969; Green *et al.*, 1970; Lucas and Ginsberg, 1971) and apparently the transcription of about 50% of the early mRNAs, the so-called class I early mRNAs (Lucas and Ginsberg, 1971; Craig *et al.*, 1975), ceases or is markedly reduced, although there is also not complete agreement on these findings (Thomas and Green, 1969; Tibbetts *et al.*, 1974).

The apparent discrepancies in the data describing the proportion of the genome transcribed at any given time, and hence the nature of regulation of transcription, may follow from the differences in techniques employed. Fundamentally, two methods are used: (1) liquid hybridization of excess RNA to a small amount of radioactively labeled DNA and (2) DNA–RNA hybridization with varying amounts of denatured DNA stabilized on a filter. In the former technique, the reaction is driven by a large amount of RNA and therefore even sparse species of complementary RNAs are detected. In contrast, the filter hybridization procedure, which can distinguish different species of RNA by sequential hybridization competition, readily differentiates unique RNA species, but abundant transcripts are primarily detected. The biological significance of rarely transcribed RNAs in the replication process, particularly under conditions of very high multiplicity of infection (10^3 or more viral particles per cell), is unclear at present.

The reactions that regulate the limited but not localized transcription of the parental viral genome, the onset of late transcription, and the switching of transcription from one strand to the other during late transcription (Tibbetts et al., 1974; Fujinaga and Green, 1970; Tibbetts and Pettersson, 1974) are still unknown. Indeed, there are several reactions by which the original transcripts are modified to produce functional mRNAs, and their mechanisms and controls are also uncertain: (1) the primary transcripts are considerably larger than the polysomal mRNAs (McGuire et al., 1972; Wall et al., 1972), which are also heterogeneous in size, varying from 9 S to 27 S (Parsons and Green, 1971; Lindberg et al., 1972; Philipson et al., 1973; Craig et al., 1975); (2) only 70–80% of the RNA transcribed is processed and transported into the cytoplasm (McGuire et al., 1972; Lucas and Ginsberg, 1972); (3) the 3′ terminus of most, if not all, viral mRNAs is polyadenylated in the nucleus after transcription (Philipson et al., 1971); and (4) the 5′ ends of the mRNAs are methylated (Moss, personal communication). It is noteworthy that the heterogeneity and processing of adenovirus-specific RNAs resemble the characteristics of the uninfected host cell's heterogeneous (hn) RNAs, and hence investigation of transcription of adenovirus mRNAs offers another convenient probe for study of the molecular biology of eukaryotic cells.

1.2.3. DNA Replication

In productive infections, under conditions of multiple infection of each cell, replication of type 5 viral DNA begins about 6 h after infection, reaching a maximum about 18 h after viral attachment (Ginsberg *et al.,* 1967; Piña and Green, 1969). Because viral DNA has a higher G + C content than that of the host, the two species can be effectively separated (Ginsberg *et al.,* 1967; Piña and Green, 1969). Accordingly, it is noted that synthesis of host DNA begins to decline about 6 h after infection, when replication of viral DNA commences, and production of host DNA is effectively blocked by 12 h (Ginsberg *et al.,* 1967). But prior synthesis of DNA, host or viral, is not essential for the inhibition of host DNA replication (Ginsberg *et al.,* 1967), which implies that the shutoff is mediated by an early viral event or by a component of the infecting viral particle.

Like replication of most linear DNA molecules, little is known about the precise mechanism of duplicating adenovirus DNA. Although protein synthesis is required for the initiation of viral DNA replication (Wilcox and Ginsberg, 1963*b*), there is no evidence to indicate whether the DNA polymerase is host or viral coded. Continued protein production, however, is not needed after replication of viral DNA is established (Horwitz *et al.,* 1973). Van der Vliet and Levine (1973) have identified in type 5-infected cell extracts proteins of 72,000 and 48,000 daltons which bind preferentially to single-stranded DNA (so-called DNA-binding proteins), similar to the T4 phage gene-32 protein (Alberts and Frey, 1970). Peptide maps of the two suggest, however, that the 48,000 dalton polypeptide is a proteolytic breakdown product of the 72,000 dalton protein (Levine, personal communication). Whether both proteins are functional is uncertain. Like T4 gene-32 protein (Alberts and Frey, 1970), the DNA-binding protein in adenovirus-infected cells appears to be a viral gene product which is present in large numbers of copies per cell, and is essential for DNA replication (van der Vliet *et al.,* 1975). Type 12-infected cells contain similar proteins of 60,000 and 48,000 daltons (Rosenwirth *et al.,* 1975).

There are present in virus-infected cells replicative forms of viral DNA which sediment more rapidly and are denser than mature virion DNA (Bellett and Younghusband, 1972; van der Vliet and Sussenbach, 1972; van der Eb, 1973; Pettersson, 1973). These replicative intermediates can also be isolated by the so-called M-band (Sarkosyl) technique (Pearson and Hanawalt, 1971; Shiroki *et al.,* 1974; Yamashita and Green, 1974). In each instance, the replicative intermediate appears to consist of double-stranded DNA with single-stranded branches (Bellett and Younghusband, 1972; van der Vliet and Sussenbach, 1972; van der Eb, 1973; Pettersson, 1973). Studying viral DNA replication in nuclei from infected cells, Sussenbach and colleagues have presented data which indicate that the DNA is replicated semiconservatively but asymmetrically, that the strand which has the greater buoyant density in alkaline CsCl is initially replicated, displacing the complementary strand, and that the lighter strand is then copied in discontinuous segments which are subsequently joined (Sussenbach *et al.,* 1972, 1973; Ellens *et al.,* 1974). Recent unpublished data, however, suggest that DNA replication can be initiated at either end of the molecule and that either strand can be displaced (Pettersson *et al.,* 1973; Winnacker, personal communications; Lavelle *et al.,* 1975). It should be stressed that although each viral DNA strand has the structure to generate a single-stranded circle (i.e., the strands have inverted terminal repetitious ends, as described above), such single-strand "circles" have not been observed in the replication complexes (Pettersson, 1973; Ellens *et al.,* 1974).

1.2.4. Protein Synthesis

Like host nuclear proteins, adenovirus proteins, whose transcripts are also made in the nucleus, are produced in the cytoplasm and rapidly transported into the nucleus for assembly (Velicer and Ginsberg, 1968, 1970). Evidence clearly demonstrates that synthesis of early proteins precedes and is mandatory for replication of viral DNA (Wilcox and Ginsberg, 1963b; Horwitz *et al.,* 1973). Thus far, only the T (Pope and Rowe, 1964; Gilead and Ginsberg, 1965) and P (Russell and Knight, 1967) antigens and the DNA-binding protein (van der Vliet and Levine, 1973; Rosenwirth *et al.,* 1975) have been identified as probable early viral gene products. Translation of late proteins, which primarily consist of virion components, occurs on cytoplasmic polyribosomes of 180–200 S (Velicer and Ginsberg, 1968; Thomas and Green, 1966) and requires 1–2 min per polypeptide (Velicer and Ginsberg, 1970; White *et al.,* 1969). Kinetic data suggest that after completion and release from polyribosomes the nascent polypeptide chains are rapidly transported into the nucleus, where they are assembled into immunologically reactive multimeric capsid proteins (Velicer and Ginsberg, 1970). However, cytoplasmic assembly of newly made protomers into capsid proteins can occur, as will be noted below with certain temperature-sensitive mutants (Kauffman and Ginsberg, 1976). Indeed, nascent polypeptides made *in vitro* can even self-assemble into capsid proteins in a cell-free reaction mixture (Wilhelm and Ginsberg, 1972).

Hexon protein, the major viral protein, is the first capsid protein to appear in the cell and is made in greatest amounts. All the capsid proteins, however, are produced in relative abundance since only about 10–20% of each of the proteins synthesized is assembled into virions (Green, 1962; Wilcox and Ginsberg, 1963c). The excess viral proteins (often termed "soluble antigens"), along with similar amounts of excessive viral DNA, are the constituents of the characteristic intranuclear inclusion bodies seen in adenovirus-infected cells (Boyer et al., 1957, 1959; Morgan et al., 1960).

1.2.5. Assembly

It was generally accepted until several years ago that the capsid of isometric viruses self-assembled around previously formed viral nucleoprotein cores. Evidence has accumulated, however, showing that an RNA-deficient poliovirus procapsid may be initially assembled as the precursor of the infectious virion (Maizel et al., 1967; Phillips et al., 1968). With insertion of the viral RNA, a procapsid protein is processed to form the stable capsid (Jacobson and Baltimore, 1968). Incomplete particles of SV40 have also been described as putative precursors of intact virions (Ozer, 1972; Ozer and Tegtmeyer, 1972). King and his collaborators, studying the assembly of the Salmonella typhimurium phage P22, reported convincing evidence that formation of a prohead is an initial phase of virion assembly. The prohead is a shell consisting of the capsid protein and a "scaffolding protein," which exits from the precursor shell in concert with encapsidation of viral DNA (King and Casjens, 1974). The P22 proheads are similar to the T4 τ particles which are precursors to T4 heads (Kellenberger et al., 1968; Simon, 1972).

Data have been recently presented reporting that incomplete adenovirus particles (i.e., empty capsids) are also assembled as precursors into which viral DNA is inserted (Sundquist et al., 1973a; Ishibashi and Maizel, 1974a). With final assembly, two or three precursor viral proteins appear to be processed by cleavage, and at least one disappears from the putative precursor particle (Sundquist et al., 1973a; Ishibashi and Maizel, 1974a; Anderson et al., 1973).

Evidence obtained from the experiments summarized above, as well as from studies of abortive infections produced by elevated temperatures (Okubo and Raskas, 1971), arginine deprivation (Rouse and Schlesinger, 1972; Everitt et al., 1971), and temperature-sensitive mutants (Williams et al., 1974; Ensinger and Ginsberg, 1972), implies that assembly is controlled at several junctures during viral replication: (1) transport of nascent polypeptide chains or capsomers, (2) assembly of protomers into capsomers, (3) formation of capsids, and (4) incorporation of viral nucleoprotein cores into virions.

2. ADENOVIRUS MUTANTS

2.1. Types of Mutants

A priori, the following classes of mutants might be sought in adenoviruses.

Temperature-restricted mutants: in particular, the so-called temperature-sensitive (*ts*) mutants that fail to replicate at a higher, non-permissive temperature while doing so at a lower, permissive one.

Host range mutants: both those with an increased and those with a restricted host-cell range compared to wild type. In some circumstances, where a function is required for replication in only one of the hosts, restricted mutants may display an absolute, as opposed to a conditional, defectiveness for the function concerned.

Plaque morphology mutants: both the size and appearance of plaques may be mutable.

Drug-resistant mutants: if drugs that act specifically on viral replication exist, mutants resistant to their action may be sought.

Virion structural mutants: both those with altered capsid proteins that affect the sensitivity of the virus to *in vitro* treatments and those with altered genomes so that the virions have an altered buoyant density. The latter might be defective, requiring a helper virus for replication.

Table 1 lists the publications describing the isolation of adenovirus mutants. It can be seen that most studies have been directed toward isolating temperature-sensitive mutants. There are several reasons for this: (1) Most genes that code for a protein product are expected to be able to mutate to a *ts* form since the temperature optimum for enzyme activity or for macromolecular folding or assembly should be mutable. In addition, since it is a reasonable assumption that most of the adenovirus genome is transcribed and translated, it is probable that *ts* mutations can occur throughout the genome. (2) *Ts* mutants are conditionally lethal and thus are suitable for functional studies since the external environment, namely, the temperature of incubation, may be manipulated to identify the time of action of the mutated gene and the consequences of a temperature shift. (3) Since *ts* mutants fail to grow at the restrictive temperature, this property may be used to select rare *ts*+ revertants or recombinants arising in a predominantly *ts* population and also to study phenotypic interactions between different *ts* mutants. (4) In certain favorable circumstances, the *ts* mutation may be proved to be in a gene specifying a particular protein product. This can be done if the protein can be isolated and proved to be chemically altered from, or functionally more thermolabile than, the wild-type protein. In the absence of such a demonstration, the assignment of mutations to particular genes is more problematic. Fortunately, despite the lack of "nonsense" mutants and the appropriate suppressor hosts in animal virus systems, other physical and biochemical methods that unambiguously ascribe mutations to particular proteins are becoming available and will be described in a later section.

While emphasis on *ts* mutants reflects concern about the use of mutants as *tools* for investigating the lytic cycle, it should be recognized that other classes of mutants are necessary for certain objectives. For example, genetic mapping is more reliable with deletion mutants or with the use of three-factor crosses involving a third marker with non-*ts* phenotype. Similarly, if mutants that are absolutely defective in nonlytic processes such as transformation exist, they would be helpful in revealing the details of the mechanisms involved.

2.2. Mutagenic Procedures

During serial passage of a virus, diverse spontaneous mutations will accumulate, giving rise to a stock of virus that is genetically heterogeneous. To reduce the amount of background genetic heterogeneity and to reduce the risk of isolating siblings of a mutation that has occurred early during viral replication, it is necessary to clone the virus, generally by a number of rounds of plaque-purification, before growing up a stock from which mutants are to be isolated. Therefore, relatively homogeneous starting material can be prepared, and since there are frequently no selective methods to isolate particular classes of mutants (see below) a variety of mutagenic treatments have been used to increase the frequency of mutants within the population (Table 1). The mutagens used have been those that will predominantly induce "missense" base-pair changes. This type of mutation is considered to be essential for the lesion that leads, for example, to a *ts* phenotype. The treatments fall into two experimental categories: (1) those used *in vitro* which are directed against the virion DNA (nitrous acid, hydroxylamine, UV irradiation) and (2) those used in the infected cell during viral replication (nitrosoguanidine, bromodeoxyuridine). Both categories have pitfalls which require caution. The mutagenic lesion induced by *in vitro* methods will be a mismatched base pair $m/+$. If the virus is plated directly, the plaques arising from viruses containing such mismatches will be genetically mixed. Many methods of mutant isolation score mixed plaques as wild type, as, for example, in the case of ts/ts^+, where the plaque may be confused with a homogeneous ts^+ unless the individual progeny arising within the plaque are in turn examined. In theory, this problem may be avoided by allowing the mutagen-treated virus to replicate a number of times to segregate the mutated and wild-type DNA strands, but this procedure may lead to errors associated with treatments of type 2. In practice, mutant viruses have been isolated without a prior growth cycle (as, for example, in Williams *et al.*, 1971; Ledinko, 1974; Bégin and Weber, 1975). This implies either that $m/+$ mismatches are repaired, in some cases, to m/m before the first round of DNA replication reaches them, or perhaps that during the first round of replication the $+$ strand is displaced and occasionally lost in the single-strand displacement mechanism of DNA replication characteristic of adenoviruses (Sussenbach *et al.*, 1972; Ellens *et al.*, 1974). The reasons for this apparent anomaly are unknown, but it may yield clues as to the processes of adenovirus-DNA repair or replication. The errors associated with treatments directed against virus replicating *in vivo* arise from the fact that mutations occurring early during the treatment will be replicated, and "separate" mutants isolated from the mutagenized stock may prove to be clonally related. Since the aim is to obtain a range of different mutants, the isolation of related ones is a waste of materials and time, and, moreover, could lead to false conclusions concerning the mutation frequency of certain gene functions. The problem may be avoided by isolating single mutants from a number of independently treated stocks. Even where this precaution has not been taken, separate mutants isolated from one stock may prove to be different. For example, Lundholm and Doerfler (1971) isolated ten *ts* mutants from a nitrosoguanidine-treated stock of type 12 adenovirus, and several of the mutants displayed different degrees of "leakiness" at the nonpermissive temperature, which suggests that they were not clonally related.

The frequency of mutants and the degree of inactivation or reduction in viral yield induced by the various mutagens are listed in Table 1. From the data on mutant frequencies which have been published so far, it is difficult to assess the optimal dose of, or length of treatment with, a particular mutagen for the induction of mutations. This is partly because treatment conditions have varied among the different laboratories, but more importantly because methods of screening for rare *ts* mutants among predominantly ts^+ populations are inadequate to give statistically reliable dose–response curves, even where several hundred plaques have been examined (Suzuki *et al.,* 1972). Technically, it is much easier to study the relationship between mutagen treatment and mutant frequency in the reversion of *ts* mutants to *ts*$^+$. This has been examined using SV40 *ts* mutants (Cleaver and Weil, 1975) and, in principle, could be studied in adenoviruses. It is clear from Table 1 that many of the mutants isolated are derived from populations that have undergone extensive mutagenesis. Therefore, it is likely that each mutant contains several base-pair differences from wild type in conjunction with the one that leads to the particular phenotype being sought. The consequences of this will be dealt with in Section 2.4.

2.3. Isolation of Mutants

All of the phenotypic changes sought result from "forward" mutations, i.e., mutations from wild to mutant phenotype. In general, the change involves the loss or restriction of some function: for example, the ability to replicate in a certain host cell or at a particular temperature. Consequently, in these circumstances, it is impossible to select directly for the mutant phenotype among a population composed overwhelmingly of wild-type virus. Thus all searches for mutants of this kind involve picking individual plaques that are screened for the desired phenotype. Semiselective methods, however, are available to help speed the screening procedures and some have been exploited in the search for adenovirus mutants.

Potentially, the most powerful method involves an adaptation of the mutant enrichment technique first devised by Davis (1948) in which, under restrictive conditions, nongrowing mutants avoid incorporating a toxic substance, such as an amino acid or base analogue, while the wild type, which grows under the test conditions, incorporates it and is destroyed, or may be killed by subsequent treatment (e.g., UV irradiation of virus containing bromodeoxyuridine). Hence the proportion of mutants in the population is increased and fewer individual plaque isolates have to be screened to obtain the desired number of mutants. As yet, no reports of attempts to use this approach have been published. However, several other techniques have been used to make the screening procedure itself quicker so that large numbers of plaque isolates from mutagenized stocks could be screened rapidly: (1) Most commonly, samples of plaque isolates were plated under permissive and nonpermissive conditions, at low multiplicities of infection, to determine whether or not they were capable of producing cytopathic effects (CPE) under the latter conditions. Isolates that failed to do so were characterized further. This technique has been used by Suzuki and Shimojo (1971), Shiroki *et al.* (1972), Takahashi (1972), Ledinko (1974), and Bégin and Weber (1975) in their searches for *ts* mutants and by Takahashi (1972) for host range mutants. (2) A second approach has been used by Ensinger and Ginsberg (1972) and by Bégin and Weber (1975) in the isolation of *ts* mutants. Mutagenized virus was propagated at the permissive temperature and after small plaques had appeared each was circled and the plates were then shifted to the restrictive temperature. Plaques that failed to enlarge were picked and characterized further either by a CPE test (Ensinger and Ginsberg, 1972) or by checking the plaque isolate for efficiency of plating at the two temperatures (Bégin and Weber, 1975). (3) Bégin and Weber (1975) have also screened isolates at the two temperatures for their ability to form the microscopically visible inclusion bodies which are characteristic of the wild-type infection.

Various attempts also have been made to miniaturize the screening procedures so that culture materials may be handled more easily and efficiently. Thus Lundholm and Doerfler (1971), in a CPE test, transferred samples of plaque isolates by means of sterile toothpicks to culture plates already overlaid with agar. CPE was thus confined to a small area of the plate, allowing several plaques to be screened per dish. Bégin and Weber (1975) performed CPE screening tests in microtest tissue culture plates that contained 60 wells per plate.

While these methods certainly speed the screening procedures, all are expected to underestimate the frequency of *ts* mutants in the population because (1) "leaky" mutants will give false positive results in the tests (for example, CPE might be extensive at the restrictive temperature), (2) the input virus itself may cause CPE, especially if the input multiplicity is 1 PFU or greater per cell, and (3) the cytocidal effects of defective virus or of viral proteins released by the abortive infections may produce plaque enlargement. To obviate these risks, several investigators have decided to screen plaque isolates directly by comparing their efficiency of plating under permissive and restrictive conditions. Hence the plaques screened by Williams *et al.* (1971) were classified as *ts* if the ratio of the efficiency of plating at 31°C and 38.5°C was greater than 50:1. Similar procedures were carried out by Ishibashi (1971) and Grodzicker *et al.* (1974a) in their searches for CELO adenovirus *ts* mutants and host range mutants of the nondefective SV40–adenovirus type 2 hybrid Ad2⁺ND1, respectively.

So far, only two reports have appeared that deal with direct selection of mutant phenotypes. Takemori *et al.* (1968) isolated cytocidal mutants from type 12 adenovirus by virtue of their characteristic plaque morphology, easily distinguishable from that induced by the wild type. A heat-stable mutant of type 5 adenovirus has been described (Young and Williams, 1975), whose isolation involved three rounds of selection by heat inactivation.

2.4. Genetic Constitution of the Mutants

Where mutagenesis has been employed to enhance the frequency of the mutant sought, the level of viral inactivation employed inevitably led to more mutational lesions than the one giving rise to the desired phenotype. The means to eliminate these extraneous and confusing mutations is to cross the mutant with wild type repeatedly, until it is certain that the final isolate has a wild-type genetic constitution except for the single lesion underlying the phenotype being selected. In adenovirus, because of the extended growth cycle, this procedure is technically impossible, but fortunately there are a number of ways to clarify the nature of the mutational event that causes the phenotype.

A good example of the complexity of the phenotypes of certain mutants is provided by H5ts125, isolated by Ensinger and Ginsberg (1972). This strain is temperature sensitive for the initiation of DNA synthesis in the lytic cycle, is more heat labile than the wild type when inactivated *in vitro,* and at both the permissive and restrictive temperatures transforms rat embryo cells at a higher frequency than does the wild type. Similarly, H5ts36 cannot replicate its DNA and has a low transformation efficiency at the restrictive temperature (Williams *et al.,* 1974). Clearly, it is important to decide whether these phenotypes are pleiotropic effects of one mutation or are caused by several mutations. One way to check is to isolate ts^+ revertants. If all phenotypic characteristics simultaneously revert to wild type, it is likely that they are caused by a single mutation. Formally, the only alternative is that an external suppressor mutation has caused all mutational effects to be simultaneously reversed, thus giving a spurious impression of a single pleiotropic mutation in the original mutant. If the phenotypic characteristics are separable by reversion, the situation is much less clear. The mutant may have separate mutations, but, equally, the ts^+ revertants may have "second-site" mutations that are capable of suppressing only the ts phenotype. Such second-site mutations have been detected by physical means in ts^+ revertants of SV40 ts mutants (Shenk *et al.,* 1975). In addition, the original mutant base pair may have mutated, not back to wild type, but to another non-wild-type base pair that is sufficient to restore ts^+ phenotype but not the other wild-type characteristics. If the phenotypes are separable by recombination, there is an absolute certainty that they arise from more than one mutation. The failure to detect separation, however, merely sets an upper limit on the distance separating any two mutations.

In addition to the problems arising from a heterogeneous background, another potentially serious source of confusion rests in the isolation of mutants whose phenotype results from multiple mutations of the same type. For example, in a population where, following mutagenic treatment, 10% of the survivors are *ts,* 10% of the mutants are expected to have double *ts* mutations (Ishibashi, 1971; Williams and Ustacelebi, 1971*b*). A number of techniques help to uncover this situation. Thus the frequency of reversion from *ts* to *ts*$^+$ is expected to be very low since both *ts* mutations would have to revert simultaneously. Furthermore, attempts to place the mutant in an appropriate complementation group or to assign it to a specific genetic location by recombination may reveal the double nature of the mutation.

3.   CHARACTERISTICS OF THE ADENOVIRUS GENETIC SYSTEM

3.1.   Aims of Genetic Analysis

The interactions between differently marked input adenovirus genomes have been exploited in two ways. The first was of practical importance and involved the classification of the available mutants both into discrete functional groupings and into the order of their genetic location one to another. The second involved the use of mutants to study the nature of the interactions between different genomes. Together, the two approaches aim to give a complete description of the organization of the genome and of the interactions between separate genomes. To date, most studies of adenovirus genetics have used complementation and recombination for classification of mutants, but adenoviruses appear to offer unusual promise for investigating the mechanisms of genetic interaction. While this section is primarily concerned with strictly genetic techniques, it is also appropriate to discuss physical methods for mapping the adenovirus genome and the correlations that can be drawn between physical and genetic maps.

3.2.   Complementation

Complementation tests are tests of gene function; they are designed to show whether or not two mutants have mutations lying in the same or in different genes. They are applicable only where the mutant phenotypes arise from a loss or restriction of function, and in which the gene products can act in *trans*. Fortunately, these constitute a majority of the mutants tested in adenoviruses. For complementation analysis, two such mutants are used to establish a double infection which is maintained under restrictive conditions to determine if there is a greater production of infectious virus than in either of the infections with a single mutant. In most cases, if such an increase occurs, the conclusion may be drawn that the mutations are in separate genes; if no increase is observed, it is implied that the mutations are allelic. Exceptions to these rules occur and will be discussed in the next subsection.

3.2.1. Complementation between Mutants of the Same Serotype

Apart from a brief comment concerning complementation tests between *cyt* mutants in type 12 adenovirus (Takemori *et al.*, 1969; Takemori, 1972), all the complementation analyses within adenovirus serotypes have been performed with *ts* mutants. Although experimental details have varied among the different investigations, essentially the tests have been conducted in the following way: Cells were infected with each mutant at a multiplicity sufficient to ensure that each cell was doubly infected. As controls, parallel cultures were infected with each mutant alone. After a period of incubation at the restrictive temperature, cells were harvested and the viral yields assayed at the permissive temperature to compare the amount of virus produced by the double and single infections. Ideally, either the yields are also titrated at the restrictive temperature, or numerous plaques produced at the permissive temperature are tested at the restrictive temperature, to ensure that any increase observed in the double infections is not caused by wild-type revertants or recombinants. The latter do occur (Williams and Ustacelebi, 1971a; Suzuki *et al.*, 1972) and are a potential source of confusion, especially where the increase in yield in the double infection is small. As yet, adenovirus complementation tests have not been performed by comparing the frequency of infectious centers produced by doubly infected and singly infected cells at the restrictive temperature. This has been a successful technique in analyzing *ts* mutants of HSV-2 (Timbury, 1971) and HSV-1 (Brown *et al.*, 1973). Similarly, attempts have not been made to use qualitative methods of analysis, for example, by screening mixed infections for the ability to induce CPE at the restrictive temperature, in the manner described by Chou and Martin (1974) for *ts* mutants of SV40.

Since quantitative methods of analysis have been used, it has been possible to estimate the efficiency of complementation in several ways. Thus some authors (Russell *et al., 1972a*; Suzuki *et al., 1972*; Ledinko, 1974; Bégin and Weber, 1975) have calculated the ratio between the mixed infection yields and those from the single infections to obtain a "complementation index" (CI). (Different authors have used slightly different formulas depending on whether corrections for statistical fluctations and for wild-type virus present in the yields were made, and also on whether the sum or the higher of the two single infection yields was used as the denominator.) Many CIs have been very high, for example, 10^6 (Williams and Ustacelebi, 1971*a*). Similarly, the double infection yield has been shown to be as high as 50% of the yield of wild type grown at the restrictive temperature (Ledinko, 1974), or up to 40% of the yield of either mutant grown at the permissive temperature (Williams and Ustacelebi, 1971*a*). All of these comparisons indicate that complementation with many mutants is an extremely efficient process. This implies that under conditions of mixed infection there is little compartmentalization of the steps of replication and assembly specified by different input genomes. Confirmation of this comes from an analysis of the time course of complementation (Ensinger and Ginsberg, 1972) in which it was found that the viral yield in the mixed infection rose as quickly as that of a parallel wild-type culture.

The distribution of *ts* mutants into complementation groups, proposed by the various investigators, is summarized in Table 2. Several important points can be drawn from these reports:

1. Williams *et al.* (1974), using a CI $\geq$ 10 as indicative of positive complementation, proposed that the type 5 adenovirus mutants isolated in their laboratory could be arranged into 16 nonoverlapping complementation groups. Whether or not all of these groups represent separate gene functions is still a moot point, however, for the following reasons. Five of the groups gave low but positive complementation among themselves, and their phenotypes were shown to affect some aspects of hexon transport, assembly, or synthesis. (The exact gene functions are still undecided, as will be discussed in Section 4.) In complementation studies using mutants from the two laboratories (Kauffman and Ginsberg, unpublished), members of three of these groups fell into the unique group of *ts* "hexon" mutants isolated by Ensinger and Ginsberg (1972). Thus it is possible, as Williams *et al.* (1974) pointed out, that members of at least some of these groups are involved in interallelic (intracistronic) complementation; i.e., each mutant

TABLE 2
Complementation Groups and Their Phenotypic Defects

| Virus | Complementation tests | | Mutants with single phenotypic defects[a] | | | | | | References |
	Number of mutants	Number of groups	DNA synthesis	"Hexon"	"Hexon transport"	Fiber	Penton base	"Assembly"	
Ad2	15	13	0	0	0	0	3 (1, 1, 1)[b]	8 (6 × 1; 2 × 2)	Bégin and Weber (1975), Weber et al. (1975)
Ad5	51	12[c]	1 (3)	1 (24)[c]	1 (7)[c]	3 (3, 2, 1)	0	4 (3, 2, 1, 1)	Russell et al. (1972a, 1974), Williams et al. (1974), Wilkie et al. (1973)
	15	6	2 (1, 1)	1 (6)	1 (1)	1 (1)	0	1 (5)	Ensinger and Ginsberg (1972), Ginsberg et al. (1974a)
	3	3	1 (1)	1 (1)	0	0	0	1 (1)	Rubenstein and Ginsberg (1974)
Ad12	34	13	3 (5, 3, 3)	0	1 (2)	1 (2)	1 (2)	3 (6, 1, 1)	Shiroki et al. (1972), Shiroki and Shimojo (1974)
	10	6	2 (1, 1)	1 (1)	—	—	—	1 (1)	Ledinko (1974)
Ad31	12	8	3 (1, 1, 1)	0	0	1 (1)	0	2 (2, 2)	Suzuki et al. (1972)
CELO	—	—	(1)[d]	—	(16)	—	—	(22)	Ishibashi (1971)

[a] Some complementation groups have more than one phenotypic defect and are not included in this table (with the exception of DNA synthesis mutants which fail to synthesize hexon, fiber, and penton base). Not all complementation groups have been examined phenotypically.

[b] Numbers in parentheses refer to the numbers of mutants in each complementation group, e.g., 2 (1, 1) indicates two complementation groups with one mutant each and (6 × 1) indicates six groups with one mutant each. Not all mutants in each group have been examined phenotypically.

[c] The publication by Williams et al. (1974) classified these mutants as hexon, 2 (1, 1), and hexon transport, 4 (20, 7, 1, 1). The reassignment is based on preliminary complementation data, as explained in the text (see Section 3.2.1).

[d] Complementation was not performed with the CELO is mutants.

has a single defect differently located in the same polypeptide, whose native form is multimeric. Each defect can be corrected by the wild-type counterpart from the other mutant to give a partially active structure akin to the native multimeric form (for a review, see Fincham, 1966). Hence some alleles complement each other and others do not, depending on their locations. The former leads to interallelic complementation and the sum of the complementation analyses often gives rise to overlapping complementation groups. The problem of deciding whether or not positive complementation indicates separate gene functions arises because of the very sensitive nature of the measurement of yield increase, so that any complementation, arising from whatever mechanism, is readily detectable, and because the assignment of a particular CI value for positive complementation is arbitrary. Moreover, the criterion for such complementation can be manipulated to give nonoverlapping complementation groups (Bégin and Weber, 1975). Thus the number of complementation groups can be varied and, correspondingly, the number of apparent gene functions will fluctuate.

2. Irrespective of whether the number of complementation groups is equal to the number of genes that have *ts* mutations located in them, it is possible to ask how many more complementation groups remain to be discovered. Most investigators have demonstrated the accumulation of mutants within certain complementation groups, the most extreme example being one group with at least 20 "hexon" mutants (Williams *et al.*, 1974). The increase from 22 mutants allocated into 14 groups (Russell *et al.*, 1972a) to 51 mutants in 16 groups (Williams *et al.*, 1974) illustrates the magnitude of the task of classifying any new mutants without rapid qualitative tests, since each mutant must be complemented with representatives of the 16 existing groups. It is not clear whether the approach to saturation observed by Williams *et al.* (1974) followed because the mutagenic procedures used selected for certain genes, whether some gene functions are intrinsically more mutable than others, or, indeed, whether most genes have been mutated already in the studies carried out.

3. Some *ts* mutants fail to complement representatives from more than one complementation group (Suzuki *et al.*, 1972; Bégin and Weber, 1975), and it seems probable that they arise

from multiple mutations. No mutations comparable to SV40 *ts**101 (Robb and Martin, 1972), which fails to complement with any other mutant because of a failure to uncoat at the restrictive temperature (Chou and Martin, 1975), have been discovered in adenoviruses.

Hence complementation analysis has been of value since it has provided a broad functional classification of the mutants. This classification is empirically useful in that it limits the number of mutants that must be tested physiologically to gain a clear picture of the range of mutational lesions in the available mutants. Since alleles have been defined also, they may be examined if it is desired to see whether a particular defect is allele specific or complementation group specific (Ensinger and Ginsberg, 1972; Russell *et al.*, 1972*a*; Shiroki *et al.*, 1972; Weber *et al.*, 1975). Furthermore, complementation analysis has demonstrated the presence of interallelic complementation, and therefore a combined genetic and physiological study of the functioning of a particular polypeptide is now possible. Lastly, complementation has been of predictive value in recombination analysis since mutants in the same complementation group are expected to map closely together.

3.2.2. Complementation between Mutants of Different Serotypes

The numerous serotypes of adenoviruses fall into three groups depending on several properties (see Section 1.1.3). One way to study the functional differences between serotypes is to perform heterotypic complementation tests in order to determine which replicative functions and which structures can be substituted by one serotype for another. Furthermore, heterotypic complementation broadens the classification of adenovirus-specific gene functions and permits comparisons to be drawn between viruses, regardless of the mutants' serotypes.

Heterotypic complementation analysis has been performed between type 5 adenovirus, a member of the so-called nononcogenic group, and type 12 adenovirus, a member of the highly oncogenic group (Williams *et al.*, 1975*b*). Williams *et al.* (1975*b*) used a wild-type strain of type 12 (1131) that failed to produce plaques on HeLa cells, although capable of infecting and producing cell-associated virus. In addition, type 12 did not inhibit, nor was its replication inhibited by, replication of type 5. These characteristics allowed the construction of a nonreciprocal complementation test in which it could be determined whether or not a type 12 function could substitute for a *ts* type 5 function at the restrictive temperature. The reverse relationship, i.e., whether type 5 functions could substitute in type 12 replication, could not be tested in these experiments. Eight complementation groups from type 5 could be complemented while seven others could not. The groups that were not complemented included those involved in the production of antigenically reactive fiber, in DNA synthesis, and in two of the four "assembly" groups. Mutants representing all groups displaying hexon phenotypic defects were complemented. Furthermore, it could be shown that monospecific neutralizing antisera directed against type 5 or type 12 adenovirus neutralized the yield from some, but not all, infections that showed positive complementation. This suggests that phenotypic mixing of serotypically different hexons had occurred and had still produced infectious virus. Progeny from individual plaques obtained from titration of the mixed infections proved to be genetically type 5 and *ts*, so the mixed nature of the virions was solely phenotypic. In this context, it is worth pointing out that no evidence for genetic recombination could be obtained in these crosses. There was no increase in type 5 *ts*$^+$ progeny occurring in the mixed infections, compared with the single infection controls, whether the crosses were performed at 38.5°C or at a lower, permissive temperature, 32.5°C. Thus type 5 and 12 adenoviruses, as well as being serotypically different, are genetically separated in that genetic exchange is limited. They are thus evolving separately, which may account, in part, for the large proportion of type 5 functions that cannot be substituted by corresponding type 12 functions. A useful comparison may be drawn with the lambdoid phages, in which divergence of the immunity region at the DNA level is accompanied by an absolute divergence at the functional level (see Hershey, 1971). Hyman *et al.* (1973) have pointed out that even a limited degree of DNA heterology leads to a failure to recombine in the T3, T7, ΦII group of bacteriophages.

Earlier reports (Ginsberg *et al.*, 1974*a,b*) of heterotypic complementation between type 5 and 12 adenoviruses are now invalid, since the type 12 *ts* mutants used in the study (Rubenstein and Ginsberg, 1974) have recently been shown to be of type 5 serotype and also to have the restriction endonuclease fragment pattern characteristic of type 5 (Wu and Ginsberg, unpublished).

Heterotypic complementation *within* adenovirus subgroups, where the extent of DNA homology is considerable (Bartok *et al.*, 1974), has been used to classify *ts* mutants of one serotype with respect to *ts* mutants with known phenotypic defects of another related serotype. Shiroki and Shimojo (1974) used a *ts* mutant of type 31 with a defect in

DNA synthesis to classify mutants of type 12. In conjunction with mapping studies, *ts* mutants of type Ad2⁺ND1 have been complemented with type 5 *ts* mutants (Grodzicker *et al.*, 1974*b*; Williams *et al.*, 1975*a*).

3.3. Recombination and Mapping of the Adenovirus Genome

Many animal viruses can undergo genetic recombination, either by reassortment of genome subunits or by intramolecular exchange. The latter mechanism allows very closely linked mutations to be recombined. Experimentally, recombination may be exploited in many ways, the resolving power of the system being limited only by the technical necessity of being able to select rare recombinants from a population of parental types and by the intrinsic rates of mutation of the parental types themselves. Among the possible uses of recombinational analysis are the following: (1) the construction of genetic maps so that mutants may be located with respect to each other; (2) the construction of novel genotypes for particular experimental purposes; (3) the determination of whether or not the phenotypic characteristics of a particular mutant are separate or arise from a single pleiotropic mutation; (4) the investigation of whether or not all mutants in one complementation group are separate alleles; (5) the study of the process of recombination itself using mutants as markers of the molecular events involved. Adenovirus mutants have been used in all of these ways, but our primary concern in the following subsection will be to examine mapping studies using *ts* mutants.

3.3.1. Genetic Mapping of Adenovirus *ts* Mutants

It is generally considered that genetic maps reveal the underlying arrangement of genes in the genome and that this arrangement is relevant to the way in which gene control is exercised. The methods for constructing such maps vary, but in many organisms it has been possible to use deletions or multifactorial-cross analysis. Where a set of overlapping deletion mutants is available, a completely unambiguous map position may be assigned to a particular mutant, within limits set by the size and extent of overlap of the various deletions. Defective adenoviruses, with deleted genomes, have been characterized biologically and biochemically (Mak, 1971; Burlingham *et al.*, 1974), but attempts have not been made to clone them for use in genetic studies.

In multifactorial analysis, the frequencies with which unselected markers are distributed among selected recombinants may be determined and, in most cases, their relative positions can be located unambiguously. *Cyt* mutants (Takemori *et al.,* 1968) and host range mutants (Takahashi, 1972) are potentially useful unselected third markers in *ts* × *ts* crosses. A heat-stable mutant has been used as an unselected third marker in *ts* × *ts* crosses, but the task of screening each *ts*⁺ plaque for the heat stability of the progeny virus was very laborious (Young and Williams, 1975). Ideally, unselected third markers should be detectable either by visual inspection, i.e., plaque morphology mutants, or by rapid screening techniques. In the absence of more precise genetic mapping methods for adenoviruses, two-factor *ts* × *ts* crosses have been used to construct genetic maps. The ordering of mutants by this method depends solely on the recombination frequencies (r.f.) between pairs of mutants, so that any experimental and statistical variations contribute greatly to the difficulty of establishing an unambiguous order. In addition, some mutants may have intrinsic effects on the r.f.

Recombination tests have normally been arranged as follows: cells were infected with both parental strains of virus and parallel cultures of cells were infected with each virus alone. The infected cells were incubated for several days at the permissive temperature and the yields titrated at both restrictive and permissive temperatures to select for *ts*⁺ recombinants and to measure total yield, respectively. The recombination frequency is normally expressed as a percentage based on the following formula:

$$\frac{\text{titer at the restrictive temperature}}{\text{titer at the permissive temperature}} \times 2 \times 100$$

In general, the frequency of *ts*⁺ revertants in the parental controls has been so low as to make a correction for reversion in the mixed infection unnecessary. The factor of 2 in the expression is included to take account of the reciprocal recombinant class, expected to arise at an equal frequency to the *ts*⁺ class (Ensinger and Ginsberg, 1972; Williams *et al.,* 1974). The presence of this doubly mutant class has never been established in adenoviruses as it is extremely difficult to screen for them. Limited data from crosses involving a heat-stable mutant, however, suggest that reciprocal recombinants arise at approximately equal frequency in adenovirus recombination (Young and Williams, 1975). Since the double *ts* recombinants have not been scored, Ledinko (1974) and Bégin and Weber (1975) preferred to restrict the r.f. value to the frequency of *ts*⁺. Some points of practical importance should be emphasized. (1) The r.f. values for a particular cross vary over a considerable range (Williams and Ustacelebi, 1971a; Williams et al., 1974), and thus to obtain a reliable statistic several independent tests should be run. The experimental variability has many components, of which the most important is probably the accuracy of the restrictive temperature assay for ts^+ recombinants, since it is difficult on occasion to keep monolayers alive and morphologically intact for a time sufficient to allow growth and scoring of plaques—for example, 9–10 days. (2) It is important to establish that the virus in plaques appearing at the restrictive temperature is genotypically ts^+ and is not a complementing mixture of different ts mutants. Ensinger and Ginsberg (1972) showed that this could be a serious disturbance to r.f. values in some crosses. In most investigations, however, this has not been observed, since plaque progeny proved to have an equal plating efficiency at both permissive and restrictive temperatures, i.e., were genotypically ts^+ (Williams and Ustacelebi, 1971a; Ledinko, 1974; Bégin and Weber, 1975). (3) The mixed infections should be incubated until the exponential phase of viral replication is completed, since r.f. increases with viral increase and then reaches a plateau (Williams et al., 1974).

So far, very few attempts have been made to construct genetic maps using the adenovirus mutants now available. However, two groups (Williams et al., 1974; Ensinger, Kauffman, Cheng, and Ginsberg, unpublished) dealing with ts mutants of type 5 adenovirus, which have been isolated and characterized independently, have produced genetic maps that are compared in Fig. 4. Both maps have been constructed in approximately the same way, using data obtained from two-factor crosses performed in a similar manner. These data have been accumulated over a number of years: the geometric mean values for the various r.f.'s have been calculated, and the maps have been drawn up to produce as few anomalies of r.f. additivity as possible. It is not yet clear whether those anomalies which are observed occur because of the effects of specific markers which alter the r.f.'s, whether certain regions of the genome undergo more or less recombination than others, whether some mutants are multiply ts, or, indeed, whether the effects are merely artifactual.

The comparison between the maps (Fig. 4) brings out several points: (1) The order of markers in corresponding complementation groups is identical and the r.f.'s between them are very similar. Not all possible complementations between the two sets of mutants have been performed, so there remain some areas of doubt—for instance, in the order of assembly groups. (2) In both maps, early and late functions are

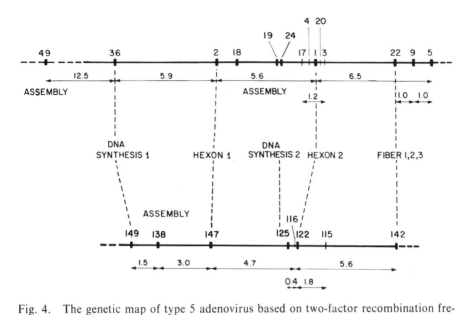

Fig. 4.   The genetic map of type 5 adenovirus based on two-factor recombination frequencies between pairs of *ts* mutants. Adapted from Williams *et al.* (1974), upper line, and Ensinger *et al.* (unpublished), lower line. (———|————|———) mutant positions on map: **|** mutant representative of a complementation group. | other alleles of one of the complementation groups displaying an altered "hexon" phenotype. (←————→) recombination frequency between two mutants. (FIBER) mutant phenotype; vertical dashed lines indicate that complementation tests have been performed between mutants isolated in the laboratories of J. F. Williams and H. S. Ginsberg and the mutants have been assigned to particular complementation groups (Kauffman, Cheng, and Ginsberg, unpublished).

interspersed, and there is no absolute segregation of blocks of early and late gene functions. Biochemical studies on the distribution of early and late mRNAs confirm the genetic evidence (Craig *et al.*, 1975*). (3) Mutants within complementation groups map closely together and at approximately the same distance from alleles in other genes. This is expected if r.f.'s reflect physical distances.

   Recombination studies with type 2 *ts* mutants have ordered the markers approximately (Bégin and Weber, 1975). A direct comparison with the type 5 maps is hard to make, however, since the characteriza-

* See also Note Added in Proof, p. 76.

tion of the type 2 *ts* mutants is only just beginning (Weber *et al.*, 1975) and complementation analysis between type 2 and type 5 mutants has not been done. Some of the mutants are unlinked since values for the frequency of *ts*$^+$ recombinants were found to be as high as 38%. Ledinko (1974), using type 12 *ts* mutants, has also shown very high levels of recombination (18% *ts*$^+$) between two DNA synthesis defective mutants, again probably demonstrating the dispersal of early functions in the genome.

Mapping studies have yielded important information about the disposition of mutants with distinct phenotypic defects. With the advent of biochemical methods (see below) that directly locate genes, specifying particular polypeptides, on the adenovirus genome (Lewis *et al.*, 1975), the value of recombinational analysis in the future may rest in the resolving power of the system. For example, mutants within a gene can be ordered and used to dissect the functional regions of a specific polypeptide. In other words, fine-structure analysis of an adenovirus gene and its product is now feasible. The nature of the recombinational process itself, however, is an area that is still relatively unexplored. Some of the parameters that affect the r.f. values have been examined (Williams *et al.*, 1974), but the molecular events involved remain to be discovered.

3.3.2. Physical Mapping of the Adenovirus Genome and Its Products

The genomes of many adenovirus serotypes have been investigated using a variety of site-specific restriction endonucleases. The characteristic DNA fragments that are produced may be ordered to construct a physical map (Mulder *et al.*, 1974*a,b*). With the development of hybridization techniques for selecting messenger RNAs that bind to specific fragments, and of systems to translate such exogenous messengers *in vitro*, it is possible to map early and late transcripts and to locate genes for specific viral polypeptides. Using these techniques, Lewis *et al.* (1975) have been able to determine the genomic location of ten distinct type 2 polypeptides specified by mRNAs extracted at late times from infected-cell cytoplasm (Fig. 5). Although several of the polypeptides could not be oriented with respect to one another, especially those located in the large *Eco* · RI "A" fragment, given a sufficient number of different endonuclease fragments and the ability to extract, hybridize, and translate the appropriate mRNA, it should be possible to order all the structural genes of adenovirus.

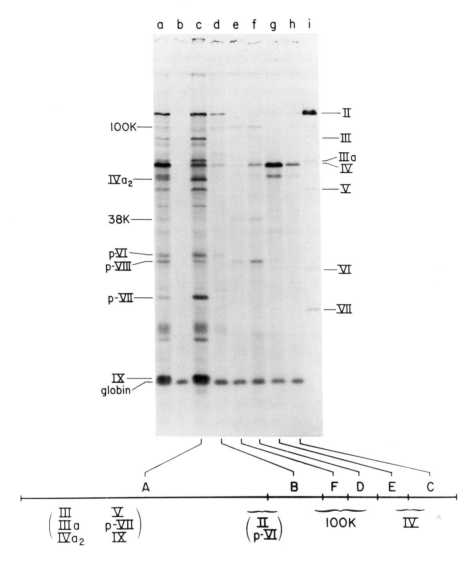

Fig. 5. Biochemical mapping of late adenovirus genes by cell-free translation of mRNAs selected by hybridization to the $Eco \cdot RI$ restriction fragments of type 2 adenovirus. Autoradiogram of products of *in vitro* protein synthesis electrophoresed on 17.5% polyacrylamide gel containing sodium dodecylsulfate. The mRNAs used for translation were selected by hybridization to (a) intact type 2 adenovirus DNA, (b) λ plac DNA, (c) $Eco \cdot RI$ A fragment of Ad2 DNA, (d) B fragment, (e) F fragment, (f) D fragment, (g) E fragment, and (h) C fragment. (i) represents an autoradiogram of disrupted, purified virions. At the bottom of the figure, the genes for ten late viral polypeptides are associated with the $Eco \cdot RI$ fragments to which the specific mRNA hybridized (Lewis *et al.*, 1975).

3.3.3. Correlations between Genetic and Physical Maps

The value of genetic mapping rests on the assumption that the genetic order corresponds to the physical order of mutations in the genome. Such an assumption has proved to be correct in most other organisms, but if genetic mapping is to be a useful predictive tool it must be demonstrated for adenoviruses as well.

The question can be approached in two ways. As noted in the previous subsection, the physical order of several genes is now known. Furthermore, the phenotypes of several *ts* mutants suggest that the mutations underlying them may be in genes specifying particular polypeptides. Thus it is possible to compare the biochemical with the phenotypic map. The drawback to this approach is that the mutation may *not* be in the structural gene for the polypeptide whose phenotype appears to be affected. In very few cases has it been possible to demonstrate the functional thermolability of a particular polypeptide specified by an adenovirus *ts* mutant. In view of this difficulty, a more direct approach must be used that correlates a mutation with a specific genomic position. Recently, a novel way to solve this problem has been developed (Grodzicker *et al.,* 1974*b*; Williams *et al.,* 1975*a*) based on the finding that *ts* mutants in type 2 and 5 adenoviruses are sufficiently homologous to allow complementation and recombination to occur between them, and that the genomes can be identified because they are cleaved by restriction endonucleases into distinguishable DNA fragments (Fig. 2) (Mulder *et al.,* 1974*a,b*). These characteristics allow the selection of *ts*[+] recombinants from heterotypic *ts* × *ts* crosses, and the contribution of each parental virus to the recombinant may be determined physically.

The tests involved *ts* mutants of type 5 adenovirus and of the nondefective adenovirus–SV40 hybrid Ad2[+]ND1. Types 2 and 5 are in the same virus subgroup and display a considerable DNA/DNA homology as measured by studies on heteroduplexes (Bartok *et al.,* 1974). In Ad2[+]ND1, some 17% of the SV40 genome replaces approximately 5.5% of the type 2 genome at a position about 15% from the conventional right-hand end of the molecule (Kelly and Lewis, 1973). Moreover, the SV40 fragment apparently supplies a helper function that allows the hybrid to plaque equally well on human and monkey cells (Lewis *et al.,* 1969). The degree of nonhomology is not enough to prevent viable recombinants being formed between *ts* mutants of type 5 and Ad2[+]ND1, although the r.f.'s are not as high as in homotypic type 5 crosses (Grodzicker *et al.,* 1974*b*; Williams *et al.,* 1975*a*). The crosses were analyzed in two ways: (1) Viral yields were plated on both human and monkey cells at the restrictive temperature. The ratio between the two yields revealed the frequency of ts^+ recombinants that contained the SV40 fragment necessary for growth on monkey cells. Therefore, the fragment was acting as a selected third marker, but the data presented suggest that, for reasons unknown, it was not distributed in a consistent way. (2) Ts^+ recombinants were picked from both human and monkey cell assay plates and the genomes of the recombinants and of the two parents were analyzed using restriction enzymes $Eco \cdot RI$ and HpaI. An alteration in the fragment pattern from those of the parents indicated that one or more crossovers from one parent to the other had taken place to generate the recombinant. Furthermore, the positions of the crossovers could be deduced. When several ts^+ recombinants from a particular cross were compared, those crossovers that were found to be present in all of them were taken to be necessary for the production of this type of recombinant. The positions of these invariant crossovers set limits on the positions of the ts markers that entered the cross. Using this technique to locate the positions of three mutants of type 5 and one of Ad2$^+$ND1, the orders and distances of the physical map corresponded remarkably well with the genetic map (Fig. 4) previously obtained (Williams *et al.*, 1974). Recently, this correspondence has also been found to hold for one of the DNA synthesis-defective mutants, H5ts125 (Sambrook and Ginsberg, personal communication). There are two possible limitations to the technique: (1) Double crossovers within the limits of a pair of adjacent, heterotypic, endonucleolytic cleavages are not observed. This could lead to ambiguities if they bracket the position of one of the ts mutants in all the recombinants examined. (2) Certain constraints may be placed on the distribution and frequency of crossovers by the various regions of nonhomology between type 5 and Ad2$^+$ND1. *A priori,* one would expect no crossovers in these regions, but whether or not the frequency of recombination is affected in adjacent regions is not clear. This is important if it increases the frequency of "cryptic" double crossovers. Although not necessarily a source of confusion in the mapping analysis, it is conceivable that the regions of nonhomology between type 2 and type 5 include inversions of genetic sequences; thus certain recombinant molecules might be nonviable owing to addition or deletion of DNA.

The analysis of heterotypic recombinants has been invaluable in demonstrating that the genetic and physical maps are approximately colinear. But it is equally useful as a physical technique for locating gene function on the genome, independent of whether or not mutations occur in the functions to be mapped (Grodzicker *et al.,* 1974*b*). Provided that recombinants are available (and of course *ts* mutants are useful in allowing them to be selected), the genomic contribution of each parent to the recombinant may be determined. If the polypeptides specified by the two parental serotypes are distinguishable, then the recombinants may be defined in terms of the polypeptides they specify. Hence it has been possible to characterize *ts*$^+$ recombinants, by using monospecific antisera directed against hexon and fiber of type 2 and 5 adenoviruses, to locate the position of the respective structural genes (Mautner *et al.,* 1975). When the size of polypeptides differs between serotypes, this may be distinguished on SDS-polyacrylamide gels and, as Mautner *et al.* (1975) note, recombinants may be compared with the parental viruses.

   Restriction endonuclease analysis of recombinants may be used also to examine the frequency and distribution of genetic exchange in animal viruses. From the analysis of 17 recombinants from various crosses (Mautner *et al.,* 1975), it is possible to deduce that at least ten have more than one crossover. The figure may be greater than this since some crossovers may not be observed in the 30% at the left-hand end of both the Ad2$^+$ND1 and type 5 genomes, where distinguishable endonuclease cuts were not made.

   Other methods that might be used for physical location of mutations also involve the use of restriction endonucleases. It is now known that adenovirus DNA is infectious (Graham and van der Eb, 1973). It may be possible to use this property to perform marker rescue experiments using specific fragments of wild-type DNA to complement or recombine with *ts* mutants. This approach has been used successfully with *ts* mutants of SV40 (Lai and Nathans, 1974). Alternatively, if deletion mutants become available, they may be used to determine which mutants fail to recombine with them and which fragment(s) are missing or altered from the normal endonuclease pattern, thus defining the limits within which the mutants must lie.

4. PHENOTYPES OF ADENOVIRUS MUTANTS

4.1. Temperature-Sensitive Mutants

   More than 20 virus-induced, possibly virus-coded, proteins have been detected in extracts of adenovirus-infected cells; of those noted, the virion proteins are the predominant species (Maizel *et al.,* 1968*a,b*; Anderson *et al.,* 1973; Everitt *et al.,* 1973) (Fig. 1). Several proteins are precursors of virion proteins, for example, pVI and pVIII (Sundquist *et* *al.*, 1973*a*; Anderson *et al.*, 1973; Ishibashi and Maizel, 1974*a*), and a few minor components have not yet been shown to be unique polypeptides. Hence at least 12–15 putative primary gene products have been identified (Maizel *et al.*, 1968*a*,*b*; Everitt *et al.*, 1973; Anderson *et al.*, 1973), with a total molecular mass of about 792,500 daltons, which accounts for about 70% of the coding capacity of the viral genome. Of the known viral gene products, only a few appear to be altered in the large number of adenovirus temperature-sensitive mutants which have now been characterized (Table 2). Perhaps this can be attributed to the fact that the precise function and immunological properties of the native proteins have been identified only for the major viral proteins, and these are the viral products that appear to be represented in most of the phenotypes thus far described. Thus the most common and the best-characterized protein phenotypes listed in Table 2 represent lesions in the most easily studied and assayed capsid proteins, the hexon and fiber proteins. It is inexplicable that penton mutants have been infrequently isolated, except for those reported by Weber *et al.* (1975). As noted earlier, however, the precise relationship is not always clear between the apparent phenotype and the gene in which the viral protein is encoded. For example, two complementation groups (Table 2 and Fig. 4) contain mutants which display either defective hexon structure or function ranging from those that are immunologically unreactive and unassembled to fully assembled trimers that are immunologically as reactive as wild-type hexons but unable to be transported into the nucleus (Russell *et al.*, 1972*a*; Ensinger and Ginsberg, 1972; Kauffman and Ginsberg, 1976). Although the latter mutants (for example, H5*ts*147) make hexons which appear physically normal, two physical mapping techniques imply that these mutants have defective hexon genes. In contrast, the former mutants, which may not produce either immunologically or physically detectable hexons (for example, H5*ts*115), are said to have unaffected hexon genes but rather map in that region of the genome in which the 100K nonvirion protein is encoded (Figs. 1 and 5) (Mautner *et al.*, 1975; Lewis *et al.*, 1975). The biological function of the 100K protein is unknown. Although the explanation is not clear for this disparity between the apparent phenotype and the gene responsible for production of hexon protein, the basis for a marked variation in the phenotypic expression of a mutation in the hexon gene is explicable. The amino acid substitution resulting from the missense mutation may be so critically located that the affected polypeptide chain could not fold appropriately, and hence the interchain interactions could not ensue to permit the trimer hexon assembly. As a consequence, the phenotype of this mutation would fail to produce hexons which could be detected either immunologically or physically [e.g., H5ts10 (Russell *et al.,* 1972a; Luciw and Ginsberg, unpublished)]; but the defective polypeptide chains could react with antibodies directed against isolated wild-type hexon polypeptide chains (Stinski and Ginsberg, 1975). Or the defect in the hexon protomer could be so strategically situated as to interfere variably with intra- and interchain folding so that imperfect or essentially perfect hexons could be assembled to permit a varying degree of immunological reactivity. But the immunologically reactive but imprecisely formed hexon might be incapable of movement into the nucleus for virion assembly [e.g., H5ts2 (Russell *et al.,* 1972a)]. It is further possible, however, that another gene product may be required for hexon transport from its cytoplasmic site of synthesis into the nucleus (to be discussed below).

Fiber mutants fall into three nonoverlapping complementation groups (Fig. 4), which suggests that each of the three polypeptide chains is unique (Dorsett and Ginsberg, 1975). None of the fiber mutants makes immunologically reactive proteins (Russell *et al.,* 1972a; Ensinger and Ginsberg, 1972), and in at least one class of mutants (H5ts142) the fiber is not glycosylated (Cheng and Ginsberg, unpublished). It is perhaps surprising that fiber mutants that are immunologically reactive but untransportable have not been detected.

The so-called assembly mutants constitute a large proportion of the *ts* mutants classified, but the specific defect has not yet been identified in a single mutant of the several complementation groups identified. These mutants are said to represent assembly-defective phenotypes, because at the nonpermissive temperature all identifiable proteins are synthesized and all of the proteins that can be assayed are immunologically functional (Russell *et al.,* 1972a; Ensinger and Ginsberg, 1972). The assembly mutants may represent defects in one of the minor virion components or in a nonvirion protein that is essential for modulating the assembly process. If the "assembly" mutants represent a melange of mutations in a number of genes coding for nonvirion proteins, such as the 100K, 50K, 27K, 26K, or virion proteins VIII–XII (Fig. 1), a comparable number of complementation groups should have been identified. Instead, a maximum of five "assembly" complementation groups for type 5 *ts* mutants have been described (until mutants isolated in different laboratories are compared, the precise number of complementation groups remains uncertain). The type 2 "assembly" mutants are said to present a rather unusual phenotype as compared to type 5 mutants: eight mutants, each reported to represent a distinct complementation group, are described as forming noninfectious virions containing viral DNA at the nonpermissive temperature (39°C) (Weber et al., 1975).

Two of the putative assembly mutants belonging to different complementation groups also fail to induce interferon in chick embryo fibroblasts (CEF) at the nonpermissive temperature (Ustacelebi and Williams, 1972). Since interferon is not a virus-coded product, nor is its induction viral specific, one simple interpretation of this observation is that the uncoating of these two mutants does not proceed to completion in CEF at the nonpermissive temperature because structural components of the capsid are altered. Consistent with this hypothesis are the findings that the mutants did complement in the infectious cycle in HeLa cells, although they failed to complement in the induction of interferon in CEF (Ustacelebi and Williams, 1972), and that the induction of interferon was thermosensitive only during the first 6 h after infection, while the *ts* lesion blocked the production of virus in HeLa cells at late times during infection (Ustacelebi, 1973). In addition, both mutants were found to be considerably more thermolabile than wild-type virus *in vitro* (Ustacelebi, 1973; Young and Williams, 1975), which is not unexpected for *ts* mutations in capsid structural components (Fenner, 1969). Thermolability has also been observed in other type 5 *ts* mutants (Ensinger and Ginsberg, 1972), in some *ts* mutants of type 12 (Shiroki et al., 1972), and in some type 2 adenovirus *ts* mutants (Weber et al., 1975).

During viral replication, adenovirus DNA can be separated from host cell DNA by virtue of its higher $G + C$ content (Piña and Green, 1969; Ginsberg et al., 1967). Thus it has been a relatively simple task to screen *ts* mutants for the ability to synthesize DNA at the restrictive temperature. So far, mutants with DNA synthesis defects have been isolated in type 5 (Ensinger and Ginsberg, 1972; Wilkie et al., 1973), type 12 (Ledinko, 1974; Shiroki and Shimojo, 1974), type 31 (Suzuki et al., 1972), and CELO (Ishibashi, 1971) adenoviruses. The mutants studied indicate that at least three viral genes are essential for initiation of DNA replication, but no mutant defective in DNA chain elongation has yet been detected. Several DNA-defective mutants have also been examined for alteration in the frequency of transformation of rat or hamster embryo cells; these investigations will be discussed later.

It is noteworthy that only a single mutant has been described that appears to replicate its DNA at the restrictive temperature but is incapable of synthesizing late capsid proteins (Weber et al., 1975). These data imply that a viral protein is required for either late transcription or translation of late proteins.

4.2. Plaque Morphology and Host Range Mutants

Takemori *et al.* (1968) isolated a large number of type 12 adenovirus mutants which gave plaques that were larger and clearer than those given by wild-type virus on early passage human embryo kidney (HEK) cells. Some of the mutants ("*cyt-kb*") failed to propagate in one line of KB cells (KB-1), while these cells supported the multiplication of others ("*cyt-kb*$^+$"); both mutant types propagated in KB-2 cells (Takemori *et al.*, 1969). *Cyt* mutants were discovered to be of low tumorigenicity in newborn hamsters and failed to transform newborn hamster kidney cells *in vitro*. Although there is evidence that the product of the *cyt* gene is diffusible (see Section 5.4), as yet it is not known what viral product is involved.

Takahashi (1972) and Harrison and Williams (personal communication) have isolated host range mutants of human type 5 adenovirus which are capable of growing on human cells but are unable to multiply in hamster cells. As yet, a specific lesion has not been identified, but it is clear, from analysis on SDS-polyacrylamide gels, that in hamster cells all virus-specific proteins are made, but in reduced quantities (Harrison and Williams, personal communication). It is striking that unlike wild-type virus the conditionally lethal mutants, host range and temperature sensitive, which are unable to replicate in hamster cells, can transform them (Williams, 1973; Takahashi *et al.*, 1974) (see Section 5.4).

As mentioned previously, the nondefective adeno-SV40 hybrid Ad2$^+$ND1 is capable of growing on both human and monkey cell lines (Lewis *et al.*, 1969). It was thought that host range mutants that fail to grow on monkey cells would be mutated in the integrated SV40 fragment which presumably promotes adenovirus lytic cycle functions in the normally semipermissive monkey cells. Accordingly, Grodzicker *et al.* (1974a) selected such mutants and examined the polypeptides made in both human cells (HeLa) and monkey cells (CV1 clone of AGMK) infected with Ad2$^+$ND1 wild type, a host range mutant, and Ad2. In the HeLa cell line, a protein product of 30,000 daltons which is characteristic of Ad2$^+$ND1 infection was absent in both the Ad2-infected and the host range mutant infected cells. In CV1 cells, the characteristic underproduction of adenovirus late proteins was observed in both Ad2 and host range mutant infections. The authors also examined the production of the perinuclear SV40 U antigen and found that in permissive cells infected with the host range mutant the appearance of maximal detectable antigen was delayed, while in CV1 cells very few nuclei ever displayed antigen. Whether or not the host range mutation lies in the structural gene for the 30,000 dalton protein or in a viral gene which induces a host cell protein is not clear.

As noted previously (Section 2.1), host range mutants can be absolutely defective if the function(s) that are mutable are required only for replication of the virus in the restrictive host. This is perhaps unlikely in the hamster/human type 5 mutants, but is a distinct possibility in the Ad2+ND1 host range mutants. Absolute defectives are of considerable value, since they include deletion mutants which may be used for mapping purposes; if they delete part of a gene so that only a fragment of the polypeptide is made, they may be used to identify specific gene products.

5. FUNCTIONAL STUDIES USING ADENOVIRUS MUTANTS

Since, during replication, conditionally lethal temperature-sensitive mutants can be conveniently shifted from conditions that permit full expression of the viral genome to nonpermissive conditions that do not allow expression of a defective gene, the gene product affected can be identified and its functional role in viral synthesis can be explored. This approach to the study of viral replication and its regulation has had noteworthy success with bacterial viruses and offers similar promise for unraveling the intricacies of adenovirus synthesis. Studies taking advantage of adenovirus *ts* mutants are in effect just beginning and significant progress has been made only in investigating three central areas in viral replication: DNA synthesis (Suzuki and Shimojo, 1974; Shiroki and Shimojo, 1974; van der Vliet *et al.*, 1975; Levine *et al.*, 1974; Ginsberg *et al.*, 1974a), transcription (Carter and Ginsberg, 1976), and transport of viral proteins (Kauffman and Ginsberg, 1976). In addition, both *ts* and absolute mutants are being employed to explore the mechanisms underlying the establishment and maintenance of adenovirus transformation (Ledinko, 1974; Ginsberg *et al.*, 1974a,b; Williams *et al.*, 1974; Takemori *et al.*, 1968; Takahashi *et al.*, 1974).

5.1. Viral DNA Replication

Genes responsible for early adenovirus functions appear to be uncommonly mutated, and therefore there have been relatively few isolations of mutants that cannot replicate their DNA under the restrictive conditions. The mutants presently available are encompassed in two complementation groups for type 5 virus (Williams *et al.*, 1974; Ginsberg *et al.*, 1974a,b), three groups for type 12 virus (Shiroki and

Shimojo, 1974; Ledinko, 1974), and one group for type 31 adenovirus (Suzuki and Shimojo, 1971; Suzuki *et al.,* 1972).

It is noteworthy that all of the mutants studied appear to be defective in initiation. That is, when infected cells are shifted from the permissive to the restrictive temperature (which stops DNA replication at varying rates depending on the mutant), intermediate, replicative forms of viral DNA do not accumulate, and the replicative intermediates are completed to form mature viral DNA molecules (Shiroki and Shimojo, 1974; Ginsberg *et al.,* 1974a; van der Vliet and Sussenbach, personal communication). The methods employed, however, do not distinguish between a mutant that cannot initiate replication and one that can elongate but not engage in a final reaction which may be required to terminate the synthesis of a complementary strand in order to initiate a new round.

At least three virus-coded gene products, therefore, appear to be essential for adenovirus DNA replication, and each is probably required for a reaction in chain initiation. An early, nonvirion, infected-cell-specific protein, which binds preferentially to single-stranded DNA (van der Vliet and Levine, 1973) in a similar manner to the T4 gene-32 protein (Alberts and Frey, 1970), has been shown to be defective in H5*ts*125 (van der Vliet *et al.,* 1975) and H12*ts*275 (Rosenwirth *et al.,* 1975). Moreover, the so-called DNA-binding protein made in H5*ts*125-infected cells is degraded at 39.5°C and dissociates from single-stranded DNA at lower temperatures than the wild-type protein (van der Vliet *et al.,* 1975), findings which strengthen the interpretation that this 72,000 dalton protein is a viral gene product. Presumably H31*ts*13, which heterotypic complementation analysis shows is mutated in the same cistron as H12*ts*275 (Suzuki and Shimojo, 1974), is also defective in the DNA-binding protein. The function of the DNA-binding protein in DNA replication is uncertain, but since the adenovirus replicating form contains extensive single-stranded regions (Sussenbach *et al.,* 1972, 1973; Ellens *et al.,* 1974; Pettersson, 1973) the binding protein could serve to maintain the single strands and thus permit effective copying of the displaced strand (van der Vliet *et al.,* 1975). The gene products represented by H12*ts*B and *ts*C mutants and H5*ts*36/*ts*149 have not yet been identified.

5.2. Transcription of the Viral Genome

Evidence obtained using pyrimidine analogues to inhibit DNA replication showed that *only* early mRNAs could be transcribed, from the infecting parental genome, and that late transcripts could be made only after DNA synthesis was begun (Bello and Ginsberg, 1969; Lucas and Ginsberg, 1971). However, since it was not possible to demonstrate unambiguously that the chemicals employed (i.e., 5-fluoro-2-deoxyuridine and arabinosylcytosine) did not affect any other intracellular biosynthetic reactions, these data were accepted with some uneasiness. With the availability of appropriate mutants, it became possible to investigate more rigorously the relationship between viral DNA replication and viral transcription. Two DNA$^-$ mutants, H5*ts*125 and H5*ts*149, were used to infect KB cells at a nonpermissive temperature (41°C) and hybridization techniques were employed to measure DNA replication and RNA transcription (Carter and Ginsberg, 1976). In confirmation of the earlier studies, the data obtained showed that no late transcripts appeared if onset of DNA replication was not permitted, and that under the restrictive conditions all early class I and II mRNAs (Lucas and Ginsberg, 1971) were transcribed. It was further shown that both class I and II mRNAs continued to be transcribed as long as 15 h after infection at 41°C, indicating that the shutoff of class I mRNA required a late gene function. It is also striking to note that although the onset of DNA replication was essential for the switch to transcription of late messages, the continuous replication of viral DNA was not necessary for late transcripts to be made: when cells were infected with H5*ts*125 or H5*ts*149 at 32°C for 25 h and then shifted to 41°C, the rate of DNA synthesis decreased rapidly for H5*ts*125 and slowly for H5*ts*149, but the rate of viral RNA synthesis after the shiftup did not change for 3–4 h for *ts*125 and even continued to increase for *ts*149; within the limits of the hybridization-competition techniques employed, the data indicated that the mRNAs made consisted of all the late sequences and the class II early RNAs.

5.3. Transport of the Hexon Protein

As noted earlier, adenovirus proteins are synthesized on cytoplasmic polyribosomes and rapidly transported into the nucleus (Velicer and Ginsberg, 1968, 1970), where about 10% are assembled into virions (Wilcox and Ginsberg, 1963c). The mechanism of protein transport has been difficult to investigate, however, owing to the marked leakiness of the infected nucleus for viral proteins (Velicer and Ginsberg, 1968), although it was considered likely that host cell functions played a major role. The discovery of *ts* mutants in which one or more capsid proteins were made but accumulated in the cytoplasm rather than moving into the nucleus under nonpermissive conditions (Ishibashi, 1970, 1971; Shiroki *et al.*, 1972; Russell *et al.*, 1972a; Ginsberg *et al.*, 1974a,b) suggested that these may offer an opportunity to study the process of protein transport. Mutants of one complementation group, whose hexon proteins specifically cannot move into the nucleus (Russell *et al.*, 1972*a*; Ginsberg *et al.*, 1974*a,b*; Kauffman and Ginsberg, 1976), appeared to be of particular value for this purpose. With the appropriate mutant (e.g., H5*ts*147), the hexon made, like the other capsid proteins, is immunologically fully active and folds into its native, multimeric structure, but only the hexon is not transported (Kauffman and Ginsberg, 1976). These so-called hexon transport mutants are clearly distinct from mutants which cannot produce immunologically detectable hexons (e.g., H5*ts*115) since genetic recombination analysis shows that at least one other gene separates their respective gene loci. Biochemical, immunological, and physical studies of H5*ts*147 indicate that unaffected hexons are assembled and accumulate in the cytoplasm at 39.5°C; and that upon shiftdown to 32°C the preformed, cytoplasmic hexons can be transported into the nuclei and assembled into virions if protein synthesis is permitted (Kauffman and Ginsberg, 1976). This evidence suggests that a distinct viral gene product is essential for hexon transport and/or assembly, and the precursor (pVI) to protein VI (Anderson *et al.*, 1973), a putative hexon-associated protein (Everitt *et al.*, 1973), is degraded at 39.5°C in H5*ts*147-infected cells (Kauffman and Ginsberg, 1976). Whether the small (27,000 daltons) pVI protein has a precise function is still unknown.

Contrary to this interpretation, however, is the evidence that H5*ts*2 (Williams *et al.*, 1971), which cannot complement H5*ts*147 (Kauffman and Ginsberg, unpublished), is a mutant in the hexon gene (Mautner *et al.*, 1975). These two sets of data leading to apparently conflicting conclusions emphasize further the handicaps in identification of phenotypes and specific gene localization using *ts* mutants.* These ambiguities may yet be clarified, however, with further experimentation to determine (1) whether pVI or protein VI is obligatory for hexons to function as virion structural proteins, (2) whether there exist still obscure problems in the use of heterotypic (e.g., Ad5 × Ad2) recombination for physical mapping of the genome (see Section 3.3.3), and (3) whether the gene orders of the type 2 and 5 genomes are identical.

5.4. Transformation

Conditionally lethal *ts* mutants are being employed with the expectation that specific gene product(s) that effect cellular transformation

* See Note Added in Proof, p. 76.

can be identified and characterized, provided that these products are essential not only for viral replication but also for transformation. This optimistic note appears to have some validity since specific temperature-sensitive mutants of Rous sarcoma virus (for a review, see Tooze, 1973) and SV40 (Martin and Chou, 1975; Tegtmeyer, 1975; Brugge and Butel, 1975; Osborn and Weber, 1975) either cannot transform or cannot maintain the transformed state at the nonpermissive condition. The results of transformation studies with adenovirus *ts* mutants have not yet clearly identified a specific gene function directly concerned with transformation. However, two sets of DNA⁻ mutants, which are members of different complementation groups, do strikingly affect transformation. The alleles H5*ts*36 and H5*ts*37 (Wilkie *et al.,* 1973) transform rat embryo cells at a ten- to twentyfold lower frequency than wild-type virus at the nonpermissive temperature, although cells transformed at 32.5°C do not lose their transformed characteristics when grown at 38.5°C (Williams *et al.,* 1974). (One clone of such transformed cells, however, has the curious property of being unable to grow at 38.5°C, although it still maintains its transformed morphology.) The failure of the cells of all such clones to revert to a normal morphology on shiftup to the nonpermissive temperature suggests that H5*ts*36 and 37 are defective in the initiation, rather than in the maintenance, of transformation (Williams *et al.,* 1974). Temperature-shift experiments, during the establishment of transformation, suggest that the temperature-sensitive step occurs before 48 h growth at 32.5°C (Williams *et al.,* 1974). It should be noted that H5*ts*149, which is in the same complementation group as H5*ts*36 and 37, transforms cells with the same frequency as wild-type virus at either 32°C or 39.5°C (Ginsberg *et al.,* 1974*a,b*).

In sharp contrast, three independently isolated DNA-minus mutants, H5*ts*125 (Ginsberg *et al.,* 1974*a,b*), H5*ts*107* (Rubenstein and Ginsberg, 1974), and H12*ts*401 (Ledinko, 1974), transform 2–8 times more rat embryo cells than type 5 or 12 wild viruses. It is striking that the portion of the genome that contains the H5*ts*125 gene (Sambrook and Ginsberg, unpublished), which codes for a DNA-binding protein (van der Vliet *et al.,* 1975), and perhaps that which contains the H5*ts*36 gene (Sambrook *et al.,* unpublished) are not present in that minimum segment of the viral genome that has been detected in adenovirus-transformed cells (Gallimore *et al.,* 1974). This finding, in contradiction of the report by Gilead *et al.* (1975), suggests that the T antigen, which is almost always present in transformed cells, is distinct from the DNA-binding protein. Thus only 14% or less of the left terminus of the

* Previously designated H12*ts*307 (see Table 1).

$Eco \cdot RI$ restriction endonuclease-generated "A" fragment (Fig. 2) (Mulder *et al.,* 1974*a,b*) appears to be necessary to maintain the transformed state (Gallimore *et al.,* 1974; Sambrook *et al.,* 1974). Whether, under conditions of viral infection, all or only a small portion of the genome is initially integrated to induce cell transformation is unknown, but transformation can be effected by only a fragment of the viral DNA, representing as little as 5% of the viral genome and consisting of a small piece which is present at the left-hand end of the large $Eco \cdot RI$ "A" fragment (Graham *et al.,* 1974). The finding that H5*ts*125, as well as related type 5 and type 12 DNA-minus *ts* mutants, transforms at an increased frequency suggests that the DNA-binding protein may normally play a role that modulates the viral genome–cell interaction to reduce the opportunity for transformation, perhaps for DNA integration. These more efficient transforming mutants clearly demonstrate that transformation is not dependent on replication of the viral DNA. To relate unambiguously, however, the DNA$^-$ phenotype, defective DNA-binding protein, and increased transformation frequency requires evidence that the three characteristics result from a single mutation (see Section 2.4).

Type 5 adenovirus *ts* mutants have also been used to transform hamster embryo cells, which are normally permissive for Ad5 (Williams, 1973). By performing the transformation at 38.5°C, *ts* mutants were unable to enter the lytic cycle and transformed clones were obtained. The clones were found to be highly oncogenic in newborn hamsters (Williams, 1973), and, furthermore, sera taken from such animals were found by indirect immunofluorescence techniques to react with the transformed cell nuclei (Williams *et al.,* 1974). Another approach to restricting the usual lytic cycle of type 5 adenovirus infection in hamster cells has been taken by Takahashi *et al.* (1974) and Harrison and Williams (personal communication). They have demonstrated that host range mutants that fail to replicate in hamster cells nevertheless can transform them.

The use of nonconditional mutants of defined genotype to study transformation has so far been restricted to the *cyt* mutants of human adenovirus type 12 (Takemori *et al.,* 1968). These mutants, which gave larger and clearer plaques on early passage HEK cells than did the parental wild-type strain, were found to have lost the ability to transform hamster cells *in vitro* and to cause tumors in newborn hamsters. The mutants cooperated with low tumorigenic *cyt*$^+$ field strains of type 12 and the weakly tumorigenic type 3 and 7 adenoviruses to produce high levels of tumorigenicity, which suggested that the *cyt*$^+$ gene product was diffusible and that the *cyt* mutants did not elaborate an antitumorigenic factor (Takemori *et al.,* 1968). The *cyt* mutants have also been examined for the percentage of defective particles which they and the parental strain generated, to determine whether there was a positive correlation between the frequency of transformation and the proportion of defectives (Ezoe and Mak, 1974). No such correlation could be found. This does not rule out the possibility, however, that a specific class of defectives is the agent of transformation. Such a demonstration may have to await the development of methods for cloning virus of known defective constitution, in ways analogous to those devised for SV40, in which specific deletion mutants were complemented by specific *ts* mutants at the restrictive temperature (Brockman and Nathans, 1974).

It should be pointed out that all mutants that have been examined for transforming abilities were selected primarily for alterations in the lytic cycle and only secondarily for changes in transformation. This method of screening precludes mutants that are deficient only in transformation, if, indeed, such exist.

5.5. Helper Function

Adeno-associated viruses (AAV) are defective agents whose complete multiplication is totally dependent on coinfection with an adenovirus. Presumably, an adenovirus gene product functions to permit synthesis of the AAV-specific macromolecules: DNA, RNA, and structural proteins (Rose, 1974). Conditionally lethal *ts* mutants of adenoviruses, each defective in a single viral function, offered promise of assistance in identifying the flaw in the AAV genome. Two different DNA-minus mutants, H5*ts*125 and H5*ts*149, served as complete helpers of AAV, although unable to replicate their own DNA, transcribe late mRNAs, or synthesize late proteins at 39.5°C (Straus *et al.,* 1976). It is important to note that, under the experimental conditions employed, replication of adenovirus DNA could not be detected with either mutant. H31*ts*13, a DNA⁻ mutant which heterotypic complementation analysis (Suzuki and Shimojo, 1974) suggests indirectly may be in the same complementation group as H5*ts*125, also provides a helper function at the restrictive temperature (Ito and Suzuki, 1970). Unfortunately, H31*ts*13 is a "leaky" mutant and adenovirus functions were not measured. These data indicate that either (1) the adenovirus merely serves to induce a cryptic host cell function necessary for AAV replication or (2) the adenovirus helper function is an early protein which is still unidentified. The latter conclusion is the more appealing since it permits the hypothesis that the unique type of terminal repetition common to the genomes of both viruses (Garon *et al.*, 1972; Koczot *et al.*, 1973) serves a functional role, for which an early adenovirus protein is required, in AAV DNA replication.

6. CRITIQUE AND PERSPECTIVES

Studies of adenovirus genetics, although still in their formative stages, serve notice that they will provide data to satisfy the classical roles of microbial genetics, revealing the processes of genetic interaction and exposing the molecular mechanisms which regulate biosynthesis and assembly of viral macromolecules. The reports reviewed in this chapter show that genetic recombination between adenovirus genomes is an effective event which permits localization of viral genes and the relationship between a mutation and a defective viral function; that complementation is an efficient phenomenon which demonstrates the interchange of viral proteins and its use for classification of conditionally lethal mutants; and that the appropriate mutants permit functional studies which expose the reactions driving viral replication.

Despite the intense interest in, and early success of, adenovirus genetics, the studies have not been without disappointments and problems. For example, a relatively large number of mutants have been isolated but comparatively few corresponding viral gene functions have been identified. Thus the viral proteins chemically detected represent about 70% of the genome's coding capacity, which may, in fact, account for all of the usable mRNAs, since about 30% of the transcripts never leave the nucleus (Lucas and Ginsberg, 1972; McGuire *et al.*, 1972). But only four of these proteins (i.e., the hexon, fiber, penton base, and DNA-binding proteins) have been identified with the phenotypes of the *ts* mutants. And, as was noted earlier, correlation of the phenotype with the physical map of the viral genome may be difficult. The *ts* mutants thus far characterized affect the major capsid proteins, assembly of the virion, and DNA replication. Perhaps the large number of mutants, which appear to belong to an undetermined number of complementation groups, reflect defective minor virion proteins or even nonstructural proteins. Only three mutants in early gene functions, DNA replication mutants, have been characterized, but at least six early mRNAs and their associated early viral proteins have been identified (Craig *et al.*, 1975; Lewis *et al.*, personal communication). It is not clear why mutants affecting the numerous other viral gene products occur so rarely or have not even been isolated, but there are several possibilities: (1) the target size of the genes may be small; (2) associated proteins or folding may protect the viral DNA from mutagenic agents; (3) repair mechanisms may be so effective that damage is efficiently corrected; or (4) certain genes can perhaps not be mutated to give a temperature-sensitive product.

It should also be emphasized that identification of a faulty viral protein may be difficult in conditionally lethal *ts* mutants. Such missense mutants synthesize a defective polypeptide, and recognition depends on the structural effect of a single amino acid substitution. The mutated protein may be distinguished if it does not assume its appropriate secondary and tertiary structures and therefore is not immunologically reactive or cannot form its native shape, or if it is degraded at the nonpermissive temperature. But even degradation at the restrictive condition, which has been demonstrated for several mutated adenovirus proteins (Russell *et al.*, 1974; van der Vliet *et al.*, 1975; Kauffman and Ginsberg, 1976), is not an absolute criterion of a defective protein. For instance, Kauffman (personal communication) has demonstrated that, in cells infected with some type 5 hexon-minus mutants (e.g., H5*ts*115), not only hexon polypeptides are degraded at 39.5°C, but also pV1 and perhaps some minor proteins are unstable (recombination and complementation analyses showed that the mutant studied resulted from a single-site mutation).

Recombinational analysis is now allied with a variety of physical and chemical tools, and it is reasonable to assume that within a short time the location of most of the structural genes for adenovirus-specified proteins will be determined. It is clear already that there is not an apparent functional order to the gene array. Therefore, it remains to be seen whether or not the display of this architectural plan will help to understand how control of the expression of the gene functions is exercised.

In spite of the handicaps imposed by the problems described, the mutants of adenoviruses generated have served well in functional studies, which have usually been the primary objective for their isolation. Although the specific gene product mutated has been identified for only one of the three unique types of DNA⁻ mutants (van der Vliet *et al.*, 1975; Rosenwirth *et al.*, 1975), studies with these three groups of mutants have already clearly indicated that at least three viral proteins are essential for initiation of DNA replication (Shiroki and Shimojo, 1974; Ginsberg *et al.*, 1974a; van der Vliet and Sussenbach, personal communication). These DNA⁻ mutants have also proved to be invaluable for investigating the regulation of transcription (Carter and Ginsberg, 1976) and the transformation of cells (Williams *et al.*, 1974; Ginsberg *et al.*, 1974*a,b*; Ledinko, 1974). The use of *ts* mutants to study structure and function of viral proteins and assembly of the virions is just beginning, but encouraging data are already emerging.

Genetics is not the fount from which will flow solutions to all problems of viral functions and their controls, although during certain investigative periods it may receive "favored discipline status." But if used rigorously and as a strong partner with other basic sciences, viral genetics offers a powerful tool to further knowledge of viral replication, regulation of cell growth, and gene interactions.

7. NOTE ADDED IN PROOF

Since this review was written, several important papers of direct relevance have been published. We wish to draw particular attention to those that have contributed to our understanding of the gene maps of adenoviruses. In addition, some studies on characterization of *ts* mutants will be summarized, and the list of mutants isolated will be updated.

The mapping of viral cytoplasmic RNAs to specific regions and strands of the genome has been an area of active interest. The general picture for both adenovirus serotypes studied is one of strand switching and interspersing of late and early messages. For an up-to-date review, the paper by Sharp and Flint (1976) is recommended.

Lewis *et al.* (1976), using the technique of selecting RNA by hybridization to specific endonuclease fragments, and subsequent *in vitro* translation, have extended their studies to localize the genes encoding the polypeptides specified at early times in the infectious cycle of type 2 adenovirus. Six polypeptides have been translated *in vitro*. Their apparent molecular weight and the locations on the genome within which they lie are as follows:

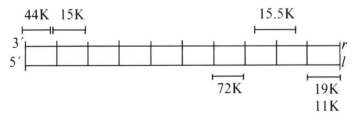

The 44K and 15K polypeptides are located in the region of the genome known to be required for cellular transformation of rodent cells by adenoviruses.

The physical mapping of *ts* mutants by heterotypic recombination analysis has been extended by Sambrook *et al.,* (1975) and now includes the positioning of three mutants on the Ad2⁺ND1 genome and six mutants on the Ad5 genome. The correspondence between the physical maps and the recombination maps has been maintained. The extensiveness of the analysis, involving five different endonucleases with fifteen distinguishable cuts in the DNA, confirms the notion that this technique has great resolving power, especially in the right half of the adenovirus genome where distinguishable endonuclease cuts have been determined in the two parents. Using the heterotypic recombination-endonuclease technique, various mutants described previously as "hexon transport" and "assembly," have been mapped in the hexon polypeptide region of the genome (Luciw and Ginsberg, unpublished). Coupled with immunochemical examination of the hexon polypeptides made in the various mutants, the data suggest that mutants mapping in the "hexon 1" region of the genome (Figure 4) are located in the hexon structural gene; by inference, those mutants mapping in "hexon 2" region, whatever their phenotype, are in the gene for the 100K protein.

Characterization studies of interest include an analysis of the viral RNAs found in the cytoplasm of cells infected with H5*ts* mutants and maintained at the restrictive temperature (Berget *et al.,* 1976). "Late" mutants, with one exception, induced the wild type concentrations of all cytoplasmic RNA species. The exception was H5*ts*2, a mutant in the hexon gene (Sambrook *et al.,* 1975): Species of RNA that hybridized to viral DNA between 40.9 and the right-hand end of the genome were present in excess at the restrictive temperature. The most pronounced increases were in viral RNAs derived from between 40.9 and 70.7. Such studies may yield clues to transcriptional control mechanisms.

Other phenotypic characterizations include an analysis of H2*ts*1, a "late" mutant (Weber, 1976). This mutant is defective in processing virion polypeptides VI–XII at the restrictive temperature. Non-infectious virions that contain uncleaved polypeptides accumulate, but, on shift-down, they are processed to yield the mature polypeptide complement, even in the absence of protein synthesis. The phenotype described implies that the virus codes for a protein that either acts as a protease or induces a host protease, or serves as a component in a polypeptide processing cascade.

The pace of isolation of mutants has slackened but a new group of mutants has been isolated from type 2 adenovirus (Kathmann *et al.,* 1976). The fourteen mutants were classified in seven complementation groups. Of special interest were the three mutants defective in DNA synthesis, which fell into three separate complementation groups, one of which was distinct from the two so far characterized in the closely related Ad5 serotype. Recent data suggest that this third group may represent an uncoating function that is defective (W. Doerfler, personal communication).

8. REFERENCES

Alberts, B., and Frey, L., 1970, T4 bacteriophage gene 32: A structural protein in the replication and recombination of DNA, *Nature (London)* **227:**1313.

Anderson, C. W., Baum, P. R., and Gesteland, R. F., 1973, Processing of adenovirus 2-induced protein, *J. Virol.* **12:**241.

Bartok, K., Garon, C. F., Berry, K. W., Fraser, M. J., and Rose, J. A., 1974, Specific fragmentation of adenovirus heteroduplex DNA molecules with single-strand specific nucleases from *Neurospora crassa, J. Mol. Biol.* **87:**437.

Bégin, M., and Weber, J., 1975, Genetic analysis of adenovirus type 2. I. Isolation and genetic characterization of temperature-sensitive mutants, *J. Virol.* **15:**1.

Bellett, A. J. D., and Younghusband, H. B., 1972, Replication of the DNA of chick embryo lethal orphan virus, *J. Mol. Biol.* **72:**691.

Bello, L. J., and Ginsberg, H. S., 1969, Relationship between deoxyribonucleic acid synthesis and inhibition of host protein synthesis in type 5 adenovirus-infected KB cells, *J. Virol.* **3:**106.

Berget, S. M., Flint, S. J., Williams, J. F., and Sharp, P. A., 1976, Adenovirus transcription IV. Synthesis of viral-specific RNA in human cells infected with temperature-sensitive mutants of adenovirus 5, *J. Virol.* **19:**879–889.

Boyer, G. S., Leuchtenberger, C., and Ginsberg, H. S., 1957, Cytological and cytochemical studies of HeLa cells infected with adenoviruses, *J. Exp. Med.* **105:**95.

Boyer, G. S., Denny, F. W., Jr., and Ginsberg, H. S., 1959, The sequential cellular changes produced by types 5 and 7 adenoviruses in HeLa cells and in human amniotic cells: Cytological studies aided by fluorescein-labelled antibody, *J. Exp. Med.* **110:**827.

Brockman, W. W., and Nathans, D., 1974, The isolation of simian virus 40 variants with specifically altered genomes, *Proc. Natl. Acad. Sci. USA* **71:**942.

Brown, S. M., Ritchie, D. A., and Subak-Sharpe, J. H., 1973, Genetic studies with herpes simplex virus type 1: The isolation of temperature-sensitive mutants, their arrangement into complementation groups and recombination analysis leading to a linkage map, *J. Gen. Virol.* **18:**329.

Brugge, J. S., and Butel, J. S., 1975, Role of simian virus 40 gene *A* function in maintenance of transformation, *J. Virol.* **15:**619.

Burlingham, B. T., Brown, D. T., and Doerfler, W., 1974, Incomplete particles of adenovirus. I. Characteristics of the DNA associated with incomplete adenovirions of types 2 and 12, *Virology* **60:**419.

Carter, T. H., and Ginsberg, H. S., 1976, Viral transcription in KB cells infected by temperature sensitive "early" mutants of adenovirus type 5, *J. Virol.* **18:**156.

Chardonnet, Y., and Dales, S., 1970, Early events in the interaction of adenoviruses with HeLa cells. I. Penetration of type 5 and intracellular release of the DNA genome, *Virology* **40**:462.

Chou, J. Y., and Martin, R. G., 1974, Complementation analysis of simian virus 40 mutants, *J. Virol.* **13**:1101.

Chou, J. Y., and Martin, R. G., 1975, Products of complementation between temperature sensitive mutants of simian virus 40, *J. Virol.* **15**:127.

Cleaver, J. E., and Weil, S., 1975, UV-induced reversion of a temperature-sensitive late mutant of simian virus 40 to a wild-type phenotype, *J. Virol.* **16**:214.

Cornick, G., Sigler, P. B., and Ginsberg, H. S., 1973, Mass of protein in the asymmetric unit of hexon crystals—A new method, *J. Mol. Biol.* **73**:533.

Craig, E. A., Zimmer, S., and Raskas, H. S., 1975, Analysis of early adenovirus 2 RNA using EcoR-R1 viral DNA fragments, *J. Virol.* **15**:1202.

Crick, F. H. C., and Watson, J. D., 1956, Structure of small viruses, *Nature (London)* **177**:473.

Dales, S., 1962, An electron microscope study of the early association between two mammalian viruses and their hosts, *J. Cell Biol.* **13**:303.

Davis, B. D., 1948. Isolation of biochemically deficient mutants of bacteria by penicillin, *J. Am. Chem. Soc.* **70**:4267.

Doerfler, W., and Kleinschmidt, A. K., 1970, Denaturation pattern of the DNA of adenovirus type 2 as determined by electron microscopy, *J. Mol. Biol.* **50**:579.

Doerfler, W., Hellman, W., and Kleinschmidt, A. K., 1972, The DNA of adenovirus type 12 and its denaturation pattern, *Virology* **47**:507.

Dorsett, P. H., and Ginsberg, H. S., 1975, Characterization of type 5 adenovirus fiber protein, *J. Virol.* **15**:208.

Ellens, D. J., Sussenbach, J. S., and Jansz, H. S., 1974, Studies on the mechanism of replication of adenovirus DNA. III. Electron microscopy of replicating DNA, *Virology* **61**:427.

Ensinger, M. J., and Ginsberg, H. S., 1972, Selection and preliminary characterization of temperature-sensitive mutants of type 5 adenovirus, *J. Virol.* **10**:328.

Everett, S. F., and Ginsberg, H. S., 1958, A toxinlike material separable from type 5 adenovirus particles, *Virology* **6**:770.

Everitt, E., Sundquist, B., and Philipson, L., 1971, Mechanism of the arginine requirement for adenovirus synthesis. I. Synthesis of structural proteins, *J. Virol.* **8**:742.

Everitt, E., Sundquist, B., Pettersson, U., and Philipson, L., 1973, Structural proteins of adenoviruses. X. Isolation and topography of low-molecular-weight antigens from the virion of adenovirus type 2, *Virology* **52**:130.

Ezoe, H., and Mak, S., 1974, Comparative studies on functions of human adenovirus type 12 and its low oncogenic mutant virions, *J. Virol.* **14**:733.

Fenner, F., 1969. Conditional lethal mutants of animal viruses, *Curr. Top. Microbiol. Immunol.* **48**:1.

Fincham, J. R. S., 1966, *Genetic Complementation,* Benjamin, New York.

Franklin, R. M., Pettersson, U., Akervall, K., Strandberg, B., and Philipson, L., 1971, Structural proteins of adenovirus. V. Size and structure of the adenovirus type 2 hexon, *J. Mol. Biol.* **57**:383.

Fujinaga, K., and Green, M., 1970, Mechanism of viral carcinogenesis by DNA mammalian viruses. VII. Viral genes transcribed in adenovirus type 2 infected and transformed cells, *Proc. Natl. Acad. Sci. USA* **65**:375.

Gallimore, P. H., Sharp, P. A., and Sambrook, J., 1974, Viral DNA in transformed cells. II. A study of the sequences of adenovirus 2 DNA in nine lines of transformed rat cells using specific fragments of the viral genome, *J. Mol. Biol.* **89**:49.

Garon, C. F., Berry, K. W., and Rose, J. A., 1972, A unique form of terminal redundancy in adenovirus DNA molecules, *Proc. Natl. Acad. Sci. USA* **69**:2391.

Garon, C. F., Berry, K. W., Hierholzer, J. C., and Rose, J. A., 1973, Mapping of base sequence heterologies between genomes from different adenovirus serotypes, *Virology* **54**:414.

Gilead, Z., and Ginsberg, H. S., 1965, Characterization of a tumorlike antigen in type 12 and type 18 adenovirus-infected cells, *J. Bacteriol.* **90**:120.

Gilead, Z., Arens, M. Q., Bhaduri, S., Shanmugam, G., and Green, M., 1975, Tumour antigen specificity of a DNA-binding protein from cells infected with adenovirus 2, *Nature (London)* **254**:533.

Ginsberg, H. S., 1969, Biochemistry of adenovirus infection, in: *The Biochemistry of Viruses* (H. B. Levy, ed.), pp. 329–359, Dekker, New York.

Ginsberg, H. S., Pereira, H. G., Valentine, R. C., and Wilcox, W. C., 1966, A proposed terminology for the adenovirus antigens and virion morphological subunits, *Virology* **28**:782.

Ginsberg, H. S., Bello, L. J., and Levine, A. J., 1967, Control of biosynthesis of host macromolecules in cells infected with adenoviruses, in: *The Molecular Biology of Viruses* (J. S. Colter and W. Paranchych, eds.), pp. 547–572, Academic Press, New York.

Ginsberg, H. S., Ensinger, M. J., Kauffman, R. S., Mayer, A. J., and Lundholm, U., 1974a, Cell transformation: A study of regulation with types 5 and 12 adenovirus temperature sensitive mutants, *Cold Spring Harbor Symp. Quant. Biol.* **39**:419.

Ginsberg, H. S., Ensinger, M. J., Rubenstein, F. E., and Kauffman, R. S., 1974b, Adenovirus genes and cancer, in: *Viruses, Evolution and Cancer* (E. Kurstak and K. Maramorosch, eds.), pp. 167–181, Academic Press, New York.

Graham, F. L., and van der Eb, A. J., 1973, A new technique for the assay of infectivity of human adenovirus 5 DNA, *Virology* **52**:456.

Graham, F. L., van der Eb, A. J., and Heijneker, H. L., 1974, Size and location of the transforming region in human adenovirus type 5 DNA, *Nature (London)* **251**:687.

Green, M., 1962, Studies on the biosynthesis of viral DNA. IV. Isolation, purification and chemical analysis of adenovirus, *Cold Spring Harbor Symp. Quant. Biol.* **27**:219.

Green, M., 1970, Oncogenic viruses, *Annu. Rev. Biochem.* **39**:701.

Green, M., Piña, M., Kimes, R., Wensink, P. C., MacHattie, L. A., and Thomas, C. A., Jr., 1967, Adenovirus DNA. I. Molecular weight and conformation, *Proc. Natl. Acad. Sci. USA* **57**:1302.

Green, M., Parsons, J. T., Piña, M., Fujinaga, K., Caffier, H., and Landgraf-Leurs, I., 1970, Transcription of adenovirus genes in productively infected and in transformed cells, *Cold Spring Harbor Symp. Quant. Biol.* **35**:803.

Grodzicker, T., Anderson, C., Sharp, P. A., and Sambrook, J., 1974a, Conditional lethal mutants of adenovirus 2–simian virus 40 hybrids. I. Host range mutants of Ad2$^+$ND1, *J. Virol.* **13**:1237.

Grodzicker, T., Williams, J., Sharp, P., and Sambrook, J., 1974b, Physical mapping of temperature-sensitive mutations of adenoviruses, *Cold Spring Harbor Symp. Quant. Biol.* **39**:439.

Hedgpeth, J., Goodman, H. M., and Boyer, H. W., 1972, DNA nucleotide sequence restricted by the R1 endonuclease, *Proc. Natl. Acad. Sci. USA* **69**:3448.

Hershey, A. D. (ed.), 1971, *The Bacteriophage Lambda,* Cold Spring Harbor Laboratory, Cold Spring Harbor, N.Y.

Hilleman, M. R., and Werner, J. R., 1954, Recovery of new agent from patients with acute respiratory illness, *Proc. Soc. Exp. Biol. Med.* **85**:183.

Horwitz, M. S., Brayton, C., and Brown, S. G., 1973, Synthesis of type 2 adenovirus DNA in the presence of cycloheximide, *J. Virol.* **11**:544.

Huebner, R. J., Casey, M. J., Chanock, R. M., and Schell, K., 1965, Tumors induced in hamsters by a strain of adenovirus type 3: Sharing of tumor antigens and "neoantigens" with those produced by adenovirus type 7 tumors, *Proc. Natl. Acad. Sci. USA* **54**:381.

Hyman, R. W., Brunovskis, I., and Summers, W. C., 1973, DNA base sequence homology between coliphages T7 and ϕII and between T3 and ϕII as determined by heteroduplex mapping in the electron microscope, *J. Mol. Biol.* **77**:189.

Ishibashi, M., 1970, Retention of viral antigen in the cytoplasm of cells infected with temperature-sensitive mutants of an avian adenovirus, *Proc. Natl. Acad. Sci. USA* **65**:304.

Ishibashi, M., 1971, Temperature-sensitive conditional lethal mutants of an avian adenovirus (CELO), *Virology* **45**:42.

Ishibashi, M., and Maizel, J. V., Jr., 1974a, The polypeptides of adenovirus. V. Young virions, structural intermediates between top components and aged virions, *Virology* **57**:409.

Ishibashi, M., and Maizel, J. V., Jr., 1974b, The polypeptides of adenovirus. VI. Early and late glycopolypeptides, *Virology* **58**:345.

Ito, M., and Suzuki, E., 1970, Adeno-associated satellite virus growth supported by a temperature-sensitive mutant of human adenovirus, *J. Gen. Virol.* **9**:243.

Jacobson, M. F., and Baltimore, D., 1968, Morphogenesis of poliovirus. I. Association of the viral RNA with coat protein, *J. Mol. Biol.* **33**:369.

Kasel, J. A., Huber, M., Loda, F., Banks, P. A., and Knight, V., 1964, Immunization of volunteers with soluble antigens of adenovirus type 1, *Proc. Soc. Exp. Biol. Med.* **117**:186.

Kathmann, P., Schick, J., Winnacker, E-L., and Doerfler, W. 1976. Isolation and Characterization of temperature-sensitive mutants of adenovirus type 2, *J. Virol.* **19**:43–53.

Kauffman, R. S., and Ginsberg, H. S., 1976, Characterization of a temperature-sensitive, hexon transport mutant of type 5 adenovirus, *J. Virol.* **19**:643.

Kellenberger, E., Eiserling, F. A., and Boy de la Tour, E., 1968, Studies on the morphogenesis of the head of phage T-even. III. The cores of head-related structures, *J. Ultrastruct. Res.* **21**:335.

Kelly, T. J., Jr. and Lewis, A. M., Jr., 1973, Use of non-defective adenovirus–simian virus 40 hybrids for mapping the simian virus 40 genome, *J. Virol.* **12**:643.

King, J., and Casjens, S., 1974, Catalytic head assemblying protein in virus morphogenesis, *Nature (London)* **251**:112.

Kjellén, L., and Pereira, H. G., 1968, Role of adenovirus antigens in the induction of virus neutralizing antibody, *J. Gen. Virol.* **2**:177.

Koczot, F. J., Carter, B. J., Garon, C. F., and Rose, J. A., 1973, Self-complementarity of terminal sequences within plus or minus strands of adenovirus-associated virus DNA, *Proc. Natl. Acad. Sci. USA* **70**:215.

Lai, C.-J., and Nathans, D., 1974, Mapping temperature-sensitive mutants of simian virus 40: Rescue of mutants by fragments of viral DNA, *Virology* **60**:466.

Lavelle, G., Patch, C., Khoury, G., and Rose, J., 1975, Isolation and partial characterization of single-stranded adenoviral DNA produced during synthesis of adenovirus type 2 DNA, *J. Virol.* **16**:775.

Laver, W. G., 1970, Isolation of an arginine-rich protein from particles of adenovirus type 2, *Virology* **41**:488.

Lawrence, W. C., and Ginsberg, H. S., 1967, Intracellular uncoating of type 5 adenovirus deoxyribonucleic acid, *J. Virol.* **1**:851.

Ledinko, N., 1971, Inhibition by α-amanitin of adenovirus 12 replication in human embryo kidney cells of adenovirus transformation of hamster cells, *Nature (London) New Biol.* **233**:247.

Ledinko, N., 1974, Temperature-sensitive mutants of adenovirus type 12 defective in viral DNA synthesis, *J. Virol.* **14**:457.

Levine, A. J., and Ginsberg, H. S., 1967, Mechanism by which fiber antigen inhibits multiplication of type 5 adenovirus, *J. Virol.* **1**:747.

Levine, A. J., van der Vliet, P. C., Rosenwirth, B., Rabek, J., Frenkel, G., and Ensinger, M., 1974, Adenovirus-infected, cell-specific, DNA-binding proteins, *Cold Spring Harbor Symp. Quant. Biol.* **39**:559.

Lewis, A. M., Jr., Levin, M. J., Wiese, W. H., Crumpacker, C. S., and Henry, P. H., 1969, A nondefective (component) adenovirus–SV40 hybrid isolated from the Ad.2-SV40 hybrid population, *Proc. Natl. Acad. Sci. USA* **63**:1128.

Lewis, J. B., Atkins, J. F., Anderson, C. W., Baum, P. R., and Gesteland, R. F., 1975, Mapping of late adenovirus genes by cell-free translation of RNA selected by hybridization to specific DNA fragments, *Proc. Natl. Acad. Sci. USA* **72**:1344.

Lewis, J. B., Atkins, J. F., Baum, P. R., Solem, R., and Gesteland, R. F., 1976, Location and identification of the genes for adenovirus type 2 early polypeptides, *Cell* **7**:141–151.

Lindberg, U., Persson, T., and Philipson, L., 1972, Isolation and Characterization of adenovirus messenger ribonucleic acid in productive infection, *J. Virol.* **10**:909.

Lonberg-Holm, K., and Philipson, L., 1969, Early events of virus–cell interaction in an adenovirus system, *J. Virol.* **4**:323.

Lucas, J. J., and Ginsberg, H. S., 1971, Synthesis of virus-specific ribonucleic acid in KB cells infected with type 2 adenovirus, *J. Virol.* **8**:203.

Lucas, J. J., and Ginsberg, H. S., 1972, Transcription and transport of virus-specific ribonucleic acids in African green monkey kidney cells abortively infected with type 2 adenovirus, *J. Virol.* **10**:1109.

Lundholm, U., and Doerfler, W., 1971, Temperature-sensitive mutants of human adenovirus type 12, *Virology* **45**:827.

Maizel, J. F., Jr., Phillips, B. A., and Summers, D. F., 1967, Composition of artificially produced and naturally occurring empty capsids of poliovirus type 1, *Virology* **32**:692.

Maizel, J. V., Jr., White, D. O., and Scharff, M. D., 1968*a*, The polypeptides of adenovirus. I. Evidence for multiple protein components in the virion and a comparison of types 2, 7A, and 12, *Virology* **36**:115.

Maizel, J. V., Jr., White, D. O., and Scharff, M. D., 1968*b*, The polypeptides of adenovirus. II. Soluble proteins, cores, top components and the structure of the virion, *Virology* **36**:126.

Mak, S., 1971, Defective virions in human adenovirus type 12, *J. Virol.* **7**:426.

Martin, R. G., and Chou, J. Y., 1975, Simian virus 40 functions required for the establishment and maintenance of malignant transformation, *J. Virol.* **15**:599.

Mautner, V., Williams, J., Sambrook, J., Sharp, P. A., and Grodzicker, T., 1975, The location of the genes coding for hexon and fiber proteins in adenovirus DNA, *Cell* **5**:93.

McGuire, P. M., Swart, C., and Hodge, L. D., 1972, Adenovirus messenger RNA in mammalian cells: Failure of polyribosome association in the absence of nuclear cleavage, *Proc. Natl. Acad. Sci. USA* **69**:1578.

Morgan, C., Godman, G. C., Breitenfeld, P. M., and Rose, H. M., 1960, A correlative study by electron and light microscopy of the development of type 5 adenovirus. I. Electron microscopy, *J. Exp. Med.* **112**:373.

Morgan, C., Rosenkranz, H. S., and Mednis, B., 1969, Structure and development of viruses as observed in the electron microscope. X. Entry and uncoating of adenovirus, *J. Virol.* **4**:777.

Mulder, C., Arrand, J. R., Delius, H., Keller, W., Pettersson, U., Roberts, R. J., and Sharp, P. A., 1974a, Cleavage maps of DNA from adenovirus types 2 and 5 by restriction endonucleases *Eco · R1* and *Hpa1*, *Cold Spring Harbor Symp. Quant. Biol.* **39**:397.

Mulder, C., Sharp, P. A., Delius, H., and Pettersson, U., 1974b, Specific fragmentation of DNA of adenovirus serotypes 3, 5, 7 and 12 and adenosimian virus 40 hybrid virus Ad2⁺ND1 by restriction endonuclease R · *Eco · R1*, *J. Virol.* **14**:68.

Neurath, A. R., Rubin, B. A., and Stasny, J. T., 1968, Cleavage by formamide of intercapsomer bonds in adenovirus types 4 and 7 virions and hemagglutinins, *J. Virol.* **2**:1086.

Norrby, E., 1968, Biological significance of structural adenovirus components, *Curr. Top. Microbiol. Immunol.* **43**:1.

Norrby, E., 1969, The structural and functional diversity of adenovirus capsid components, *J. Gen. Virol.* **5**:221.

Norrby, E., and Skaaret, P., 1967, The relationship between soluble antigens and the virion of adenovirus type 3. III. Immunological identification of fiber antigen and isolated vertex capsomer antigen, *Virology* **32**:489.

Okubo, C. K., and Raskas, N. J., 1971, Thermosensitive events in the replication of adenovirus type 2 at 42°, *Virology* **46**:175.

Osborn, M., and Weber, K., 1975, Simian virus 40 gene *A* function and maintenance of transformation, *J. Virol.* **15**:636.

Ozer, H. L., 1972, Synthesis and assembly of simian virus 40. I. Differential synthesis of intact virions and empty shells, *J. Virol.* **9**:41.

Ozer, H. L., and Tegtmeyer, P., 1972, Synthesis and assembly of simian virus 40. II. Synthesis of the major capsid protein and its incorporation into viral particles, *J. Virol.* **9**:52.

Parsons, J. T., and Green, M., 1971, Biochemical studies on adenovirus multiplication. XVIII. Resolution of early virus-specific RNA species in Ad2 infected and transformed cells, *Virology* **45**:154.

Pearson, G. D., and Hanawalt, P. C., 1971, Isolation of DNA replication complexes from uninfected and adenovirus-infected HeLa cells, *J. Mol. Biol.* **62**:65.

Pereira, H. G., 1958, A protein factor responsible for the early cytopathic effect of adenoviruses, *Virology* **6**:601.

Pereira, H. G., 1960, Antigenic structure of non-infectious adenovirus materials, *Nature (London)* **186**:571.

Pettersson, U., 1973, Some unusual properties of replicating adenovirus type 2 DNA, *J. Mol. Biol.* **81**:521.

Pettersson, U., and Höglund, S., 1969, Structural proteins of adenoviruses. III. Purification and characterization of the adenovirus type 2 penton antigen, *Virology* **39**:90.

Pettersson, U., Mulder, C., Delius, H., and Sharp, P. A., 1973, Cleavage of adenovirus type 2 DNA into six unique fragments by endonuclease R-R1, *Proc. Natl. Acad. Sci. USA* **70**:200.

Philipson, L., and Lindberg, U., 1974, Reproduction of adenoviruses, in: *Comprehensive Virology,* Vol. 3 (H. Fraenkel-Conrat and R. R. Wagner, eds.), pp. 143–227, Plenum Press, New York.

Philipson, L., and Pettersson, U., 1973, Structure and function of virion proteins of adenoviruses, *Progr. Exp. Tumor Res.* **18**:1.

Philipson, L., Lonberg-Holm, K., and Pettersson, U., 1968, Virus–receptor interaction in an adenovirus system, *J. Virol.* **2**:1064.

Philipson, L., Wall, R., Glickman, G., and Darnell, J. E., 1971, Addition of polyadenylate sequences to virus-specific RNA during adenovirus replication, *Proc. Natl. Acad. Sci. USA* **68**:2806.

Philipson, L., Lindberg, U., Persson, T., and Vennström, B., 1973, Transcription and processing of adenovirus RNA in productive infection, in: *Advances in the Biosciences,* Vol. 11 (G. Raspé, ed.) pp. 167–183, Pergamon Press, Vieweg: Braunschweig.

Phillips, B. A., Summers, D. F., and Maizel, J. V., Jr., 1968, *In vitro* assembly of poliovirus-related particles, *Virology* **35**:216.

Piña, M., and Green, M., 1965, Biochemical studies on adenovirus multiplication. IX. Chemical and base composition analysis of 28 human adenoviruses, *Proc. Natl. Acad. Sci. USA* **54**:547.

Piña, M., and Green, M., 1969, Biochemical studies on adenovirus multiplication. XIV. Macromolecule and enzyme synthesis in cells replicating oncogenic and nononcogenic human adenovirus, *Virology* **38**:573.

Pope, J. H., and Rowe, W. P., 1964, Immunofluorescent studies of adenovirus 12 tumors and of cells transformed or infected by adenoviruses, *J. Exp. Med.* **120**:577.

Prage, L., and Pettersson, U., 1971, Structural proteins of adenoviruses. VII. Purification and properties of an arginine-rich core protein from adenovirus type 2 and type 3, *Virology* **45**:364.

Price, R., and Penman, S., 1972, Transcription of the adenovirus genome by an α-amanitin-sensitive ribonucleic acid polymerase in HeLa cells, *J. Virol.* **9**:621.

Robb, J. A., and Martin, R. G., 1972, Genetic analysis of simian virus 40. III. Characterization of a temperature-sensitive mutant blocked at an early stage of productive infection in monkey cells, *J. Virol.* **9**:956.

Robinson, A. J., Younghusband, H. B., and Bellett, A. J. D., 1973, A circular DNA–protein complex from adenoviruses, *Virology* **56**:54.

Rose, J. A., 1974, Parvovirus reproduction, in: *Comprehensive Virology,* Vol. 3 (H. Fraenkel-Conrat and R. R. Wagner, eds.) pp. 1–61, Plenum Press, New York.

Rosen, L., 1960, A hemagglutination-inhibition technique for typing adenoviruses, *Am. J. Hyg.* **71**:120.

Rosenwirth, B., Shiroki, K., Levine, A. J., and Shimojo, H., 1975, Isolation and characterization of adenovirus type 12 DNA binding proteins, *Virology* **67**:14.

Rouse, H. C., and Schlesinger, R. W., 1972, The effects of arginine starvation on macromolecular synthesis in infection with type 2 adenovirus. I. Synthesis and utilization of structural proteins, *Virology* **48**:463.

Rowe, W. P., Huebner, R. J., Gilmore, L. K., Parrott, R. H., and Ward, T. G., 1953, Isolation of a cytopathogenic agent from human adenoids undergoing spontaneous degeneration in tissue culture, *Proc. Soc. Exp. Biol. Med.* **84**:570.

Rubenstein, F. E., and Ginsberg, H. S., 1974, Transformation characteristics of temperature-sensitive mutants of type 12 adenovirus, *Intervirology* **3**:170.

Russell, W. C., and Knight, B. E., 1967, Evidence for a new antigen within the adenovirus capsid, *J. Gen. Virol.* **1**:523.

Russell, W. C., McIntosh, K., and Skehel, J. J., 1971, The preparation and properties of adenovirus cores, *J. Gen. Virol.* **11**:35.

Russell, W. C., Newman, C., and Williams, J. F., 1972a, Characterization of temperature-sensitive mutants of adenovirus type 5—Serology, *J. Gen. Virol.* **17**:265.

Russell, W. C., Skehel, J. J., Machado, R., and Pereira, H. G., 1972b, Phosphorylated polypeptides in adenovirus-infected cells, *Virology* **50**:931.

Russell, W. C., Skehel, J. J., and Williams, J. F., 1974, Characterization of temperature-sensitive mutants of adenovirus type 5: Synthesis of polypeptides in infected cells, *J. Gen. Virol.* **24**:247.

Sambrook, J., Botchan, M., Gallimore, P., Ozanne, B., Pettersson, U., Williams, J., and Sharp, P. A., 1974, Viral DNA sequences in cells transformed by simian virus 40, adenovirus type 2 and adenovirus type 5, *Cold Spring Harbor Symp. Quant. Biol.* **39**:615.

Sambrook, J., Williams, J., Sharp, P. A., and Grodzicker, T., 1975, Physical mapping of temperature-sensitive mutations of adenoviruses, *J. Mol. Biol.* **97**:369–390.

Schlesinger, R. W., 1969, Adenoviruses: The nature of the virion and of controlling factors in productive or abortive infection and tumorigenesis, *Adv. Virus Res.* **14**:1.

Sharp, P. A., and Flint, S. J., 1976, Adenovirus transcription, *Curr. Top. Microbiol. Immunol.* **74**:137–166.

Shenk, T. E., Rhodes, C., Rigby, P. W. J., and Berg, P., 1975, Biochemical method for mapping mutational alterations in DNA with S1 nuclease: The location of deletions and temperature-sensitive mutations in simian virus 40, *Proc. Natl. Acad. Sci. USA* **72**:989.

Shiroki, K., and Shimojo, H., 1974, Analysis of adenovirus 12 temperature-sensitive mutants defective in viral DNA replication, *Virology* **61**:474.

Shiroki, K., Irisawa, J., and Shimojo, H., 1972, Isolation and preliminary characterization of temperature sensitive mutants of adenovirus 12, *Virology* **49**:1.

Shiroki, K., Shimojo, H., and Yamaguchi, K., 1974, The viral DNA replication complex of adenovirus 12, *Virology* **60**:192.

Simon, L., 1972, Infection of *Escherichia coli* by T2 and T4 bacteriophages as seen in the electron microscope: T4 head morphogenesis, *Proc. Natl. Acad. Sci. USA* **69**:907.

Steenbergh, P. H., Sussenbach, J. S., Roberts, R. J., and Jansz, H. S., 1975, The 3′-terminal nucleotide sequences of adenovirus types 2 and 5 DNA, *J. Virol.* **15**:268.

Stinski, M. F., and Ginsberg, H. S., 1975, Hexon peptides of types 2, 3 and 5 adenoviruses and their relationship to hexon structure, *J. Virol.* **15**:898.

Straus, S. E., Ginsberg, H. S., and Rose, J. A., 1975, DNA minus temperature-sensitive mutants of adenovirus type 5 help adenovirus-associated virus replication, *J. Virol.* **17**:140.

Sundquist, B., Everitt, E., Philipson, L., and Höglund, S., 1973a, Assembly of adenoviruses, *J. Virol.* **11**:449.

Sundquist, B., Pettersson, U., Thelander, L., and Philipson, L., 1973b, Structural proteins of adenoviruses. IX. Molecular weight and subunit composition of adenovirus type 2 fiber, *Virology* **51**:252.

Sussenbach, J. S., 1967, Early events in the infection process of adenovirus type 5 in HeLa cells, *Virology* **33**:567.

Sussenbach, J. S., van der Vliet, P. C., Ellens, D. J., and Jansz, H. S., 1972, Linear intermediates in the replication of adenovirus DNA, *Nature (London) New Biol.* **239**:47.

Sussenbach, J. S., Ellens, D. J., and Jansz, H. S., 1973, Studies on the mechanism of replication of adenovirus DNA. II. The nature of single-stranded DNA in replicative intermediates, *J. Virol.* **12**:1131.

Suzuki, E., and Shimojo, H., 1971, A temperature-sensitive mutant of adenovirus 31, defective in viral deoxyribonucleic acid replication, *Virology* **43**:488.

Suzuki, E., and Shimojo, H., 1974, Temperature-sensitive formation of the DNA replication complex in adenovirus 31-infected cells, *J. Virol.* **13**:538.

Suzuki, E., Shimojo, H., and Moritsugu, Y., 1972, Isolation and a preliminary characterization of temperature sensitive mutants of adenovirus 31, *Virology* **49**:426.

Takahashi, M., 1972, Isolation of conditional lethal mutants (temperature sensitive and host dependent mutants) of adenovirus type 5, *Virology* **49**:815.

Takahashi, M., Minekawa, U., and Yamanishi, K., 1974, Transformation of a hamster embryo cell line (Nil) with a host-dependent mutant of adenovirus type 5, *Virology* **57**:300.

Takemori, N., 1972, Genetic studies with tumorigenic adenoviruses. III. Recombination in adenovirus type 12, *Virology* **47**:157.

Takemori, N., Riggs, J. L., and Aldrich, C., 1968, Genetic studies with tumorigenic adenoviruses. I. Isolation of cytocidal (*cyt*) mutants of adenovirus type 12, *Virology* **36**:575.

Takemori, N., Riggs, J. L., and Aldrich, C. D., 1969, Genetic studies with tumorigenic adenoviruses. II. Heterogeneity of *cyt* mutants of adenovirus type 12, *Virology* **38**:8.

Tegtmeyer, P., 1975, Function of simian virus 40 gene *A* in transforming infection, *J. Virol.* **15**:613.

Thomas, D. C., and Green, M., 1966, Biochemical studies on adenovirus multiplication. XI. Evidence of a cytoplasmic site for the synthesis of viral coded proteins, *Proc. Natl. Acad. Sci. USA* **56**:243.

Thomas, D. C., and Green, M., 1969, Biochemical studies on adenovirus multiplication. XV. Transcription of the adenovirus type 2 genome during productive infection, *Virology* **39**:205.

Tibbetts, C., and Pettersson, U., 1974, Complementary strand-specific sequences from unique fragments of adenovirus type 2 DNA for hybridization-mapping experiments, *J. Mol. Biol.* **88**:767.

Tibbetts, C., Pettersson, U., Johansson, K., and Philipson, L., 1974, Relationship of mRNA from productively infected cells to the complementary strands of adenovirus type 2 DNA, *J. Virol.* **13**:370.

Timbury, M. C., 1971, Temperature-sensitive mutants of herpes simplex virus type 2, *J. Gen. Virol.* **13**:373.

Tooze, J. (ed.), 1973, *The Molecular Biology of Tumour Viruses,* Cold Spring Harbor Laboratory, Cold Spring Harbor, N.Y.

Ustacelebi, S., 1973, Induction of interferon in chick embryo cells infected by adenovirus type 5 and polyoma virus, Ph.D. thesis, University of Glasgow.

Ustacelebi, S., and Williams, J. F., 1972, Temperature-sensitive mutants of adenovirus defective in interferon induction at non-permissive temperature, *Nature (London)* **235**:52.

Valentine, R. C., and Pereira, H. G., 1965, Antigens and structure of the adenovirus, *J. Mol. Biol.* **13**:13.

van der Eb, A. J., 1973, Intermediates in type 5 adenovirus DNA replication, *Virology* **51**:11.

van der Eb, A. J., van Kesteren, L. W., and van Bruggen, E. F. G., 1969, Structural properties of adenovirus DNA's, *Biochim. Biophys. Acta* **182**:530.

van der Vliet, P. C., and Levine, A. J., 1973, DNA-binding proteins specific for cells infected by adenovirus, *Nature (London) New Biol.* **246**:170.

van der Vliet, P. C., and Sussenbach, J. S., 1972, The mechanism of adenovirus-DNA synthesis in isolated nuclei, *Eur. J. Biochem.* **30**:584.

van der Vliet, P. C., Levine, A. J., Ensinger, M. J., and Ginsberg, H. S., 1975, Thermolabile DNA binding proteins from cells infected with a temperature-sensitive mutant of adenovirus defective in viral DNA synthesis, *J. Virol.* **15**:348.

Velicer, L., and Ginsberg, H. S., 1968, Cytoplasmic synthesis of type 5 adenovirus capsid proteins, *Proc. Natl. Acad. Sci. USA* **61**:1264.

Velicer, L. F., and Ginsberg, H. S., 1970, Synthesis, transport, and morphogenesis of type 5 adenovirus capsid proteins, *J. Virol.* **5**:338.

Wall, R., Philipson, L., and Darnell, J. E., 1972, Processing of adenovirus specific nuclear RNA during virus replication, *Virology* **50**:27.

Weber, J., 1976, Genetic analysis of adenovirus type 2. III. Temperature sensitivity of processing of viral proteins. *J. Virol.* **17**:462–471.

Weber, J., Bégin, M., and Khittoo, G., 1975, Genetic analysis of adenovirus type 2. II. Preliminary phenotypic characterization of temperature-sensitive mutants, *J. Virol.* **15**:1049.

White, D. O., Scharff, M. D., and Maizel, J. V., Jr., 1969, The polypeptides of adenovirus. III. Synthesis in infected cells, *Virology* **38**:395.

Wilcox, W. C., and Ginsberg, H. S., 1961, Purification and immunological characterization of types 4 and 5 adenovirus-soluble antigens, *Proc. Natl. Acad. Sci. USA* **47**:512.

Wilcox, W. C., and Ginsberg, H. S., 1963a, Production of specific neutralizing antibody with soluble antigens of type 5 adenovirus, *Proc. Soc. Exp. Biol. Med.* **114**:37.

Wilcox, W. C., and Ginsberg, H. S., 1963b, Protein synthesis in type 5 adenovirus-infected cells: Effect of p-fluorophenylalanine of synthesis of protein, nucleic acids, and infectious virus, *Virology* **20**:269.

Wilcox, W. C., and Ginsberg, H. S., 1963c, Structure of type 5 adenovirus. I. Antigenic relationship of virus-structural proteins to virus-specific soluble antigens from infected cells, *J. Exp. Med.* **118**:295.

Wilcox, W. C., Ginsberg, H. S., and Anderson, T. F., 1963, Structure of type 5 adenovirus. II. Fine structure of virus subunits. Morphologic relationship of structural subunits to virus-specific soluble antigens from infected cells, *J. Exp. Med.* **118**:307.

Wilhelm, J. M., and Ginsberg, H. S., 1972, Synthesis *in vitro* of type 5 adenovirus capsid proteins, *J. Virol.* **9**:973.

Wilkie, N. M., Ustacelebi, S., and Williams, J. F., 1973, Characterization of temperature-sensitive mutants of adenovirus type 5: Nucleic acid synthesis, *Virology* **51**:499.

Williams, J. F., 1973, Oncogenic transformation of hamster embryo cells *in vitro* by adenovirus type 5, *Nature (London)***243**:162.

Williams, J. F., and Ustacelebi, S., 1971*a*, Complementation and recombination with temperature-sensitive mutants of adenovirus type 5, *J. Gen. Virol.* **13**:345.

Williams, J. F., and Ustacelebi, S., 1971*b*, Temperature-restricted mutants of human adenovirus type 5, in: *Strategy of the Viral Genome* (G. E. W. Wolstenholme and M. O'Connor, eds.), Ciba Foundation Symposium, Churchill Livingstone, London.

Williams, J. F., Gharpure, M., Ustacelebi, S., and McDonald, S., 1971, Isolation of temperature-sensitive mutants of adenovirus type 5, *J. Gen. Virol.* **11**:95.

Williams, J. F., Young, C. S. H., and Austin, P. E., 1974, Genetic analysis of human adenovirus type 5 in permissive and nonpermissive cells, *Cold Spring Harbor Symp. Quant. Biol.* **39**:427.

Williams, J. F., Grodzicker, T., Sharp, P., and Sambrook, J., 1975*a*, Adenovirus recombination: Physical mapping of crossover events, *Cell* **4**:113.

Williams, J. F., Young, H., and Austin, P., 1975*b*, Complementation of human adenovirus type 5 *ts* mutants by human adenovirus type 12, *J. Virol.* **15**:675.

Wolfson, J., and Dressler, D., 1972, Adenovirus-2 DNA contains an inverted terminal repetition, *Proc. Natl. Acad. Sci. USA* **69**:3054.

Yamashita, T., and Green, M., 1974, Adenovirus DNA replication. I. Requirement for protein synthesis and isolation of nuclear membrane fractions containing newly synthesized viral DNA and proteins, *J. Virol.* **14**:412.

Yoshimori, R. N., 1971, A genetic and biochemical analysis of the restriction and modification of DNA by resistance transfer factors, Ph.D. thesis, University of California, San Francisco Medical Center.

Young, C. S. H., and Williams, J. F., 1975, Heat-stable variant of human adenovirus type 5: Characterization and use in three-factor crosses, *J. Virol.* **15**:1168.

CHAPTER 3

Genetics of Herpesviruses

John H. Subak-Sharpe and Morag C. Timbury

Institute of Virology
University of Glasgow
Scotland G11 5JR

1. INTRODUCTION

Herpes simplex virus (HSV) is the prototype of a large group of animal viruses with common morphological and biochemical features. An important preliminary for genetic consideration of herpes simplex virus is familiarity with the structure and composition of the virion and its genetic information content, the virus growth cycle, and the capability of the virus to induce latency *in vivo* and to transform cells in culture. The biochemical and structural complexity of the particle of herpes simplex virus (HSV), which contains 33–36 separable polypeptides (Heine *et al.*, 1974; Marsden *et al.*, 1976), has recently been reviewed, as has the virus growth cycle (Kaplan, 1973; Roizman and Furlong, 1975).

There is general agreement that the herpesvirus genome consists of a double-stranded DNA molecule of approximately 100×10^6 daltons (Becker *et al.*, 1968; Kieff *et al.*, 1971). The DNA molecule is infectious (Lando and Ryhiner, 1969), and it is unusual in that it often contains some alkali-labile interruptions in the linear sequence of either or both single strands. The claim (Frenkel and Roizman, 1972) that the interruptions are in unique sites has been disputed (Wilkie, 1973). In an important recent paper, Sheldrick and Berthelot (1974) recognized some unusual features of intact single strands of HSV DNA by electron microscopy. Although some details have been corrected, their general conclusions have been confirmed and extended both by electron microscopy of single-stranded and partially denatured double-stranded HSV DNA (Roizman *et al.,* 1975; Delius and Clements, 1976) and by restriction enzyme analysis of native HSV DNA (Wadsworth *et al.,* 1975; Clements *et al.,* 1976) which detected the regular generation of quarter- and half-molar fragments which is implicit in their model. The native HSV DNA molecule is now considered to have the following arrangement: a terminal repeat sequence (TR$_S$ $\sim$ 4 $\times$ 10^6) at the left end of the molecule is succeeded by a short unique sequence (S $\sim$ 10 $\times$ 10^6), after which comes the inverted left terminal repeat sequence (IR$_S$ $\sim$ 4 $\times$ 10^6); then follows the inverted right terminal repeat sequence (IR$_L$ $\sim$ 6 $\times$ 10^6), a long unique sequence (L $\sim$ 70 $\times$ 10^6), and, finally, the right-end repeat sequence (TR$_L$ $\sim$ 6 $\times$ 10^6). The left (TR$_S$) and right (TR$_L$) terminal repeat sequences differ (Wadsworth *et al.,* 1975), but share a common sequence at their respective ends (indicated by a 1 in Fig. 1). The structure of the molecule is given diagrammatically at the top of Fig. 1. Fig. 1Bi,ii illustrates how a reciprocal crossing over between the internal repeat IR$_S$ and the terminal repeat sequence TR$_S$ would lead to the inversion of the short unique sequence (S) relative to the long unique sequence (L). A reciprocal crossing-over event between IR$_L$ and TR$_L$ would similarly invert the L unique sequence. (As shown in Fig. 1Ai,ii,iii, a single-strand cross-over event would lead to a different set of molecules, which, however, cannot be discussed here.) Figure 2 illustrates the complete set of four sequentially different but inversion-related molecules that are expected to be generated as a result of intramolecular reciprocal crossing over between the internal repeat and the terminal repeat sequences. The observation of the half-and quarter-molar fragments in the DNA of seven freshly prepared single-plaque isolates demonstrates (1) that the crossing-over events are frequent and (2) that the four genome structures have already reached equilibrium proportions after sufficient replicative cycles for the production of a stock of virus (Clements *et al.,* 1976).

If it is additionally postulated that all four genome structures are equally infective and in equilibrium in each infected cell when genetic recombination takes place, then the genome of HSV exhibits features which carry unique implications: First, the complete genetic information content of HSV may reside in any one of four biochemically distinguishable DNA molecules (Fig. 2). Second, all genes in the long unique sequence will map in the standard linear way relative to one

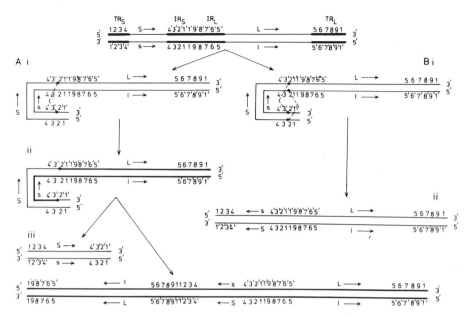

Fig. 1. Top: A molecule of herpes simplex virus double-stranded DNA showing the terminal repeat (TR$_S$) and its inverted form (IR$_S$) with the short unique region (S) between them, then the inverted other terminal repeat (IR$_L$), the long unique region (L), and the terminal repeat (TR$_L$). Different sequences in the repeat regions are indicated by different numbers and their complements by the prime of the same numbers. The complements of the unique regions S and L, are denoted by s and l, respectively. The terminal redundant sequence is denoted by 1. Ai and Bi, respectively, indicate the position of an intramolecular crossover and a reciprocal intramolecular crossover between the TR$_S$ and IR$_S$ regions. Aii indicates by thick and thin lines the points of break and subsequent reunion which after replication of each strand would result in the two molecules (one deficient in and the other duplicated in IR$_L$, L, and TR$_L$) shown in Aiii. Bii shows how a molecule inverted in the S region relative to the L region has been generated as a consequence of the intramolecular reciprocal crossover indicated in Bi.

another, and, similarly, the genes in the short unique region will map linearly relative to each other; however, as demonstrated by Table 1, every gene in the long unique region will map equidistantly from every gene in the short region. Should crossovers occur with constant probability along the HSV DNA molecule, then the common map distance will correspond to the sum of half the length of each unique region plus the two internal inverted repeat sequences. If the internal inverted repeat sequences constitute a region of locally increased or free recombination, then the long and short unique regions will behave as though loosely linked or unlinked. This last case would produce genetic results suggesting that the HSV genome consists of two "chromosomes."

It is evident that herpesvirus poses many interesting genetic problems. For example, why does HSV possess—and presumably need—so much genetic information, i.e., 100×10^6 daltons of double-stranded DNA (Becker *et al.*, 1968; Kieff *et al.*, 1971), sufficient to code for 100 average-sized (i.e., 500 amino acids long, 55,000 molecular weight) polypeptides? What are the functions of the virus-specified proteins—especially of the many nonstructural polypeptides observed only in the infected cell? Is all the genetic information in the DNA molecule essential for successful reproduction? What information is required for the initiation, maintenance, and control of latency (Stevens and Cook, 1971, Stevens, 1975), transformation, and oncogenicity (Duff and Rapp, 1971a; Rapp and Li, 1974)? How does HSV's genetic information control the consecutive or parallel expression of HSV genes? Which HSV genes are involved, at what levels of transcription and translation do they operate, and in what way do they interact? What is the strategy of the HSV genome, and particularly to what extent does its genetic information control recombination? At present, complete

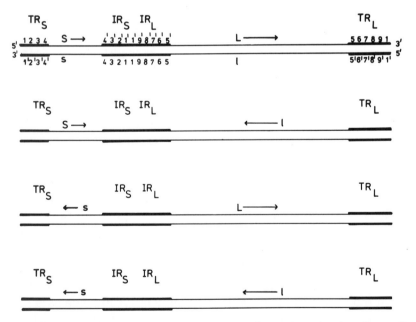

Fig. 2. Diagram of structure of herpes simplex virus DNA showing the predicted inversion-related molecules resulting from recombination between the internal and terminal repeated sequences.

TABLE 1

Recombination between Any Locus in the Long Unique Region and Any Locus in the Short Unique Region

Given that the genome arrangement is as shown in Fig. 1, then the short unique region (S) consists of loci s_1 to s_m extending from the terminal repeat (TR_S) to this inverted repeat region (IR_S); similarly, the long unique region (L) consists of loci l_1 to l_n extending from the other terminal repeat (TR_L) to this inverted repeat region (IR_L). The internal inverted region consisting of $IR_S + IR_L$ is complementary and equal in length to the sum of the terminal repeats $TR_S + TR_L$. Consider recombination between any locus s_b (in the short unique region) and any locus l_a (in the long unique region). In terms of the four possible genome arrangements shown in Fig. 2, the distances between these loci can be written as

$$(1) = s_m - s_b + IR_S + IR_L + l_n - l_a$$
$$(2) = s_m - s_b + IR_S + IR_L + l_a$$
$$(3) = s_b + IR_S + IR_L + l_n - l_a$$
$$(4) = s_b + IR_S + IR_L + l_a$$

Assuming the presence of the four genome arrangements in equal amount and equally infectious in each infected cell at the time of recombination, the average distance between loci s_b and l_a will be

$$\tfrac{1}{4}\,[(1) + (2) + (3) + (4)] = \tfrac{1}{2}\,(s_m + l_n) + IR_S + IR_L$$

Thus every locus in the short unique region will map equidistantly from every locus in the long unique region.

answers cannot be given to any of these questions, but this chapter will consider relevant information arising from the various genetic studies on HSV that have been undertaken which provides partial and preliminary answers. Where appropriate, reference will also be made to observations made in other herpesvirus systems.

2. VIRUS MUTANTS

The genetic information contained in the viral genome is at present best studied by the isolation and characterization of mutants, which enable individual genes to be identified and their functions discovered. Two major categories of HSV mutants have been used for this, namely, specialized mutants and nonspecialized conditional lethal mutants.

2.1. Specialized Mutants

Specialized mutants are mutants with a defect in an individual gene. The result is either (1) a change in plaque morphology or in plaque size, (2) altered virus host range (e.g., allowing growth in normally unsusceptible cells), or (3) resistance to a toxic compound.

2.1.1. Plaque Morphology Mutants

It has long been known that mutants of HSV-1 can be isolated which produce cell fusion—or syncytia—instead of the individual cell rounding associated with the normally observed cytopathic effect (Roizman, 1962; Ejercito et al., 1968). It has been suggested that syncytium formation results from the initially infected cell recruiting surrounding uninfected cells by successive breakdown of their cell wall. The changed biochemical function in the syncytium-forming mutant (*syn*) is not understood but is thought to involve defective glycosylation of one or more virus polypeptides (Keller et al., 1970). Incubation in the presence of 2-deoxyglucose can produce phenotypic—but not genetic—reversion from *syn* to *syn*⁺ in the case of herpes simplex virus type 1 (HSV-1) but not of type 2 (HSV-2) (Gallacher et al., 1973: Timbury et al., 1974; M. C. Timbury, R. Reid, and L. Calder, unpublished observations). Brown et al. (1973) have described a *syn* mutant of HSV-1 strain 17 which reverts spontaneously with low frequency to the wild-type *syn*⁺. In doubly infected cells, *syn*⁺ is dominant, but as a plaque grows, *syn* and *syn*⁺ segregate and form sectors. The data are compatible with the following general interpretations. In wild type virus, two genes act in series: the product of the first induces cell fusion, but that of the second blocks the fusion mechanism going to completion so that the final phenotype is nonsyncytial (*syn*⁺). In *syn* mutants, the second gene product is inactive or missing, so that the first gene's product acts continuously to cause syncytium formation.

2.1.2. Host Range Mutants

HSV-1 does not replicate in dog kidney cells (Aurelian and Roizman, 1964). However, virus mutants which are able to do so (*dk*⁺) have been selected after several weeks continuous propagation following infection with the wild-type *dk*⁻ virus (Roizman and Aurelian, 1965). In dog kidney cells infected with *dk*⁻ virus, envelopment of the viral nucleocapsids does not occur, and this is associated with failure of reduplication of the cell nuclear membrane and defective viral protein synthesis (Spring et al., 1968).

2.1.3. Mutants Resistant to Toxic Compounds

Two types of situation warrant consideration: first, where the host cells are not affected by concentrations of a compound such as phosphonoacetic acid, which blocks HSV replication. Under these circumstances, resistant mutants can be directly selected. Where a compound is toxic to the normal host cells as well as blocking HSV replication, cell mutants must first be obtained, and then virus mutants must be selected for growth in the resistant cells in the presence of the compound. Resistance to bromodeoxyuridine or to cytosine arabinoside are examples of this second type of situation.

2.1.3a. Phosphonoacetic Acid-Resistant Mutants

Phosphonoacetic acid is a powerful inhibitor of herpes-specified DNA polymerase activity *in vitro* (Mao *et al.*, 1973, 1975) which also inhibits growth of herpes virus *in vivo* (Shipkowitz and Bower, 1973). Recently, Hay and Subak-Sharpe (1976) have isolated phosphonoacetic acid-resistant mutants of HSV-1 and HSV-2 and have shown that the DNA polymerase of the virus mutants is more resistant to phosphonoacetic acid than the wild-type HSV enzyme. This indicates that the resistance of the mutants is due to an alteration in the structural polypeptide of the enzyme.

2.1.3b. Mutants Resistant to Bromodeoxyuridine and Cytosine Arabinoside

Cells lacking thymidine kinase (TK$^-$) are able to grow in the presence of 5-bromodeoxyuridine. HSV does not replicate in such cells in the presence of the inhibitor, but virus mutants that can do so (HSV TK$^-$) were first described by Kit and co-workers (Kit *et al.*, 1963; Kit and Dubbs, 1963; Dubbs and Kit, 1964), who cited this as evidence of a virus-specified but dispensable thymidine kinase. Later, this interpretation was confirmed by the isolation of temperature-sensitive TK$^-$ mutants (Aron *et al.*, 1973).

In normal BHK cells, both bromodeoxyuridine and cytosine arabinoside, although not toxic in themselves, are converted into toxic nucleotides by two separate enzymes—thymidine kinase in the case of bromodeoxyuridine and deoxycytidine kinase in the case of cytosine arabinoside. A BHK-derived cell line lacking both thymidine kinase and deoxycytidine kinase activities has been isolated (Jamieson *et al.,* 1974). HSV mutants selected in this TK⁻, dCK⁻ cell line for resistance to either bromodeoxyuridine or cytosine arabinoside invariably became simultaneously resistant to both compounds, suggesting that one HSV-specified enzyme has both thymidine kinase and deoxycytidine kinase activity. The viral ability to code for thymidine kinase activity has always been assumed to be an inessential or "luxury" function, as normal cells have thymidine kinase activity (Kit and Dubbs, 1963; Dubbs and Kit, 1964). However, this function becomes essential for viral replication in serum-starved or resting cells (Jamieson *et al.,* 1974). The cells of the intact animal initially infected by herpesvirus are probably resting and it may be that under natural conditions the ability to code for thymidine kinase activity is in fact an indispensable function.

2.2. Nonspecialized Mutants: Conditional Lethals

Conditional lethal mutants are due to defects which can occur in a large proportion if not all of the viral genes coding for macromolecules with essential functions. There are two general types of conditional lethal systems which have been exploited with great success in the study of bacteria and bacteriophages. One system—suppressible nonsense codon mutations (Campbell, 1961; Epstein *et al.,* 1963; Watson, 1970)—has not so far become available for mammalian cells and viruses, although a suggestion that this approach may be possible has recently emerged from the work of Summers *et al.* (1975). But the other type of system, the temperature-restricted mutants, has been widely used in animal virology in general (for a review, see Fenner, 1969) and with HSV in particular. These mutants will therefore be discussed in detail. In this context, the heat sensitivity of virus particles (due to an altered capsid component) must be distinguished from temperature sensitivity manifested in the viral replication cycle. Temperature sensitivity of viral replication is usually due to a functional defect, at either high or low temperatures, in virus-specified polypeptides, although it could be caused by virus-specified RNA with altered secondary structure (Smith *et al.,* 1970). Mutants with impaired function at raised temperatures have been the mainstay of the HSV genetic studies.

Normally, temperature sensitivity is regarded as due to a codon alteration in the messenger RNA caused by the replacement of one base by another within the reading frame on the DNA of the gene;

translation then results in a corresponding amino acid change in the sequence of the polypeptide.

An amino acid (missense) substitution need not—or may only slightly—affect the function of the polypeptide even when the electrophoretic mobility is altered. In other instances, the missense substitution might prevent function of the polypeptide at any physiological temperature, although a mutation of this sort would normally be detected only in a dispensable function. In a proportion of cases, however, a missense substitution impairs the polypeptide function only slightly, if at all, at one temperature, but eliminates the function at a higher temperature at which the wild-type polypeptide is fully active. This class defines the temperature-sensitive (*ts*) mutations with which the rest of this chapter is mainly concerned.

2.3. Temperature-Sensitive Mutants

Operationally, *ts* virus is able to replicate at one temperature (the permissive temperature or PT) but not another higher temperature (the nonpermissive temperature or NPT). Biochemically, a protein with changed sequences and thus temperature-impaired function has been produced. As a consequence of a functionally inactive protein at NPT, the following situations could arise:

1. The protein is at the end of a biosynthetic chain and has no regulatory function, so that all other virus-specified polypeptides and other macromolecules are made, although infectious virus is not produced. The pattern of virus-specified polypeptide bands on SDS-acrylamide gels, in which fractionation is by size rather than charge, would either be indistinguishable from wild type or—rarely, where the defective polypeptide is degraded in the infected cell—show a reduction in the one band containing the affected polypeptide. The missense substitution may also change the polypeptide's ability to be cleaved or modified (e.g., by glycosylation, phosphorylation, or sulfation) and thus alter the position of the polypeptide in gels.
2. The function of the protein directly or indirectly controls the synthesis of one or more other virus-specified polypeptides or their processing, so that multiple changes in the polypeptide pattern in gels at NPT result. R. J. Watson and J. B. Clements (personal communication) have shown that certain HSV-1 *ts*

mutants at NPT block the production of some viral RNA transcripts.

3. The function of the protein directly or indirectly controls the regulation of host cell polypeptide or RNA synthesis, so that changes in the pattern of host proteins superimposed on the pattern of virus-specified polypeptide bands will be produced.
4. The function of the protein directly or indirectly affects viral DNA synthesis, causing a block in DNA synthesis at NPT.
5. The affected protein is an essential component of the mature virus particle, so that irrespective of the protein's possible other functions a virus particle is made even at PT which has altered stability to heat, pH, or chemical reagents.

Theoretically, *ts* mutants can be obtained for every gene product with an indispensable function for virus production. The affected gene may have conceivably a primary (RNA) or usually a secondary (polypeptide) product with a secondary or tertiary structure in which missense substitutions result in retained function at PT but loss of function due to structural collapse at NPT. For two polypeptides of similar size, the relative proportions of each sequence subject to possible missense substitution may differ considerably. The frequency with which *ts* mutants in different genes are isolated may therefore also vary considerably.

It must be appreciated that the range of substitutions resulting from single base changes is limited by the nature of the genetic code. For example, alanine (GCU, GCC, GCG, and GCA) would be changed by substitution of the first base to serine, proline, or threonine, and by substitution of the second base to valine, glycine, and either asparagine or glutamine (depending on the third base); no change in the third base would result in an amino acid substitution. It should also be noted that many aminoacid substitutions (e.g., alanine by proline) may prove incompatible with function. Missense substitution may loosen the configuration of the polypeptide, with consequent loss of function at higher temperature, or tighten the configuration, with possible impaired function at lower temperature.

2.3.1. Leakiness

Ts mutants produce gene products which function at PT but are inactive at NPT. However, the precise cutoff point below the chosen NPT will differ for different mutants and may be affected by physiological conditions: thus some functional gene products may in certain circumstances be made at NPT. As a result, some viable virus with unaltered (*ts*) genotype may be produced at NPT, which is known as *leakiness*. Leakiness is expected more commonly when the *ts* gene product is an enzyme with catalytic function than when it is a structural polypeptide with stoichiometric function. In addition, leakiness derives from the nature of the missense substitution in the primary sequence of the polypeptide. The leak-through product, once formed, may be functional and stable or have a shortened half-life. Leakiness at some temperature point is a widespread and intrinsic property of temperature-restricted mutants. When only nonleaky mutants are selected by the investigator, this must restrict the range and *a priori* exclude many genes from the experimental analysis. Leak at NPT can often be distinguished from true reversion because most leak-through plaques are smaller, but the two can always be differentiated by progeny tests since the progeny of leak-through plaques are of unchanged genotype and consist of *ts* virus, whereas revertant plaques have an altered genotype and contain *ts*$^+$ or wild-type virus.

2.3.2. Reversion

Mutability is in the nature of genetic material. The genes of *ts* mutants are therefore subject to further single-base substitutions, both in the originally affected base and elsewhere in their sequence. These further single-base substitutions may result in a gene product with restored function at NPT; this is usually called *reversion*. Revertants may be of four main types:

1. True revertants which arise from restitution of the original wild-type base sequence.
2. Revertants in which change to a base different from that in the original wild-type codon (but in that codon) results in another amino acid substitution. However, the gene product may again function like the wild-type polypeptide, although differing in one amino acid.
3. Functional revertants which may be produced by a change in a codon different from the first one affected. A second amino acid is therefore substituted in the sequence of the polypeptide and this may restore function at NPT, partially or completely. This polypeptide will differ from the wild-type polypeptide in two amino acids, which may or may not be adjacent in the primary sequence.
4. Rarely, more complex changes such as duplications or defi-

ciencies, etc., which may restore "pseudowild" polypeptide function at NPT.

Irrespective of the *molecular mechanism* involved, the end result of reversion is the production of a stable genetically altered genome expressed as ts^+ phenotype. Reversion rates of ts mutants of HSV appear to vary widely, but no careful measurements of reversion rates have been published. A mutant which never appears to revert represents a strong suggestion that the defect is due to a deletion or multiple change rather than to a single-base substitution.

2.3.3. Mutagenization

Spontaneous ts mutations are rare, but ts mutants can readily be isolated following mutagenic treatment. Most workers have therefore mutagenized stocks of virus or virus-infected cells with a variety of agents before attempting to isolate ts mutants. If preexisting ts mutants are assumed to be absent from the original virus preparation, then every ts mutant isolated as a result of direct mutagenesis of virus particles (e.g., with hydroxylamine or nitrous acid) must have arisen from an independent genetic event. However, if infected cells are treated with a mutagen (e.g., with bromodeoxyuridine or nitrosoguanidine), then the altered genetic material can replicate and produce clonally related mutant progeny. The number of ts progeny in such a clone will depend on the number of genome replications subsequent to the genetic change, and the isolation of several mutants from the same treated stock does not therefore guarantee that the individual isolates have been derived independently. Independent origin in these cases has to be confirmed by complementation test or ensured by isolating only one ts mutant from each treated stock of virus—as has been done by Brown *et al.* (1973) and Schaffer *et al.* (1973).

2.3.4. Multiple Mutations

The mode of action of various mutagenic agents and the process and measurement of mutation have been described elsewhere in this volume, as well as by others (Freese, 1959; Krieg, 1963; Hayes, 1968) and will not be discussed here. Mutagenic treatment of a virus suspension usually kills a sizable proportion of the virus population—when there are only 1% survivors, this suggests an average of 4.6 lethal hits per genome. Similarly, when infected cells are treated, the yield of virus is usually greatly reduced, although the intervening DNA replications complicate precise analysis. Mutagenic treatment will yield lethal, conditional lethal, deleterious, morphological, and silent mutations; thus one has to keep in mind the chance of isolating a *ts* mutant differing by more than one base change from the original *ts*$^+$ genome.

Clearly, there will be many base changes which do not result in *ts* mutants or are lethal: for instance, the majority of base substitutions in the third position of codons do not alter the amino acid sequence of the polypeptide produced. Other base changes will result in amino acid changes which do not appreciably affect the function of the polypeptide, and still others will lead to the loss of a dispensable gene function like thymidine kinase activity.

It follows that a high proportion of the *ts* mutants isolated as a result of mutagenesis can be expected to have more than one base-pair change in the HSV genome sequence of 167,000 base pairs potentially coding for 55,000 amino acids. The relevance of these other mutations will depend on the particular questions asked; in most cases, they can be neglected. Virus geneticists who focus on particular *ts* mutants are mainly concerned with two problems related to the likelihood of multiple mutations. First, is the *ts* mutant due to more than one base change in the same gene, and, second, is the phenotypic temperature sensitivity due to two or more different genes having simultaneously but independently become *ts* mutated? Whenever a *ts* mutant reverts to *ts*$^+$ with reasonable frequency, both these possibilities are unlikely and can be discounted. But for a *ts* mutant which never reverts, the two explanations cannot be ruled out. The first (i.e., two or more missense substitutions in the same gene) could be detected biochemically, if the affected polypeptide is known, by investigating the amino acid sequence; the second could be demonstrated genetically if a particular mutant fails to complement with two or more *ts* mutants in different complementation groups. The presence of occasional double *ts* mutants in any collection of *ts* mutants cannot usually be ruled out, but will be unlikely whenever the *ts* mutants are isolated at a low frequency (no more than 1–2%) from the mutagenized stock. As a rough yardstick, the frequency of double *ts* mutants will approximate the square of the incidence of *ts* mutants isolated.

2.3.5.   Isolation of *ts* Mutants

The isolation of HSV-1 and HSV-2 *ts* mutants has been reported from several laboratories using various different mutagenic treatments, and their numbers and origin are given in Table 2. Different laboratories have unfortunately chosen different wild-type strains of HSV for

TABLE 2
Isolation of *ts* Mutants of Herpesviruses

Wild-type virus strain	Mutagen[a]	NPT	PT	Number of mutants isolated	Reference
HSV-1					
17	BrdUrd	38°C	31°C	9	Subak-Sharpe (1969), Brown *et al.* (1973)
KOS	BrdUrd, NTG, UV	39°C	34°C	39	Schaffer *et al.* (1970, 1973)
13	BrdUrd	40°C	35°C	6	Manservigi (1974).
HSV-2					
HG 52	BrdUrd	38°C	31°C	33	Timbury (1971)
IPB2	HNO$_2$	38.5°C	35°C	3	Zygraich and Huygelen (1973)
186	BrdUrd	38°C	34°C	8	Esparza *et al.* (1974)
UW-268	BrdUrd	38.5°C	32°C	42	Takahashi and Yamanishi (1974)
333	BrdUrd, NTG	39°C	33°C	4	Koment and Rapp (1975)
Pseudorabies virus	BrdUrd	41°C	37°C	10	Pringle *et al.* (1973)

[a] BrdUrd, 5-bromodeoxyuridine; NTG, nitrosoguanidine; UV, ultraviolet irradiation; HNO$_2$, nitrous acid.

isolation of *ts* mutants, and, moreover, different PT and NPT have been used. Most workers have taken precautions to avoid the isolation of clonally related *ts* mutants. The precise methods varied, but that used by one of us is described here briefly as illustration.

The wild-type HSV-1 strain 17 was genetically cleaned by three successive single-plaque purifications, and a stock of virus was prepared. Many single plaques were picked at 38°C from this starting stock and grown into substocks, each of which was independently mutagenized with bromodeoxyuridine at 31°C (PT); under these conditions, the 24-h yield of virus was reduced to between 1% and 0.1%. The mutagenized virus was titrated and then replated at PT to obtain plates with only one or very few well-separated plaques. Progeny in individual plaques were then picked and mixed with cells in suspension, of which half were plated at PT and the rest at NPT (38°C). Plaques containing progeny which grew at PT but not at NPT (putative *ts* mutants) were repurified at PT and rechecked for stability with regard to temperature sensitivity. To ensure independent origin, only one *ts* mutant was isolated from each stock.

2.3.6. Complementation

After a number of *ts* mutants have been isolated, they must first be examined to see if the lesions are in the same or different genes. This is best done by complementation analysis, after which biochemical and virological characterization can proceed. Theoretically, complementation is a nongenetic interaction between the products of the different genomes in cells simultaneously infected with two *ts* mutants. Complementation takes place at NPT when the missing essential function of the defective gene product of one *ts* mutant is compensated by the active gene product provided by the same but nondefective gene of the other mutant (Fig. 3). The second mutant possesses a *ts* lesion in a different gene, which in turn is compensated by the functional product of this unimpaired gene in the first mutant. Complementing essential genes can be identified without knowledge of their precise physiological function.

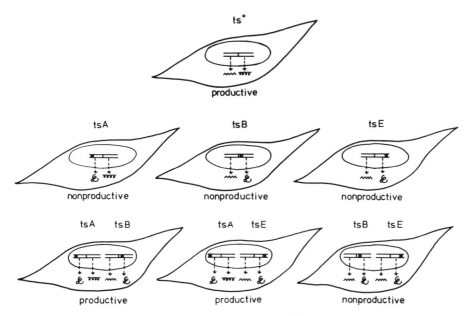

Fig. 3. Diagram of complementation showing positive complementation reactions between pairs of mutants, *ts*A and *ts*B and *ts*A and *ts*E, where the *ts* mutations are in different genes; and lack of complementation with mutants *ts*B and *ts*E, where the *ts* mutations are in the same gene. "Productive" and "nonproductive" refer to the ability and inability, respectively, to produce a yield of progeny at NPT. By definition, the *ts*⁺ infection is productive and the single-mutant infections with any of the *ts* mutants are nonproductive. & denotes defective gene products, while ∿∿ and ∽∽∽ denote active gene products.

Ts mutants can be assigned to functionally different complementation groups on the basis of positive complementation tests. These complementation groups define cistrons which can be equated with genes (Benzer, 1961). When two *ts* mutants do not complement, they are assigned to the same complementation group, with the provisional implication that the two independent mutations occurred in the same gene. The polypeptide product of a gene may function as such, but often activity depends on the formation of dimers or multimers of identical subunits. In some of these multimeric proteins, subunits with defects in different regions of their sequence may be able to compensate each other, restoring some activity to the multimer by intracistronic complementation (Crick and Orgel, 1964). Intracistronic complementation is a rare, weak complementation reaction which for herpesviruses has been reported only with HSV-specified thymidine kinase (Jamieson, 1973).

Four different complementation tests have been used with herpes viruses. First is the yield complementation test, in which the yield from mixedly infected cells after one growth cycle at NPT is compared to the yields from cells infected with each mutant alone under the same conditions. The yields are titrated at both PT and NPT in order to correct for leakiness and reversion. The complementation index for yield with respect to two *ts* mutants X and Y is calculated from the formula

$$\frac{(X + Y)^{\text{PT}} - (X + Y)^{\text{NPT}}}{\frac{1}{2}(X^{\text{PT}} + Y^{\text{PT}})}$$

For computational reasons, X^{PT} and Y^{PT} each have a minimum value of 1 (Brown *et al.*, 1973). A complementation index reproducibly greater than 2.0 is regarded as indicative of complementation. This test is the classic complementation test and has been frequently employed in other virus systems.

A second test which depends on infectious center formation has proved very useful with herpes simplex virus. In this test, the capability of mixedly infected cells to form plaques on uninfected monolayers after incubation for 36–48 h at NPT is compared with that of cells singly infected with each mutant. Replicate samples are also plated at PT and measure the efficiency of infectious center production. The complementation index is calculated from the formula

$$\frac{(X + Y)^{\text{NPT}}/(X + Y)^{\text{PT}}}{\frac{1}{2}(X^{\text{NPT}}/X^{\text{PT}} + Y^{\text{NPT}}/Y^{\text{PT}})}$$

Again, for computational reasons, X^{NPT} and Y^{NPT} have minimum values of 1.

In this test, there is opportunity for recombination within the infectious centers formed by mixedly infected cells. This does not invalidate the test, for progeny tests have shown that in plaques in which recombinants can be demonstrated, *ts* mutant progeny are also present (L. I. Messer, personal communication). Clearly, the mutants could only have been produced at NPT as a result of complementation.

A third qualitative test can occasionally be used with two *ts* mutants which additionally differ in a morphological marker—for example, if one mutant is *syn* and the other *syn$^+$*. Even when only a few infectious centers are produced by the mixedly infected cells, the formation at NPT of mixed-morphology plaques (which have both syncytial and nonsyncytial sectors) indicates complementation (Brown *et al.*, 1973).

A fourth very useful qualitative test has recently been described by Chu and Schaffer (1975). In this test, mixtures of two *ts* mutants are inoculated onto cell monolayers by means of filter paper disks. After adsorption, the disks are removed, and incubation is continued at NPT. The area of clearing produced at the disk site is compared with the corresponding areas at the sites of the disks with *ts* mutant controls. Complementation is demonstrated when the reaction produced by mixed infection is greater than that observed in the controls. This test, which is simple to perform and economical in both virus and cell cultures, is particularly useful for screening large numbers of newly isolated mutants for complementation. It is worth noting that only the yield test is based on a single cycle of virus replication. In the other tests, complementation is detected after multiple cycles of replication.

Effective complementation at 36°C has been described for some combinations of mutants which showed little or no complementation at 38°C (Brown *et al.*, 1973). This interesting observation does not seem to have been further investigated and there is at present no satisfactory theoretical explanation of complementation at 36°C rather than at 38°C with particular combinations of *ts* mutants.

The number of complementation groups reported in their material by different laboratories is listed in Table 3. A collaborative study to compare HSV-2 *ts* mutants isolated in different laboratories has also been carried out (Timbury *et al.*, 1976) and Table 4 summarizes the results of this.

3. CHARACTERIZATION OF MUTANTS

Once a number of genes with essential functions have been identified by complementation tests on a collection of *ts* mutants, the

TABLE 3

Complementation Tests on *ts* Mutants of Herpesviruses

Virus	Number of *ts* mutants	Number of comple- mentation groups	Comple- mentation tests used	Reference
HSV-1	9	8	Yield, infectious center, plaque morphology	Brown *et al.* (1973)
HSV-1	39	15	Yield	Schaffer *et al.* (1973)
HSV-2	33	13	Infectious center	Timbury (1971), Hallibur- ton and Timbury (1976)
HSV-2	8	7	Yield	Esparza *et al.* (1974)
HSV-2	4	2	Not stated	Koment and Rapp (1975)
Pseudorabies	10	9	Yield	Pringle *et al.* (1973)

TABLE 4

Complementation Groups Identified in a Collaborative Study of *ts* Mutants of HSV-2[a]

Complementation group No.	*ts* mutants		Phenotype (38°C) viral DNA
	Glasgow[b]	Houston[c]	
1	*ts*1		−
2		*ts*H9	−
3	*ts*6	*ts*B 5	−
4	*ts*9		−
5	*ts*10	*ts*C2	−
6	*ts*11		−
7		*ts*A8	−
8	*ts*2		−
9	*ts*8		−
10	*ts*3		+
11	*ts*4		+
12	*ts*5		+
13	*ts*12		+
14	*ts*13		+
15		*ts*D6	+
16		*ts*E7	+
17		*ts*F3	+
18		*ts*G4	+

[a] Timbury *et al.* (1976).
[b] Timbury (1971), Halliburton and Timbury (1976).
[c] Esparza *et al.* (1974).

time is ripe to study these genetically tagged functions. This involves the characterization of the individual *ts* mutants at both PT and NPT. The mutants can be tested at NPT for synthesis of viral DNA, of viral RNA, and of known virus-specified enzymes; the effect of each mutation on the pattern of viral RNA transcripts and of viral polypeptides produced can be studied in gels; the consequences for host macromolecular synthesis can be monitored; and particle or defective particle production can be investigated, as can the heat stability of particles formed at PT. Furthermore, upshift and downshift experiments can be carried out to determine the time of onset of the defective function, the length of time for which the function is needed, and the stability of the product.

3.1. Viral DNA Synthesis

The great disparity in $G + C$ content, and therefore in buoyant density, between the DNA of HSV-1 (66.8%) or HSV-2 (69%) (Goodheart *et al.*, 1968; Halliburton *et al.*, 1975) and cell DNA (41–42%) provides a ready test for viral DNA production in DNA preparations from infected cells. By this approach, it is also possible to measure the shutoff of host DNA synthesis. Using [^{3}H]thymidine as label and infection both at PT and NPT, *ts* mutants isolated from HSV-1 and HSV-2 have been classified as DNA positive or DNA negative by several laboratories (Table 5). A number of pseudorabies virus *ts* mutants have also been characterized in this way. If it is assumed that the *ts* mutations give an unbiased indication of the HSV genome

TABLE 5
DNA Phenotype of *ts* Mutants of HSV

Virus	Number of complementation groups	Number of complementation groups containing DNA⁻ mutants	Reference
HSV-1	15	4	Aron *et al.* (1975), Benyesh-Melnick *et al.* (1974)
HSV-1	15	9	Marsden *et al.* (1976)
HSV-2	13	8	Halliburton and Timbury (1973, 1976)
HSV-2	7	3	Esparza *et al.* (1974)

constitution, then these data show that a surprisingly large proportion—about half—of the indispensable genes code for functions that directly or indirectly affect viral DNA synthesis. This is in marked contrast to the situation with adenovirus type 5 *ts* mutants, in which only 2 of 17 cistrons are DNA synthesis negative (Williams *et al.,* 1974; Ginsberg *et al.,* 1974), and adenovirus type 2, where Weber (personal communication) has found that the *ts* mutants from 13 cistrons did not affect DNA synthesis. There is no sound reason at present to suspect strong bias in *ts* mutant distribution over the HSV genome. As it seems unlikely that viral DNA synthesis *per se* is much more complex with HSV than with other viruses, the frequency of DNA⁻ cistrons furnishes a first hint that many herpes simplex virus genes may affect viral DNA synthesis indirectly through control mechanisms. As will be seen, other evidence also supports this view.

3.2. Virus-Specified Enzymes

Herpes simplex virus specifies a new DNA polymerase (Keir *et al.,* 1966) which is relatively easy to assay in crude extracts of infected cells: the viral enzyme has optimal activity at high monovalent cation concentrations at which the DNA polymerase of the cell is virtually inactive. It should be appreciated that the *in vivo* production at NPT of DNA polymerase activity—which is then assayed under standard conditions—is used as a test system. Thus the finding that particular genes switch on or shut off production of DNA polymerase does not indicate that this is their sole or even main function; the function of such genes may well simultaneously control the appearance or shutoff of several unassayed virus-specified polypeptides. In contrast, production of an *in vivo* temperature-sensitive polymerase (rapidly inactivated in upshift experiments) and of an *in vitro* temperature-sensitive polymerase indicates that the studied gene directly affects the structure of the enzyme. The eight *ts* mutants representing different DNA-negative cistrons of HSV-2 (Halliburton and Timbury, 1973, 1976) which were isolated by Timbury have been checked for production at NPT of active DNA polymerase by Hay *et al.* (1976). Production is normal in only three of the eight. Polymerase activity in cells infected with mutant *ts*6 is temperature sensitive *in vivo* as demonstrated by upshift and downshift experiments (Timbury and Hay, 1975). The two genes tagged by *ts*9 and *ts*11 appear to control the production of DNA polymerase, although the enzyme, once synthesized, is as thermostable as that made by wild-type virus. Cells infected with mutant *ts*1 continue to maintain DNA polymerase activity at NPT at a higher level than the *ts*⁺ virus control, suggesting that this gene controls shutoff. Lastly, the *ts*10 mutation results in reduced polymerase activity at NPT.

Thus of eight "DNA$^-$" HSV-2 cistrons discovered through *ts* mutations, one appears to make a polymerase polypeptide and four others affect the polymerase indirectly. Purifoy and Benyesh-Melnick (1975) have reported four "DNA$^-$" *ts* mutants of HSV-2, one of which produced a thermolabile enzyme *in vivo*, while at NPT two others resulted in absence of polymerase activity. Aron *et al.* (1975) have reported that *ts* mutants in two different genes of HSV-1 (*ts*C and *ts*D) synthesize DNA polymerase at PT which is more thermolabile than the wild-type enzyme. This suggests that the enzyme must be complex and contain at least two different polypeptide subunits. *Ts* mutants in three other complementation groups show reduced polymerase activity at NPT (Aron *et al.*, 1975). Crombie (1975) has isolated a HSV-1 *ts* mutant (H) which makes thermolabile DNA polymerase. The phosphonoacetic acid resistant mutant isolated by Hay and Subak-Sharpe (1976) recombines with H and appears to map some distance from it: this suggests two different, polypeptide subunits are involved. Two of the *ts* mutants of HSV-1, K and J, lack or have reduced polymerase activity at NPT (Crombie, 1975).

One DNA-positive mutant of the 13 HSV-2 mutants described by Halliburton and Timbury (1976) shows an interesting *ts* defect in that, at NPT, *ts*13 fails to produce HSV-specified deoxyribonuclease (J. Hay, unpublished observations). Thus this enzyme appears not to be essential for DNA synthesis *per se* and the gene's unidentified product must exert some other indispensable function.

3.3. Shutoff of Host Cell DNA Synthesis

Mutants *ts*9 and *ts*11 of HSV-2, which fail to switch on DNA polymerase activity, also fail to shutoff host cell DNA synthesis at NPT, but both blocks can be reversed by downshift experiments (Halliburton and Timbury, 1976). As *ts*9 and *ts*11 belong to different complementation groups, this suggests that at least two HSV-2 gene functions are implicated in the shutdown of host cell DNA synthesis.

Mutant *ts*K of HSV-1 is also reported not to shutoff host DNA synthesis at NPT (Crombie, 1975).

3.4. Proteins

The spectrum of polypeptides induced by HSV has been extensively investigated by autoradiography of SDS-polyacrylamide slab gels containing electrophoretically separated polypeptides from cells variously labeled after infection (Honess and Roizman, 1973; Courtney and Benyesh-Melnick, 1974; Subak-Sharpe *et al.*, 1974). This not only has allowed the identification and enumeration of the HSV-1 and HSV-2 polypeptides, but also has provided essential information about their order of appearance and kinetics of synthesis (Roizman *et al.*, 1974; Marsden *et al.*, 1976). The slab gel method has also been used to identify and enumerate the virion polypeptides and compare them with infected cell polypeptides.

The pattern of polypeptide bands produced by the wild type of any strain is characteristic and can be compared with the corresponding pattern produced at PT and NPT by *ts* mutants of that strain. The remainder of this section is concerned with this type of analysis.

Schaffer *et al.* (1971) first described abnormalities of polypeptide production by a *ts* mutant of HSV-1 when they found that a mutant of complementation group A showed absence of a major envelope glycoprotein and defective glycosylation of a number of other virus-specified glycoproteins at NPT. Bone and Courtney (1974) and Courtney and Benyesh-Melnick (1974) found that mutants of two more complementation groups of HSV-1 (B and C) at NPT also displayed multiple polypeptide defects: in one case, that of *ts*B2, a polypeptide of high molecular weight (VP 175) accumulated, which was detectable only in small amounts at PT. Immunofluorescence tests demonstrated that the protein was type specific (Benyesh-Melnick *et al.*, 1974). Schaffer (1975) has reported the accumulation of more than one polypeptide at NPT with several mutants and also that DNA-negative *ts* mutants of HSV-1 show more polypeptide defects than DNA-positive mutants.

Subak-Sharpe *et al.* (1974) reported the comparative analysis at PT and NPT of the polypeptide pattern for six HSV-1 *ts* mutants, and Marsden *et al.* (1976) have made an extensive and detailed analysis (using SDS-polyacrylamide gradient gel slabs) of polypeptide production at NPT by 16 *ts* mutants of HSV-1. Their experiments demonstrated that

1.   Most *ts* mutants gave rise at NPT to multiple changes in the pattern of polypeptide bands, with the individual affected bands either missing, reduced, or boosted in amount. Ten of the mutants were DNA synthesis negative; one appeared to be very early (*ts*K) and produced only very few detectable virus-specified polypeptides at NPT, while the other nine affected between 21 and 12 of the bands. Furthermore, three of the six DNA-positive *ts* mutants affected the appearance of ten,

seven, and four polypeptides. These findings imply that many of the HSV genes identified by *ts* mutations exert control at different points over the established order of expression of the viral genome.

2. Many bands were dependent on the function of varying numbers of different genes (e.g., eight polypeptide bands were affected by at least 11 mutations, three different bands exclusively by DNA⁻ mutants, nine others by at least two different mutants, five by only one mutant, and over 20 bands by no mutant other than K). The production of polypeptides affected by many different *ts* mutants must be nearly the last of an orderly sequence of essential steps which is directly or indirectly controlled by every one of these viral genes. It follows that the production of polypeptides affected by only one or two *ts* mutants will depend on the function of very few or no viral genes except the gene coding their primary amino acid sequence; such polypeptides may—but need not—have a control function affecting other polypeptides.

Marsden *et al.* (1976) reported five *ts* mutants which at NPT accumulated VP 175—like *ts*B2 of Courtney and Benyesh-Melnick (1974)—and that the synthesis of four other high molecular weight polypeptides was similarly boosted by several *ts* mutations. They, like Schaffer (1975), found that the DNA⁻ *ts* mutants consistently exhibited more defects at NPT than DNA⁺ mutants; and they could discern nine classes of correlation between their spectrum of 16 *ts* mutants and individual polypeptides. In addition, they showed that structural polypeptides were much more frequently affected than nonvirion polypeptides and concluded that the observed *ts* mutant effects imply a complex system of interlocking cascade controls. Honess and Roizman (1973, 1974) investigated the control of protein synthesis in cells infected with wild-type HSV-1 by extensively analyzing the kinetics of appearance and disappearance of the different polypeptide bands. Their studies, with or without added inhibitors, led to the description of five patterns of synthesis, and to the proposal that viral polypeptides form at least three groups (α, β, γ) whose synthesis is sequential and coordinately regulated (Roizman *et al.*, 1975) with abundance control superimposed. They infer the existence of a "complex multilevel regulatory system": thus both the biochemical and the genetic experiments have led to many similar conclusions.

The profiles of electrophoretically separated polypeptides of the virions from different HSV-1 strains have been reported to differ in various bands (Heine *et al.,* 1974). This interstrain variation in polypeptide size indicates that HSV subpopulations in nature harbor considerable genetic variability.

3.5. Particles

Production of heat-labile particles by *ts* mutants has been reported by Schaffer *et al.* (1974*b*) for three HSV-1 and three HSV-2 mutants, and by Subak-Sharpe *et al.* (1974) for one HSV-1 mutant. Halliburton and Timbury (1973, 1976) found two *ts* mutants of HSV-2 markedly less heat stable than wild-type virus at 39°C, while four other DNA⁻ mutants and one DNA⁺ mutant were somewhat less stable at 52°C.

Production of particles in *ts* mutant-infected cells at NPT was studied by electron microscopy by Schaffer *et al.* (1974*b*), who recognized eight morphologically different structures. They found that some DNA⁺ and DNA⁻ mutants made no detectable nucleocapsids, whereas others produced empty nucleocapsids; some mutants of complementation group C formed not only empty but also enveloped nucleocapsids and some had dense cores. Particles in the nucleus of cells infected with DNA⁻ and DNA⁺ *ts* mutants have also been observed by Mechie (1974) and Dargan and Subak-Sharpe (to be published).

3.6. Temperature-Shift Experiments

Schaffer *et al.* (1971) reported the results of upshift and downshift experiments with a mutant in complementation group A. The times after infection when the functions of eight *ts* mutants are required have been investigated by upshift and downshift experiments by Mechie (1974), who found that this varied with different mutants from 0 to 5 h postinfection. She was also able to show that different mutant products varied in their stability at NPT, and that particular gene products were needed for only a short time while others were necessary throughout the growth cycle.

3.7. Effect of Host Cells on *ts* Mutant Phenotype

A recent publication demonstrates that the temperature sensitivity of HSV *ts* mutant products can be host dependent. Koment and Rapp

(1975) have studied the ability of four HSV-2 *ts* mutants (from two complementation groups) to replicate at PT and NPT in different epithelioid and fibroblastoid cells. They found that all four mutants were host-dependent *ts* mutants which were temperature sensitive in fibroblasts of rodents but able to replicate at PT and NPT in epithelioid cells of rodents and also in both fibroblastoid and epithelioid cells of rabbit and man.

3.8. *ts* Mutants *in Vivo*

Zygraich and Huygelen (1973) isolated three *ts* mutants of HSV-2 and compared their neuropathogenicity in rabbits and mice with the parental wild-type strain. The *ts* mutants exhibited reduced pathogenicity with a much lower incidence of paralysis than wild-type virus. Surviving animals were resistant to challenge with virulent virus, although they had no circulating antibody to HSV-2.

4. RECOMBINATION

For any species of virus, recombination is a process of immense evolutionary significance, for it allows the bringing together of separately occurring genetic variation into single stable lineages of descent.

Wildy first reported recombination between two different strains of HSV in 1955, but the markers and system used were not easy to score or analyze so that the work was not continued.

When two different *ts* mutants are crossed, the wild-type (ts^+) recombinant, but not the double mutant *ts*X *ts*Y recombinant, can be easily selected at NPT; this provides a very favorable system. Ts^+ recombinants from crosses between *ts* mutants were first demonstrated for HSV by Subak-Sharpe (1969); since this time, a number of laboratories have published the results from recombination analyses involving *ts* mutants (Table 6). Linear linkage maps have now been obtained with several herpesviruses: for example, HSV-1 (Brown *et al.*, 1973; Schaffer *et al.*, 1974*a*), HSV-2 (Benyesh-Melnick *et al.*, 1974; Timbury and Hay, 1975; Timbury and Calder, 1976), and pseudorabies virus (Pringle *et al.*, 1973).

The most elaborate recombination analysis undertaken with HSV *ts* mutants was based on reciprocal three-factor crosses using the *syn* and *syn*$^+$ allele differences as an additional unselected marker (Brown

TABLE 6

Recombination Analysis of Herpesviruses

Virus strain	Number of mutants	Number of complementation groups represented	Tests used	Reference
HSV-1				
17	9	8	3-factor crosses	Brown et al. (1973)
KOS	11	7	2-factor crosses	Schaffer et al. (1974ab)
HSV-2				
186	8	7	2-factor crosses	Benyesh-Melnick et al. (1974)
HG52	9	9	3- and 2-factor crosses	Timbury and Calder (1976)
Pseudorabies	9	8	2-factor crosses	Pringle et al. (1973)

et al., 1973). Inclusion of the plaque morphology marker allows the arrangement of any pair of ts mutants in terms of their relative proximity to the syn locus for every cross; by combining the data and also by taking into account the recombination frequencies between ts mutants, they can then be placed in unambiguous order on a linear map. The nine ts mutants of Brown et al. (1973) had originally been isolated from the same ts^+ syn stock of strain 17 as tsx syn; hence the isolation of syn^+ revertants from the syn stocks of every ts mutant made all ts mutants available in combination with syn as well as syn^+. The three-factor crosses could therefore be carried out reciprocally in isogenic material.

Brown et al. (1973) found that the reciprocal three-factor crosses carried out on the same day and in the same cells agreed closely; they were able to correct the position of one marker in a preliminary map published earlier (Hay et al., 1971). Their published linkage map spans 25–30 recombination units, but they pointed out that recombination frequencies between any two markers could vary considerably in tests performed at different times and in different cells, although relative positions on the map were unchanged. They noted that about 5% of the progeny in recombination experiments presented as plaques with mixed syn and syn^+ morphology.

A linkage map for HSV-1 prepared by Schaffer et al. (1974a) was based on two-factor crosses but showed excellent additivity. Benyesh-Melnick *et al.* (1974) have published a HSV-2 linkage map also based on two-factor crosses, and Pringle *et al.* (1973) have prepared a map on the same basis for pseudorabies virus. Timbury and Calder (1976) employed three-factor crosses on a limited scale, as only one mutant stock carried the third marker, but have obtained a linkage map for 9 of 13 *ts* mutant HSV-2 cistrons.

Three general points emerge from the results of the various groups. First, *ts* mutants which complement recombine efficiently, while mutants with lesions in the same cistron neither complement nor recombine (or, if they do recombine, do so with a very low frequency). Second, most recombination results—especially if obtained in the same cells at the same time—are additive, so that a linkage map can be constructed, but the clustering of DNA⁻ mutants on the published linkage maps has become less clear-cut as more loci have been added. Third, the *ts* mutants do not appear to be evenly distributed over the map, but the anomalous recombination behavior predicted between mutants in the large and the small unique regions of the DNA has not been reported.

5. EFFECTIVE GENOMES

Inclusion of the *syn* alleles as unselected third markers bestows additional important advantages: it allows precise evaluation of the relative input of genetically effective parental genomes into a cross.

The problem of effective genome input in genetic experiments with animal viruses arises as follows: cells infected with 5 PFU of a mutant stock in which the particle/PFU ratio is 6:1 are infected with 30 particles; if these cells are also infected with 5 PFU of a second mutant stock but with particle/PFU ratio 50:1, then the particle input for this second mutant would be 250 per cell. Depending on the parameter used, the theoretical multiplicity of infection would be either 5:5 or 30:250. But does either estimate evaluate the genetically active input? By measuring the ratio of *syn* to *syn⁺* progeny in the output, the relative proportions of *effective* genomes in the input can be evaluated—assuming that viral DNA molecules replicate at similar rates irrespective of which *syn* allele they encode. The output monitored at PT thus gives the relative proportion of effective genomes in the input virus.

Brown *et al.* (1973) observed that the effective genome input varied with different stocks, indicating the importance of checking input by output. Use of the independent (i.e., non-*ts*) *syn/syn⁺* marker also enabled the interesting mixed-morphology plaques to be detected and analyzed as discussed later.

6. VALIDITY OF RECOMBINATION ANALYSIS

Implicit in genetic recombination analysis (Subak-Sharpe *et al.*, 1973) are the following assumptions: (1) the observed ts^+ plaques are recombinants; (2) double mutant recombinants are formed with statistically equal frequency to ts^+ recombinants; and (3) the average number of genome matings in all crosses incorporated in the analysis is not significantly different.

Recombinants are usually scored as the plaques observed at NPT where neither the two parental *ts* mutants nor the double *ts* mutant can grow. However, as already discussed, two other classes of virus may grow under these conditions, namely, revertants and leak-through virus. Parental *ts* mutant controls, usually included in recombination tests to allow correction for these potential sources of error, are not fully adequate. There are additional possibilities of growth at NPT due to virus aggregates or multiploid particles containing both genomes or heterozygous particles being formed as a consequence of topography or other conditions in the mixedly infected cells. Putative recombinants must therefore be tested by progeny analysis to obtain an estimate of the proportion of true recombinants.

Brown *et al.* (1973) found that 90–95% of the putative recombinants in several crosses were true recombinants. Brown and Ritchie (1975b) demonstrated that double *ts* recombinants arose with the same frequency as ts^+ recombinants. Another problem is the time, place, and frequency with which recombinants are generated. For example, are recombinants generated only during a short period of the replicative cycle or are there continuous recombination events throughout the cycle so that the proportion of recombinants rises with time? Subak-Sharpe *et al.* (1973) reported that the proportion of recombinants increased with time over several hours before attaining a plateau level, while the ratio of *syn* to *syn*+ alleles in the progeny of the same three-factor cross remained constant. This strongly suggests that the infecting genomes undergo successive rounds of mating (Visconti and Delbrück, 1953) during a single infectious cycle and makes it unlikely that asynchrony of virus infection or of viral genome replication could explain the increase in recombinants with time. Multiple rounds of mating not only imply an increasing recombinant fraction but also the production of individual recombinant molecules comprising genetic information from more than two parental genomes. When this possibility was tested in the cross *ts*F *ts*G *syn* × *ts*G *syn*+ × *ts*F *syn*+, the looked-for triparental recombinant + + *syn* was reproducibly isolated, providing good evidence for multiple rounds of mating (Subak-Sharpe *et al.*, 1974). A second means of achieving triparental progeny could be one molecule simultaneously recombining with two others, but such double events are not likely to offer the sole explanation since recombination depends on genetically different molecules having the opportunity to come together in the possibly compartmentalized nucleus. The opportunity to recombine could also be contingent on compartmentally sequestered genome pools fusing—an event likely to become more probable with time. Lastly, by analogy with bacteriophages (Visconti and Delbrück, 1953), multiple rounds of mating can influence precise recombination values, particularly if the number of effective rounds varies in different cells with different physiological and environmental conditions.

7. THE GENES OF HSV

Brown *et al.* (1973) found the first nine *ts* mutants of HSV-1 to fall into eight complementation groups, with one cistron containing two *ts* mutants. Calculating on the basis of Poisson distribution considerations, this suggests that the HSV genome codes for at least 30 indispensable genes in each of which *ts* mutations can arise. This minimum estimate is fully consonant with the proposition that most of the 100×10^6 daltons of HSV DNA codes for such genes. There exists at present no evidence that an appreciable part of the genome is either inconsequential or coding for inessential functions under the experimental conditions employed.

8. MIXED-MORPHOLOGY PLAQUES

A small proportion (about 5%) of the recombinant plaques in three-factor crosses manifested mixed morphology (*syn/syn*+) (Brown *et al.*, 1973; Subak-Sharpe *et al.*, 1974). Brown and Ritchie (1975a) analyzed the genesis of mixed-morphology plaques and found by reconstruction experiments that they were not due to overlapping of *syn* and *syn*+ plaques; sedimentation analysis on neutral sucrose density gradients, together with studies using ultraviolet irradiation, heat inactivation, and sonication, showed that the particles producing mixed-morphology plaques were physically indistinguishable from the general population of particles. The results also suggested that mixed-morphology plaques were unlikely to be due to clumped or multiploid particles. Progeny testing demonstrated that the majority of progeny plaques produced from mixed-morphology plaques were either purely *syn* or *syn*[+], but again a minority of about 5% exhibited mixed morphology. Genetic analysis of segregants from mixed-morphology plaques (formed in two-factor crosses with various individual *ts* mutants) revealed that frequently all the *syn* and *syn*[+] segregants from the same plaque bred true for one and the same allele at the unselected *ts* locus. This implies that the genome which gave rise to the mixed-morphology plaque was heterozygous for the *syn* locus, but already homozygous for the *ts*-tagged locus. This situation has been met before in bacteriophage.

Hershey and Chase (1951) and Levinthal (1959) have described particles with single genomes which, while homozygous for one allele at a nonselected locus, are heterozygous for the alleles at a plaque morphology locus. The alleles at this locus then segregate at the next replication. Such partial heterozygotes are now called "hets." Although the analysis of *syn/syn*[+] mixed-morphology plaques is not complete, all the data are consistent with the interpretation that these plaques are due to partially heteroduplex but otherwise standard DNA molecules generated as a result of the events leading to recombination. The average length of the heteroduplex region and the distribution of heteroduplex regions over the genome are not yet known. Mixed-morphology plaques have not so far been described in other animal virus systems.

8.1. Infectious DNA and Marker Rescue

Lando and Ryhiner (1969) and Sheldrick *et al.* (1973) first demonstrated that HSV DNA is infectious, and this was confirmed by Graham *et al.* (1973) using a different technique. Wilkie *et al.* (1974) then developed a marker rescue technique which combined the use of herpes DNA and superinfection with virus. By exploiting different combinations of genetic markers they showed that the infectious DNA bred true and produced progeny with the same markers as the stock of origin, but that the infectivity of the DNA was destroyed by shearing. By exposing cells to fragments of sheared wild-type DNA and superinfecting with *ts* mutants, they then demonstrated successful marker rescue of various *ts* loci and of the *syn* locus. With one *ts* marked gene which was closely linked to the *syn* locus, both markers were rescued together in a proportion of cases. Recently, a more efficient marker rescue technique has been developed, which combines the use of infectious DNA and DNA fragments (N. Stow, personal communication).

8.2. Thymidine Kinase

Kit and Dubbs (1963) and Dubbs and Kit (1964) first described mutants of HSV deficient in thymidine kinase activity (TK⁻). Later, Hay *et al.* (1971) described HSV-induced deoxycytidine kinase activity and produced preliminary evidence that both activities were lost simultaneously as a result of the same mutational event. These observations were extended by Jamieson *et al.* (1974), who showed that, irrespective of the selective system used, more than 40 independently isolated *ts* mutants always lost both activities simultaneously. Three strains of HSV-1 and one of HSV-2 behaved identically, but pseudorabies and vaccinia virus were found to code only for thymidine kinase activity, while the two strains of equine abortion virus examined did not code for either enzyme activity. Jamieson *et al.* (1974) failed to devise a selective system able to select for only one of these two activities of HSV. They concluded that the HSV gene codes for deoxypyrimidine kinase activity; although this gene is not essential for virus replication under normal laboratory conditions, they could demonstrate that its function was indispensable for virus growth in serum-starved cells.

Double infection of thymidine kinase-less and deoxycytidine kinase-less cells by different HSV-1 TK⁻ mutants was investigated by autoradiography (Jamieson, 1973). The HSV-1 TK⁻ mutants fell into at least two groups which complemented each other significantly but failed to do so when TK⁻ mutants belonging to the same group were tested together (Jamieson, 1973). The accumulated evidence is consistent and implies that the HSV-specified deoxypyrimidine kinase activity is composed of a multimer of identical polypeptide subunits coded by a single viral gene; the observation of significant complementation by different HSVTK⁻ mutants thus appears to be the first demonstration of intragenic complementation with HSV or indeed with any animal virus.

Aron *et al.* (1973) found that two of 18 *ts* mutants of HSV-1 were *ts* in the production of thymidine kinase activity at NPT and a third mutant synthesized a heat-sensitive thymidine kinase. This suggests that at least two additional genes of HSV control the production of thymidine kinase activity; the mutant which produced heat-sensitive thymidine kinase activity provides evidence that the enzyme is virus coded. Esparza *et al.* (1974) found that *ts* mutants from two of seven complementation groups of HSV-2 lacked thymidine kinase activity at NPT, which again suggests two control genes. Recently, Crombie (1975) showed that three different HSV-1 *ts* mutations (K, D, T) were involved in the switch-on of deoxypyrimidine kinase activity at NPT.

8.3. Intertypic Complementation and Recombination

Intertypic complementation was first described by Timbury and Subak-Sharpe (1973), who used seven *ts* mutants of HSV-1 which belonged to six complementation groups and ten *ts* mutants of HSV-2 all from different complementation groups. Good complementation was observed in many combinations, but a number of pairs of mutants failed to complement. However, the observation that individual mutants of one type failed to complement two or more *ts* mutants of the other type, which themselves clearly belonged to different complementation groups, suggested that intertypic complementation data must be interpreted with caution. While positive complementation clearly indicates that the *ts* mutations are in different genes, failure to complement does not necessarily imply that the lesions are in exactly equivalent genes in the two types of virus. Later, Benyesh-Melnick *et al.* (1974) reported similar experiments involving seven *ts* mutants belonging to five HSV-1 complementation groups and seven *ts* mutants all from separate complementation groups of HSV-2. Only three instances of noncomplementation were found, and as the pairs of mutants in these three crosses also failed to recombine they concluded that the noncomplementing *ts* mutants of HSV-1 and HSV-2 were defective in functionally common or equivalent genes. Schaffer (1975) then further analyzed these data, and in view of the phenotypic differences between noncomplementing mutants concluded that the theoretical basis for failure of mutants to complement in intertypic tests is so far unknown.

Both groups of investigators (Timbury and Subak-Sharpe, 1973; Benyesh-Melnick *et al.*, 1974) were able to obtain recombinants. Timbury and Subak-Sharpe made three main observations: (1) some of the putative recombinants segregated and continued to segregate over three successive single-plaque purifications for both the *ts* and *syn* markers; (2) some intertypic recombinants bred true (and when later tested immunologically were shown to have both HSV-1 and HSV-2 type-specific antigens: R. A. Killington, R. E. Randall, and D. H. Watson, personal communication); and (3) a number of segregants exhibited novel *ts* phenotypes. Schaffer (1975) reported decreased frequencies of recombination and lack of additivity of recombination frequencies in intertypic recombination tests. She concluded that these results reflect the limited homology between the DNAs of HSV-1 and HSV-2 (Kieff *et al.*, 1972; Ludwig *et al.*, 1972) as well as differences in the genetic organization of the two viruses. Schaffer (1975) also discussed the probability of finding type-specific genes with essential functions but the data did not identify any such gene.

It is perhaps useful to discuss type-specific antigens at this point. As a result of evolutionary divergence from a common ancestor, the DNAs of HSV-1 and HSV-2 have come to differ by 2.2% in gross base composition (Subak-Sharpe, 1973); it seems not unreasonable to suppose that, as they diverged, there must have taken place numerous amino acid substitutions in the sequences of originally identical polypeptides so that ultimately the polypeptides differed in many sections of their sequence while retaining similar function. Not only amino acid substitutions but also deletions or duplications causing either decrease or increase in the size of the polypeptides would be expected.

Depending on the constraints on polypeptide variability exerted by the selection pressures which operate on the virus, antigenic divergence of the same functional polypeptide in HSV-1 and HSV-2 may be (1) absent (type-common), (2) very limited (also classed as type-common), (3) partial (possessing both type-specific and type-common determinants) (Thouless, 1972; Savage *et al.*, 1972; Sim and Watson, 1973), or (4) complete (type-specific with no cross-reaction). The substitution of a gene specifying a type-specific polypeptide in one genome by the equivalent type-specific gene from the other genome is not precluded, provided that the substitution is compatible with the formation of a viable particle. Such type-specific genes can therefore take part in intertypic complementation. Substitution of type-specific genes in the genetic background of the other HSV type has been detected in two recombinants from a cross between HSV-1 and HSV-2 (Timbury and Subak-Sharpe, 1973; R. A. Killington, R. E. Randall, and D. H. Watson, personal communication).

However, there may exist another class of type-specific gene which has a function uniquely required by that type only (Benyesh-Melnick *et al.*, 1974). A *ts* mutation in this kind of type-specific gene could not be complemented by any *ts* mutant of the other type. Neither Timbury and Subak-Sharpe (1973) nor Schaffer (1975) appear to have identified such a mutant.

9.   TRANSFORMATION

LMTK.⁻ cells are mouse cells lacking thymidine kinase activity, which were originally derived from the LM (TK⁺) cell line by Kit *et al.* (1963). Such LMTK⁻ cells are unable to grow in HAT medium (Szybalski and Szybalska, 1962). The genetic transformation of LMTK⁻ cells after exposure to HSV-1 or HSV-2 inactivated by exposure to ultraviolet irradiation has been reported by Munyon *et al.* (1971), who selectively eliminated all but the transformed clones of LMTK⁺ (HSV) cells in HAT medium and identified HSV thymidine kinase electrophoretically (Munyon *et al.*, 1972).

Munyon *et al.* (1971) have shown that multipassage cultures of these genetically transformed LMTK⁺ (HSV) cells continue to express HSV-specific thymidine kinase activity, while Davidson *et al.* (1973) demonstrated that the viral enzyme activity could be suppressed by selective passaging and then again reactivated. Type specificity of the thymidine kinase activity was demonstrated by Davis *et al.* (1974), who found in the LMTK⁺ (HSV) cells the characteristic differences in heat stability of the thymidine kinases expected for HSV-1 and HSV-2 (Thouless, 1972). HSV type specificity has since been confirmed in independently produced LMTK⁺ (HSV) cells by Jamieson *et al.* (1976), who identified the transformed cell enzyme activity as deoxypyrimidine kinase activity. The LMTK⁺ (HSV) cells appeared to contain only a small fragment of the HSV genome. HSV-specific antigens could also be demonstrated in the cells transformed by Munyon *et al.* by immunofluorescence (Chadka and Munyon, 1975). Genetic transformation of thymidine kinase-less cells by other animal viruses has not been reported.

Morphological transformation of hamster embryo cells by ultraviolet-irradiated HSV-2, and later HSV-1, was first reported by Duff and Rapp (1971*a,b*). They showed by immunofluorescence that transformed cells expressed HSV-specific antigens both on the cell surface and in the cytoplasm, and that cells transformed by both types of virus produced tumors after inoculation into hamsters. Macnab (1974) confirmed these observations with hamster embryo cells and also developed a transformation assay system in rat embryo cells obtained from inbred rats (Table 7). Transformation was demonstrated not only

TABLE 7

Transformation by *ts* Mutants of HSV

Number of mutants tested	Number of mutants showing transformation	Cells transformed	Phenotype of transforming mutants		Reference
			DNA$^+$	DNA$^-$	
HSV-1					
9	4	Rat embryo	3	1	Macnab (1975)
5	1	Hamster embryo	1	0	Kimura *et al.* (1975)
HSV-2					
13	5	Rat embryo	3	2	Macnab (1974)
12	3	Hamster embryo	Not stated		Takahashi and Yamanishi
	1	Human embryo lung	Not stated		(1974)
6	2	Hamster embryo	1	1	Kimura *et al.* (1975)

with ultraviolet-irradiated virus but also with *ts* mutants of HSV-1 and HSV-2 at NPT (Macnab, 1974, 1975). Later, Wilkie *et al.* (1974) showed that rat embryo cells could also be transformed with the DNA of *ts* mutants and even with DNA randomly fragmented to a size of 5–7 × 10^6 daltons. In these studies, both DNA$^+$ and DNA$^-$ *ts* mutants were able to transform successfully. So far, no *ts* mutant has been positively identified as unable to transform at NPT, but negative results have been obtained with many *ts* mutants where only preliminary experiments have been completed. Transformation of hamster embryo cells with *ts* mutants of HSV-1 and HSV-2 has also been reported by Kimura *et al.* (1975), and transformation of both hamster embryo cells and human embryo lung cells with *ts* mutants of HSV-2 has been described by Takahashi and Yamanishi (1974). Induction of tumors in hamsters following inoculation of *in vitro* transformed cells has been demonstrated by four groups of workers (Duff and Rapp, 1971*a,b*; Macnab, 1974; Takahashi and Yamanishi, 1974; Kimura *et al.*, 1975). Macnab (1975, 1976) has also induced tumors with *ts* mutant-transformed rat embryo cells both in immunosuppressed and in untreated rats of the same inbred strain. Macnab *et al.* (1977) have found that HSV-2-specific thymidine kinase activity is expressed not only in the rat cells transformed by the HSV-2 mutant, *ts* 1, but also in the cells of about 50% of the tumors obtained a year later from rats injected as newborns with the transformed cells. The sera from some of the tumor-bearing rats contained not only virus-specific antibodies demonstrated by immunofluorescence but also anti-thymidine kinase activity and virus-neutralizing activity. Kimura *et al.* (1975) also found that hamster embryo fibroblasts transformed by *ts* mutants induced tumors after injection into newborn hamsters and confirmed the observation of Duff and Rapp (1971*b*) that some of the sera from the tumor-bearing hamsters contained HSV-specific neutralizing antibody.

Kimura *et al.* (1974) carried out experiments with two cell lines transformed by ultraviolet-irradiated HSV-2 to see if the genetic information present could promote the replication of eight *ts* mutants of HSV-2 at NPT. They found that the growth of two DNA$^+$ mutants was significantly enhanced and suggested that the function of residual HSV genetic material in the transformed cells had assisted the replication of the mutants by complementation mechanisms. Macnab and Timbury (1976) used rat embryo cells transformed by the HSV-2 mutant *ts*1 and tested their ability to support the growth of *ts* mutants in 13 different complementation groups of HSV-2 (including the mutant *ts*1 originally used to transform the cells). Only three mutants, two DNA positive and one DNA negative, were significantly complemented. It therefore appears that cells transformed by *ts*1 continue to express the genetic information of at least some DNA$^+$ and DNA$^-$ cistrons.

10. LATENCY

Very recently Lofgren *et al.* (1977) tested the wild type and five *ts* mutants of HSV-1 strain 17 for ability to establish latent infection in the brain of the mouse. The wild type and four *ts* mutants were shown to produce latent infections, but one *ts* mutant (*ts*I) was not able to do so. Any trivial explanation depending on leakiness could be ruled out. This marks the beginning of investigation into the genetic control of herpesvirus latency.

The reader will rightly conclude that the genetic study of HSV-1 and HSV-2 has only begun to get under way. The results already achieved suggest that herpes simplex virus represents extremely favorable and at the same time challenging material for critical investigation of the strategy of the viral genome as presented by a large, DNA-containing animal virus. There can be no doubt that our knowledge of virus as a genetic system will expand rapidly in the next few years as our understanding of viral strategy increases. Our insight into the phenomena of HSV latency and HSV tumorigenic transformation—which in both cases is rudimentary—will doubtless be increased and advanced by genetic attack. Lastly, it should be more widely appreciated that the formal genetic study of HSV *per se* constitutes an important and interesting problem likely to prove of considerable relevance to our comprehension of the genetic systems of all animal viruses.

ACKNOWLEDGMENTS

Thanks are due Dr. D. A. Ritchie for helpful discussion and for kindly making the drawings of Figs. 1 and 3. We are grateful to Miss Helen Moss for drawing Fig. 2.

11. REFERENCES

Aron, G. M., Schaffer, P. A., Courtney, R. J., Benyesh-Melnick, M., and Kit, S., 1973, Thymidine kinase activity of herpes simplex virus temperature-sensitive mutants, *Intervirology* **1**:96.

Aron, G. M., Purifoy, D. J. M., and Schaffer, P. A., 1975, DNA synthesis and DNA polymerase activity of herpes simplex virus type 1 temperature-sensitive mutants, *J. Virol.* **16**:498.

Aurelian, L., and Roizman, B., 1964, The host range of herpes simplex virus: Interferon, viral DNA and antigen synthesis in abortive infection of dog kidney cells, *Virology* **22**:452.

Becker, Y., Dym, H., and Sarov, I., 1968, Herpes simplex virus DNA, *Virology* **36**:184.

Benyesh-Melnick, M., Schaffer, P. A., Courtney, R. J., Esparza, J., and Kimura, S., 1974, Viral gene functions expressed and detected by temperature-sensitive mutants of herpes simplex virus, *Cold Spring Harbor Symp. Quant. Biol.* **39**:731.

Benzer, S., 1961, On the topography of the genetic fine structure, *Proc. Natl. Acad. Sci. USA* **47**:403.

Bone, D. R., and Courtney, R. J., 1974, A temperature-sensitive mutant of herpes simplex virus type 1 defective in the synthesis of the major capsid polypeptide, *J. Gen. Virol.* **24**:17–27.

Brown, S. M., and Ritchie, D. A., 1975a, Genetic studies with herpes simplex virus type 1. Analysis of mixed-plaque forming virus and its bearing on genetic recombination, *Virology* **64**:32.

Brown, S. M., and Ritchie, D. A., 1975b, Genetic studies with herpes simplex virus type 1: Quantitative analysis of the products from two-factor crosses, *Virology* **64**:281.

Brown, S. M., Ritchie, D. A., and Subak-Sharpe, J. H., 1973, Genetic studies with herpes simplex virus type 1: The isolation of temperature-sensitive mutants, their arrangement into complementation groups and recombination analysis leading to a linkage map, *J. Gen. Virol.* **18**:329.

Campbell, A., 1961, Sensitive mutants of bacteriophage λ, *Virology* **14**:22.

Chadka, K. C., and Munyon, W., 1975, Presence of herpes simplex virus-related antigens in transformed L cells, *J. Virol.* **15**:1475.

Chu, C.-T., and Schaffer, P. A., 1975, Qualitative complementation test for temperature sensitive mutants of herpes simplex virus, *J. Virol.* **16**:1131.

Clements, J. B., Cortini, R., and Wilkie, N. M., 1976, Analysis of herpes virus DNA substructure by means of restriction endonucleases, *J. Gen. Virol.* **30**:243.

Courtney, R. J., and Benyesh-Melnick, M., 1974, Isolation and characterisation of a large molecular weight polypeptide of herpes simplex virus type 1, *Virology* **62**:539.

Crick, F. H. C., and Orgel, L. E., 1964, The theory of interallelic complementation, *J. Mol. Biol.* **8**:161.

Crombie, I. K., 1975, Genetic and biochemical studies with herpes simplex virus type 1, Ph.D. thesis.

Davidson, R. L., Adelstein, S. J., and Oxman, M. N., 1973, Herpes simplex virus as a source of thymidine kinase for thymidine kinase-deficient mouse cells: Suppression and reactivation of the viral enzyme, *Proc. Natl. Acad. Sci. USA* **70**:1912.

Davis, D. B., Munyon, W., Buchsbaum, R., and Chawda, R., 1974, Virus type-specific thymidine kinase in cells biochemically transformed by herpes simplex virus types 1 and 2, *J. Virol.* **13**:140.

Delius, H., and Clements, J. B., 1976, A partial denaturation map of herpes simplex virus type 1 DNA: Evidence for inversions of the two unique DNA regions, *J. Gen. Virol.* **33**:125.

Dubbs, D. R., and Kit, S., 1964, Mutant strains of herpes simplex deficient in thymidine kinase inducing activity, *Virology* **22**:493.

Duff, R., and Rapp, F., 1971*a*, Oncogenic transformation of hamster cells after exposure to herpes simplex virus type 2, *Nature (London) New Biol.* **233**:48.

Duff, R., and Rapp, F., 1971*b*, Properties of hamster embryo fibroblasts transformed *in vitro* after exposure to ultra-violet irradiated herpes simplex virus type 2, *J. Virol.* **8**:469.

Ejercito, P. M., Kieff, E. D., and Roizman, B., 1968, Characterization of herpes simplex virus strains differing in their effects on social behaviour of infected cells, *J. Gen. Virol.* **2**:357.

Epstein, R. H., Bolle, A., Steinberg, C. M., Kellenberger, E., Boy de la Tour, E., Chevalley, R., Edgar, R. S., Susman, M., Denhardt, G. H., and Lielausis, A., 1963, Physiological studies of conditional lethal mutants of bacteriophage T4D, *Cold Spring Harbor Symp. Quant. Biol.* **28**:375.

Esparza, J., Purifoy, D. J. M., Schaffer, P. A., and Benyesh-Melnick, M., 1974, Isolation, complementation and preliminary phenotypic characterisation of temperature-sensitive mutants of herpes simplex virus type 2, *Virology* **57**:554.

Fenner, F., 1969, Conditional lethal mutants of animal viruses, *Curr. Top. Microbiol. Immunol.* **48**:1.

Freese, E., 1959, The specific mutagenic effect of base analogues on phage T4, *J. Mol. Biol.* **1**:87.

Frenkel, N., and Roizman, B., 1972, Separation of the herpesvirus deoxyribonucleic acid duplex into unique fragments and intact strand on sedimentation in alkaline gradients, *J. Virol.* **10**:565.

Gallacher, W. R., Levitan, D. B., and Blough, H. A., 1973, Effect of 2-deoxy-D-glucose on cell fusion induced by Newcastle disease and herpes simplex viruses, *Virology* **55**:193.

Ginsberg, H. S., Ensinger, M. J., Kauffman, R. S., Mayer, A. J., and Lundholm, U., 1974, Cell transformation: A study of regulation with types 5 and 12 adenovirus temperature-sensitive mutants, *Cold Spring Harbor Symp. Quant. Biol.* **39**:419.

Goodheart, C. R., Plummer, G., and Waner, J. L., 1968, Density difference of DNA of human herpes simplex viruses types 1 and 2, *Virology* **35**:473.

Graham, F. L., Veldhuisen, G., and Wilkie, N. M., 1973, Infectious herpesvirus DNA, *Nature* (*London*) *New Biol.* **245**:265.

Halliburton, I. W., and Timbury, M. C., 1973, Characterization of temperature sensitive mutants of herpes simplex virus type 2: Growth and DNA synthesis, *Virology* **54**:60.

Halliburton, I. W., and Timbury, M. C., 1976, Temperature-sensitive mutants of herpes simplex virus type 2: Description of three new complementation groups and studies on the inhibition of host cell DNA synthesis, *J. Gen. Virol.* **30**:207.

Halliburton, I. W., Hill, E. A., and Russell, G. J., 1975, Identification of strains of herpes simplex virus by comparison of the density of their DNA using the preparative ultracentrifuge, *Arch. Virol.* **48**:157.

Hay, J., and Subak-Sharpe, J. H., 1976, Mutants of herpes simplex virus types 1 and 2 that are resistant to phosphonoacetic acid induce altered DNA polymerase activities in infected cells, *J. Gen. Virol.* **31**:145.

Hay, J., Perera, P. A. J., Morrison, J. M., Gentry, G. A., and Subak-Sharpe, J. H., 1971, Herpes virus-specified proteins, in: *Strategy of the Viral Genome: A CIBA Foundation Symposium* (G. E. W. Wolstenholme and M. O'Connor, eds.), p. 355, Churchill Livingstone, Edinburgh.

Hay, J., Moss, H., Jamieson, A. T., and Timbury, M. C., 1976, Herpesvirus proteins: DNA polymerase and pyrimidine deoxynucleoside kinase activities in temperature-sensitive mutants of herpes simplex virus type 2, *J. Gen. Virol.* **31**:65.

Hayes, W., 1968, *The genetics of bacteria and their viruses,* 2nd ed., p. 302, Blackwell, Oxford.

Hayward, G. S., Frenkel, N., and Roizman, B., 1975, Anatomy of herpes simplex virus DNA; strain differences and heterogeneity in the locations of restriction endonuclease cleavage sites, *Proc. Natl. Acad. Sci. USA* **72**:1768.

Heine, J. W., Honess, R. W., Cassai, E., and Roizman, B., 1974, Proteins specified by herpes simplex virus XII: The virion polypeptides of type 1 strains, *J. Virol.* **14**:640.

Hershey, A. D., and Chase, M., 1951, Genetic recombination and heterozygosis in bacteriophage, *Cold Spring Harbor Symp. Quant. Biol.* **16**:471.

Honess, R. W., and Roizman, B., 1973, Proteins specified by herpes simplex virus. XI. Identification and relative molar rates of synthesis of structural and non-structural herpes virus polypeptides in the infected cell, *J. Virol.* **12**:1347.

Honess, R. W., and Roizman, B., 1974, Regulation of herpesvirus macromolecular synthesis. I. Cascade regulation of the synthesis of three groups of viral proteins, *J. Virol.* **14**:8.

Jamieson, A. T., 1973, *In vivo* and *in vitro* studies on herpes virus-induced deoxypyrimidine kinase activity, Ph.D. thesis.

Jamieson, A. T., and Subak-Sharpe, J. H., 1974, Biochemical studies on the herpes simplex virus-specified deoxypyrimidine kinase activity, *J. Gen. Virol.* **24**:481.

Jamieson, A. T., Gentry, G. A., and Subak-Sharpe, J. H., 1974, Induction of both thymidine and deoxycytidine kinase activity by herpes viruses, *J. Gen. Virol.* **24**:465.

Jamieson, A. T., Macnab, J. C. M., Perbal, B., and Clements J. B., 1976, Virus-specified enzyme activity and RNA species in herpes simplex virus type 1 transformed mouse cells, *J. Gen. Virol.* **32**:493.

Kaplan, A. S., 1973, *The Herpesviruses,* Academic Press, New York.

Keir, H. M., Subak-Sharpe, J. H., Shedden, W. I. H., Watson, D. H., and Wildy, P.,

1966, Immunological evidence for a specific DNA polymerase produced after infection by herpes simplex virus, *Virology* **30**:154.

Keller, J. M., Spear, P. G., and Roizman, B., 1970, Proteins specified by herpes simplex virus. III. Viruses differing in their effects on the social behaviour of infected cells specify different membrane glycoproteins, *Proc. Natl. Acad. Sci. USA* **65**:865.

Kieff, E. D., Bachenheimer, S. L., and Roizman, B., 1971, Size, composition and structure of the deoxyribonucleic acid of subtypes 1 and 2 herpes simplex virus, *J. Virol.* **8**:125.

Kieff, E. D., Hoyer, B., Bachenheimer, S. L., and Roizman, B., 1972, Genetic relatedness of type 1 and type 2 herpes simplex viruses, *J. Virol.* **9**:738–745.

Kimura, S., Esparza, J., Benyesh-Melnick, M., and Schaffer, P. A., 1974, Enhanced replication of temperature-sensitive mutants of herpes simplex virus type 2 (HSV-2) at the non-permissive temperature in cells transformed by HSV-2, *Intervirology* **3**:162.

Kimura, S., Flannery, V. L., Levy, B., and Schaffer, P. A., 1975, Oncogenic transformation of primary hamster cells by herpes simplex virus type 2 (HSV-2) and an HSV-2 temperature-sensitive mutant, *Int. J. Cancer* **15**:786.

Kit, S., and Dubbs, D. R., 1963, Nonfunctional thymidine kinase cistron in bromodeoxyuridine resistant strains of herpes simplex virus, *Biophys. Biochem. Res. Commun.* **13**:500.

Kit, S., Dubbs, D. R., Piekarski, L. J., and Hsu, T. C., 1963, Deletion of thymidine kinase activity from L cells resistant to bromodeoxyuridine, *Exp. Cell Res.* **31**:297.

Koment, R. W., and Rapp, F., 1975, Variation in susceptibility of different cell types to temperature-sensitive host range mutants of herpes simplex virus type 2, *Virology* **64**:164.

Krieg, D. R., 1963, Specificity of chemical mutagenesis, *Prog. Nucl. Acid Res.* **2**:125.

Lando, D., and Ryhiner, M. L., 1969, Pouvoir infectieux du DNA d'Herpesvirus hominis en culture cellulaire, *Comp. Rend. Acad. Sci. (Paris)* **269**:527.

Levinthal, C., 1959, Bacteriophage genetics, in: *Animal Viruses,* Vol. 2 (F. M. Burnet and W. M. Stanley, eds.), p. 281, Academic Press, New York.

Lofgren, K. W., Stevens, J. G., Marsden, H. S., and Subak-Sharpe, J. H., 1977, Temperature sensitive mutants of herpes simplex virus differ in the capacity to establish latent infections in mice, *Virology* **76**:440.

Ludwig, H. O., Biswal, N., and Benyesh Melnick, M., 1972, Studies on the relatedness of herpesviruses through DNA-DNA hybridization, *Virology* **49**:95.

Macnab, J. C. M., 1974, Transformation of rat embryo cells by temperature-sensitive mutants of herpes simplex virus, *J. Gen. Virol.* **24**:143.

Macnab, J. C. M., 1975, Transformed cell lines produced by temperature sensitive mutants of herpes simplex types 1 and 2, in: *Oncogenesis and Herpesviruses,* p. 227, Proceedings of a Symposium held in Nuremberg, 1974, IARC, Lyon.

Macnab, J. C. M., 1976, Tumour production of HSV-2 transformed lines in rats and the varying response to immunosuppression, submitted for publication.

Macnab, J. C. M., and Timbury, M. C., 1976, Complementation of HSV-2 *ts* mutants by a *ts* mutant transformed cell line, *Nature (London)* **261**:233.

Macnab, J. C. M., Visser, L., Jamieson, A. T., and Hay, J., 1977, Specific viral antigens in rat cells transformed by herpes simplex virus type 2 and in tumours induced in rats by inoculation of transformed cells, manuscript in preparation.

Manservigi, R., 1974, Method for isolation and selection of temperature-sensitive mutants of herpes simplex virus, *Appl. Microbiol.* **27**:1034.

Mao, J. C.-H., Robishaw, E. E., Schleicher, J. B., Shipkowtiz, N. L., Ructer, A., and Overby, L. R., 1973, Abstract 144, 13th Conference Antimicrobial Agents and Chemotherapy, Washington D.C.

Mao, J. C.-H., Robishaw, E. E., and Overby, L. R., 1975, Inhibition of DNA polymerase from herpes simplex virus-infected Wi-38 cells by phosphonoacetic acid, *J. Virol.* **15**:1281.

Marsden, H. S., Crombie, I. K., and Subak-Sharpe, J. H., 1976, Control of protein synthesis in herpesvirus-infected cells: Analysis of the polypeptides induced by wild-type and sixteen temperature-sensitive mutants of HSV strain 17, *J. Gen. Virol.* **31**:347.

Mechie, M., 1974, A biological and biochemical characterisation of *ts* mutants of herpes simplex virus type 1, Ph.D. thesis.

Munyon, W., Kraiselburd, E., Davis, D., and Mann, J., 1971, Transfer of thymidine kinase to thymidine kinaseless L cells by infection with ultraviolet-irradiated herpes simplex virus, *J. Virol.* **7**:813.

Munyon, W., Buchsbaum, R., Paoletti, E., Mann, J., Kraiselburd, E., and Davis, D., 1972, Electrophoresis of thymidine kinase activity synthesized by cells transformed by herpes simplex virus, *Virology* **49**:683.

Pringle, C. R., Howard, D. K., and Hay, J., 1973, Temperature-sensitive mutants of pseudorabies virus with differential effects on viral and host DNA synthesis, *Virology* **55**:495.

Purifoy, D. J. M., and Benyesh-Melnick, M., 1975, DNA polymerase induction by DNA-negative temperature-sensitive mutants of herpes simplex virus type 2, *Virology* **68**:374.

Rapp, F., and Li, J.-L. H., 1974, Demonstration of the oncogenic potential of herpes simplex viruses and human cytomegalovirus, *Cold Spring Harbor Symp. Quant. Biol.* **39**:747.

Roizman, B., 1962, Polykaryocytosis: Results from fusion of mononucleated cells, *Cold Spring Harbor Symp. Quant. Biol.* **27**:327.

Roizman, B., and Aurelian, L., 1965, Abortive infection of canine cells by herpes simplex virus. 1. Characterisation of viral progeny from cooperative infection with mutants differing in capacity to multiply in canine cells, *J. Mol. Biol.* **11**:528.

Roizman, B., and Furlong, D., 1975, The replication of herpesviruses, in: *Comprehensive Virology*, Vol. 3 (H. Fraenkel-Conrat and R. R. Wagner, eds.), p. 229, Plenum Press, New York.

Roizman, B., Kozak, M., Honess, R. W., and Hayward, G., 1974, Regulation of herpesvirus macromolecular synthesis: Evidence for multilevel regulation of herpes simplex 1 RNA and protein synthesis, *Cold Spring Harbor Symp. Quant. Biol.* **39**:687.

Roizman, B., Hayward, G., Jacob, R., Wadsworth, S., Frenkel, N., Honess, R. W., and Kozak, M., 1975, Human herpesviruses I: A model for molecular organisation and regulation of herpesviruses—A review, in: *Oncogenesis and Herpesviruses II*, p. 3, Proceedings of a Symposium, Nuremberg, 1974, IARC, Lyon.

Savage, T., Roizman, B., and Heine, J. W., 1972, Immunological specificity of the glycoproteins of herpes simplex virus sub-types 1 and 2, *J. Gen. Virol.* **17**:31.

Schaffer, P. A., 1975, Genetics of herpesviruses—A review, in: *Oncogenesis and Herpesviruses II*, p. 195, Proceedings of a Symposium, Nuremberg, 1974, IARC, Lyon.

Schaffer, P. A., Vonka, V., Lewis, R., and Benyesh-Melnick, M., 1970, Temperature-sensitive mutants of herpes simplex virus, *Virology* **42**:1144.

Schaffer, P. A., Courtney, R. J., McCombs, R. M., and Benyesh-Melnick, M., 1971, A temperature-sensitive mutant of herpes simplex virus defective in glycoprotein synthesis, *Virology* **46**:356.

Schaffer, P. A., Aron, G. M., Biswal, N., and Benyesh-Melnick, M., 1973, Temperature-sensitive mutants of herpes simplex virus type 1: Isolation, complementation and partial characterization, *Virology* **52**:57.

Schaffer, P. A., Tevethia, M. J., and Benyesh-Melnick, M., 1974*a*, Recombination between temperature-sensitive mutants of herpes simplex virus type 1, *Virology* **58**:219.

Schaffer, P. A., Brunschwig, J. P., McCombs, R. M., and Benyesh-Melnick, M., 1974*b*, Electron microscopic studies of temperature-sensitive mutants of herpes simplex virus type 1, *Virology* **62**:444.

Sheldrick, P., and Berthelot, N., 1974, Inverted repetitions in the chromosome of herpes simplex virus, *Cold Spring Harbor Symp. Quant. Biol.* **39**:667.

Sheldrick, P., Laithier, M., Lando, D., and Ryhiner, M. L., 1973, Infectious DNA from herpes simplex virus: Infectivity of double-stranded and single-stranded molecules, *Proc. Natl. Acad. Sci. USA* **70**:3621.

Shipkowitz, N. L., and Bower, R., 1973, Phosphonoacetic acid: A new antiherpesvirus agent II: *in vivo* activity, Abstract 145, 13th Conference of Antimicrobial Agents and Chemotherapy, Washington, D.C.

Sim, C., and Watson, D. H., 1973, The role of type-specific and cross-reacting structural antigens in the neutralization of herpes simplex virus types 1 and 2, *J. Gen. Virol.* **19**:217.

Smith, J. D., Barnett, L., Brenner, S., and Russell, R. L., 1970, More mutant tyrosine transfer ribonucleic acids, *J. Mol. Biol.* **54**:1.

Spring, S. B., Roizman, B., and Schwartz, J., 1968, Herpes simplex virus products in productive and abortive infection. II. Electron microscopic and immunological evidence for failure of virus envelopment as a cause of abortive infection, *J. Virol.* **2**:384.

Stevens, J. G., 1975, Latent herpes simplex virus and the nervous system. *Curr. Top. Microbiol. Immunol.* **70**:31.

Stevens, J. G., and Cook, M. L., 1971, Latent herpes simplex virus in spinal ganglia of mice, *Science* **173**:843.

Subak-Sharpe, J. H., 1969, *Proceedings of the First International Congress for Virology, Helsinki, 1968* (J. L. Melnick, ed.), p. 252, Karger, Basel.

Subak-Sharpe, J. H., 1973, The genetics of herpesviruses, *Cancer Res.* **33**:1385.

Subak-Sharpe, J. H., Brown, S. M., Ritchie, D. A., Timbury, M. C., and Halliburton I. W., 1973, Herpesvirus genetics, in: *Advances in the Biosciences,* Vol. 11, p. 205, Schering Workshop on Virus–Cell Interactions, Pergamon Press, Braunschweig.

Subak-Sharpe, J. H., Brown, S. M., Ritchie, D. A., Timbury, M. C., Macnab, J. C. M., Marsden, H. S., and Hay, J., 1974, Genetic and biochemical studies with herpesvirus, *Cold Spring Harbor Symp. Quant. Biol.* **39**:717.

Summers, W. P., Wagner, M., and Summers, W. C., 1975, Possible peptide chain termination mutants in thymidine kinase gene of a mammalian virus, herpes simplex virus, *Proc. Natl. Acad. Sci. USA* **72**:4081.

Szybalski, W., and Szybalska, E. H., 1962, Drug sensitivity as a genetic marker for human cell lines, in: *Approaches to the Genetic Analysis of Mammalian Cells,* p. 11, University of Michigan Press, Ann Arbor.

Takahashi, M., and Yamanishi, K., 1974, Transformation of hamster embryo and human embryo cells by temperature-sensitive mutants of herpes simplex virus type 2, *Virology* **61**:306.

Thouless, M. E., 1972, Serological properties of thymidine kinase produced in cells infected with type 1 or type 2 herpes virus, *J. Gen. Virol.* **17**:307.

Timbury, M. C., 1971, Temperature-sensitive mutants of herpes simplex virus type 2, *J. Gen. Virol.* **13**:373.

Timbury, M. C., and Calder, L., 1976, Temperature-sensitive mutants of herpes simplex virus type 2: A provisional linkage map based on recombination analysis, *J. Gen. Virol.* **30**:179.

Timbury, M. C., and Hay, J., 1975, Genetic and physiological studies with herpes simplex virus type 2 temperature-sensitive mutants, in: *Oncogenesis and Herpesviruses II,* p. 219, Proceedings of a Symposium, Nuremberg, 1974, IARC. Lyon.

Timbury, M. C., and Subak-Sharpe, J. H., 1973, Genetic interactions between temperature-sensitive mutants of types 1 and 2 herpes simplex viruses, *J. Gen. Virol.* **18**:347.

Timbury, M. C., Theriault, A., and Elton, R. A., 1974, A stable syncytial mutant of herpes simplex type 2 virus, *J. Gen. Virol.* **23**:219.

Timbury, M. C., Hendricks, M. L., and Schaffer, P. A., 1976, A collaborative study of temperature-sensitive mutants of herpes simplex virus type 2, *J. Virol.* **18**:1139.

Visconti, R., and Delbrück, M., 1953, The mechanism of genetic recombination in phage, *Genetics* **38**:5.

Wadsworth, S., Jacob, R. J., and Roizman, B., 1975, Anatomy of herpes simplex virus DNA. II. Size, composition and arrangement of inverted terminal repetitions, *J. Virol.* **15**:1487.

Watson, J. D., 1970, *Molecular Biology of the Gene,* 2nd ed., Benjamin, New York.

Wildy, P., 1955, Recombination with herpes simplex virus, *J. Gen. Microbiol.* **13**:346.

Wilkie, N. M., 1973, The synthesis and substructure of herpesvirus DNA, the distribution of alkali-labile single strand interruptions in HSV-1 DNA, *J. Gen. Virol.* **21**:453.

Wilkie, N. M., Clements, J. B., Macnab, J. C. M., and Subak-Sharpe, J. H., 1974, The structure and biological properties of herpes simplex virus DNA, *Cold Spring Harbor Symp. Quant. Biol.* **39**:657.

Williams, J. F., Young, C. S. H., and Austin, P. E., 1974, Genetic analysis of human adenovirus type 5 in permissive and nonpermissive cells, *Cold Spring Harbor Symp. Quant. Biol.* **39**:427.

Zygraich, N., and Huygelen, C., 1973, *In vivo* behaviour of a temperature-sensitive (*ts*) mutant of herpesvirus hominis type 2, *Arch Virusforsch.* **43**:103.

CHAPTER 4

Genetics of Picornaviruses

Peter D. Cooper

Department of Microbiology
John Curtin School of Medical Research
Australian National University
Canberra, Australia

1. INTRODUCTION

Picornaviruses have long seemed to have many genes. The size of the genome compared with the "average" gene product suggested about ten for poliovirus (Fenner, 1968), which causes at least a dozen synthetic and degenerative changes in the host cell. Many viral polypeptides are found, originally about 14 (Summers *et al.*, 1965) and now more than 34 (Abraham and Cooper, 1975*a*). Other picornaviruses are very similar.

This chapter attempts to set out current knowledge on the structure and function of the picornavirus genome in terms of a balance sheet between total genetic information and genetic function, with emphasis on methods and results of genetic analysis. A few years ago, such an attempt seemed premature, although a tentative scheme could be suggested (Cooper *et al.*, 1971). A more complete attempt (which resembles the earlier one) is now possible, despite some important remaining gaps. However, the new evidence leads to a much simpler concept of the genetic makeup of picornaviruses. In contrast to the initial appearance of complexity, they now seem to have only three or four "genes."

This substantial simplification allows us a birds-eye view of the strategy of the picornavirus genome. Unfortunately, although we have used the term, the classical concept of "gene"—one gene, one polypeptide chain—does not really apply to picornaviruses, raising a semantic and conceptual problem that is considered in terms of a novel genetic element, the "schizon." Much of the evidence is derived from poliovirus, for which the earlier genetic studies have been discussed (Cooper, 1969). The establishment of a family such as Picornaviridae, although based mainly on virion structure, nevertheless implies that fundamental properties such as genetics will be common to all members, and aspects of relatedness within this large family are accordingly considered under "classification" (Section 4). However, new genetic and molecular results are becoming available for the aphthoviruses (foot-and-mouth disease viruses: Greek, *aphtha*, vesicles in the mouth; Fenner *et al.*, 1974), cardioviruses, and rhinoviruses which closely resemble those for poliovirus. Apart from certain detailed differences in makeup and function of structural protein, the picornaviruses do indeed have much in common.

2. DEFINITION OF A PICORNAVIRUS

The following properties have been found in all picornaviruses looked at in sufficient detail.

A naked, ether-resistant icosahedral nucleocapsid, 20–40 nm in diameter, is composed of 60 fundamental structural units; probably because of the composition of this structural unit, the appearance of 32 or 42 capsomeres is sometimes presented, but usually the surface is featureless. Each structural unit is usually comprised of several different polypeptides whose size (and number) can vary even between closely related strains, but whose aggregate molecular mass lies between 80 and 140 kilodaltons (kdal). Besides protein, virus particles contain only RNA, in one linear, single-stranded piece, of 2.3–2.9×10^6 daltons, probably close to 2.6×10^6. The RNA is infectious and is the message for protein translation. Multiplication occurs on cytoplasmic membranes, and functional proteins are mainly or entirely produced by posttranslational cleavage of an unpunctuated precursor polyprotein. A low but reproducible amount of intra-RNA genetic recombination occurs. The only genetically separable functions so far identified are (in order from the 5′ end) for structural protein and for one or two RNA replicases or replicase factors, although these "genes" may have secondary activities.

3. THE SCHIZON

Via the idea of one gene–one enzyme, the gene has become generally equated with the cistron (Benzer, 1957), that functional genetic unit defined by the *cis–trans* complementation test and specifying the initiation, continuation, and punctuation of a single polypeptide's translation. Unfortunately, there are now many genetic instances to which the concept of "cistron" does not really apply, as the functional polypeptide is produced by subdivision of the primary translation product. These may be parts of otherwise orthodox cistron systems (Hershko and Fry, 1975) or can comprise whole systems in themselves. Poliovirus is a good example of the latter: its genome contains several functionally distinct genetic elements for which, however, the terms "gene" and "cistron" are confusing or incorrect in their current connotation. For this novel unit of genetic function, therefore, the term "schizon" (Greek, *schizein*, to cleave) will be used in what follows. Picornavirus RNAs behave ostensibly as mono- (possibly di-) cistronic, polyschizonic messengers.

Definitions. Schizon: the genetic information coding for a polypeptide created by posttranslational cleavage. A component of a particular class of cistron that codes for a possibly functionless precursor (e.g., proinsulin) later subdivided by such cleavage. In operation analogous to a cistron, but differing in that (1) adjacent schizons may overlap, may be totally contained in other schizons, or may not directly meet at all, (2) initial and terminal sequences may not be uniquely defined, and (3) signals for initiation and punctuation of translation products are not usually included. *Schizomer:* a particular polypeptide created by posttranslational cleavage.

The schizon's boundaries are probably determined by certain amino acid sequences plus the overall conformation of the primary translation product of its parental cistron in reaction with the proteolytic specificities of its environment, rather than by any particular signal within the genetic material. Indeed, the schizon is a genetic element defined substantially by its phenotype, which may vary in different environments. The inconstant nature of this entity has naturally raised difficulties not only in terminology but also conceptually and in practical investigation, especially for genetic analysis.

4. CLASSIFICATION OF PICORNAVIRUSES

There is a case (Cooper, 1974) for including within a particular family only those viruses having fundamentally identical overall schemes of gene replication and function ("genome strategies"). While no picornavirus strategy is yet fully understood, it is nevertheless clear that those of entero-, cardio-, aphtho-, and rhinovirus must be quite similar. This follows from the common properties of picornaviruses (Section 2), coupled with the apparent restrictions on translation and punctuation of polycistronic RNA messages in animal cells (Fenner *et al.*, 1974). It would be very surprising indeed to find divergence in principle of gene replication and function in a group of viruses with such similar properties as the Picornaviridae.

The Study Group on Picornaviridae of the International Committee on Taxonomy of Viruses (Melnick *et al.*, 1974) recommends that, for the present, the aphthoviruses and the equine rhinovirus be included in the genus *Rhinovirus,* and the cardioviruses in the genus *Enterovirus,* possibly placing them later in separate genera. However, criteria for this grouping are arbitrarily selected characters of capsid protein (see below), and there seems more value in separating them at this stage into "natural" clusters of similar biology. The family Picornaviridae is therefore suggested to include at least four genera of equal status (Table 1), namely *Enterovirus, Cardiovirus, Rhinovirus,* and *Aphthovirus.* Unclassified viruses with many of the properties given in the definition are known, including some from insects. Ribophages are excluded as having a quite distinct strategy, as are plant viruses because their particle structure usually differs, and their strategies remain almost totally obscure.

The caliciviruses are relegated to a genus for possible inclusion in Picornaviridae (Melnick *et al.*, 1974) as they do not conform in some respects, raising the question of whether they should comprise a separate family (Burroughs and Brown, 1974). The most important difference is that only one major polypeptide, of 60–65 kdal, is resolved in gel electrophoresis of purified virus. There is no evidence for post-translational cleavage of vesicular exanthema virus proteins in infected cells (Black and Brown, 1976) and it is probable that caliciviruses have a different genome strategy and should not, accordingly, be considered as picornaviruses. The question is not answered, therefore, as to whether or not the information in this chapter applies to caliciviruses. No direct genetic experiments for this group are yet available.

TABLE 1
Distinguishing Features of Picornavirus Genera

Property	Enterovirus	Cardiovirus	Rhinovirus	Aphthovirus	?Calicivirus[a] (possible genus)	Probably others
Main members	Polio-, echo-, and coxsackievirus	Columbia SK group	Common cold	Foot-and-mouth disease	Vesicular exanthema (pigs), "picorna" (cats)	?Equine ?"Rhinovirus," others
Serotypes	Many	One or few	>90	Several	Several	
Main hosts	Human, vertebrate	Human, rodent, vertebrate	Human vertebrate	Rodents, ungulates	Pig, cat, sea lion	Horses, insects, ?others
Host range and tissue tropisms of individual strains	Narrow	Wide	Narrow	Wide	Wide (pig), narrow (cat)	
Main habitat	Gut	CNS, heart	Upper respiratory tract	Generalized	Generalized (pig), respiratory (cat)	
pH 3	Stable	Stable	Labile	Labile	Labile	
pH 5–6	Stable	Labile in 0.1 M halide	Stable	Becoming labile	Variable	
Ceiling temperature	High	High	Usually low	High	High	
EM: surface diameter (nm)	Featureless 24–28	Featureless 24–30	Featureless 20–30	Featureless 23–25	Large "cups" 30–40	
RNA: C	20–24	24–26	19	28	25	
A	27–30	25–27	35	25	29	
G	23–28	23–24	19	24	21	
U	23–25	24–27	27	22	25	
Virion %	29	31	30	31.5	22–24	
CsCl density	1.33–1.35	1.34	1.38–1.43	1.43	1.37–1.38	

[a] Recent work indicates that caliciviruses are probably not picornaviruses.

Almost all of the differences used to distinguish the genera or possible genera of Picornaviridae that are listed in Table 1 (serology, acid lability, CsCl density, tissue and host tropisms, percentage content of RNA, size of particle, and electron microscopic appearance) primarily reflect differences in capsid structure. [This follows from the constant size of the RNA ($2.3–2.9 \times 10^6$) coupled with its infectivity and its loss of tissue specificity when the capsid is removed or changed by transcapsidation.] Such differences are useful and quite valid, but they all are likely to depend solely on the conformation, cohesiveness, and permeability of the unique fundamental structural unit. More than any other gene product, this unit is extremely vulnerable to evolutionary pressure, and as these differences can often be visualized as being (in some cases actually are) manipulable in the laboratory by mutational or environmental changes, they seem less significant than strategy as a primary classification criterion. There seems no particular merit in selecting any one of them for secondary groupings either. The "biological" groupings comprising the genera of Table 1 embody various combinations of capsid properties.

Having considered the likely relationships within the family Picornaviridae, it must now be emphasized that genetic studies, with which this chapter is concerned, have been made extensively only with poliovirus and some other picornaviruses. So far, there are no fundamental differences, and a major value of classification schemes is to predict common properties from a well-studied example. Nevertheless, it is desirable to test the assumption of genetic homogeneity with examples from other genera.

5. GENETIC METHODS

Many of the methods and some 40 of the selective and nonselective markers used for genetic experiments with picornaviruses have been summarized previously (Cooper, 1969), together with a discussion of the problems of reversion and penetrance (leak rate) of *ts* mutants and of pleiotropism or covariance. The main tests are discussed in detail later (recombination test, Sections 6.1 and 7; complementation test, Section 6.2; tests for physiological defect, Section 8; detection of gene products by differential labeling of viral polypeptides followed by polyacrylamide gel electrophoresis, and "mapping" with pactamycin, Section 9).

5.1. Markers and Mutant Isolation

The markers most useful for genetic analysis are temperature sensitivity (*ts*) and resistance to certain antiviral inhibitors (Ghendon, 1972; Sergiescu *et al.*, 1972). Cold-sensitive (*cs*) poliovirus mutants have been described (Wright and Cooper, 1974*b*). These are all selective markers, that is, markers for or against which the assay system can be arranged to select specifically. The mutagenic treatment used to obtain *ts* mutants has been growth in the presence of 5-fluorouracil (Cooper, 1964*a*; Pringle, 1968; la Bonnardière, 1971; MacKenzie *et al.*, 1975; Lake *et al.*, 1975) or nitrosoguanidine (Cooper *et al.*, 1975; Bond and Swim, 1975), or treatment of virus or free RNA with nitrous acid (Cooper *et al.*, 1971, 1975) or hydroxylamine (Lake *et al.*, 1975). Some isolates appeared to be spontaneous mutants (Cooper *et al.*, 1971). The mutagenic treatment had no detectable effect on mutant properties. The mutation rates were kept low (isolation rates < 3%)—if possible, selecting only one clone from each culture after a single growth cycle—in order to minimize the isolation of sister mutants. Other mutagenic procedures for picornaviruses are summarized by Sergiescu *et al.* (1972), together with an extensive treatment of the methods for use of suitable viral inhibitors in picornavirus genetic analysis (see also Section 10).

The *ts* isolates were routinely assayed and cloned by monolayer or agar cell-suspension plaque methods, and were frequently enriched during isolation by temperature-shift incubation and detected by spot test (Cooper *et al.*, 1966; la Bonnardière, 1971; Lake and MacKenzie, 1973), or by replica plating (Bond and Swim, 1975). The method of Lake and MacKenzie (1973) allows direct identification of *ts* plaques.

5.2. Covariant Reversion

The use of revertants to confirm the location of mutations in specific gene functions merits special mention. Changes are often found that seem to be associated with the mutation under study; for example, many *ts* mutants produce a virion that is less thermostable than wild type. Although this might be held to identify the gene in which the *ts* defect lies as structural protein, one cannot assume that the two mutations are necessarily in the same gene, as they may have arisen by independent mutational events. Sometimes the changed property seems unrelated to the primary lesion; for example, some *ts* mutants are covariantly resistant to certain antiviral inhibitors (Cooper *et al.*, 1974). Whether or not the change (e.g., heat lability or inhibitor resistance) and the primary lesion (e.g., *ts* mutation) lie in the same functional gene product can be tested by comparing the properties of a number of revertants, in this case selected for *ts*$^+$, thermostable, or inhibitor-sensitive characters. The covariation of two characters in a substantial proportion (not necessarily all) of the revertants can virtually rule out double mutation as a cause of their association, and indicates that they do occur in the same gene product. This useful proposition is elaborated elsewhere (Cooper *et al.*, 1970*a*; Steiner-Pryor and Cooper, 1973), where it was used to confirm that guanidine sensitivity and repression of host protein synthesis of poliovirus were both determined by the configuration of a product of the structural protein schizon.

5.3. Temperature-Shift Experiments

The temperature-shift method has not proved of much value in genetic analysis of picornaviruses (Cooper, 1969). The intracellular replication of some viruses can be subdivided into "early" or "late" phases by shifting cultures infected with *ts* mutants to or from restrictive temperature at various times in the growth cycle: mutants with defects in the early phase will not be affected by a shift to the restrictive temperature after that phase is passed, and so on. However, picornaviruses behave as though all genes operate throughout the cycle. Most of their *ts* mutants register as "late"; i.e., their functions are still needed for new virus formation at a time when virus maturation has begun (Cooper *et al.*, 1966; Pringle *et al.*, 1970; Mikhejeva *et al.*, 1973; Bond and Swim, 1975). Although a few *ts* mutants seem to have an "early" defect, there is no invariable correlation between physiological lesion and this property. The "early" mutant of Cooper *et al.* (1966), *ts*23, was defective in replicase I, as were six "late" mutants: presumably, the defective gene product of *ts*23 was *ts* only if synthesized at restrictive temperature, and growth was aborted if infection was not established at an early stage by synthesis of the cRNA strand. Quantitative comparisons of the yields of RNA and hemagglutinin from the "early" mutants of Bond and Swim (1975) suggest that their defects lie in structural protein and lead to a substantial but not complete impairment of uncoating, a function that could possibly be examined by direct means.

6. INTERACTIONS OF PICORNAVIRUS GENOMES

This section deals with interactions between picornavirus and other virus genomes inside mixedly infected cells.

6.1. Genetic Recombination

Mixed infection by viruses with mutations in different loci may produce some genetic recombinant progeny with characters from both parents. Novel combinations of DNA genetic material may arise either by reassortment of large linkage groups such as chromosomes or by "molecular" recombination within linkage groups. In the latter case, the DNA pieces are covalently broken and rejoined by enzymes. With one known exception, "recombination" of RNA genetic material (which is found only among viruses) either does not occur or seems to arise by simple reassortment of unlinked pieces of RNA analogous to very small chromosomes ("segmented genomes"). Picornaviruses provide the unique exception, for which a phenomenon with the appearance of genetic recombination is well established. It may be mentioned that the genetic information of RNA tumor viruses, which is also held in a piece of RNA of 2.5×10^6 daltons, has a more complex pathway of replication, and their high frequency of genetic recombination is likely to be effected by enzymes making DNA rather than RNA (Cooper and Wyke, 1974).

6.1.1. Properties of Genetic Recombination in Picornaviruses

As in many instances in biology, the existence of genetic recombination in picornaviruses (Hirst, 1962; Ledinko, 1963b; Pringle, 1968; Cooper, 1968) can only be inferred from the observation of double mutants in the progeny of a cross in significant excess over spontaneous mutation. For poliovirus (Cooper, 1968), the proportion of excess double mutants is high (up to 30 times the spontaneous reversion background), reproducible, and characteristic of the parental pair and the genetic map derived from it has many properties (mentioned below) that give confidence in this inference.

6.1.2. Time of Occurrence of Recombination

Recombination between picornavirus genomes appears to be an early event. Although there is some increase in the proportion of poliovirus recombinants during growth, judging by assays of progeny harvested at intervals during the phase of maturation (Ledinko, 1963*b*; Cooper, 1968), still 68% of the recombinational events have occurred by the time that only 25% of the replicative events have taken place (Cooper, 1968). Similarly, the recombinant content of aphthovirus crosses as a percentage of total yield does not increase significantly during the period of infectivity increase (Pringle, 1968; MacKenzie *et al.*, 1975; Lake *et al.*, 1975). This is the converse of expectations from topographical factors, and presumably reflects some change in, or decrease in the accessibility of, templates during growth. Both vRNA and cRNA strands are expected to be involved because of the precise alignments mentioned below; in support of this, the presence of guanidine (which increases the cRNA strand content, Cooper *et al.*, 1970*b*; Caliguiri and Tamm, 1968) early in the cycle approximately doubles the recombination frequency (P. D. Cooper, unpublished).

6.1.3. Reciprocity of Recombination

The additivity of recombination frequencies in polio- and aphthovirus could not in theory be obtained without equal and reciprocal involvement of both parental strands. Direct evidence for this is so far lacking.

6.1.4. Recombination Frequencies

The frequencies for picornaviruses seem low in comparison with recombination of other RNA viruses (influenza, reo-, RNA tumor viruses), but these either have segmented genomes allowing a high degree of reassortment of discrete genetic elements or replicate via more complex mechanisms involving DNA. The genome of picornaviruses is small, and their recombination frequencies per codon are not in fact very different from those of conventional DNA systems, raising the possibility of some similarity in mechanism. In poliovirus, the total recombination frequency (assuming reciprocal crossovers) between the most distant markers averages 2.2%, equivalent to 1% per 1250 nucleotide pairs of the double-stranded form (Cooper *et al.*, 1975). Aphthovirus is similar (Lake *et al.*, 1975), but in addition presents evidence for a very low level of genetic recombination between different serotypes (MacKenzie and Slade, 1975). In phage T4 and *Escherichia coli,* the recombination frequencies are 1% per 200 nucleotide pairs (involving multiple rounds of mating) and 1% per 1750 nucleotide pairs, respectively (Hayes, 1968).

6.1.5. Possible Artifacts in the Recombination Test

A number of spurious effects that might conceivably have given rise to the appearance of recombination have been examined and ruled out. Reconstruction experiments (Cooper, 1968) showed that the recombinant type (ts^+) was not selected for or against during mixed growth with mutants at 37°C. Mutant virus in artificial mixtures with ts^+ had no effect on ts^+ plating efficiencies at 10 times its normal content in assays at restrictive temperature. Similarly, mixtures of mutants assayed at restrictive temperature gave the sum of the ts^+ contents of each assayed singly, so that no recombination or complementation occurred in the assay plate. This is indeed to be expected, as its cells were not mixedly infected and poliovirus recombination and complementation frequencies are by nature low.

The same applies to interactions that might occur between particles in a clump. Some poliovirus progeny are released in small aggregates, probably linked by membranous material, but are dispersed by pH 2.5 glycine buffer (Fenwick and Cooper, 1962). All assays included a dilution through this buffer (Cooper, 1968), and both sucrose rate zonal sedimentation analysis and UV light inactivation of progeny from a cross, of both parental and recombinant types, showed that clumps were not participating in the assays (Cooper et al., 1974). All virus stocks were also disaggregated by glycine buffer before the crosses were made.

The observed effect (increase in proportion of double mutants during mixed infection) might in theory not reflect genetic recombination but result from some increase in reversion frequency. (As mentioned, there is no *selective* enhancement of such revertants during the test.) This would be a function of mixed infection, since reversion frequencies in single infection are reasonably constant. However, evidence against reversion enhancement was provided by comparison of a property of revertants and recombinants (Cooper et al., 1974). The property was resistance to a synthetic growth inhibitor, 2-(3-chloro-p-tolyl)-5-ethyl-1,3,4-oxadiazole. The mutant $ts3$ was resistant, while ts^+ was sensitive, and ts^+ revertants from $ts3$ were covariantly sensitive. Such covariation is a useful test for mutations in the same schizon (Section 5.2), usually reflecting a second amino acid replacement elsewhere in the same schizomer (informational or internal suppression, Gorini and Beckwith,

1966) that partly or completely restores the conformation required for correct gene function. However, because the originally changed amino acid is rarely precisely replaced, the restored function is seldom identical to the original. Thus a range of revertants usually has a range of phenotypes that only approximates to the original wild type. When 29 ts^+ recombinants from the cross $ts3 \times ts20$ ($ts20$ is oxadiazole sensitive like ts^+) were compared with ts^+ (and $ts20$), all were equally sensitive to the oxadiazole. In marked contrast, ts^+ revertants from $ts3$ showed the wide range of sensitivities expected from internal suppression. The ts^+ recombinants seemed to have derived the oxadiazole-sensitive schizon (the structural protein region) *en bloc* from $ts20$ by crossing over, and not by reversion of the oxadiazole-resistant schizon of $ts3$

6.1.6. The Mechanism of Recombination in Picornaviruses

The characters of the recombinant particles enable us to consider the ways in which these characters could have arisen (Cooper *et al.*, 1974). Recombinant and parental particles were compared in the progeny of the cross $ts3 \times 28g$ by sucrose rate zonal centrifugation, by CsCl gradient centrifugation, and by UV inactivation. In all respects (S value, density, and UV inactivation kinetics), parental and recombinant types were identical. These tests should distinguish RNA contents that differed by 10–15%. Next, genetic segregation of one parental (ts) phenotype in a ts^+ recombinant stock was looked for. Gross ts segregation did not occur, but any small ts content could not be distinguished from spontaneous mutation, and so advantage was taken of parental mutants that were resistant to several inhibitors (guanidine, a synthetic thiopyrimidine, and the synthetic oxadiazole already mentioned). These would allow the detection of a very small amount of genetic segregation, or of gene duplication of the drug-resistant schizon. However, none (< 0.1%) was found among the progeny of 53 recombinant clones. Finally, the vRNA extracted from recombinant particles was the same size as parental or wild-type RNA.

These tests enable us to discard most of the ways in which pieces of vRNA could theoretically come together in a recombinant particle to provide a full set of genetic information. These include two or more full genomes, one full genome plus a fragment, two overlapping fragments (covalently joined or not), and two separate fragments whose sequences do not overlap. The only model remaining is of two covalently joined fragments closely similar to normal vRNA. In other words, the recombinants were entirely conventional virus particles containing one piece of normal vRNA.

The recombinant vRNA should indeed not occur in fragments, for the following independent reasons: (1) Wild-type infective RNA is one single-stranded piece (Baltimore, 1969), inactivated with a single hit by UV (Norman, 1960), by ionizing radiation (Ohlbaum et al., 1970), or by ribonuclease (Holland et al., 1960). (2) Fragments or inactive whole genomes generated by UV inactivation do not complement genetically even in large excess (Drake, 1958). (3) Complementation even between intact genomes is not very effective (Cooper 1965), provided that growth of both is restricted. (4) Translation of poliovirus RNA is initiated only at one or perhaps two sites (Section 9.7), so that random fragments are unlikely to be accurately translated; in any case, much overlapping of genetic material would be required to provide entire schizomers, involving a substantial excess of RNA in the recombinant particle.

These factors, and the self-consistent nature of the genetic map (Sections 7 and 8) argue strongly in favor of a precisely ordered molecular exchange or "crossing over" for genetic recombination in poliovirus, similar in end result to that of DNA systems (Hotchkiss, 1971). An obstacle to the acceptance of this idea has been the lack of suitable host enzymes for analogous processing of RNA, but recent research has turned up several candidates (Závadová, 1971; Béchet, 1972; Silber et al., 1972; Cranston et al., 1973; Pérez-Bercoff et al., 1974a,b,).

However, one is not obliged to assume the involvement of enzymes for breakage–reunion of RNA systems. Because of the limited base pairing in the poliovirus replication complex (Öberg and Philipson, 1971), it is possible that template dissociation *in vivo* could be appreciable. Thus poliovirus recombinants could well arise by reassortment of nascent chains plus replicase between templates, followed by precise realignment and continued replicase action on the new template. This is a form of copy choice. The relatively small double-stranded regions also raise problems for breakage–reunion models. The question of the mechanism of crossing over in poliovirus seems open for the present.

6.2. Genetic Complementation

Mixed infection by viruses with defects in different genes (i.e., cistrons) can in many cases allow virus growth, as each mutant contributes a functional gene product for the defective one made by the other. However, the degree of genetic complementation between picornavirus strains under conditions where neither can replicate is very inefficient. One pair of poliovirus *ts* mutants (*ts*5 × *ts*19, Cooper, 1965) was studied in some detail, using light-sensitive inocula to destroy uneclipsed virus. Complementation reproducibly occurred, up to 14 times the background of leak rate but only to some 0.1% of *ts*$^+$ yields, and only one strain appeared in the yield. The efficiency was lower or equally low between all other pairs of mutants tested (unpublished results), and in the hindsight of the grouping now obtained by means of the recombination map and its physiological characterization (Sections 7 and 8) there was no correlation with gene function. Those few pairs of mutants that failed to show complementation were exhibiting "interference-without-multiplication" (Section 6.7). Thus the concept of "cistron" cannot be applied to picornaviruses (Section 3). A similar lack of complementation has been stated to exist between a substantial number of *ts* mutants with different phenotypes from mengovirus (Bond and Swim, 1975) and from aphthovirus (Lake *et al.*, 1975).

The direct interpretation of these findings is that all mutants lie in the same complementation group or cistron, despite their different phenotype. This is indeed the implication of posttranslational cleavage in this system (Section 9), but it is not quite so simple, as separate functional units or schizomers are produced. Presumably a misfolding in one part of the primary translation product will induce an error in cleavage elsewhere, so that more than one schizomer will be incorrect. Intracistronic complementation of variable efficiency does occur in other systems, particularly for multimeric proteins (Fincham, 1966), but it seems that the polar effects on translation of polyschizonic systems introduce too many allelic defects to allow substantial intracistronic complementation. Multiple errors in configuration and cleavage caused by a single *ts* defect probably occur sometimes in one locus and sometimes in another in different cells, so that average cleavage patterns may not noticeably be changed, although some gross *ts* changes are found (Cooper *et al.*, 1970c; Garfinkle and Tershak, 1972; Bond and Swim, 1975).

A form of genetic "complementation" between enteroviruses can be efficient (Wecker and Lederhilger, 1964a; Agol and Shirman, 1964; Cords and Holland, 1964c; Cole and Baltimore, 1973a), provided that one strain can grow. This situation is not one of mutual assistance by complementary gene functions, but of asymmetrical rescue, and may not consist of more than a special case of phenotypic mixing (Section 6.4), since the defects involved are all in structural protein. Because phenotypic mixing is quite efficient between enteroviruses (as also is genetic recombination when account is taken of the small genome, Section 6.1.4.), the poor efficiency of complementation is not due to compartmentalization either of gene products or of replicating units.

6.3. Genetic Reactivation

Multiplicity reactivation of UV-inactivated poliovirus has been reported to occur at a very low frequency (Drake, 1958). However, although certain alternatives were ruled out, the probable contribution of clumps to the very small effect found has not been investigated.

6.4. Phenotypic Mixing

Mixed infection of serologically distinct picornavirus strains, within the enterovirus genus at least, allows a free mixing of subunits in progeny capsids (Ledinko and Hirst, 1961), amounting in some cases to complete transcapsidation or genomic masking, and alteration of the host specificity of the particle (Cords and Holland, 1964*b*; Wecker and Lederhilger, 1964*b*). This phenomenon indicates a substantial degree of homology between capsid structural units, and might be used with advantage to explore degrees of relatedness between picornavirus genera. Whether it occurs within or between structural units (e.g., whether VP1 from one strain is found within the same structural unit as VP2, VP3, and VP4 from the other strain, or whether each structural unit is derived from one strain only) has not been investigated, but consideration of the cleavage mechanism suggests that the latter is the case (Section 9.2). Phenotypic mixing between different serotypes of aphthovirus is rare, however (Pringle and Slade, 1968; Pringle, 1969).

6.5. Homologous Interference-with-Multiplication

Live poliovirus strains interfere markedly with each other in mixed infection (Ledinko, 1963*a*); this is not established until after the interfering virus has penetrated. UV-inactivated poliovirus does not induce interference (Drake, 1958), neither is there interference between equal multiplicities of different enteroviruses unless the interfering virus replicates for about 1 h before the challenge (Cords and Holland, 1964*a*). This does not indicate that some interfering event occurs at 1 h

postinfection, but rather that the interfering process needs a head start
of 1 h. Interference induced by a guanidine-sensitive enterovirus is
reversible when challenged with a resistant strain in presence of guanidine, and the same is true if the resistant challenge is of a different
genus (McCormick and Penman, 1968). The presence of molecules
involved in early virus synthesis does not accelerate the growth of a
guanidine-resistant challenge in presence of guanidine.

The nature of this interference, particularly its increase with head
start in replication or input messenger templates, suggests a competition for some limiting factor. Picornavirus RNA replication is self-
limiting in that the final yield of RNA is the same irrespective of
multiplicity of infection (Baltimore *et al.*, 1966). The reasons for this
are not known, but a likely explanation can be based on the half-life of
replicase and its kinetics of formation (Section 11). The change of
replication kinetics at about midcycle from exponential to linear
increase of vRNA (Baltimore *et al.*, 1966) means that viral proteins
now increase linearly instead of exponentially. The increase of any
labile component will then fail to keep pace with its spontaneous inactivation (which remains exponential), so that its pool size starts to
decrease about one half-life later. The half-life of poliovirus replicase
activity is about 15 min *in vivo* (Ehrenfeld *et al.*, 1970; Cooper *et al.*,
1975); the pool size of replicase may be quite large, but will bear a
constant relation to the amount of vRNA made at the time of change
of kinetics (which in turn is held to depend on the pool size of the
hypothetical regulator, Section 11), and will run down in a constant
time. Thus the total quantity of vRNA made will also be constant, as it
depends solely on the amount of vRNA made at the time of change of
kinetics and on the half-life of replicase activity *in vivo,* and not on the
makeup of the input vRNA. Interference between replicating vRNAs
accordingly seems to result from simple competition for this total pool
of vRNA, which is limited by the overall kinetics of replication.

6.6   Defective Interfering (DI) Particles

As with many viruses, repeated passage at high multiplicity
produces poliovirus particles in which portions of the genome are
deleted (Cole *et al.*, 1971; Cole and Baltimore, 1973*a*) and which
interfere with the growth of parental virus. Poliovirus requires a relatively large number of passes (>20), compared with, for example,
vesicular stomatitis virus (2–4, Cooper and Bellett, 1959). The defective
genomes are lacking up to one-third of the structural protein schizon,

and can only be isolated by rescue in mixed infection with standard parental virus, which provides normal capsid protein. This is a form of one-sided complementation. Interference between DI and standard virus (Cole and Baltimore, 1973*b*) appears to result from the same mechanism as that outlined for homologous interference-with-multiplication (Section 6.5), namely, that the total yield of vRNA made per cell is constant, and DI vRNA, being able to replicate normally, competes with standard vRNA in proportion to its input multiplicity. The DI virus would not be obtained without some selective advantage for the DI vRNA, which is observed to be enriched about 8% in each passage. The cause of this enrichment is not known, but may simply be that the cellular limit is on total mass of vRNA rather than number of molecules. Since the total mass of DI vRNA made at high multiplicity is about the same as that of standard vRNA (Cole and Baltimore, 1973*a*), and the molecular weight of the DI vRNA is some 10% less than that of standard vRNA, more DI vRNA molecules appear in the yield.

6.7.   Homologous Interference-without-Multiplication

A different situation exists in what has been called "interference-without-multiplication" (Pohjanpelto and Cooper, 1965). In this case, interference that can be even more effective than interference-with-multiplication can be induced by certain poliovirus strains under restrictive conditions, in which multiplication of the interfering virus and its RNA is largely prevented. Thus interference is not due to competition in vRNA replication. The restrictive conditions are either high growth temperature (interference induced by certain *ts* mutants with *ts*$^{+}$ as challenge) or the presence of guanidine (interference induced by guanidine-sensitive strains, with guanidine-resistant strains as challenge). Again, this is not a cell-surface phenomenon. A further study (Cooper *et al.*, 1970*a*) showed that it was the RNA replication of the challenge that was blocked, and that the temperature-induced interference property was restricted to those mutants that had been shown to have a single *ts* defect in structural protein. Only certain *ts* structural protein mutants had this interfering property, however. As the guanidine-resistance locus was also shown to lie in structural protein (Cooper, 1968; Cooper *et al.*, 1970*a*), it was concluded that vRNA replication depended on the configuration of structural protein, and that this was an instance of a genetically dominant inhibition by a misfolded product of the structural protein schizon. This conclusion has been interpreted to demonstrate the involvement of a product of the structural protein schizon in the regulation of poliovirus RNA replication (Cooper *et al.*, 1973, and Section 11.1).

6.8. Heterologous Interference

In mixed infection with viruses of other families (NDV, Marcus and Carver, 1967; Ito *et al.*, 1968; herpesvirus, Saxton and Stevens, 1972; VSV, Doyle and Holland, 1972; adenovirus, Bablanian and Russell, 1974), poliovirus rapidly and completely dominates unless given a substantial time and multiplicity handicap. This is not a matter simply of faster replication. In the case of VSV and herpesvirus, poliovirus interferes by shutting off synthesis of challenge virus polypeptides and inducing disaggregation of its polysomes even if added some hours after, when the challenge VSV or herpesvirus is committed to massive protein synthesis. Challenge virus nucleic acid synthesis is unaffected, and only translation, not replication, of poliovirus RNA is required. Poliovirus coinfection markedly reduces the quantity and rate of adenovirus message translation and consequent particle formation, but as adenovirus needs some early host protein synthesis, poliovirus also reduces its DNA replication. By restricting poliovirus replication with guanidine, cell proteins are selectively repressed, unmasking the VSV and adenovirus proteins.

In contrast, the maturation of SV5 in a firmly established 16-h infection was found to be little affected by poliovirus, which itself grew normally (Choppin and Holmes, 1967). Conceivably, poliovirus proteins and the late maturation proteins of SV5 were made by different machinery. Presumably, poliovirus would dominate as usual in simultaneous infection. Mutual interference occurred between vaccinia and mengovirus in simultaneous infection (Freda and Buck, 1971), but in the case of vaccinia the inhibition of host protein synthesis is probably effected by a preformed virion component (Moss, 1968). In general, the mengovirus predominated; Dales and Silverberg (1968) found that it dominated completely. Again, interference mainly affected vaccinia proteins made after 2–3 h rather than DNA synthesis.

The properties and kinetics of heterologous interference by picornaviruses are so similar to those of their repression of host cell protein synthesis (Section 8.2.1) that these activities seem likely to be one and the same. If the effect of poliovirus is to supply a component like an initiation factor with a high, perhaps irreversible, affinity for the 45 S ribosomal subunit (Cooper *et al.*, 1973), then this would override a virus that does not supply one, or would compete successfully with one of less avidity.

6.9. Interferon

Enteroviruses are not good inducers of interferon synthesis. A chick embryo-attenuated type 2 poliovirus was effective (Ho and Enders, 1959), and there was an inverse correlation between ability to replicate and interferon production (Ho, 1973). This may be expected from the marked repression of host protein synthesis when these viruses grow vigorously, which also seems likely to prevent the development of interference if picornavirus and interferon are added together.

Perhaps for this reason, picornaviruses are not good subjects for study of interferon action either. As with viruses of other families, interferon represses or delays synthesis of mengovirus proteins (Gordon *et al.*, 1966; Miner *et al.*, 1966), possibly by preventing association of vRNA with ribosomes (Levy and Carter, 1968). However, interferon does not block mengovirus cytopathic effect or repression of host protein synthesis (Levy, 1964; Joklik and Merigan, 1966) except in very large doses (Haase *et al.*, 1969), despite its interference with replication at much lower doses. This provides a paradox for the idea that the ribosome is the target both for interferon and for repression of host protein synthesis by picornaviruses. Conceivably, interferon and the picornavirus repressor molecule interact with different sites of ribosome function.

6.10. Implications for Gene Function

Section 8 will consider what gene functions can be ascribed to the picornavirus genome, as part of the attempt to define its activities completely. It is worth surveying the preceding paragraphs (Section 6) at this stage for the same purpose. The properties of genetic recombination have not suggested any novel function of the virus (e.g., a "recombinase") and can well be accounted for either by cellular enzymes or by copy choice of the known viral replicases. Genetic complementation and multiplicity reactivation are virtually absent, and phenotypic mixing appears to involve only the known viral structural unit. The several forms of interference can all be explained ultimately in terms of properties already predicted for the regulator (Section 11.1), either by its effect in limiting the size of the vRNA pool, or its effect (in a misfolded form) on vRNA replication, or its repression of host-protein synthesis. Thus there is no compulsion to involve any novel gene function to account for the various interactions of picornavirus genomes described above.

7. THE GENETIC RECOMBINATION MAP OF PICORNAVIRUSES

7.1. Obtaining a Map for Poliovirus

Early searches for genetic recombination in picornaviruses using poliovirus were not successful (Dulbecco, 1961; McBride, 1962). We now know that the markers then available were too closely linked, or too frequently covariant because they were in the same schizomers (structural protein). Recombination between poliovirus strains was reproducibly obtained by Hirst (1962) and Ledinko (1963*b*), using three noncovariant markers (*ho, bo,* and *g*, resistance to inhibition by certain batches of horse or bovine serum or by guanidine, respectively; Section 10). The equally spaced sequence *g-ho-bo* was determined by the appropriate crosses. Bengtsson (1968) has shown certain Δ (thermolability) and *m* (resistance to inhibition by dextran sulfate) markers to be close to *ho*, but the recombination frequencies were variable. All these markers unfortunately are in structural protein.

The isolation of poliovirus *ts* mutants (Cooper, 1964*a*) made possible a more extensive map, but quantitative mapping was not feasible until the system was more rigorously defined (Cooper, 1968). The most important factors were that (1) inocula for crosses and their progeny at the time of assay were not aggregated, (2) the revertant contents of the stocks used were kept very low by selection and limited passage, (3) assay conditions were closely controlled, and (4) double mutants were identified, mainly by reversion and recombination characteristics. Variation in recombination frequencies between assays was minimized by normalizing the frequencies (after a small subtraction for spontaneous reversion) in terms of concurrent standard crosses. This reduced the standard deviation to about 10% of the mean, and allowed the construction of a genetic map that was both additive and linear. The frequencies between a few main mutants were first accurately determined and the remaining mutants worked out from these a few at a time. Mapping was greatly helped by use of a guanidine-resistant strain (*ts28g*), giving some sequences unambiguously by three-factor crosses and allowing the site of the *g* locus to be accurately identified (Cooper, 1969).

These studies all used mutants isolated by mild mutagenization with 5-fluorouracil (Cooper *et al.*, 1966). Fresh isolations were made after mutagenization with HNO_2 (treating both intact virus and free RNA) and *N*-nitrosoguanidine, and with procedures that might be expected to mutagenize preferentially the 5′ and 3′ ends of the genome (Section 9.4) (Cooper *et al.*, 1971, 1975). Isolates were again mapped a few at a time, and in each case their physiological properties correlated exactly with their position in the existing map. The completed version of the poliovirus genetic map is given in Fig. 1.

7.2. Properties of the Genetic Map of Poliovirus

The recombination frequencies from crosses between mutants that gave other evidence of singularity were additive (Fig. 1). Their additivity gave sequences that were identical to those obtained with the guanidine three-factor crosses, and this has now been repeated using resistance to dextran sulfate and to two synthetic inhibitors, ethyl-2-methylthio-4-methyl-5-pyrimidine carboxylate (or S-7) and 2-(3-chloro-*p*-tolyl)-5-ethyl-1,3,4-oxadiazole (Cooper *et al.*, 1974, 1975).

The additivity also implies a linear map, as is expected from the linear nature of poliovirus vRNA, but the appearance of linearity could arise from a circular map if only a small contiguous part of it was covered by the mutants used. Some kind of circular structure still might be involved in the replication of picornavirus RNA (Brown and Martin, 1965; Agol *et al.*, 1972). However, studies on the scale of the poliovirus *ts* map (Section 7.3) indicated that it probably covered more than 80% of the genome, and was thus not a small part of a larger circular one but was in fact linear. As mentioned (Section 6.1.4), the recombination efficiencies obtained with poliovirus are comparable to conventional DNA systems in terms of the size of the genome.

The map showed an entirely self-consistent correlation with physiological defect (Section 8). These properties showed a gradation termed "asymmetrical covariation" (Cooper *et al.*, 1966; Cooper, 1969) in that mutants to the left of the map (replicase region) were defective in a larger number of properties than those to the right (structural protein region). This is now seen as probably reflecting a gradation in the amount of mRNA formed because of the nature of the defects: the mutants on the left make no RNA (double or single stranded), those in the middle make double-stranded RNA plus some single-stranded (messenger) vRNA, while those on the right make a good deal of vRNA.

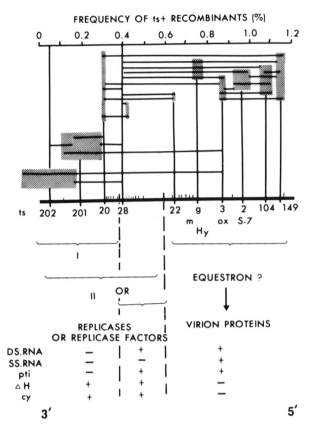

Fig. 1. Genetic recombination map of poliovirus temperature-sensitive mutants. The horizontal bars (top half) show the mean standardized recombination frequencies between the main mutants (*ts*202, etc.), and the hatched boxes show the maximum discrepancies in additivity. The loci for resistance to five inhibitors of poliovirus are also shown: *m*, dextran sulfate; *Hy,* 5-methyl-5-3,4-dichlorophenylhydantoin; *ox,* 2-(3-chloro-*p*-tolyl)-5-ethyl-1,3,4-oxadiazole; *S-7,* ethyl-2-methylthio-4-methyl-5-pyrimidine carboxylate; *g*, guanidine. The lower half summarizes the main tests on which the identification of map position with gene function is based, namely, synthesis of double-stranded (DS) and single-stranded (SS) RNA, prevention of host DNA synthesis (*pti*), thermal lability (Δ*H*), and cystine dependence (*cy*); + and − indicate wild-type or mutant response, respectively, at restrictive temperature. The 5′ end of the map is to the right.

7.3. Scale of the *ts* Map of Poliovirus

The first genetic map of poliovirus, comprised of 19 *ts* mutants, revealed a surprisingly small number of gene functions—three in all, prompting the suspicion that it may represent only a small portion of the genome. Such a possibility was examined in two independent ways:

(1) by a chemical estimation of the scale of the map and (2) by a second mutant isolation series designed in particular to extend the boundaries of the map.

7.3.1. The Chemical Approach

The coding potential of the poliovirus RNA was first redefined as accurately as possible. Earlier estimates of the molecular weight of poliovirus RNA ($1.2-2 \times 10^6$) by sedimentation velocities were much affected by secondary structure. Gel electrophoresis minimized these effects (Tannock *et al.*, 1970), and in comparison with several standard RNAs gave a molecular weight of $2.56 \pm 0.13 \times 10^6$, equivalent to 7320 ± 372 nucleotides and coding for a maximum of 2300–2600 amino acids. Centrifugation in denaturing solvents supported this value. In an electron microscopic study using only R17 RNA as a standard (Granboulan and Girard, 1969), the length of poliovirus double- and single-stranded RNA was equivalent to 7500 ± 400 nucleotides, or 2.6×10^6 daltons. Similar studies with other picornaviruses and comparison of their RNA contents, $A_{260:280}$ ratios, S_{20} values, particle diameters, and partial specific volumes with those of poliovirus (Rueckert, 1971; Newman *et al.*, 1973; Burroughs and Brown, 1974; Paucha *et al.*, 1974; Todd and Martin, 1975) indicate that all picornaviruses studied have RNAs of closely similar size. Estimates range from 2.3 to 2.9×10^6; the most probable value is close to 2.6×10^6, so that the maximum coding potential of all of them may be a little under 2600 amino acids.

The second step was to determine the size of a known segment of the poliovirus genetic map, i.e., of a particular gene in terms of its gene product. The most suitable was structural protein, as individual polypeptides in purified virions can be sized by gel electrophoresis. Unfortunately, their production by possibly ambiguous posttranslational cleavage (Section 9) (Cooper *et al.*, 1970c) allows the chance of overlapping amino acid sequences. Thus the total molecular mass of unique sequences, i.e., the total amount of genetic information in structural protein, can only be predicted to lie between 180 kdal (the total molecular mass of all structural proteins found) and 30 kdal (the molecular mass of VP1, the largest unit found in infective virus particles; Abraham and Cooper, 1975a).

This uncertainty was bypassed by comparing a count of tryptic peptides from purified virus, containing either methionine or histidine label, with its methionine or histidine content (Cooper and Bennett,

1973). These peptides should be largely independent of ambiguous cleavage, and the method assumes only that each segment of the coat protein sequence is evenly represented. A two-dimensional "fingerprint" should recover more label than column chromatography, and resolution of the theoretical total of 90 peptides was simplified by use of rare amino acids.

Reproducible peptide patterns, characteristic of each amino acid, showed that there were at least 21 and 25 (or integral multiples thereof) uniquely placed residues of histidine and methionine, respectively, in poliovirus structural protein of type 1, strain Mahoney. Their proportions, redetermined after correction for certain losses, were, respectively, 21 and 27 residues per 1000 amino acids recovered, indicating 1000 and 930 as the total of amino acids in the structural protein schizomer. In confirmation, tryptic peptide fingerprints of VP1, VP2, and VP3 (total molecular mass 84.5 kdal) are distinct, but together largely make up the fingerprint of the structural protein precursor NCVPIA (110 kdal) (Abraham and Cooper, 1975a,b). The possibility of integral multiples (2000 or 3000 amino acids) is ruled out by the limited coding capacity of poliovirus RNA.

Semiquantitative assay of the N-terminal amino acids in purified Mahoney virions with [^{125}I] p-iodophenylisothiocyanate in a modified Edman procedure gave a virtually identical result (Burrell and Cooper, 1973). N-Terminal aspartate, glycine, and serine were recovered in amounts equivalent to about 60 molecules of each per particle. The molecular mass of poliovirus RNA (2.6×10^6 daltons) and the RNA per particle (29% by N:P ratio, Schaffer and Schwerdt, 1965) then indicates 6.0–6.4×10^6 daltons of protein per virion, equivalent to 100–108 kdal or just under 1000 amino acids for the repeating structural unit.

As the coding capacity of poliovirus RNA is rather less than 2600 amino acids, the proportion of the genome occupied by the coat protein schizon is about 40%. The proportion of the genetic map represented by coat protein mutants is 48% (Cooper $et\ al.$, 1971, 1975). If the mutation sites are randomly distributed and map distance is approximately proportional to genetic distance, it follows that the genetic map covers a major portion of the genome.

7.3.2. Saturation with ts Mutants

The second mutant isolation series (Cooper $et\ al.$, 1971, 1975) used a variety of mutagenic procedures to obtain a further 18 ts mutants suitable for mapping. A particular effort was made to mutagenize preferentially either the 3′ or the 5′ ends of the genome and thus to extend the map (Section 9.4). However, virtually doubling the number of mutants in the map only extended its boundaries by 25%. No new physiological class of *ts* mutant was found by any mutagenic procedure, as the second set of mutants corresponded precisely with the first in physiological defect and map position.

Thus the *ts* map of poliovirus (Fig. 1) appears substantially saturated, again indicating (if all poliovirus genes are essential for viability) that the genetic map represents the major part of the genome.

7.4. The Genetic Map of Aphthovirus

As with poliovirus, a genetic recombination map of aphthovirus was not feasible (Pringle *et al.*, 1970) until sources of variation were more closely controlled (MacKenzie *et al.*, 1975; Lake *et al.*, 1975). Again, the most useful devices were three-factor crosses with guanidine-resistant *ts* mutants, and recombination frequencies normalized in terms of concurrent standard crosses. The result was a linear additive map, with the *g* locus near the middle (Fig. 2) (Lake *et al.*, 1975). Like poliovirus (Cooper *et al.*, 1974), the *ts*$^+$ recombinants bred true with no evidence of segregation. The recombination map of aphthovirus is stated to be correlated with physiological defect in that RNA production was limited to mutants on one side of the map (the right-hand side of Fig. 2). Increased lability at pH 6.6, an indication of mutation in structural protein, was also restricted to mutants on the same side of the map (MacKenzie *et al.*, 1975), including one mutant (*ts*16) mapping very close to the *g* locus. This mutant strongly supported the position of the *g* locus in the presumptive structural protein region, as it was itself guanidine resistant. Evidence on singularity or on covariant reversion with the *ts* defect is not yet available to confirm that this is the structural protein region. In general, the results are very similar to those of poliovirus.

8. RELATION OF GENETIC MAP TO GENE FUNCTIONS

8.1. The "Primary" Gene Functions of Poliovirus

Certain functions of picornaviruses are accepted as being carried out by polypeptides specified from the information in the viral genome. These are concerned with the formation of virion components, namely, the capsid and viral RNA, and comprise the structural protein and

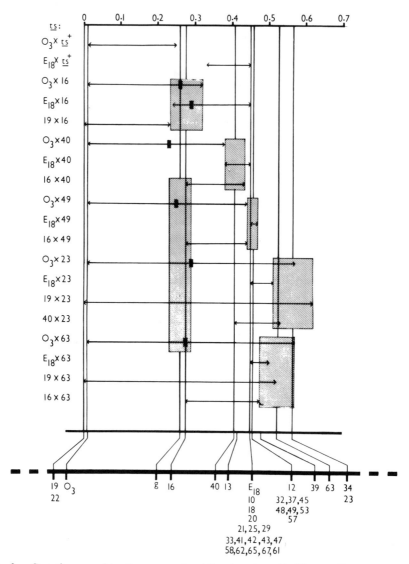

Fig. 2. Genetic recombination map of aphthovirus type O. The results are expressed as in Fig. 1. Mutants *ts*16, 10, 25, 29, 12, and 23 are labile at pH 6.6 (MacKenzie *et al.*, 1975). From Lake *et al.* (1975).

replicase schizons. They are referred to here as the *primary* gene functions of picornaviruses. Their detailed function (virion structure, RNA replication mechanisms, etc.) will not be considered. The evidence that the primary functions are indeed virus specified rests on their absence from uninfected cells, their induction (even in cells blocked in host syntheses) on addition of purified virus or its RNA, and their exhibition of specific mutations after mutagenic treatments of purified virus or its RNA, as detailed below.

The RNA is made by virus-coded RNA-dependent RNA polymerases (replicases), which are genetically separable (Cooper *et al.*, 1970*b*) into an activity (replicase I) to make the complementary or cRNA strand from invading vRNA templates and another (replicase II) to make progeny vRNA from cRNA templates. In confirmation of this two-step synthesis, two distinct RNA replication complexes with different activities have been separated from cells infected with aphthovirus (Arlinghaus and Polatnick, 1969) and poliovirus (Caliguiri, 1974). For both viruses, the smaller complex (20–70 S) contained and synthesized mainly double-stranded RNA, and therefore corresponded with replicase I activity. The larger complex (100–300 S) contained only a small amount of cRNA, synthesized mainly vRNA, and therefore corresponded with replicase II activity. Their sizes were in proportion to their activity *in vivo,* where much more vRNA is made than cRNA.

The *ts* genetic map of poliovirus has been related to gene function by studies of the physiological defects of the mutants. Many such tests have been made (Cooper, 1969). The most immediately useful was for a thermolabile virion (McCahon and Cooper, 1970; Mikhejeva *et al.*, 1970; Ghendon *et al.*, 1970), since (assuming that a single base change in the RNA is unlikely to affect its stability in the intact particle) this is almost certain to reflect a mutation in structural protein. Most of the mutants mapping in the right-hand half (Fig. 1 and Table 2) were found to be significantly less stable than ts^+ at 45°C (McCahon and Cooper, 1970), provided that cystine stabilization was avoided (Pohjanpelto, 1958). These mutants therefore had a change in structural protein. The linking of this stability defect with *ts* lesion to show that both occurred in the same schizomer was confirmed by covariant reversion studies (Section 5.2), in which three out of five ts^+ revertants were covariantly revertant to thermostability. Not all of the right-hand mutants were thermolabile but the thermostable ones all had some defect in maturation or assembly (Wentworth *et al.*, 1968), as they converted infectious RNA to infectious virions with low efficiency. None of the left-hand single mutants was thermolabile or had a defect in assembly.

These studies unequivocally identified the right-hand half of the map with structural protein. Many of the structural protein mutants required cystine for growth at the permissive temperature (Table 2), an interesting correlation that is not in all cases explicable in terms of defects in maturation and assembly and hints at some other role for structural protein (Section 11.1) This correlation was also confirmed by

TABLE 2
Significant Characters of Poliovirus Single *ts* Mutants[a]

Character of virus		Left (3')				Center									Right (5')							*ts*[+]
		202	201	20	81	28	46	96	44	150	94	22[b]	89	155	147	151	123	3	2	104	149	
Repression of host DNA synthesis	*pti*	−	−	−	−	+	+	+	+	+	+	+	+	+	·	·	+	+	+	+	+	+
Damage to cell chromatin	*chr*	·	·	−	−	+	·	·	·	·	·	+	+	·	·	·	·	+	+	·	·	+
Damage to cell membrane	*tb*	−	−	−	−	+	·	+	·	+	+	+	+	·	·	·	+	·	+	+	+	+
Replicase I activity	ssRNA	−	−	−	−	−	·	·	·	·	·	·	·	·	·	·	·	·	+	+	+	+
Replicase II activity	dsRNA	−	−	−	−	+	·	·	·	·	·	·	·	·	·	·	·	·	+	+	+	+
Infectious RNA production	iRNA	·	·	−	+	+	+	+	+	+	+	+	+	+	·	·	+	+	+	+	+	+
Interference with *ts*[+] at 39.5°C		·	·	+	·	+	+	+	+	+	+	−	−	+	+	+	+	+	+	+	−	+
iRNA maturation efficiency		·	·	·	+	+	+	+	+	+	−	−	−	−	−	−	−	−	−	+	−	+
Thermostability	ΔH 45°C	+	+	+	+	+	+	+	+	+	+	+	+	−	−	−	·	−	−	+	+	+
Cystine dependence	*cy*	+	+	+	+	+	+	+	+	+	−	−	+	−	−	−	−	−	−	−	−	+
Sensitive to 120 μg/ml guanidine	*g/120*	·	·	·	+	+	+	+	+	+	−	−	−	−	−	−	+	+	+	+	+	+
Sensitive to 10 μg/ml S-7	S-7	+	+	+	+	+	+	+	+	+	−	+	+	·	·	·	+	+	+	+	+	+
Repression of host protein synthesis	*psr*	+	+	+	·	+	·	·	·	+	+	+	+	+	−	·	·	+	−	+	·	+
"Early" or "late"		L	L	L	L	L	L	L	·	L	L	L	L	L	·	·	·	·	·	·	L	L

[a] +, Wild type; −, mutant at restrictive temperature; ·, not determined.
[b] *Ts22* is a double mutant, but both defects lie in structural protein.

showing a covariation of reversion from cystine requirement to cystine independence with reversion to ts^+ character (McCahon and Cooper, 1970).

Mutants in the left-hand half failed to show any structural protein defect but were defective in RNA synthesis (Wentworth *et al.*, 1968; Cooper *et al.*, 1970*b*, 1975). All seven mutants at the extreme left produced neither single- nor double-stranded RNA. Since at least several of these (listed in Table 2) gave good evidence of being single mutants, such covariation implies the involvement of this portion of the genome in the production of both cRNA from vRNA templates (replicase I activity) and progeny vRNA from cRNA templates (replicase II activity).

In contrast, mutant *ts*28, mapping in the middle, showed no defect in structural protein amd made double-stranded RNA efficiently, but made very little progeny vRNA. Thus the center region of the map is concerned with replicase II activity only. The evidence for two (genetically) separable replicase activities is based on this dichotomy. It does not indicate whether or not the two activities reside in the same molecule, i.e., whether the activities are chemically separable; neither can the abovementioned existence of two replication complexes indicate this until their viral proteins are identified. More mutants in this small central region should be tested, but suitable ones are rare.

Many poliovirus mutants mapping in the structural protein region are also somewhat defective in production of vRNA (Table 2). In fact, the *ts* mutants of all picornaviruses studied, not only poliovirus (Wentworth *et al.*, 1968; Cooper *et al.*, 1970*b*; Mikhejeva *et al.*, 1970; Fiszman *et al.*, 1970) but also aphthovirus (Pringle *et al.*, 1970) and mengovirus (Bond and Swim, 1975), show a wide range of defects in RNA synthesis, and some RNA-defective mutants are certainly also defective in structural protein. In the case of poliovirus, at least, this cannot be interpreted in terms of double mutations for the structural protein mutants, but is linked with the interference-without-multiplication effect (Table 2 and Section 6.7) and is suggested to be another expression of the dependence of viral RNA synthesis on the configuration of structural protein (Cooper *et al.*, 1970*a*). This aspect is considered in Section 11.1 in terms of the equestron hypothesis for the regulation of poliovirus replication.

8.2.   The Secondary Gene Functions of Poliovirus

Section 8.1 shows that the entire genetic map is taken up by the three primary gene functions of poliovirus, specifying structural protein, replicase I, and replicase II activities. Section 7.3 shows that this map represents most or all of the genome. Nevertheless, poliovirus has many other well-documented effects on cells, which are accordingly not accounted for by this map. The most prominent are the early or midcycle prevention of host protein, RNA, and DNA synthesis, and a variety of later changes culminating in cell membrane rupture and release of virus. In addition, poliovirus growth kinetics and logistics indicate a compelling need for a regulator (Section 11.1). The next sections summarize recent genetic evidence that most, if not all, of these are secondary effects arising from additional activities of two of the primary gene functions.

8.2.1. Early Metabolic Repressions by Poliovirus

The change first seen in cells infected by most picornaviruses is the repression of host protein synthesis (psr^+ character), which occurs 1–4 h after infection. It is more rapid with higher virus input, and depends on a virus protein that prevents entry of host mRNA into polysomes (Leibowitz and Penman, 1971, and references in Steiner-Pryor and Cooper, 1973). The nature of this protein might be shown by means of defective mutants, but searches for them have previously failed (Cooper, 1969; Cooper et al., 1971). However, since the psr^+ character is expressed fully in the presence of guanidine (Penman and Summers, 1965) when very little virus protein is made (Summers et al., 1965), only small amounts of the repressor protein are needed. Thus the "leak" (small synthesis of functional gene product at restrictive temperature) that is always present with ts mutants may well suffice to mask the repressor defect.

Fortunately, the finding of a product of the structural protein schizon associated with the smaller ribosomal subunit (Wright and Cooper, 1974a), and the implication of some control by structural protein of vRNA replication embodied in the equestron concept (Section 11.1), allowed the prediction that psr mutants might also be defective in structural protein. This turned out to be the case (Steiner-Pryor and Cooper, 1973): when leak was minimized by the presence of guanidine, the absence of cystine, and low virus input, ts defects in the psr^+ character were revealed and were confined to mutants defective in structural protein (Table 2). All six structural protein ts mutants tested were psr, while all five mutants (ts182 is not included in Table 2) ts in nonstructural functions were psr^+. This association of the psr^+ character with the structural protein schizon was confirmed by showing that three out of four independent ts^+ revertants from a structural protein ($psr \cdot ts$) mutant were also psr^+.

Despite the fact that picornavirus double-stranded RNA strongly inhibits protein translation *in vitro* (Ehrenfeld and Hunt, 1971) and *in vivo* (Cordell-Stewart and Taylor, 1973a), poliovirus *ts* mutants that are very defective in production of double-stranded RNA are not defective at all in the psr^+ character (Table 2) (Steiner-Pryor and Cooper, 1973). Thus double-stranded RNA is not the *in vivo* effector of host protein synthesis repression, as expected from the very small amounts found at the early times that repression becomes fully expressed. A similar conclusion was reached by Collins and Roberts (1972) for mengovirus, on the basis of drug inhibition of cytopathic effect and double-stranded RNA production but not host protein synthesis repression.

Accordingly, the repression of host protein synthesis by poliovirus appears as a secondary function of the schizon whose primary function is the specification of structural protein.

The repression of host RNA synthesis by poliovirus follows shortly after that of protein (Fenwick, 1963; Zimmerman *et al.*, 1963). Its cause is still unknown, but because puromycin stops the synthesis of RNA soon after that of protein in HeLa cells (Holland, 1963), these two effects of the virus are probably also linked. No direct association of viral protein with the DNA was found, although both DNA-dependent RNA polymerases I and II were affected (Garwes *et al.*, 1975). Mitochondrial RNA synthesis was not affected (Vesco and Penman, 1969). However, RNA synthesis is sometimes stopped sufficiently quickly to suggest some other cause; an interesting lipid induced by poliovirus that inhibits RNA synthesis (Ho and Washington, 1971) may be linked with changes in cell lipid metabolism (Section 8.2.4).

8.2.2. Late Cytological Changes

The secondary activity of the structural protein schizon in repressing host protein and probably RNA synthesis, as part of its proposed role as regulator (Section 11.1), offers a plausible explanation of the early effects of poliovirus growth. Another group of effects occurs later, comprised of repression of host DNA synthesis (pti^+ character), various visual changes (including some in chromatin, the chr^+ character), and rupture of the cell membrane as measured by uptake of trypan blue (the tb^+ character). They appear to depend on accumulation of some gene product distinct from that effecting the early changes

(Bablanian, 1972). This distinction is based on two findings: (1) duplication of the early effects (repression of host protein and RNA synthesis) in uninfected cells with puromycin or actinomycin does not duplicate the cytopathic effects, and (2) inhibition of virus by guanidine permits the early changes but not the late ones.

Cordell-Stewart and Taylor (1971, 1973ab) have shown that purified picornavirus double-stranded RNA is cytotoxic under conditions of no protein synthesis. This material rapidly reproduces the membrane damage typical of late picornavirus growth. The rate of cytopathic effect induced by virus growth is greater with higher yields of double-stranded RNA. Garwes et al. (1975) report the inverse correlation, namely that ts defects in membrane damage are restricted to poliovirus mutants specifically ts in making double-stranded RNA (Table 2). This is not due to the complete absence of all gene products under these conditions, since sufficient product is made to inhibit cell protein synthesis (Steiner-Pryor and Cooper, 1973). These results, briefly reviewed earlier (Cooper 1969), appear to provide the functional test to confirm that the membrane changes are directly caused by double-stranded RNA in vivo.

If double-stranded RNA is the in vivo effector of the late cytopathic effects, they are seen as a secondary activity of the replicase I schizon. This is a genetic function distinct from that causing the early effects, thus satisfying the requirement of the inhibitor studies. Certain alternatives, notably gross activation of lysosomal enzymes, do not show the required correlation and are probably an effect rather than the cause of the membrane changes.

8.2.3. Repression of DNA Synthesis

Poliovirus begins to prevent host DNA synthesis by 4 h after infection, i.e., later than host protein and RNA synthesis but much earlier than the membrane changes. Garwes et al. (1975) showed that the DNA effect does not result from the earlier ones, since antibiotic inhibition of protein and RNA synthesis only slowly affects DNA synthesis. Neither does the DNA effect cause the membrane changes, since addition of fluorodeoxyuridine to uninfected cells does not affect the membrane. Nevertheless, ts defects in repression of host DNA synthesis (pti) are exclusively associated with all the ts mutants that are defective in double-stranded RNA synthesis (Table 2) (Cooper et al., 1966). These mutants are also those exclusively defective in the chromatin changes (Table 2) (chr character), which may well be linked with the pti character. The DNA and chromatin effects are therefore also functions of the replicase I schizon. The effect of viral double-stranded RNA on DNA synthesis is not reported, although the DNA repression occurs before much double-stranded RNA has accumulated. Alternatively, replicase I may make use of, and sequester, cellular core enzymes relating to the *initiation* (the stage affected by picornaviruses, Ensminger and Tamm, 1970) of DNA synthesis, which happens to depend on an RNA polymerase (Kornberg, 1974).

8.2.4. Membranes and Lipid Metabolism

A maturation factor of poliovirus was suggested previously (Cooper *et al.*, 1971) by the enhancement of assembly of 13–14 S precursors into empty capsids by infected cytoplasm (Phillips *et al.*, 1968; Phillips, 1969). Noninfected cytoplasm will not suffice. However, this probably reflects a facilitation of assembly by added membranes carrying viral proteins, apparently 14 S subunits (Phillips, 1971; Perlin and Phillips, 1973), as the "factor" has properties of a lipoprotein and the capsid precursors will self-assemble in high concentration. The added infected membranes remove the concentration dependence of the assembly process, and may simply provide an adsorptive surface.

Reactions on membranes are also important in picornavirus translation (Penman *et al.*, 1964; Roumiantzeff *et al.*, 1971) and replication (Girard *et al.*, 1967; Caliguiri and Tamm, 1970a,b), as well as in morphogenesis. The rapid progress of these processes in a large cell may directly depend on high local concentrations of reactants confined to two dimensions on an intracellular surface, especially for the first few steps in translation and replication.

Poliovirus slightly deranges cellular lipid synthesis, causing an increase (1) in choline and glycerol uptake 3–4 h after infection and (2) of intracellular membranes that continues after RNA synthesis has reached its peak (Penman, 1965; Dales *et al.*, 1965; Mosser *et al.*, 1972a,b). Although these changes favor virus growth, there is no reason to ascribe them to specific viral functions. Indeed, all the viral products (single- and double-stranded RNA and proteins) have a high affinity for membranes and are found attached to them. The cell may "notice" a growing shortage of free membrane space, and respond with a general proliferation of membranes. This occurs despite the repression of host protein synthesis and the onset of late cytopathic effects, but is stopped if viral replication is stopped by guanidine. Amako and Dales (1967) speculate that phospholipid synthesis in picornavirus-infected cells may be stimulated by some lysolipids liberated by traces of lysosomal enzymes. A slight leakiness of lysosomes could well result from attachment of the various membrane-prone products of poliovirus to the lysosomal surface.

8.2.5. Virulence

Several of the markers originally selected for the genetic study of poliovirus vaccine strains (summarized by Cooper, 1969) were naturally concerned or associated with aspects of neurovirulence. Unfortunately, the virulence of poliovirus remains undefined in molecular terms, despite the existence of a well-characterized suite of *ts* mutants. The attenuated type 1 vaccine strain LSc contains several mutations, some of which are *ts* (Cooper, 1969; Ghendon *et al.*, 1973*b*). In that *ts* mutants of many viruses are usually attenuated, there seems to be some relation between *ts* character and virulence, and this also applies to poliovirus (Sabin and Lwoff, 1959; Ghendon *et al.*, 1973*b*), to echovirus-9 (Margalith *et al.*, 1969), to EMC virus (Pérol-Vauchez *et al.*, 1962), and to aphthovirus (MacKenzie, 1975; J. R. Lake, personal communication). However, the relation as studied in mutants of high or low leak rate and in *ts*+ revertants or recombinants was not absolute. For example, some mutants that were stable and very *ts* nevertheless retained full virulence so that the *ts* phenotype did not by itself confer attenuation. Since attenuation is so readily found among *ts* mutants, it does not seem feasible to ascribe virulence to a small specific gene. Perhaps attenuation is caused by, for example, changes in structural protein that affect virus entry into certain cells *in vivo,* and the fact that these changes may also confer temperature sensitivity may be a secondary circumstance.

8.3. Host-Controlled Modification and Nonpermissive Cell Systems

Two interesting and rather similar examples of apparently host-controlled modifications of picornaviruses were reported some years ago. A mutant strain of EMC virus (Hoskins, 1959) that could grow in sarcoma 180 cells (EMC virus normally cannot) was passed in a single 12-h cycle in mouse brain. This removed its ability to replicate in sarcoma 180 cells, which was restored by a single cycle of the mouse brain material in Krebs ascites cells. It is not clear whether the RNA itself loses its infectivity for sarcoma cells or whether it is a cell-surface effect. A mutant strain of coxsackievirus A-9 (identified by forming small plaques in rhesus cells; Hsiung, 1960) that could grow in *Erythrocebus patas* cells (this virus normally cannot) was passed in a single 8-h cycle in rhesus cells or mouse brain. This produced virus yielding predominantly large plaques, in a yield too large to suggest the selection of a subpopulation of large plaque variants. These phenomena should be tested in the light of modern concepts. For example, cleavage enzymes in mouse brain may produce an EMC virus structural unit, replicase, or regulator particle that is slightly different in the variant virus strain and is nonfunctional in sarcoma cells but works in Krebs cells, in which different cleavage enzymes restore the original schizomer.

The most familiar form of restriction in picornavirus growth occurs at the cell surface, as the cellular receptors for adsorption and uncoating are highly virus-specific. Infection can fail in, and side products be made by, a variety of ways at this stage (data and references in Shirman *et al.*, 1973; Lonberg-Holm *et al.*, 1975), while free RNA may be unrestricted in infectivity. A restriction in uncoating of EMC virus by HeLa cells can be partly relieved by nonreplicating poliovirus (Shirman *et al.*, 1973) in a process apparently involving host cell gene activity and distinguishable from genetic complementation. Host gene functions are also required for poliovirus growth under some other circumstances whose cause remains unclarified (Cooper, 1966; Schaffer and Gordon, 1966).

Intracellular instances of nonpermissiveness are also known (Buck *et al.*, 1967; Sturman and Tamm, 1966). The enterovirus GDVII (or murine poliovirus) growing abortively in HeLa cells (Sturman and Tamm, 1969) yielded <1% of the infective virus formed in BHK cells, while the 35 S vRNA yield was 10–30% and cRNA (in the double strand) was almost normal. Cytopathic effects were slow but eventually complete. A variant that grew in HeLa cells showed that the defect in the normal GDVII virus was mutationally minor. This phenotype closely resembles that of *ts* structural protein mutants growing under restrictive conditions (Wentworth *et al.*, 1968; Cooper *et al.*, 1970*b*): the normal GDVII virus growing abortively in HeLa cells is defective in a factor required for efficient maturation of the vRNA that has a feedback on viral RNA synthesis. It would be interesting if HeLa$^+$ GDVII strains could be shown to have covariant changes in structural protein.

A similar mengovirus nonpermissive system (Wall and Taylor, 1969, 1970) was taken further to show that the decreased vRNA synthesis was associated with its late degradation. Early RNA synthesis was normal. Fiszman *et al.* (1970) and Mikhejeva *et al.* (1973) compared *ts* and *ts*$^+$ strains of poliovirus, and concluded that a nuclease, possibly lysosomal, was activated later in the cycle and acted on *ts* and *ts*$^+$ strains alike. However, *ts* strains were more susceptible, presumably because their RNA production was restricted at the nonpermissive temperature for other reasons and could not keep pace with nucleolysis. In these mengo- and poliovirus systems, therefore, the degradation is an effect secondary to the main restriction in RNA replication.

For both GDVII and mengovirus growth in nonpermissive cells, an interpretation in terms of a faultily cleaved, structural protein-based regulator like the equestron that acts mainly in the second half of the cycle (Section 11) would fit the data well. It is worth looking at polypeptide cleavage in all nonpermissive picornavirus systems, in the first instance at proteins associated with translation and replication complexes, with a regulator in mind.

8.4. Summary of Picornavirus Gene Functions

The entire genetic map is taken up by the *primary* gene functions of picornavirus, namely to specify replicase I and II activities and structural protein. The genetic map represents most of the genome. The replicase I schizon is also involved in replicase II activity. All other effects of the virus seem to be secondary activities of these primary functions. The repression of host protein and probably RNA syntheses are secondary functions of the structural protein schizon, as may be the regulator activity (Section 11.1). The *in vivo* effector of the late cytopathic effects, including membrane rupture and release of virus, appears to be double-stranded RNA. These are therefore secondary effects of the replicase I schizon, as also are repression of DNA synthesis and changes in chromatin.

This virtually completes the catalogue of known picornavirus gene functions. A virus-specified maturation factor appears not to be required, and some intracellular membrane changes are probably indirect effects of virus replication. The quite varied intracellular interactions of picornavirus genomes (Section 6.10) do not suggest any novel gene functions, nor do their interactions with the intact animal. The proteases involved in cleavage are probably cell coded (Section 9.8). However, as mentioned below (Section 9.7), a substantial portion of the poliovirus genome is not translated, yet is apparently needed for infectivity.

9. RELATION OF GENETIC MAP TO GENE PRODUCTS

9.1. Mode of Production of Picornavirus Polypeptides

As detailed in this section, picornavirus RNA behaves *in vivo* and *in vitro* as though it has only one or perhaps two sites for the initiation of translation, so that most of its protein is made in one continuous polypeptide chain. Individual schizomers (functional polypeptides) are generated by a series of posttranslational cleavages (Summers and Maizel, 1968; Jacobson and Baltimore, 1968*b*; Holland and Kiehn, 1968; Black, 1975), presumably by highly specific proteases. The primary cleavages are almost all "nascent"; i.e., they occur while the new protein is attached to the translating ribosome. There are two or three main primary schizomers, subdivided by many secondary cleavages into some stable products and some labile intermediates that are themselves soon cleaved. One small primary product may not be produced by cleavage but by conventional initiation of translation and punctuation (see below).

These mechanisms have made it difficult to relate gene function to the observed gene products, particularly as the polypeptides of the main class of mutants (*ts*) cannot be distinguished in gel electrophoresis from the parental type. In addition, the large number of polypeptides has made existing nomenclature clumsy. An increasing practice is to designate viral polypeptides in terms of molecular mass, e.g., p110 for a polypeptide of 110 kdal (Abraham and Cooper, 1975*a*). This will be used with the existing nomenclature in what follows, as it helps to clarify anomalies in size relationships.

9.2. Structural Proteins

The structural polypeptides of picornaviruses are unambiguously identified in the virion, which does not appear to contain lipids or glycopeptides as integral components (Rueckert, 1971; Burness *et al.*, 1973; Drzeniek and Billelo, 1974). Comparison with tryptic peptides or cyanogen bromide digests from purified virus has identified the cleavage precursor of structural protein (Jacobson *et al.*, 1970; Butterworth *et al.*, 1971; Abraham and Cooper, 1975*b*) as a primary schizomer (NCVP1 for poliovirus) of about 100 kdal that is a little larger than the sum of the molecular mass of virion polypeptides. This is cleaved with a half-life of 5–10 min via intermediates into a 6 S structural unit precursor containing two virion polypeptides (VP1 and

VP3 for poliovirus) and an intermediate (VP0). The structural units as such are slowly created with a half-life of 30 min by a final "morphogenetic" cleavage (see review by Hershko and Fry, 1975), in which VP0 is converted to VP2 plus VP4. The schemes for several picornaviruses are outlined in Section 9.5.

Most laboratories have failed to separate structural proteins such as VP0, VP1, VP2, VP3, and VP4 chemically without completely denaturing them, indicating that they are very tightly bonded in the structural unit. This tight bonding (and considerations of efficient assembly) suggests that, once the precursor NCVP1 (p110) has taken up the initial configuration that allows its specific cleavage from the nascent chain, it remains as a physically distinct, tightly bonded entity no matter how many cleavages have occurred and until it is finally assembled into the virion as a structural unit (Cooper and Bennett, 1973). This might be investigated via phenotypic mixing experiments (Section 6.4). The final cleavages may occur at slightly different loci in closely related strains (Cooper et al., 1970c).

9.3. Replicase Proteins

In contrast, purified picornavirus replicases are still undefined and so the actual polypeptides with replicase activity are not known. Since the genetic map indicates distinct regions for structural and replicase proteins (Section 7.2), the replicase polypeptides are presumably the major primary schizomers whose tryptic peptides are distinct from structural protein [for poliovirus, NCVP1B (p90) and NCVPX (p31), or cleavage products thereof; see Fig. 3].

Several viral polypeptides have been found specifically associated with various replicase activities of undefined purity. The only viral polypeptide found in a highly purified poliovirus (type 1) RNA polymerase preparation was NCVP4 (p58, Lundquist et al., 1974); p58 (of type 2 poliovirus) was labeled after pactamycin treatment as if it were a cleavage derivative of p79 or NCVP2 (see Fig. 3) (Butterworth, 1973), and so, if it is analogous to p58 of type 1 poliovirus, it is specified by the replicase region of the genome. It is not yet reported what other proteins are present, whether this preparation is equivalent to replicase I or replicase II or both, or whether it can only extend existing chains rather than initiate new ones on exogenous templates. All these activities are required of the complete enzyme(s). Predominantly NCVPX (p31) plus some NCVP2 (p79), but also a little of a peptide around 60 kdal, were found to be enriched in the smooth membrane fraction of infected cells (Caliguiri and Mosser, 1971; Wright and Cooper, 1976), which carry the RNA "factories" and comprise a crude replicase preparation. However, when freed of membranes the only polypeptides left attached to the replication complex were VP0, VP1, and VP3 (Wright and Cooper, 1976). These structural protein precursors are likely mainly to reflect virions in process of assembly (Caliguiri and Compans, 1973; Fernandez-Tomas and Baltimore, 1973), but may also include the presence of a regulator protein (Cooper *et al.,* 1973). They were not present as empty capsids. Two polypeptide aggregates could be separated by zonal electrophoresis from poliovirus-infected cytoplasms, one comprised of VP0, VP1, and VP3, and the other containing only NCVP2 and NCVPX (Korant, 1973).

A purified polycytidylate-dependent RNA polymerase from EMC virus-infected cells contained polypeptides of molecular mass 72, 65, 57, 45, and 35 kdal (Rosenberg *et al.,* 1972). Unfortunately, virus-specified proteins were not identified (e.g., by labeling with amino acids and correlation with whole cytoplasm), and so these might be host proteins unrelated to viral replicase. Their total molecular mass exceeded the virus coding capacity, and individually resembled those of subunits of $Q\beta$ replicase, which includes some host components. Poliovirus mutants *ts* in replicase I activity are all also specifically defective in repression of host DNA synthesis (Garwes *et al.,* 1975), so that host polymerase proteins might be involved with the replicase I function (Section 8.2.3).

In summary, NCVP1B or p90 [or cleavage product(s), perhaps NCVP2 or NCVP4] and NCVPX are implicated in several ways as being involved with replicase activity, possibly as replicase factors rather than complete enzymes. However, polypeptide associations with enzyme preparations must be regarded as circumstantial for the present, in the absence of rigorously purified material. It is also a pity that one often cannot be sure of the identity of polypeptides found in different laboratories because of small divergences in size estimations.

One more problem associated with cleavage needs mention. Since poliovirus or aphthovirus replicase activity is labile at 37°C *in vivo* (half-life about 15 min, Ehrenfeld *et al.,* 1970; Manor *et al.,* 1974; Cooper *et al.,* 1975) but usually not *in vitro* (G. A. Tannock and P. D. Cooper, unpublished; Manor *et al.,* 1974), the replicase itself may be undergoing cleavage. Thus one cannot assume that the polypeptides with replicase activity are stable end products like NCVP4. For this reason, and for others involving correct nucleation of nascent protein (Section 9.7), cleavage products derived from the replicase schizon (and, as they are chemically like the actual replicase schizomers, with affinity for vRNA) do not necessarily have any replicase activity.

In sum, the system is so complex that the only acceptable criterion is of individually homogeneous separated polypeptides whose reconstitution with vRNA or cRNA yields replicase I or replicase II activities, respectively.

9.4. 5′-3′ Orientation

The question of which region of the poliovirus genome is translated first, i.e., which is nearest the 5′ end, has been approached in two ways.

The approach involving the least assumptions used pactamycin to differentially inhibit the rate of label incorporation into various products of poliovirus translation (Summers and Maizel, 1971; Taber *et al.,* 1971; Rekosh, 1972). This has been referred to as "genetic mapping," although *per se* it gives information only on polypeptide products rather than on genes. At certain low concentrations, pactamycin inhibits initiation of translation much more than chain elongation: a delay in addition of label after such pactamycin treatment then allows the ribosome to move away from the 5′ end, thus decreasing the amount of label in products of the genome nearest the 5′ end. The method can be applied only to a monocistronic message comprising a single sequence of translation.

This approach has since been applied to EMC, mengovirus, and rhinovirus (Butterworth and Rueckert 1972*b*; Butterworth, 1973; Paucha *et al.,* 1974), and shows unambiguously that in each case it is the precursor of structural protein that is least heavily labeled after such delay and is accordingly nearest the 5′ end. Since the replicase schizomers are unidentified (replicase action could in theory be a secondary function of structural protein), this method does not by itself reveal the position of the replicase schizon nor of any other possible gene function.

A biological approach was taken by Cooper *et al.* (1971, 1975). Many separate attempts were made to mutagenize preferentially the 3′ or 5′ end of poliovirus RNA, by two procedures involving the addition of 5-fluorouracil under certain conditions restricting replication. A number of assumptions were involved that could not be tested directly. However, the procedure predicted to mutagenize mainly the 3′ end produced only two mutants suitable for mapping (*ts*201 and *ts*202), but both were located at the far left of the map (Fig. 1). Like all other mutants in that region, they were defective in replicase I and II activities. In contrast, the procedure predicted to mutagenize mainly the 5′ end produced many mutants, nearly all of which were defective in structural protein. Thus the biological experiments support and extend the pactamycin studies, namely, to show that the structural protein region is nearest the 5′ end and the replicase is nearest the 3′ end.

9.5. Cleavage Pathways

The cleavage patterns are predictably complex, as a small number n of cleavage sites can in theory produce $\frac{1}{2}(n + 1)(n + 2) - 1$ different schizomers (Cooper, 1969).

The use of pactamycin discussed above has been extended to the practical limit of the method to suggest the cleavage relationships for the schizomers of poliovirus, EMC virus, mengovirus, and rhinovirus (Summers and Maizel, 1971; Taber et al., 1971; Butterworth and Rueckert, 1972b; Butterworth, 1973; McClean and Rueckert, 1973; Paucha et al., 1974). Prevention of initiation with 150 mMNaCl gives the same result, but has the advantage of being reversible (Saborio et al., 1974). These pathways are summarized in Fig. 3. The results with aphthovirus are virtually identical (D. N. Black, D. V. Sangar, and D. J. Rowlands, personal communication).

5′		POLYPROTEIN (p204–216)			3′
Poliovirus (types 1 and 2)	1A (p110) 3 (p63) VP0 (p35) VP4 (p8)	VP2 (p27)	VP3 (p25)	VP1 (p31)	X (p31)	1B (p90) 2 (p79) 4 (p58)
Rhinovirus type IA	92 67 ε (p39) δ (p8)	β (p30)	γ (p25)	α (p35)	47 38	84 76 55
EMC virus	A (p100) B (p90) D1 (p65) ε (p40) δ (p9)	β (p30)	γ (p23)	α (p34)	F (p38)	C (p84) D (p75) E (p56)
Mengovirus	A (p114) B (96) ε (p40) δ (p11)	β (p30)	D2 (p58) γ (p24)	α (p33)	G (p16) F (p38) H (p16) I (p13)	C (p88) D (p77) E (p57)

Fig. 3. Pactamycin maps of the gene products of several picornaviruses (Summers and Maizel, 1971; Taber et al., 1971; Rekosh, 1972; Butterworth, 1973; Butterworth and Korant, 1974; Paucha et al., 1974).

Such studies are based on a number of assumptions, including constancy of amino acid pool sizes, equivalent amino acid composition of and random amino acid distribution in various proteins, the feasibility of quantitative assays from peak heights in gel extracts, constancy of rates of ribosomal readout, and the total lack of effect of pactamycin on chain elongation. It seems difficult to allow for the rates of labeling of intermediates of variable stability that may comigrate with stable peaks, and of schizomers of overlapping sequences produced by alternate pathways. In particular, the method assumes that there is only one site for initiation of translation; if there is a second site (the possibility of which is suggested below), the apparent location in the pactamycin or high-salt maps of the products of the second cistron will depend on its relative kinetics of initiation, of blockage of initiation, and of translation. Appropriate differences in these parameters could explain all results obtained so far, which accordingly do not rule out the presence of a second cistron.

Nevertheless, the experiments have given a similar picture for several picornaviruses, namely that there are only three main (primary) schizomers, and the largest (structural protein) primary schizomer is nearest the 5′ end, the smallest one is in the middle, and the third, almost as large as the first, is toward the 3′ end (Fig. 3). Based on the genetic map, the last two presumably include the replicase sequences. These primary schizomers may be subdivided in various ways. Because of the assumptions listed above, some reservations must be attached to the pathways summarized in Fig. 3. The nature of the experiment suggests that the most reliable assignments are to the first product in each sequence (NCVP1A in the polyprotein, VP0 in NCVP1A, and VP4 in VP0), and the last (NCVP2, NCVP4).

Attempts to follow pathways by kinetic analysis (Butterworth and Rueckert, 1972a; Abraham and Cooper, 1975a) had only limited success. The most convincing indications of pathways have been obtained by tryptic peptide analysis of electrophoretically isolated polypeptides (Jacobson et al., 1970; Butterworth et al., 1971), and for this purpose two-dimensional fingerprints of peptides labeled with a rare amino acid ([^{35}S]methionine) and detected by autoradiography have proved the most sensitive for assessing degrees of relatedness (Abraham and Cooper, 1975b) (see Fig. 5). By this means it was ascertained that, in poliovirus, NCVP1A (p110) contains the same amino acid sequence as virion protein, and NCVP1B (p90) is distinct from NCVP1A, but contains the sequences of NCVP2 (p79); VP0 is similarly confirmed as the precursor to VP2. However, additional and rather surprising information was obtained, which is discussed in Section 9.7.

Gel electrophoresis of a given purified picornavirus preparation gives polypeptide bands that can often be resolved into two or more components (Cooper *et al.*, 1970*c*; Vanden Berghe and Boeyé, 1972; Phillips and Fennell, 1973). Their combined molecular mass may be considerably greater than the apparent coding capacity of the genome for structural protein. The ts^+ poliovirus strain used for genetic analysis was derived from strain Mahoney, yet several of their virion polypeptides differ; however, an apparently single mutation in ts^+ (yielding strain *ts*2) restored a pattern very close to that of Mahoney (Cooper *et al.*, 1970*c*). This led to the concept of "ambiguous cleavage," in which the polypeptide cleavage precursors are supposed to have alternative, mutually exclusive cleavage sites situated not far apart in the amino acid sequence. Cleavage at one site in preference to another yields schizomers of different sizes, yet containing the same overall sequences. Similar findings, which are expected to have similar causes, are found in some of the normal cleavage patterns of nonstructural proteins summarized in Fig. 3 and in the slightly different electrophoretic patterns induced by different inhibitors of cleavage (Abraham and Cooper, 1975*a*).

9.6. Information from *in Vitro* Translation

The amount of separated EMC, mengo-, aphtho-, and poliovirus vRNA translated in mammalian cell-free extracts is variable and rarely complete (Smith *et al.*, 1970; Ascione and Vande Woude, 1971; Dobos *et al.*, 1971; Eggen and Shatkin, 1972; Kerr *et al.*, 1972; Boime *et al.*, 1971; Boime and Leder, 1972; Villa-Komaroff *et al.*, 1973; Esteban and Kerr, 1974). As judged by amino acid-labeled tryptic peptides, the *in vitro* products resemble the *in vivo* ones, although products of the structural protein region predominate *in vitro*. This is perhaps to be expected from its proximity to the site for initiation of translation. However, noncapsid tryptic peptides may be found in the yield (Dobos *et al.*, 1971; Kerr *et al.*, 1972; Esteban and Kerr, 1974). In general, up to 60% of the genome may be partially or completely translated *in vitro*, apparently from a common initiation site, in the correct reading phase and producing discrete polypeptides of sizes up to 140 kdal. Not much cleavage occurs and the vRNA is not broken down, but translation is prematurely terminated at unique "preferred sites" (Kerr *et al.*, 1972; Boime *et al.*, 1971; Boime and Leder, 1972). Much the same picture was found with poliovirus polysomes initiated *in vivo* but translated *in vitro* (Roumiantzeff *et al.*, 1971), although tryptic peptides were not examined. Use of an *E. coli* ribosome system did not give fidelity of initiation (Rekosh *et al.,* 1970).

Using [^{35}S]formylmethionyl-tRNA$_f$, predominantly one peptide was labeled when free vRNA was the message (Villa-Komaroff *et al.,* 1973; Smith, 1973; Öberg and Shatkin, 1972, 1974). This fMet initiation peptide forms part of a "lead-in" sequence of some 20 amino acids that includes *N*-terminal methionine and is rapidly cleaved away *in vivo*. Methionine is the initiator amino acid for poliovirus protein in intact cells (Chatterjee *et al.,* 1973).

9.7. Is Picornavirus RNA Comprised of Two Independent Translation Units?

These *in vitro* studies, and the *in vivo* cleavage patterns, all strongly imply that there is only one site for initiation of translation of picornavirus RNA, and therefore that it is comprised of only one cistron. However, none of them really rules out the possibility of a second cistron *in vivo*. In some cases (Öberg and Shatkin, 1972, 1974; Smith, 1973), up to 10% of the formylmethionine label in tryptic or chymotryptic digests was found in a second peptide, although this may have represented an overdigestion artifact. Also, the early lead-in sequence (Met-Ala-Thr-X · · ·) may be the same for each initiation site, giving only one pronase digestion peptide for two distinct sites. Most of the ribosomes ceased translation *in vitro* before the middle of the message, and the "preferred sites" for premature termination are probably particular locations of secondary structure of different avidities that stop the ribosome (it is known that poliovirus vRNA has marked secondary structure *in vitro*). Thus a second initiation site, away from the 5′ end, may be relatively inaccessible to ribosomes *in vitro*, particularly as most of these studies used "unprimed" ribosomes from noninfected cells. It is clear that any second cistron could comprise only a small portion of the genome. *In vivo*, secondary structures may be minimized by extension of the vRNA on membranous surfaces, and it would be interesting to look for *in vitro* initiation sites using rough membranes and ribosomes from infected cells.

The possibility of a second cistron has been emphasized by size estimations of poliovirus polyprotein and schizomers in relation to genome size (Abraham and Cooper, 1975a).* This study aimed at a

---

* **Note Added in Proof:** Convincing evidence for two different sites for *in vitro* initiation of translation of endogenous or exogenous poliovirus RNA has been reported by Celma and Ehrenfeld [*J. Mol. Biol.* **98**:761 (1975)].

definitive balance sheet between coding capacity of the vRNA (up to 2600 amino acids, Section 7.3.1) and amount actually translated. Particular attention was paid to molecular mass determinations in polyacrylamide gel electrophoresis, notably in the use of ^{125}I-labeled standard proteins incorporated into the same gel, more fully denaturing gel conditions, and linear relations between mobility and logarithm of molecular masses up to 210 kdal. By high-resolution autoradiography (using [^{35}S]methionine), at least 26 distinct poliovirus polypeptides were found in normal growth *in vivo,* and a total of at least 34 were found which had various modifications of cleavage. The size of the largest translation product was the same under several different conditions minimizing cleavage and was presumably the primary polyprotein (NCVP00). In many determinations under conditions suggesting full denaturation, it always migrated very close to myosin (molecular mass 200–210 kdal) and was designated p210 (Fig. 4). The two major primary schizomers, NCVP1A and NCVP1B, reproducibly had mobilities that led to the designations p110 and p90 (Fig. 4).

A value as low as 210 kdal for NCVP00 was first reported by Jacobson *et al.* (1970), with several reservations: (1) NCVP00 revealed by incorporation of amino acid analogues may have an altered electrophoretic mobility, (2) molecular mass determinations above 100 kdal may not be valid in gel electrophoresis, and (3) the molecular mass sum of the major primary schizomers (NCVP1 + NCVP2 + NCVPX = 250 kdal) exceeded that of NCVP00 (210 kdal). However, in answer to reservation (1), the migration rates of NCVP00 obtained by restraining cleavage with TPCK or TLCK, or by incubation at 43°C, or by several different amino acid analogues used separately were the same (Abraham and Cooper, 1975a). In answer to reservation (2), linearity between mobility and logarithm of molecular mass was obtained over the range 10–210 kdal, by using low gel strengths. Similar results have been obtained by Paucha *et al.* (1974) and Butterworth and Korant (1974) for the mengo-, EMC, polio-, and rhinovirus systems with different sets of marker proteins, namely, 204–216 kdal for the apparent polyprotein, and about 110, 90, and 40 kdal for the three primary schizomers analogous to NCVP1A, NCVP1B, and NCVPX, respectively. The potential coding capacity of these genomes was 250–270 kdal. But, in confirmation of reservation (3), there does not seem to be room for either NCVPX (polio) or its analogues in other picornaviruses in the primary polyproteins.

A value as low as 210 kdal for the polyprotein implies that 20% of the poliovirus genome, or 1500 nucleotides, either is not translated or is

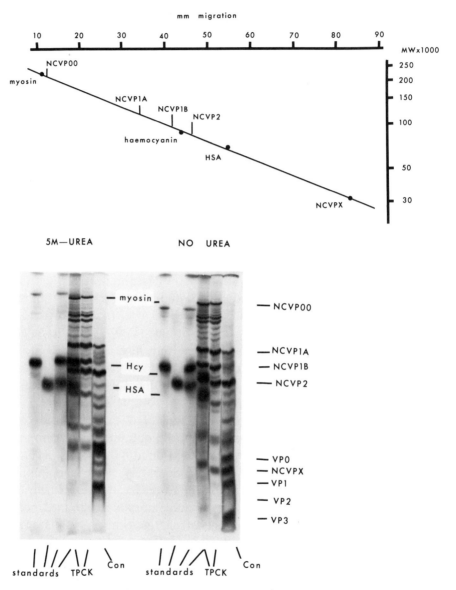

Fig. 4.   Mobility in 6% acrylamide gels, containing 5 M urea (left) or no urea (right), of the three standards myosin, hemocyanin, and human serum albumin in comparison with poliovirus-infected cytoplasms. The standards were labeled with ^{125}I and the virus proteins with [35S]methionine, which can be distinguished in a mixture by autoradiography. Cleavage was inhibited in some cultures by 0.12 mM TPCK; the fourth gel in each sequence was a coelectrophoresis of the TPCK-treated cytoplasm with the standards, in which the position of the standards is indicated (center). The graph (top) indicates the relation between mobility and molecular weight; the molecular weight of NCVPX was obtained in separate gels with other markers. From Abraham and Cooper (1975a).

in part translated as an independent cistron. Only a small portion (100–150 nucleotides) is 3′-terminal poly(A) (Yogo and Wimmer, 1973), although this appears to be necessary for infectivity (Spector and Baltimore, 1974). Despite the presence of several ribosome binding sites, only 400 nucleotides, or 10%, of the ribophage R17 RNA are not translated (Cory et al., 1972).

More compelling data are the following. When the two-dimensional tryptic fingerprints of NCVP1A (p110) and NCVP1B (p90), labeled with [^{35}S]methionine and isolated from gels, were compared, spot by spot, with that of NCVP00 (p210), it was found that the amino acid sequences of p110 and p90 had scarcely any overlap but were both contained in p210 (Abraham and Cooper, 1975b) (Fig. 5); p110 was confirmed to have the same fingerprint as virion protein, and NCVP2 (p79) was found to be contained in p90. In contrast, the fingerprint of the smallest primary gene product NCVPX (p31) was quite distinct from p210, p110, p90, p79, VP0, VP1, VP2, and VP3 and from two components (p168, p155) that contained p90 and should overlap the NCVPX region if it lay between p110 and p90. The tryptic peptide and size relationships of this study are summarized in Fig. 5.

Thus (1) the close correspondence of the molecular mass of p210 with the sum of p110 and p90, (2) the distinct nature of the peptide map of p31, and (3) the fact that p210 accounts for only 80% of the coding potential of poliovirus RNA together oblige us to consider the heterodox possibility that p31 is specified by a second cistron. The conclusions for other picornaviruses are the same, although tryptic fingerprints are not yet available. It is worth measuring the size of polyproteins of picornaviruses by an independent chemical assay, e.g., of content of N-terminal amino acid. An independent cistron for NCVPX is presumably located near the 3′ end, and as NCVPX has been implicated with replicases (Section 9.3) would not conflict with the genetic map. Although complementation tests between the main mutants of Fig. 1 failed to detect two cistrons (Section 6.2), mutants defective in a small cistron comprising only 15% of the genome at its extreme 3′ end may not have been isolated.

A need for a separate translation unit in picornavirus RNA is not clear, but let us consider the mechanisms proposed for the folding during synthesis of large proteins (Wetlaufer and Ristow, 1973), i.e., those that do not readily renature after denaturation. Their normal tertiary conformation may not represent the lowest energy state of the entire structure, but rather is probably determined by "nucleation," i.e., the folding to the lowest energy state of the first 20–30 amino acids

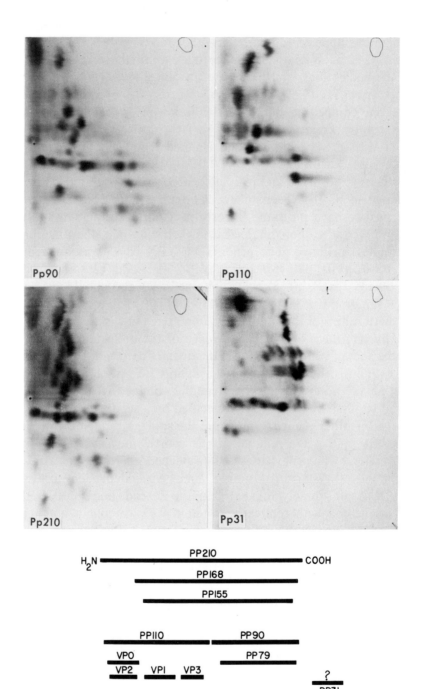

polymerized. The rest of the chain then folds along the guidelines of this nucleus. For cleavage of picornavirus polyproteins, such initial nucleation raises no problem for the first schizomer in the sequence (structural protein). In contrast, the "initiation" of the second schizomer (i.e., its cleavage from the first) is random and delayed by a variable number of amino acids from its N-terminus, which itself may not be uniquely defined. Thus its nucleus is probably variable and its conformation often "incorrect." This could explain why the main product of the poliovirus nonstructural schizon (NCVP2), although prominent in cytoplasms, is rarely found in replicase preparations. By extension, the proportion of "correct" products of any third schizon in a long translation train may be vanishingly small, and so a monocistronic message as big as picornavirus RNA may be self-limiting to two schizons only. If there is a second cistron that can be translated conventionally, it does of course raise the question of why the first cistron must be subdivided by cleavage, unless it is to achieve two replicases for the price of one, by ambiguous cleavage.

9.8. Cleavage Enzymes

The enzymes responsible for subdividing the polyprotein are highly specific, as the schizomers are of a reproducible size, with nonrandom N-termini (Laporte, 1969; Burrell and Cooper, 1973) and C-termini (Bachrach et al., 1973), and host protein is not degraded (Kiehn and Holland, 1970). A specificity pattern is emerging in that most picornavirus structural protein precursors, and other specifically cleaved serine esterase substrates such as fibrinogen, prothrombin, chymotrypsinogen, trypsinogen, and proinsulin, on cleavage yield virtually exclusively N-terminal Gly (or Ala), Asp (or Glu), Ser (or Thr), or Ile, but conformational factors are probably equally important. In one instance (ts89, Cooper et al., 1970c), a single ts defect caused many errors in the cleavage process. Larger conformational differences in the viral protein can lead to its rapid and virtually complete proteolysis

---

Fig. 5.   Relation (lower diagram) between the primary polyprotein of poliovirus (Pp210) and virion proteins (VP2, VP1, VP3), some cleavage intermediates, and the anomalous product Pp31, as indicated by tryptic peptide autoradiographs (exemplified by the four upper prints) of bands isolated from polyacrylamide gels. Pp110, NCVPIA; Pp90, NCVP1B; Pp79, NCVP2; Pp31, NCVPX. The origin is at the black dot, center left of each print; the phenol red marker is outlined at the top right of each print. From Abraham and Cooper (1975b).

(Garfinkle and Tershak, 1972; Cole and Baltimore, 1973a). Product precursor molecular mass comparisons suggest that interjacent sequences are often lost in normal cleavage.

Coxsackie B1 virus produces only one polypeptide species after 3.5 h (Kiehn and Holland, 1970). This suggests that cleavage activity may have increased during infection and thus may conceivably be virus coded. If so, it would have to be a function of the first polypeptide translated, one that could "bite its own tail off." However, such a change in polypeptide pattern has not been found with any other picornavirus and is therefore not a general property. Purified mengovirus does have some proteinase activity (Holland et al., 1972), but this seems unlikely to be related to cleavage. Many conditions inhibiting cleavage (high temperatures, amino acid analogues, serine esterase inhibitors: Jacobson et al., 1970; Garfinkle and Tershak, 1971; Summers et al., 1972; Korant, 1972; Abraham and Cooper, 1975a) usually inhibit some cleavage steps but not others, so that more than one cleavage activity is almost certainly involved. In some systems, it is very difficult to prevent cleavage with these inhibitors (Dobos and Martin, 1972; Black, 1975). Although the cleavage pattern depends on the virus rather than host cell (Holland and Kiehn, 1968), some properties of cleavage can vary with cell type (Korant, 1972) and some proteases at least are cell specified. Cell-free extracts give cleavage patterns that differ from in vivo ones (Ginevskaya et al., 1972; Korant, 1972).

In general, sufficient picornavirus genetic information is not available to code for such activities. In view of the known variety of specific proteases inside animal cells (Pine, 1972), the cleavage enzymes are probably almost all cell coded, although some may be virus induced in the sense of activation of, e.g., lysosomal proteases, and one of them might be a viral enzyme.

10. SITES OF ACTION OF VIRAL GROWTH INHIBITORS

The extensive literature on the use of certain antiviral agents in genetic studies with picornaviruses has been comprehensively reviewed by Sergiescu et al. (1972). The value of these inhibitors is that they apparently do not affect cellular processes, and that inhibitor-resistant mutants can be obtained. Thus they act specifically against the function of a particular viral gene, so that information on their action yields information on normal gene function, and vice versa. Although many potent inhibitors of picornavirus growth are reported or known, unless resistant mutants are available so that their locus can be identified by mapping or covariant reversion studies, the miscellaneous observations on their physiological effects may be difficult to interpret. As a purely technical contribution, inhibitor-resistant mutants have proved of the greatest value for genetic analysis by allowing three-factor crosses (Section 7).

Sergiescu et al. (1972) also reviewed in detail six inhibitors that have proved particularly useful for genetic analysis, and which will be summarized here briefly. Three of them act on the extracellular phase of the virus, preventing attachment and penetration in various ways, and therefore bind directly to structural protein. Two are heterogeneous antibody-like globulins found in sera of certain horses (ho) and bovines (bo), and their value in genetic studies was that, unlike antibody, poliovirus strains resistant to each could be obtained. These showed no covariation with other characters, a property that enabled genetic recombination in picornavirus to be first detected (Hirst, 1962). Their locus in the ts genetic map has not been established, but presumably they will lie in the structural protein region. The third, dextran sulfate, resembles a sulfated polysaccharide present in agar that inhibits the growth of many strains of polio-, aphtho-, coxsackie-, and cardiovirus, although their precise modes of action probably differ. Recombination between dextran sulfate-resistant (m) and other poliovirus strains has been demonstrated (Bengtsson, 1968; Sergiescu et al., 1969). One m locus has now been related to the poliovirus ts genetic map (Cooper et al., 1971, 1975) and shown, as expected, to lie in the structural protein region close to the g locus (Fig. 1).

A great deal of work has been published on the mode of inhibition of many picornavirus strains by the simple compound guanidine hydrochloride (reviewed by Sergiescu et al., 1972). It acts intracellularly, and does not affect a very early stage of replication. Guanidine-sensitive, -resistant (independent), or (for enteroviruses) -dependent strains can readily be obtained, and some simple metabolites can suppress its action. It appears to affect primarily RNA replication, preventing the release of vRNA from the replication complex. However, it also slows the cleavage of the structural protein precursor VP0 (Jacobson and Baltimore, 1968a), and guanidine resistance maps as a single locus in structural protein, (Fig. 1) (Cooper, 1968; Cooper et al., 1970a; Lake et al., 1975). It does not affect RNA replication in vitro. Guanidine in fact has many complex effects on picornavirus replication. These and several other at first sight perplexing phenomena in picornavirus replication have been unified in the equestron hypothesis (Cooper et al., 1973) (Section 11). This proposes a regulator particle controlling several processes, whose configuration and thus affinity for various sites of action are determined by the presence or absence of guanidine and other substances and conditions. The candidate for the equestron is a product of the structural protein schizon.

The synthetic inhibitor 2-(α-hydroxybenzyl)benzimidazole (HBB) has many similarities in activity to guanidine, although its site of action is not identical (Eggers and Tamm, 1966). Unfortunately, the poliovirus ts^+ strain used for the poliovirus genetic map was HBB resistant (unpublished observations) and the HBB locus has not been mapped. The antibiotic gliotoxin acts intracellularly and irreversibly blocks RNA and protein synthesis, but its resistance locus has not been mapped either, and no covariation with other markers was found (Sergiescu and Aubert-Combiescu, 1969).

The sites of action of another three specific inhibitors of poliovirus have been identified, both by covariation with resistance in *ts* mutants and by genetic mapping of resistant strains (Fig. 1). These are S-7 (ethyl-2-methylthio-4-methyl-5-pyrimidine carboxylate, Cooper *et al.*, 1975), a synthetic oxadiazole [2-(3-chloro-*p*-tolyl)-5-ethyl-1,3,4-oxadiazole, Cooper *et al.*, 1974], and a synthetic hydantoin (5-methyl-5-3,4-dichlorophenylhydantoin, D. DeLong, A. Steiner-Pryor, and P. D. Cooper, unpublished results). There was no cross-resistance of resistant mutants, but in each case the resistance locus lay well into the structural protein region, allowing a conclusion similar to that for guanidine that resistance was determined by the configuration of a product of the structural protein schizon. Not much is known of the effects on virus growth of these compounds, although S-7 appears to interact with capsid protein in the free particle to prevent viral penetration (Lonberg-Holm *et al.*, 1975).

11. THE STRATEGY OF THE PICORNAVIRUS GENOME

11.1. Regulation Mechanisms

The preceding sections consider those "primary" schizons specifying the components of picornavirus particles, and their secondary activities implied by various cellular changes. These functions fully occupy the genetic map. However, there is another aspect of picornavirus replication that must be considered.

Several details of poliovirus growth kinetics from many molecular and biological studies strongly implicate some kind of regulator (Cooper *et al.*, 1973). These include the brisk economy of the process, in which RNA and protein are made in the correct (1:60) ratio for assembly (despite the fact that RNA is innately made faster than protein), then synchronously combined without much waste, and the increase of the three pools of vRNA in the correct sequence—replication complex, translation complex, and progeny virions—for efficient replication. All this is achieved without differential translation of "genes," as the messenger RNA is polyschizonic, and in almost all picornavirus systems all gene products increase in equivalent molar ratios, at the same rate at different times of the cycle (Summers *et al.,* 1965; Abraham and Cooper, 1975*a*). One exception is mengovirus, in which capsid protein increases twice as fast as noncapsid protein (Paucha *et al.,* 1974; Lucas-Lenard, 1975), but this effect seems unlikely to represent a regulation mechanism as it is relatively small and is not common to all picornaviruses. Possibly it reflects an internal mutation with a polar effect on translation.

It can be deduced (1) that ribosomes in poliovirus-infected cells *decrease* in affinity for host mRNA while *increasing* in affinity for vRNA, (2) that the completion rate of cRNA templates becomes blocked at about midcycle, and (3) that there is a change in the regulator a little later in order not to interfere with maturation of the vRNA. The fact that these functions are seen to *change* during growth makes unlikely such simpler explanations as differences in intrinsic affinities of ribosomes for host mRNA and vRNA. As mentioned, such regulatory effects occur despite the finding that the genetic map of poliovirus is completely occupied by primary gene functions (Sections 7 and 8).

It was accordingly predicted (Cooper *et al.,* 1973) that poliovirus makes a labile regulator(s) with affinities for some ribosomal factor or subunit and for vRNA. To conserve genetic economy, this hypothetical entity is suggested to be a single particle binding both to the 45 S ribosomal subunit and to the 5′ end of vRNA, but with a half-life of 20–40 min. It was termed the "equestron," to imply a directive rider of both ribosomes and vRNA.

At this time, several data became available to suggest a candidate for the equestron. Prime among these was that a search for polioviral proteins associated with the translation complex (Wright and Cooper, 1974*a*) showed that the smaller ribosomal subunit isolated from infected cells carried the structural unit precursor proteins VP0 + VP1 + VP3, in equimolar ratio. These could not be ascribed to contamination with empty capsids or soluble protein. Disruption of the small subunit allowed these proteins to be isolated as a 6 S particle. The larger (65 S) subunit did not carry label, but the VP0 + VP1 + VP3 complex was also found associated with vRNA and with a complex of vRNA and a single ribosome; it was also associated with the membrane-free replication complex (Wright and Cooper, 1976). It accordingly was the candidate for the equestron. The proposed function of the equestron is summarized in Fig. 8, and described in Section 11.2.

This implication of structural protein in the regulation mechanism prompted a successful search for mutants defective in repression of host protein synthesis (one of the proposed functions of the equestron) in the light of known properties of mutants defective in structural protein (Section 8.2.1). It was confirmed by this means that the repression of host protein synthesis was dependent on the configuration of a product of the structural protein schizon (Steiner-Pryor and Cooper, 1973).

Finally, although the poliovirus-inhibitor guanidine has several effects on RNA synthesis, the genetic locus of resistance to guanidine lies in the structural protein schizon (Cooper, 1968, 1969). The only change seen in viral proteins is a delayed cleavage of VP0 (Jacobson and Baltimore, 1968a), implying that guanidine alters its conformation, and therefore reacts directly with it. Guanidine sensitivity is dominant for vRNA and virus replication in mixed infection of sensitive and resistant strains plus guanidine (Cooper et al., 1970a), implying that the sensitive strain makes a viral protein that slows all replicating centers equally. A single amino acid change neutralizes this effect in resistant strains, but is deduced to be in structural protein (Cooper et al., 1970a). Guanidine has most effect 2–3 h after infection (Lwoff and Lwoff, 1963; Koch et al., 1974); if present only from 0 to 2 h, it has much less effect on later growth, despite vigorous RNA replication at 0–2 h in untreated cultures (Baltimore et al., 1966). Thus guanidine cannot appreciably interact with the simple replication process; it has no effect on replicase action in vitro, although it rapidly slows vRNA production in vivo, equalizing vRNA and cRNA synthesis (Cooper et al., 1970b; Caliguiri and Tamm, 1968; Baltimore, 1968). It was concluded (Cooper et al., 1973) that guanidine is likely to interact only when replication becomes regulated. This implies that guanidine primarily affects the regulator, and therefore, from the genetic map, that such a regulator involves structural protein. Several other effective inhibitors of poliovirus intracellular replication have also been shown to involve structural protein (Section 10).

This system requires further examination. In particular, studies on the effect of purified [VP0, VP1, VP3] monomers in appropriate in vitro systems of translation and replication of picornavirus RNA are strongly indicated, but these monomers have not yet been prepared in sufficient quantity. They behave as a readily aggregated basic protein with a strong affinity for surfaces (P. D. Cooper, unpublished results). The relevant *in vitro* replication systems, in which both replicase I and II activities can polymerize RNA on exogenous templates, are not yet available either. Some early studies indicated viral "priming" of ribosomes as, in contrast to normal ribosomes, ribosomes from EMC virus-infected Krebs cells showed marked stimulation of translation as a specific response to EMC virus RNA (Kerr *et al.,* 1962). Also, Ascione and Vande Woude (1971) reported that initiation factors extracted only from aphthovirus-infected cells and added to a ribosome–viral RNA mixture could stimulate binding of aminoacylated tRNA and amino acid incorporation *in vitro*. The response was marked and was dependent on aphthovirus RNA. Ribosomal extracts from various noninfected cells were ineffective. Unfortunately, most *in vitro* studies have used only extracts from noninfected cells or from *E. coli*. Since free picornavirus RNA is infective, some translation on unprimed ribosomes must be feasible, but the above considerations imply a marked enhancement with ribosomes from infected cells.

In contrast to the results of Wright and Cooper (1974*a*), membrane-bound material containing ribosomes from EMC virus-infected cells was found to contain mainly nonstructural proteins (Medvedkina *et al.,* 1974), but its content of the large or small replication complex (Caliguiri, 1974) was apparently not examined. With regard to the postulated involvement of structural protein in RNA replication, Ghendon *et al.* (1973*a*) found that immune globulin directed specifically (Ghendon and Yakobson, 1971) against the 14 S component of poliovirus cytoplasms (which contains predominantly the structural proteins VP0, VP1, and VP3, Phillips *et al.,* 1968) could suppress *in vitro* RNA replication by a consistent if small amount. However, the antigen might also have contained replicase proteins.

Cole and Baltimore (1973*a*) give data indicating that the RNA of a poliovirus mutant with an extensive deletion in structural protein (DI virus) replicated only slightly slower than normal virus RNA. These mutants have been selected for competent RNA replication in mixed infection with standard virus. Its repression of host protein synthesis and its guanidine sensitivity were also normal in absence of helper virus, although viral polysomes were less stable. The mutant's truncated equivalent of the structural protein precursor (60 kdal) was degraded completely and failed to encapsidate the RNA; its half-life was not measured but, as label was incorporated in short pulses at least as well as into the normal precursor (NCVP1), appears comparable to that of NCVP1 (5–10 min).

Cole and Baltimore (1973a) suggest that this material is too unstable to allow any role for structural protein in regulation machinery. On the contrary, the mutant structural protein precursor may well retain ability to bind to appropriate sites on ribosome and vRNA. Its half-life is not negligible, and such binding may modify its cleavage sensitivity just as a substantial amount of VP0 remains in a form unsusceptible to cleavage up to the end of the cycle. Since this system is not obscured by the presence of capsid protein, it would be most interesting to look at its translation and replication complexes for associated viral protein with possible regulatory functions in mind.

11.2. Genome Expression

The information summarized in this chapter allows an assignment of gene expression to genetic information of picornaviruses that seems close to being complete in outline, although almost totally obscure in detail of function. The data are mainly for poliovirus, but where information is available the other picornaviruses do not differ significantly. The most important missing items are the identification of the functional replicase polypeptides, and the functions of the nontranslated portions of the genome.*

Unfortunately, there is also at present a major ambiguity (Section 9.7). The two alternatives are summarized in Fig. 6, in terms of the map distances occupied by primary and secondary gene functions, the sizes of the primary translation products and main schizomers, and the size of the poliovirus genome. The results of the tryptic peptide analyses indicate a satisfactory balance between size of translation products and coding potential, leaving the same proportion untranslated as for the ribophage R17 (10%). This assignment necessitates the presence of two cistrons.

In contrast, the pactamycin analyses leave 20% of the genome (1500 nucleotides) untranslated, and a major anomaly between the sizes of the primary polyprotein and the presumed primary schizomers. This

---

* **Note Added in Proof:** Picornavirus RNA lacks a "cap" [Hewlett et al., Proc. Natl. Acad. Sci. USA **73**:327 (1976); Nomoto et al., Proc. Natl. Acad. Sci. USA **73**:375 (1976)], the methylated guanosine of reversed polarity added to the 5′ end of almost all other mRNAs of eukaryotic cells and necessary for initiation of translation. A function of part of the untranslated portion of the picornavirus genome is therefore to provide an alternative site for initiation. The unknown function of the poly A segment, which may be encoded genetically rather than added posttranscriptionally [Dorsch-Häsler et al., J. Virol. **16**:1512 (1975)], is probably needed for replication rather than translation [Spector et al., Cell **6**:41 (1975)].

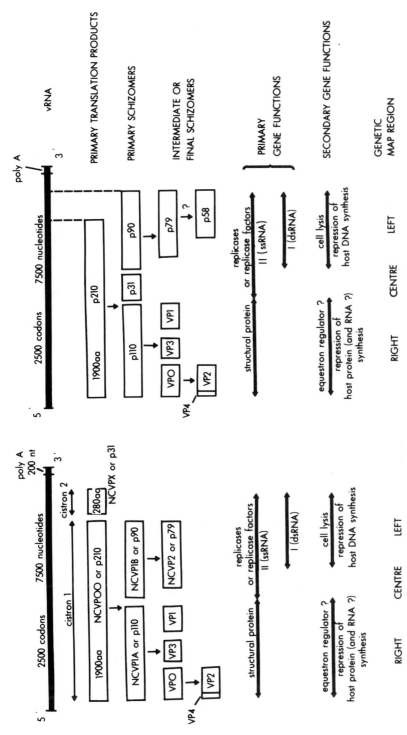

Fig. 6. Quantitative relations of the poliovirus genome RNA (top) and its primary and secondary gene functions (bottom), with the main translation and cleavage products (center), as indicated by comparisons of tryptic peptides (left) or rates of labeling in presence of pactamycin (right).

result assumes without evaluation the presence of only one cistron (among other assumptions), but it does offer a simple explanation for the difference between replicase I and II activities in terms of the latter's possession of p31 (NCVPX), as indicated by its position between p110 and p90. A decision between these alternatives cannot yet be made, although the evidence favoring the two-cistron scheme appears the stronger.

11.3.   The Growth Process as Indicated by Genetic and Other Studies

The growth process of poliovirus will now be summarized in several phases based on the suggested function of the equestron regulator, which dominates the strategy of the poliovirus genome in the form that is proposed. References and some details are given by Cooper *et al.* (1973). This summary is best read in conjunction with Fig. 7 (a flow sheet of the growth process), Fig. 8 (a detail of Fig. 7 outlining the activities proposed for the equestron), and Figs. 9 and 10 (idealized one-step growth curves).

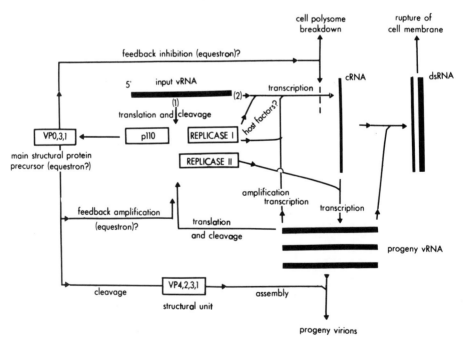

Fig. 7.   Flow sheet of the growth process of picornaviruses. The role of the equestron regulator is not yet proven.

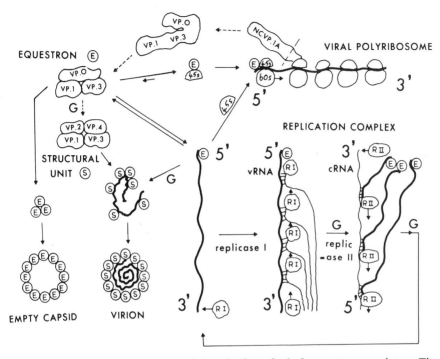

Fig. 8.   Detailed functions proposed for the hypothetical equestron regulator. The thick and thin wavy lines represent vRNA and cRNA, respectively; broken arrows represent cleavage steps, and G represents the steps blocked by guanidine. From Cooper *et al*. (1973).

Fig. 9. Idealized single-multiplicity one-step growth cycle of poliovirus. •, vRNA or total structural protein; O, total equestrons; ——, equestrons bound to 45 S ribosomal subunits; ●, virions, or virion structural units. The broken line indicates the vRNA capacity of ribosomes.

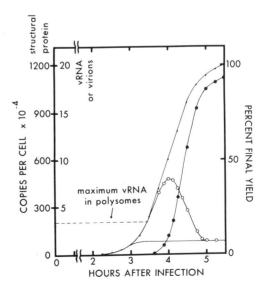

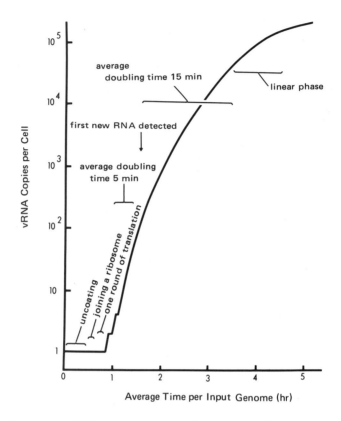

Fig. 10.   Kinetics of vRNA increase from a single-input poliovirus particle. The lag period is comprised of the average time for uncoating (Cooper, 1964*b*) plus average time predicted for first joining a ribosome (Cooper *et al.*, 1973) plus average time to complete one round of translation and transcription.

11.3.1.   Establishment of Infection: 0–2 h

The input vRNA must first join a ribosome, on average taking longer than 11 min after uncoating; the structural protein schizon is translated and an equestron produced by cleavage within a further 5–10 min. The growth process initiated by a single infectious particle includes random delays averaging 60 min, of which only 30 min can be ascribed to uncoating (Cooper, 1964*b*). Soon after the first round or two of translation (taking 20–30 min), the input vRNA must join with a replicase I molecule (liberated after its translation near the 3′ end, its site of action) making a cRNA strand in 1–2 min. If this fails to occur before the vRNA is irreversibly occupied with ribosomes, the infection is not established and must abort. The equestrons form a reversible

complex with small ribosomal subunits, with vRNA, or with both, linking them specifically like an initiation factor and speeding up vRNA
translation. More equestrons are then made in a self-accelerating
process. The 45 S–equestron complex coordinately blocks host mRNA
association with ribosomes, which progressively become almost entirely
available for viral polysome formation.

The affinity of equestrons for the small subunit must be high to be
effective at such low initial concentrations, and so the small subunits
will preferentially bind the equestrons, which will therefore infrequently
exist either free or on vRNA until the subunits approach saturation 2–3
h after infection. The level of equestrons bound to 45 S subunits shown
in Fig. 9 is based on the content of small subunits per cell
(approximately 10^6). Progeny vRNA is transcribed from the first
cRNA template by replicase II, and more cRNA from this vRNA is
transcribed by replicase I. This process is exponentially self-amplifying,
and is probably unregulated at first and will at this time outstrip protein synthesis. One vRNA transcript is completed in 1–2 min, while a
complete protein translation of the genome takes 10 min; the initial
delay of 30–60 min and the doubling time of 15 min observed after 2 h
would not yield 10^4 progeny vRNA per cell by 3 h (particularly as some
is sequestered in polysomes) without a period of some 30 min of
replication with a doubling time initially 2–3 min and averaging 5 min
(Fig. 10). This is the period when the bulk of genetic recombination
occurs (Section 6.1.2).

11.3.2. Polysome Predominance and Beginning of Regulation: 2–3.5 h

The growing pool of equestron-primed 45 S subunits takes more
and more vRNA for polysomes, shifting the balance of the vRNA pool
from replication to translation complexes. However, the amounts
transferred are quantitatively insufficient to account for the reduction
of the doubling time to 15 min, and it is probable that the regulator is
coming into action at this time (see next section).

11.3.3. Restriction on Completion of cRNA Strands: 3.5–4.5 h

When the number of equestrons becomes comparable to that of
the small subunits, an excess of equestrons becomes available to
interact with vRNA. As an initiation factor, the equestron is proposed
to bind specifically to the 5′ end, whose free time will accordingly
progressively decrease. Completion of the cRNA strands will gradually

decrease in proportion, and ultimately will stop. When this happens, the cell makes steady use of those cRNA templates already completed, and the increase of vRNA (and protein) changes from exponential to linear (Fig. 9).

11.3.4. Assembly Caused by Decay of Labile Intermediates: 3.5–6 h

Much of the protein destined to enter virions has accumulated in the form of the structural unit precursor (VP0,3,1), since its half-life (20–40 min) is greater than that of the primary schizomer NCVP1A (5–10 min). Its cleavage to the structural unit is presumably a first-order reaction, and the vRNA templates for its production have been increasing exponentially up to now; along with other viral protein, it has maintained a constant ratio to vRNA and will itself increase exponentially. However, when the vRNA increase slows to a constant rate, the increase of structural unit precursors also becomes linear, and because their cleavage will remain exponential, their concentration will drop sharply about one half-life later (Fig. 9), suddenly creating a large pool of mature structural units. The theoretical kinetics of Fig. 9 closely resemble those for incorporation of soluble antigen (probably the VP0, VP3, VP1 complex) into virions (Scharff *et al.,* 1964). At this time, almost all the cell's ribosomes (3–4×10^6/cell) are locked up in viral polyribosomes, and most of the new vRNA is available to associate with the newly created structural units. Thus the pool of vRNA shifts yet again, from translation complex to progeny virions. This corresponds with the end of the eclipse period (production of the first infectious progeny/cell).

11.3.5. Late Effects: 4 h Onward

The change of kinetics will also cause a drop, at about the same time and for the same reasons, in other labile components, one of which is the viral replicase (Section 9.3). RNA production can be expected to tail off when replicase concentration, rather than available templates, becomes the rate-limiting factor (Fig. 9). This sets a limit of vRNA molecules made per cell, as it is independent of input virus but depends on the change of kinetics (which is itself held to depend on the regulator) and on the half-life of replicase. Such a limit is suggested as the cause of homologous interference-with-multiplication (Section 6.5). Host DNA synthesis also falls off at this time, and if this is associated with the replicase (Section 8.2.3) may reflect a growing shortage of host factors for both enzymes.

Finally, although the cRNA and vRNA "factories" are held in separate replication complexes (Section 8.1), it must be expected that, later in the cycle, vRNA and cRNA molecules will now and again achieve full base pairing to the double-stranded form (RF), which will not dissociate *in vivo*. The RF is indeed found after phenol extraction, although its presence in native cytoplasm is not usually demonstrated. Nevertheless, its final accumulation appears to be the cause of membrane rupture and release of virus (Section 8.2.2), signaling the abrupt end of the replication cycle.

Thus in regulating vRNA and cRNA production the equestron destroys itself in favor of the structural unit. Posttranslational cleavage is exploited as a regulation device. Saturation of the small subunit with equestrons, and of ribosomes with vRNA, and saturation of vRNA with equestrons leading to linear growth and their decay to structural units are all stages with a fixed relation to each other, so that the system will be synchronized under a wide range of cultural conditions. The effects of guanidine (sensitivity, dependence, neutralization of inhibition by metabolites), and other intracellular inhibitory substances and conditions that appear to depend on the configuration of a product of the structural protein schizon are proposed to modify the tertiary configuration of the equestron and thus, allosterically, various of its binding affinities. The most plausible explanation for the effect of guanidine is to lock the equestron prematurely onto the 5′ end of vRNA, thus preventing release (but not synthesis) of cRNA and stopping the initiation of new vRNA synthesis.

12. CONCLUSIONS

In a previous review (Cooper, 1969), it was concluded that the small size of the poliovirus genome may reflect sophisticated internal relationships rather than intrinsic simplicity. This chapter now shows that the reality embodies both images. There are only three or four gene functions, it is true, but a substantial variety of very effectively coordinated activities is purchased for a modest investment in genetic information. Much of this sophistication depends on the changes that can be rung by posttranslational cleavage on relatively large gene products, so that the work done by almost all genetic sequences is doubled or even trebled. It seems likely that this apparently extreme example of genetic economy is only one among many to be found in small virus systems. However, in contrast to the situation outlined in the earlier review, we now have a detailed if not quite complete outline of the overall functions of the genome of picornaviruses.

13. REFERENCES

Abraham, G., and Cooper, P. D., 1975a, Poliovirus polypeptides examined in more detail, *J. Gen. Virol.* **29**:199.

Abraham, G., and Cooper, P. D., 1975b, Relations between poliovirus polypeptides as shown by tryptic peptide analysis, *J. Gen. Virol.* **29**:215.

Agol, V. I., and Shirman, G. A., 1964, Interaction of guanidine-sensitive and guanidine-dependent variants of poliovirus in mixedly infected cells, *Biochem. Biophys. Res. Commun.* **17**:28.

Agol, V. I., Romanova, L. I., Cumakov, I. M., Dunaevskaya, L. D., and Bogdanov, A. A., 1972, Circularisation and cross-linking in preparations of replicative form of EMC virus RNA, *J. Mol. Biol.* **72**:77.

Amako, K., and Dales, S., 1967, Cytopathology of mengovirus. II. Proliferation of membranous cisternae, *Virology* **32**:201.

Arlinghaus, R. B., and Polatnick, J., 1969, The isolation of two enzyme–RNA complexes involved in the synthesis of foot-and-mouth-disease virus RNA, *Proc. Natl. Acad. Sci. USA* **62**:822.

Ascione, R., and Vande Woude, G. F., 1971, Ribosomal factors effecting the stimulation of cell-free protein synthesis in the presence of foot-and-mouth disease virus ribonucleic acid, *Biochem. Biophys. Res. Commun.* **45**:14.

Bablanian, R., 1972, Mechanisms of virus cytopathic effect, in: *Microbial Pathogenicity in Man and Animals* (H. Smith and J. H. Pearce, eds.), *Symp. Soc. Gen. Microbiol.* **22**:359.

Bablanian, R., and Russell, W. C., 1974, Adenovirus polypeptide synthesis in the presence of non-replicating poliovirus, *J. Gen. Virol.* **24**:261.

Bachrach, H. L., Swaney, J. B., and Vande Woude, G. F., 1973, Isolation of the structural polypeptides of foot-and-mouth disease virus and analysis of their *C*-terminal sequences, *Virology* **52**:520.

Baltimore, D., 1968, Inhibition of poliovirus replication by guanidine, in: *Medical and Applied Virology* (M. Sanders and E. H. Lennette, eds.), pp. 340–347, Warren H. Green Inc., St. Louis.

Baltimore, D., 1969, The replication of picornaviruses, in: *The Biochemistry of Viruses* (H. B. Levy, ed.), pp. 101–176, Dekker, New York.

Baltimore, D., Girard, M., and Darnell, J. E., 1966, Aspects of the synthesis of poliovirus RNA and the formation of virus particles, *Virology* **29**:179.

Béchet, J. M., 1972, Isolement de la chaíne "moins" d'acide ribonucléique du virus de l'encephalomyocardite de la souris et étude de son infectivité, *C. R. Acad. Sci. Ser. D* **274**:1761.

Bengtsson, S., 1968, Attempts to map the poliovirus genome by analysis of selected recombinants, *Acta Pathol. Microbiol. Scand.* **73**:592.

Benzer, S., 1957, The elementary units of heredity, in: *The Chemical Basis of Heredity* (W. D. McElroy and B. Glass, eds.), pp. 70–93, Johns Hopkins Press, Baltimore.

Black, D. N., 1975, Proteins induced in BHK cells by infection with foot-and-mouth disease virus, *J. Gen. Virol.* **26**:109.

Black, D., and Brown, F., 1976, A major difference in the strategy of the calici- and picornaviruses and its significance in classification. *Intervirology* **6**:57.

Boime, I., and Leder, R., 1972, Protein synthesis directed by encephalomyocarditis virus mRNA. III. Discrete polypeptides translated from a monocistronic messenger *in vitro, Arch. Biochem. Biophys.* **153**:706.

Boime, I., Aviv, H., and Leder, P., 1971, Protein synthesis directed by EMC virus RNA. II. The *in vitro* synthesis of high molecular weight proteins and elements of the viral capsid, *Biochem. Biophys. Res. Commun.* **45**:788.

Bond, C. W., and Swim, H. E., 1975, Physiological characteristics of temperature-sensitive mutants of mengovirus, *J. Virol.* **15**:288.

Brown, F., and Martin, S. J., 1965, A new model for virus RNA replication, *Nature (London)* **208**:861.

Buck, C. A., Granger, G. A., Taylor, M. W., and Holland, J. J., 1967, Efficient, inefficient and abortive infection of different mammalian cells by small RNA viruses, *Virology* **33**:36.

Burness, A. T. H., Pardoe, I. U., and Fox, S. M., 1973, Evidence for lack of a glycoprotein in the encephalomyocarditis virus particle, *J. Gen. Virol.* **18**:33.

Burrell, C. J., and Cooper, P. D., 1973, *N*-Terminal aspartate, glycine and serine in poliovirus capsid protein, *J. Gen. Virol.* **21**:443.

Burroughs, J. N., and Brown, F., 1974, Physico-chemical evidence for the reclassification of the caliciviruses, *J. Gen. Virol.* **22**:281.

Butterworth, B. E., 1973, A comparison of the virus-specific polypeptides of encephalomyocarditis virus, human rhinovirus and poliovirus, *Virology* **56**:439.

Butterworth, B. E., and Korant, B. D., 1974, Characterisation of the large picornaviral polypeptides produced in the presence of zinc ion, *J. Virol.* **14**:282.

Butterworth, B. E., and Rueckert, R. R., 1972a, Kinetics of synthesis and cleavage of EMC virus-specific proteins, *Virology* **50**:535.

Butterworth, B. E., and Rueckert, R. R., 1972b, Gene order of encephalomyocarditis virus as determined by studies with pactamycin, *J. Virol.* **9**:823.

Butterworth, B. E., Hall, L., Stolzfus, C. M., and Rueckert, R. R., 1971, Virus-specific proteins synthesised in encephalomyocarditis (EMC) virus-infected HeLa cells, *Proc. Natl. Acad. Sci. USA* **68**:3083.

Caliguiri, L. A., 1974, Analysis of RNA associated with the poliovirus RNA replication complexes, *Virology* **58**:526.

Caliguiri, L. A., and Compans, R. W., 1973, Formation of poliovirus particles in association with the RNA replication complexes, *J. Gen. Virol.* **21**:99.

Caliguiri, L. A., and Mosser, A. G., 1971, Proteins associated with the poliovirus RNA replication complex, *Virology* **46**:375.

Caliguiri, L. A., and Tamm, I., 1968, Action of guanidine on the replication of poliovirus RNA, *Virology* **35**:408.

Caliguiri, L. A., and Tamm, I., 1970a, The role of cytoplasmic membranes in poliovirus biosynthesis, *Virology* **42**:100.

Caliguiri, L. A., and Tamm, I., 1970b, Characterization of poliovirus-specific structures associated with cytoplasmic membranes, *Virology* **42**:112.

Chatterjee, N. K., Koch, G., and Weissbach, H., 1973, Initiation of protein synthesis *in vivo* in poliovirus-infected cells, *Arch. Biochem. Biophys.* **154**:431.

Choppin, P. W., and Holmes, K. V., 1967, Replication of SV5 and the effects of superinfection with poliovirus, *Virology* **33**:442.

Cole, C. N., and Baltimore, D., 1973*a*, Defective interfering particles of poliovirus. II. Nature of the defect, *J. Mol. Biol.* **76**:325.

Cole, C. N., and Baltimore, D., 1973*b*, Defective interfering particles of poliovirus. III. Interference and enrichment, *J. Mol. Biol.* **76**:345.

Cole, C. N., Smoler, D., Wimmer, E., and Baltimore, D., 1971, Defective interfering particles of poliovirus. I. Isolation and physical properties, *J. Virol.* **7**:478.

Collins, F. D., and Roberts, W. K., 1972, Mechanism of mengovirus-induced cell injury in L cells: Use of inhibitors of protein synthesis to dissociate virus-specific events, *J. Virol.* **10**:969.

Cooper, P. D., 1964*a*, The mutation of poliovirus by 5-fluorouracil, *Virology* **22**:186.

Cooper, P. D., 1964*b*, Synchrony and the elimination of chance delays in the growth of poliovirus, *J. Gen. Microbiol.* **37**:259.

Cooper, P. D., 1965, Rescue of one phenotype in mixed infections with heat-defective mutants of type 1 poliovirus, *Virology* **25**:431.

Cooper, P. D., 1966, The inhibition of poliovirus growth by actinomycin D and the prevention of the inhibition by pretreatment of the cells with serum or insulin, *Virology* **28**:663.

Cooper, P. D., 1968, A genetic map of poliovirus temperature-sensitive mutants, *Virology* **35**:584.

Cooper, P. D., 1969, The genetic analysis of poliovirus, in: *Biochemistry of Viruses* (H. B. Levy, ed.), pp. 177–218, Dekker, New York.

Cooper, P. D., 1974, Towards a more profound basis for the classification of viruses, *Intervirology* **4**:317.

Cooper, P. D., and Bellett, A. J. D., 1959, A transmissible interfering component of vesicular stomatitis virus preparations, *J. Gen. Microbiol.* **21**:485.

Cooper, P. D., and Bennett, D. J., 1973, Genetic and structural implications of tryptic peptide analysis of poliovirus structural protein, *J. Gen. Virol.* **20**:151.

Cooper, P. D., and Wyke, J. A., 1974, The genome of RNA tumor viruses: A functional requirement for a polyploid structure? *Cold Spring Harbor Symp. Quant. Biol.* **39**:997.

Cooper, P. D., Johnson, R. T., and Garwes, D. J., 1966, Physiological characterization of heat-defective (temperature-sensitive) poliovirus mutants: Preliminary classification, *Virology* **30**:638.

Cooper, P. D., Wentworth, B. B., and McCahon, D., 1970*a*, Guanidine inhibition of poliovirus: A dependence of viral RNA synthesis on the configuration of structural protein, *Virology* **40**:486.

Cooper, P. D., Stanček, D., and Summers, D. F., 1970*b*, Synthesis of double-stranded RNA by poliovirus temperature-sensitive mutants, *Virology* **40**:971.

Cooper, P. D., Summers, D. F., and Maizel, J. V., 1970*c*, Evidence for ambiguity in the posttranslational cleavage of poliovirus proteins, *Virology* **41**:408.

Cooper, P. D., Geissler, E., Scotti, P. D., and Tannock, G. A., 1971, Further characterisation of the genetic map of poliovirus temperature-sensitive mutants, in: *Strategy of the Viral Genome* (G. E. W. Wolstenholme and M. O'Connor, eds.), pp. 75–100, Churchill Livingstone, Edinburgh.

Cooper, P. D., Steiner-Pryor, A., and Wright, P. J., 1973, A proposed regulator for poliovirus: The equestron, *Intervirology* **1**:1.

Cooper, P. D., Steiner-Pryor, A., Scotti, P. D., and Delong, D., 1974, On the nature of poliovirus genetic recombinants, *J. Gen. Virol.* **23**:41.

Cooper, P. D., Geissler, E., and Tannock, G. A., 1975, Attempts to extend the genetic map of poliovirus temperature-sensitive mutants, *J. Gen. Virol.* **29**:109.

Cordell-Stewart, B., and Taylor, M. W., 1971, Effect of double-stranded viral RNA on mammalian cells in culture, *Proc. Natl. Acad. Sci. USA* **68**:1326.

Cordell-Stewart, B., and Taylor, M. W., 1973a, Effect of viral double-stranded RNA on protein synthesis in intact cells, *J. Virol.* **11**:232.

Cordell-Stewart, B., and Taylor, M. W., 1973b, Effect of viral double-stranded RNA on mammalian cells in culture: Cytotoxicity under conditions preventing viral replication and protein synthesis, *J. Virol.* **12**:360.

Cords, C. E., and Holland, J. J., 1964a, Interference between enteroviruses and conditions affecting its reversal, *Virology* **22**:226.

Cords, C. E., and Holland, J. J., 1964b, Alteration of the species and tissue specificity of poliovirus by enclosure of its RNA within the protein capsid of Coxsackie B1 virus, *Virology* **24**:492.

Cords, C. E., and Holland, J. J., 1964c, Replication of poliovirus RNA induced by heterologous virus, *Proc. Natl. Acad. Sci. USA* **51**:1080.

Cory, S., Adams, J. M., Spahr, P. F., and Rensing, U., 1972, Sequence of 51 nucleotides at the 3′ end of R15 bacteriophage RNA, *J. Mol. Biol.* **63**:41.

Cranston, J., Malathi, V. G., and Silber, R., 1973, Further studies on RNA ligase, *Fed. Proc. Abst.* **32**:498.

Dales, S., and Silverberg, H., 1968, Controlled double infection with unrelated animal viruses, *Virology* **34**:531.

Dales, S., Eggers, H. J., Tamm, I., and Palade, G. E., 1965, Electron-microscopic study of the formation of poliovirus, *Virology* **26**:379.

Dobos, P., and Martin, E. M., 1972, Virus-specific polypeptides in ascites cells infected with encephalomyocarditis virus, *J. Gen. Virol.* **17**:197.

Dobos, P., Kerr, I. M., and Martin, E. M., 1971, Synthesis of capsid and non-capsid viral proteins in response to encephalomyocarditis virus RNA in animal cell-free systems, *J. Virol.* **8**:491.

Doyle, M., and Holland, J. J., 1972, Virus-induced interference in heterologously infected HeLa cells, *J. Virol.* **9**:22.

Drake, J. W., 1958, Interference and multiplicity reactivation in poliovirus, *Virology* **6**:244.

Drzeniek, R., and Billelo, P., 1974, Absence of glycoproteins in poliovirus particles, *J. Gen. Virol.* **25**:125.

Dulbecco, R., 1961, Poliovirus mutations seen from the point of view of molecular biology, in: *Poliomyelitis,* pp. 21–24, Fifth International Poliomyelitis Conference, Lippincott, Philadelphia.

Eggen, K. L., and Shatkin, A. S., 1972, *In vitro* translation of cardiovirus RNA by cell-free extracts, *J. Virol.* **9**:636.

Eggers, H. J., and Tamm, I., 1966, Antiviral chemotherapy, *Annu. Rev. Pharmacol.* **6**:231.

Ehrenfeld, E., and Hunt, T., 1971, Double-stranded poliovirus RNA inhibits initiation of protein synthesis by reticulocyte lysates, *Proc. Natl. Acad. Sci. USA* **68**:1075.

Ehrenfeld, E., Maizel, J. V., and Summers, D. F., 1970, Soluble RNA polymerase complex from poliovirus-infected HeLa cells, *Virology* **40**:840.

Ensminger, W. D., and Tamm, I., 1970, The step in cellular DNA synthesis blocked by Newcastle disease or mengovirus infection, *Virology* **40**:152.

Esteban, M., and Kerr, I. M., 1974, The synthesis of encephalomyocarditis virus polypeptides in infected L cells and cell-free systems, *Eur. J. Biochem.* **45**:567.

Fenner, F., 1968, *The Biology of Animal Viruses,* 1st ed., Academic Press, New York.

Fenner, F., McAuslan, B. R., Mims, C. A., Sambrook, J., and White, D. O., 1974, *The Biology of Animal Viruses,* 2nd ed., Academic Press, New York.

Fenner, F., Pereira, H. G., Porterfield, J. S., Joklik, W. K., and Downie, A. W., 1975, Family and generic names for viruses approved by the International Committee on Taxonomy of Viruses, June 1974, *Intervirology* **3**:193.

Fenwick, M. L., 1963, The influence of poliovirus infection on RNA synthesis in mammalian cells, *Virology* **19**:241.

Fenwick, M. L., and Cooper, P. D., 1962, Early interactions between poliovirus and ERK cells: Some observations on the nature and significance of the rejected particles, *Virology* **18**:212.

Fernandez-Thomas, C. B., and Baltimore, D., 1973, Morphogenesis of poliovirus. II. Demonstration of a new intermediate, the proviron, *J. Virol.* **12**:1122.

Fincham, J. R. S., 1966, *Genetic Complementation,* W. A. Benjamin, New York.

Fiszman, M. Y., Bucchini, D., Girard, M., and Lwoff, A., 1970, Inhibition of poliovirus RNA synthesis by supra-optimal temperatures, *J. Gen. Virol.* **6**:293.

Freda, C. E., and Buck, C. A., 1971, System of double infection between vaccinia virus and mengovirus, *J. Virol.* **8**:293.

Garfinkle, B. D., and Tershak, D. R., 1971, Effect of temperature on the cleavage of polypeptides during growth of LSc poliovirus, *J. Mol. Biol.* **59**:537.

Garfinkle, B. D., and Tershak, D. R., 1972, Degradation of poliovirus polypeptides *in vivo, Nature (London) New Biol.* **238**:206.

Garwes, D. J., Wright, P. J., and Cooper, P. D., 1975, Poliovirus temperature-sensitive mutants defective in cytopathic effects are also defective in synthesis of double-stranded RNA, *J. Gen. Virol.* **27**:45.

Ghendon, Y. Z., 1972, Conditional-lethal mutants of animal viruses, *Prog. Med. Virol.* **14**:68.

Ghendon, Y. Z., and Yakobson, G. A., 1971, Antigenic specificity of poliovirus related particles, *J. Virol.* **8**:589.

Ghendon, Y. Z., Babushkina, L., Mikheeva, A., and Soloviev, G. Y., 1970, Synthesis of the virus-specific proteins of a conditionally lethal mutant of poliovirus under non-permissive conditions, *Virology* **40**:595.

Ghendon, Y. Z., Babushkina, L., and Blagoveshienskaya, O., 1973a, Inhibition of poliovirus RNA synthesis in an *in vitro* system by antiserum against 14 S virus-specific structures, *Arch. Ges. Virusforsch.* **40**:47.

Ghendon, Y. Z., Marchenko, A. T., Markushin, S. G., Chenkina, D. B., Mikheeva, A. V., and Rozian, E. E., 1973b, Correlation between *ts* phenotype and pathogenicity of some animal viruses, *Arch. Ges. Virusforsch.* **42**:154.

Ginevskaya, V. A., Scarlat, I. V., Kalinina, N. O., and Agol, V. I., 1972, Synthesis and cleavage of virus-specific proteins in Krebs II carcinoma cells infected with encephalomyelitis virus, *Arch. Ges. Virusforsch.* **39**:98.

Girard, M., Baltimore, D., and Darnell, J. E., 1967, The poliovirus replication complex: Site for synthesis of poliovirus RNA, *J. Mol. Biol.* **24**:59.

Gordon, I., Ghenault, S. S., Stevenson, D., and Acton, J. D., 1966, Effect of interferon and polymerisation of single-stranded and double-stranded mengovirus RNA, *J. Bacteriol.* **91**:1230.

Gorini, L., and Beckwith, J. R., 1966, Suppression, *Annu. Rev. Microbiol.* **20**:401.

Granboulan, N., and Girard, M., 1969, Molecular weight of poliovirus ribonucleic acid, *J. Virol.* **4**:475.

Haase, A. T., Baron, S., Levy, H. B., and Kasel, J. A., 1969, Mengovirus-induced cytopathic effect in L-cells: Protective effect of interferon, *J. Virol.* **4**:490.

Hayes, W., 1968, *The Genetics of Bacteria and Their Viruses,* 2nd ed., Blackwell, Oxford.

Hershko, A., and Fry, M., 1975, Posttranslational cleavage of polypeptide chains: Role in assembly, *Annu. Rev. Biochem.* **44**:775.

Hirst, G. K., 1962, Genetic recombination with Newcastle disease virus, poliovirus and influenza, *Cold Spring Harbor Symp. Quant. Biol.* **27**:303.

Ho, M., 1973, Animal virus and interferon formation, in: *Interferon and Interferon Inducers* (N. B. Finter, ed.), p. 36, North-Holland, Amsterdam.

Ho, M., and Enders, J. F., 1959, Further studies on an inhibition of viral activity appearing in infected cell cultures and its role in chronic viral infections, *Virology* **9**:446.

Ho, P. P. K., and Washington, A. L., 1971, Evidence for a cellular RNA synthesis inhibitor from poliovirus infected HeLa cells, *Biochemistry* **10**:3646.

Holland, J. J., 1963, Depression of host-controlled RNA synthesis in human cells during poliovirus infection, *Proc. Natl. Acad. Sci. USA* **49**:23.

Holland, J. J., and Kiehn, E. D., 1968, Specific cleavage of viral proteins as steps in the synthesis and maturation of enteroviruses, *Proc. Natl. Acad. Sci. USA* **60**:1015.

Holland, J. J., McLaren, L. C., Hoyer, B. H., and Syverton, J. T., 1960, Enteroviral ribonucleic acid. II. Biological, physical and chemical studies, *J. Exp. Med.* **112**:841.

Holland, J. J., Doyle, M., Perrault, J., Kingsbury, D. T., and Etchison, J., 1972, Proteinase activity in purifying animal viruses, *Biochem. Biophys. Res. Commun.* **46**:634.

Hoskins, J. M., 1959, Host-controlled variation in animal viruses, in: *Virus Growth and Variation* (A. Isaacs and B. W. Lacey, eds.), *Symp. Soc. Gen. Microbiol.* **9**:122.

Hotchkiss, R. D., 1971, Towards a general theory of recombination in DNA, *Adv. Genet.* **16**:325.

Hsiung, G. D., 1960, Studies in variation in coxsackie A9 virus, *J. Immunol.* **84**:285.

Ito, Y., Okazaki, H., and Ishida, N., 1968, Growth inhibition of Newcastle disease virus upon superinfection with poliovirus in the presence of guanidine, *J. Virol.* **2**:645.

Jacobson, M. F., and Baltimore, D., 1968a, Morphogenesis of poliovirus. I. Association of the viral RNA with protein, *J. Mol. Biol.* **33**:369.

Jacobson, M. F., and Baltimore, D., 1968b, Polypeptide cleavage in the formation of poliovirus proteins, *Proc. Natl. Acad. Sci. USA* **61**:77.

Jacobson, M. F., Asso, J., and Baltimore, D., 1970, Further evidence on the formation of poliovirus proteins, *J. Mol. Biol.* **49**:657.

Joklik, W. K., and Merigan, T. C., 1966, Concerning the mechanism of action of interferon, *Proc. Natl. Acad Sci. USA* **56**:558.

Kerr, I. M., Martin, E. M., Hamilton, M. G., and Work, T. S., 1962, The initiation of virus protein synthesis in Krebs ascites tumor cells infected with EMC virus, *Cold Spring Harbor Symp. Quant. Biol.* **27**:259.

Kerr, I. M., Brown, R. E., and Tovell, D. R., 1972, Characterization of the polypeptides formed in response to encephalomyocarditis virus RNA in a cell-free system from mouse ascites tumor cells, *J. Virol.* **10**:73.

Kiehn, E. D., and Holland, J. J., 1970, Synthesis and cleavage of enterovirus polypeptides in mammalian cells, *J. Virol.* **5**:358.

Koch, A. S., Eremenko, T., Benedetto, A., and Volpe, P., 1974, A guanidine-sensitive step of the poliovirus RNA replication cycle, *Intervirology* **4**:221.

Korant, B. D., 1972, Cleavage of viral precurser proteins *in vivo* and *in vitro*, *J. Virol.* **10**:751.

Korant, B. D., 1973, Cleavage of poliovirus-specific polypeptide aggregates, *J. Virol.* **12**:556.

Kornberg, A., 1974, *DNA Synthesis*, Freeman, San Francisco.

la Bonnardière, C., 1971, Application de la technique de Cooper a l'isolement de mutants thermosensibles du virus de la fièvre aphteuse, *Ann. Rech. Vet.* **2**:231.

Lake, J. R., and MacKenzie, J. S., 1973, Improved technique for the isolation of temperature-sensitive mutants of foot-and-mouth disease virus, *J. Virol.* **12**:665.

Lake, J. R., Priston, R. A. J., and Slade, W. R., 1975, A genetic recombination map of foot-and-mouth disease virus, *J. Gen. Virol.* **27**:355.

Laporte, J., 1969, The structure of foot-and-mouth disease virus protein, *J. Gen. Virol.* **4**:631.

Ledinko, N., 1963*a*, An analysis of interference between active poliovirus types 1 and 2 in HeLa cells, *Virology* **20**:29.

Ledinko, N., 1963*b*, Genetic recombination with poliovirus type 1: Studies of crosses between a normal horse-serum resistant mutant and several guanidine resistant mutants of the same strain, *Virology* **20**:107.

Ledinko, N., and Hirst, G. K., 1961, Mixed infection of HeLa cells with polioviruses types 1 and 2, *Virology* **14**:207.

Leibowitz, R., and Penman, S., 1971, Regulation of protein synthesis in HeLa cells. III. Inhibition during poliovirus infection, *J. Virol.* **8**:661.

Levy, H. B., 1964, Studies on the mechanism of interferon action. II. The effect of interferon on some early events in mengovirus infection in L-cells, *Virology* **22**:575.

Levy, H. B., and Carter, W. A., 1968, Molecular basis of the action of interferon, *J. Mol. Biol.* **31**:501.

Lonberg-Holm, K., Gosser, L. B., and Kauer, J. C., 1975, Early alteration of poliovirus in infected cells and its specific inhibition, *J. Gen. Virol.* **27**:329.

Lucas-Lenard, J., 1975, Cleavage of mengovirus polyprotein *in vivo*, *J. Virol.* **14**:261.

Lundquist, R. E., Ehrenfeld, E., and Maizel, J. V., 1974, Isolation of a viral polypeptide associated with poliovirus RNA polymerase, *Proc. Natl. Acad. Sci. USA* **71**:4773.

Lwoff, A., and Lwoff, M., 1963, L'action de la guanidine sur le développement du poliovirus, *C. R. Acad. Sci.* **256**:5001.

MacKenzie, J. S., 1975, Virulence of temperature-sensitive mutants of foot-and-mouth disease virus, *Arch. Virol.* **48**:1.

MacKenzie, J. S., and Slade, W. R., 1975, Evidence for recombination between two different immunological types of foot-and-mouth disease virus, *Aust. J. Exp. Biol. Med. Sci.* **53**:251.

MacKenzie, J. S., Slade, W. R., Lake, J., Priston, R. A. J., Bisby, J., Laing, S., and Newman, J., 1975, Temperature-sensitive mutants of foot-and-mouth disease virus:

The isolation of mutants and observations on their properties and genetic recombination, *J. Gen. Virol.* **27**:61.

Manor, D., Barzilai, R., and Goldblum, N., 1974, Dependence of RNA replication on continuous protein synthesis in a temperature-sensitive mutant of foot-and-mouth disease virus, *J. Gen. Virol.* **25**:157.

Marcus, P. I., and Carver, D. H., 1967, Intrinsic interference: A new type of viral interference, *J. Virol.* **1**:334.

Margalith, M., Margalith, E., and Goldblum, N., 1969, Genetic characteristics of echovirus type 9 strains: association of mouse virulence with other genetic markers, *J. Gen. Virol.* **4**:379.

McBride, W. D., 1962, Biological significance of poliovirus mutants of altered cystine requirement, *Virology* **18**:118.

McCahon, D., and Cooper, P. D., 1970, Identification of poliovirus temperature-sensitive mutants having defects in virus structural protein, *J. Gen. Virol.* **6**:51.

McClean, C., and Rueckert, R. R., 1973, Picornaviral gene order: Comparison of a rhinovirus with a cardiovirus, *J. Virol.* **11**:341.

McCormick, W., and Penman, S., 1968, Replication of mengovirus in HeLa cells preinfected with non-replicating poliovirus, *J. Virol.* **2**:859.

Medvedkina, O. A., Scarlat, I. V., Kalinina, N. O., and Agol, V. I., 1974, Virus-specific proteins associated with ribosomes of Krebs II cells infected with EMC virus, *FEBS Lett.* **39**:4.

Melnick, J. L., Agol, V. I., Bachrach, H. L., Brown, F., Cooper, P. D., Fiers, W., Gard, S., Gear, J. H. S., Ghendon, Y., Kasza, L., La Placa, M., Mandel, B., McGregor, S., Mohanty, S. B., Plummer, G., Ruecket, R. R., Schaffer, F. L., Tagaya, I., Tyrrell, D. A. J., Voroshilova, M., and Wenner, H. A., 1974, Picornaviridae, *Intervirology* **4**:303.

Mikhejeva, A., Yakobson, E., and Soloviev, G. Y., 1970, Characterization of some poliovirus temperature-sensitive mutants and poliovirus-related particle formation under non-permissive conditions, *J. Virol.* **6**:188.

Mikhejeva, A., Yakobson, E., and Ghendon, Y. Z., 1973, Studies on temperature sensitive events in synthesis of poliovirus temperature sensitive mutants, *Arch. Ges. Virusforsch.* **43**:352.

Miner, N., Ray, W. J., and Simon, E. H., 1966, Effect of interferon on the production and action of viral RNA polymerase, *Biochem. Biophys. Res. Commun.* **24**:264.

Moss, B., 1968, Inhibition of HeLa cell protein synthesis by the vaccinia virion, *J. Virol.* **2**:1028.

Mosser, A. G., Caliguiri, L. A., Scheid, A. S., and Tamm, I., 1972a, Chemical and enzymatic characteristics of cytoplasmic membranes in poliovirus-infected HeLa cells, *Virology* **47**:30.

Mosser, A. G., Caliguiri, L. A., and Tamm, I., 1972b, Incorporation of lipid precursors into cytoplasmic membranes of poliovirus infected HeLa cells, *Virology* **47**:39.

Newman, J. F. E., Rowlands, D. J., and Brown, F., 1973, A physico-chemical sub-grouping of the mammalian picornaviruses, *J. Gen. Virol.* **18**:171.

Norman, A., 1960, Ultra-violet inactivation of poliovirus ribonucleic acid, *Virology* **10**:384.

Öberg, B., and Philipson, L., 1971, Replicative structures of poliovirus RNA *in vivo, J. Mol. Biol.* **58**:725.

Öberg, B. F., and Shatkin, A. J., 1972, Initiation of picornavirus protein synthesis in ascites cell extracts, *Proc. Natl. Acad. Sci. USA* **69**:3589.

Oberg, B. F., and Shatkin, A. J., 1974, Translation of mengovirus RNA in Ehrlich ascites cell extracts, *Biochem. Biophys. Res. Commun.* **57**:1186.

Ohlbaum, A., Figueroa, F., Grado, C., and Contreras, G., 1970, Target molecular weight of foot-and-mouth disease virus and poliovirus, *J. Gen. Virol.* **6**:429.

Paucha, E., Seehafer, J., and Colter, J. S., 1974, Synthesis of viral-specific polypeptides in mengovirus infected L-cells: Evidence for asymmetric translation of the genome, *Virology* **61**:315.

Penman, S., 1965, Stimulation of the incorporation of choline in poliovirus-infected cells, *Virology* **25**:148.

Penman, S., and Summers, D. F., 1965, Effects on host cell metabolism following synchronous infection with poliovirus, *Virology* **27**:614.

Penman, S., Becker, Y., and Darnell, J. E., 1964, A cytoplasmic structure involved in the synthesis and assembly of poliovirus components, *J. Mol. Biol.* **8**:541.

Pérez-Bercoff, R., Carrara, G., Dolei, A., Conciatori, G., and Rita, G., 1974*a, In vitro* binding of a cellular α-amanitin sensitive RNA polymerase to infectious mengovirus-induced double-stranded RNA, *Biochem. Biophys. Res. Commun.* **56**:876.

Pérez-Bercoff, R., Coié, L., Meo, P., Carrara, G., Mechali, M., Falcoff, E., and Rita, G., 1974*b*, Infectivity of mengovirus replicative form: Relationship to cellular transcription, *J. Gen. Virol.* **25**:53.

Perlin, M., and Phillips, B. A., 1973, *In vitro* assembly of poliovirus. III. Assembly of 14S particles into empty capsids by poliovirus infected HeLa cell membranes, *Virology* **53**:107.

Pérol-Vauchez, Y., Tournier, P., and Lwoff, M., 1962, Atténuation de la virulence du virus de l'encéphalomyelite de la souris par culture a basse température: Influence de l'hypo- et de l'hyperthermie sur l'évolution de la maladie expérimentale, *C. R. Acad. Sci.* **253**:2164.

Phillips, B. A., 1969, *In vitro* assembly of poliovirus. I. Kinetics of the assembly of empty capsids and the role of extracts from infected cells, *Virology* **39**:811.

Phillips, B. A., 1971, *In vitro* assembly of polioviruses. II. Evidence for the self-assembly of 14 S particles into empty capsids, *Virology* **44**:307.

Phillips, B. A., and Fennell, R., 1973, Polypeptide composition of poliovirions, naturally occurring empty capsids and 14S precursor particles, *J. Virol.* **12**:291.

Phillips, B. A., Summers, D. F., and Maizel, J. V., 1968, *In vitro* assembly of poliovirus-related particles, *Virology* **35**:216.

Pine, M. J., 1972, Turnover of intra-cellular proteins, *Annu. Rev. Microbiol.* **26**:103.

Pohjanpelto, P., 1958, Stabilization of poliovirus by cystine, *Virology* **6**:472.

Pohjanpelto, P., and Cooper, P. D., 1965, Interference between polioviruses induced by strains that cannot multiply, *Virology* **25**:350.

Pringle, C. R., 1968, Recombination between conditional lethal mutants of foot-and-mouth disease virus, *J. Gen. Virol.* **2**:199.

Pringle, C. R., 1969, Electrophoretic properties of foot-and-mouth disease virus strains and the selection of intra-strain mutants, *J. Gen. Virol.* **4**:541.

Pringle, C. R., and Slade, W. R., 1968, The origin of hybrid variants of sub-type strains of foot-and-mouth disease virus, *J. Gen. Virol.* **2**:319.

Pringle, C. R., Slade, W. R., Elsworthy, P., and O'Sullivan, M., 1970, Properties of temperature-sensitive mutants of the Kenya 3/57 strain of foot-and-mouth disease virus, *J. Gen. Virol.* **6**:213.

Rekosh, D. M., 1972, The gene order of poliovirus capsid proteins, *J. Virol.* **9**:479.

Rekosh, D. M., Lodish, H. F., and Baltimore, D., 1970, Protein synthesis in *E. coli* extracts programmed by poliovirus RNA, *J. Mol. Biol.* **54**:327.

Rosenberg, H., Diskin, B., Oron, L., and Traub, A., 1972, Isolation and subunit structure of polycytidylate-dependent RNA polymerase of encephalomyocarditis virus, *Proc. Natl. Acad. Sci. USA* **69**:3815.

Roumiantzeff, M., Summers, D. F., and Maizel, J. V., 1971, *In vitro* protein synthetic activity of membrane-bound poliovirus polyribosomes, *Virology* **44**:249.

Rueckert, R. R., 1971, Picornaviral architecture, in: *Comparative Virology* (K. Maramarosch and E. Kurstar, eds.), pp. 255–306, Academic Press, New York.

Sabin, A. B., and Lwoff, A., 1959, Relation between reproductive capacity of poliovirus at different temperatures in tissue culture and neurovirulence, *Science* **129**:1287.

Saborio, J. L., Pong, S. S., and Koch, G., 1974, Selective and reversible inhibition of initiation of protein-synthesis in mammalian cells, *J. Mol. Biol.* **85**:195.

Saxton, R. E., and Stevens, J. G., 1972, Restriction of herpes simplex virus replication by poliovirus: A selective inhibition of viral translation, *Virology* **48**:207.

Schaffer, F. L., and Gordon, M., 1966, Differential inhibitory effects of actinomycin D among strains of poliovirus, *J. Bacteriol.* **91**:2309.

Schaffer, F. L., and Schwerdt, C. G., 1965, Chemistry of the RNA viruses, in: *Viral and Rickettsial Infections of Man* 4th ed. (F. L. Horsfall and I. Tamm, eds.) p. 94, Lippincott, Pennsylvania.

Scharff, M. D., Maizel, J. V., and Levintow, L., 1964, Physical and immunological properties of a soluble precursor of the poliovirus capsid, *Proc. Natl. Acad. Sci. USA* **51**:329.

Sergiescu, D., and Aubert-Combiescu, A., 1969, Differential sensitivity to gliotoxin of virulent and attenuated poliovirus and its possible use as a genetic marker, *Arch. Ges. Virusforsch.* **27**:268.

Sergiescu, D., Aubert-Combiescu, A., and Crainic, R., 1969, Recombination between guanidine-resistant and dextran sulphate-resistant mutants of type 1 poliovirus, *J. Virol.* **3**:326.

Sergiescu, D., Horodniceanu, F., and Aubert-Combiescu, A., 1972, The use of inhibitors in the study of picornavirus genetics, *Prog. Med. Virol.* **14**:123.

Shirman, G. A., Maslova, S. V., Gavrilovskaya, I. N., and Agol, V. I., 1973, Stimulation of restricted reproduction of EMC virus in HeLa cells by non-replicating poliovirus, *Virology* **51**:1.

Silber, R., Malathi, V. G., and Hurwitz, J., 1972, Purification and properties of bacteriophage T4-induced RNA ligase, *Proc. Natl. Acad. Sci. USA* **69**:3009.

Smith, A. E., 1973, The initiation of protein synthesis directed by the RNA from encephalomyocarditis virus, *Eur. J. Biochem.* **33**:301.

Smith, A. E., Marcker, K. A., and Mathews, M. B., 1970, Translation of RNA from EMC virus in a mammalian cell-free system, *Nature (London)* **225**:184.

Spector, D. H., and Baltimore, D., 1974, Requirement of 3′ terminal poly (adenylic acid) for infectivity of poliovirus RNA, *Proc. Natl. Acad. Sci. USA* **71**:2983.

Steiner-Pryor, A., and Cooper, P. D., 1973, Temperature-sensitive poliovirus mutants defective in repression of host protein synthesis are also defective in structural protein, *J. Gen. Virol.* **21**:215.

Sturman, L. S., and Tamm, I., 1966, Host dependence of GD VII virus: Complete or abortive multiplication in various cell types, *J. Immunol.* **97**:885.

Sturman, L. S., and Tamm, I., 1969, Formation of viral RNA and virus in cells that are permissive or nonpermissive for murine encephalomyletis virus (GD VII), *J. Virol.* **3**:8.

Summers, D. F., and Maizel, J. V., 1968, Evidence for large precurser proteins in poliovirus synthesis, *Proc. Natl. Acad. Sci. USA* **59**:966.

Summers, D. F., and Maizel, J. V., 1971, Determination of the gene sequence of poliovirus with pactamycin, *Proc. Natl. Acad. Sci. USA* **68**:2852.

Summers, D. F., Maizel, J. V., and Darnell, J. E., 1965, Evidence for virus specific non-capsid proteins in poliovirus infected HeLa cells, *Proc. Natl. Acad. Sci. USA* **54**:505.

Summers, D. F., Shaw, E. N., Stewart, M. C., and Maizel, J. V., 1972, Inhibition of cleavage of large poliovirus-specific precurser proteins in infected HeLa cells by inhibition of proteolytic enzymes, *J. Virol.* **10**:880.

Taber, R., Rekosh, D., and Baltimore, D., 1971, Effect of pactamycin on synthesis of poliovirus proteins: A method for genetic mapping, *J. Virol.* **8**:395.

Tannock, G. A., Gibbs, A. J., and Cooper, P. D., 1970, A re-examination of the molecular weight of poliovirus RNA, *Biochem. Biophys. Res. Commun.* **38**:298.

Todd, D., and Martin, S. J., 1975, Determination of the molecular weight of bovine enterovirus RNA by nuclease digestion, *J. Gen. Virol.* **26**:121.

Vanden Berghe, D., and Boeyé, A., 1972, New polypeptides in poliovirus, *Virology* **48**:604.

Vesco, C., and Penman, S., 1969, Insensitivity of mitochondrial RNA synthesis to mengovirus infections in CHO cells, *Nature (London)* **224**:1021.

Villa-Komaroff, L., Baltimore, D., and Lodish, H. F., 1973, Translation of poliovirus messenger RNA in mammalian cell-free systems, *Fed. Proc. Abst.* **33**:531.

Wall, R., and Taylor, M. W., 1969, Host-dependent restriction of mengovirus replication, *J. Virol.* **4**:681.

Wall, R., and Taylor, M. W., 1970, Mengovirus RNA synthesis in productive and restrictive cell lines, *Virology* **42**:78.

Wecker, E., and Lederhilger, G., 1964a, Curtailment of the latent period by double-infection with polioviruses, *Proc. Natl. Acad. Sci. USA* **52**:246.

Wecker, E., and Lederhilger, G., 1964b, Genomic masking produced by double-infection of HeLa cells with heterotypic polioviruses, *Proc. Natl. Acad. Sci. USA* **52**:705.

Wentworth, B. B., McCahon, D., and Cooper, P. D., 1968, Production of infectious RNA and serum-blocking antigen by poliovirus temperature-sensitive mutants, *J. Gen. Virol.* **2**:297.

Wetlaufer, D. B., and Ristow, S., 1973, Acquisition of 3-dimensional structure of proteins, *Annu. Rev. Biochem.* **42**:135.

Wildy, P., 1971, *Classification and Nomenclature of Viruses*, First Report of the International Committee on Nomenclature of Viruses, *Monographs in Virology*, Vol. 5, Karger, Basel.

Wright, P. J., and Cooper, P. D., 1974a, Poliovirus proteins associated with ribosomal structures in infected cells, *Virology* **59**:1.

Wright, P. J., and Cooper, P. D., 1974b, Isolation of cold-sensitive mutants of poliovirus, *Intervirology* **2**:20.

Wright, P. J., and Cooper, P. D., 1976, Poliovirus proteins associated with the replication complex in infected cells, *J. Gen. Virol.* **30**:63.

Yogo, Y., and Wimmer, E., 1973, Poly(A) and poly(U) in poliovirus double-stranded RNA, *Nature* (*London*) *New Biol.* **242**:171.

Závadová, Z., 1971, Host cell repair of vaccinia virus and of double-stranded RNA of encephalomyocarditis virus, *Nature* (*London*) *New Biol.* **233**:123.

Zimmerman, E. F., Heeter, M., and Darnell, J. E., 1963, RNA synthesis in poliovirus-infected cells, *Virology* **19**:400.

CHAPTER 5

Genetics of Togaviruses

Elmer R. Pfefferkorn

Microbiology Department
Dartmouth Medical School
Hanover, New Hampshire 03755

1. REVIEW OF THE STRUCTURE AND REPLICATION OF GROUP A TOGAVIRUSES

Genetic analysis of togaviruses is unlikely to make any substantial new contribution to our understanding of the discipline of genetics. Rather, it should provide a fuller understanding of the structure, replication, and pathogenesis of these viruses. A brief review of the structure and biochemistry of togaviruses may be useful as a background against which both the progress and the unresolved problems of togavirus genetics can be viewed. An earlier volume in this series presents a more comprehensive survey (Pfefferkorn and Shapiro, 1974).

I shall confine my description to the group A togaviruses (alphaviruses), since nearly all togaviral genetic studies have concentrated on this group. The virion consists of an enveloped icosahedral nucleocapsid with an overall diameter of 45–75 nm (reviewed by Pfefferkorn and Shapiro, 1974). The envelope contains cholesterol and phospholipids that largely reflect the composition of the plasma membrane, which is a principal site of viral budding (Renkonen *et al.*, 1971). Cellular proteins are, at least as a first approximation, absent from the virion (Pfefferkorn and Clifford, 1964). All group A togaviruses contain two virus-specific envelope glycoproteins (E1 and E2) of molecular weight 50,000–53,000 (reviewed by Pfefferkorn and Shapiro, 1974). Semliki Forest virus has recently been shown to contain a third 10,00 dalton glycoprotein (E3) in its envelope (Garoff *et al.,* 1974). I suspect that a careful reexamination of other group A viruses will reveal a similar protein. The icosahedral nucleocapsid contains but a single protein (C) of molecular weight 30,000–32,000. Recent evidence suggests that the C protein in the virion is closely apposed to segments of the envelope glycoproteins that extend through the lipid bilayer of the envelope. Proteolytic removal of the glycoproteins of Semliki Forest virus leaves small hydrophobic polypeptide remnants of the larger glycoproteins associated with the resulting bald virion (Utermann and Simons, 1974). Furthermore, the envelope and capsid proteins can be cross-linked by exposing the intact virion to formaldehyde (Brown *et al.,* 1974) or dimethylsuberimidate (Garoff and Simons, 1974). This evidence for proximity of the capsid and the envelope proteins is critical, for a protein–protein interaction can allow an intracellular nucleocapsid to recognize that a membrane bearing viral glycoproteins is suitable for budding. Additional nucleocapsid–glycoprotein interactions can then drive the process of budding (Brown *et al.,* 1972) and serve to exclude cellular membrane proteins (Garoff and Simons, 1975).

The viral genome is a single-stranded RNA molecule with a molecular weight of approximately 4.2×10^6 (reviewed by Pfefferkorn and Shapiro, 1974). This RNA has the polarity of messenger RNA and can indeed serve as messenger in a cell-free system that yields identifiable capsid protein (Simmons and Strauss, 1974; Cancedda and Schlesinger, 1974; Smith *et al.,* 1974). However, the principal messenger RNA in infected cells is not the virion RNA but the so-called interjacent RNA (26 S) that represents about a third of the viral genome (Simmons and Strauss, 1972a). This smaller messenger RNA is probably initially translated into a precursor protein that is then proteolytically cleaved in several steps to yield all of the structural proteins of the virion. The first of the cleavages, which yields the C protein, apparently takes place before the nascent precursor is completed (reviewed by Pfefferkorn and Shapiro, 1974).

An RNA of molecular weight 4.2×10^6 can code for approximately nine proteins with an average molecular weight of 40,000. Only one-third of this genetic information, that represented in the interjacent RNA, is used in the synthesis of the structural proteins of the virion. One of the principal tasks of togavirus genetics is to decipher the function of the remaining two-thirds of the viral genome. It is of interest to note that the picornaviruses have only about as half as much of the viral genetic information devoted to nonstructural proteins even though picorna- and togaviruses appear to face the same biosynthetic problem, replication of a plus-stranded genome in the cytoplasm of an infected cell. It is possible that the additional information devoted to nonvirion proteins of togaviruses is related to their broad host range. These viruses must be able to multiply in phylogenetically diverse vertebrate and arthropod cells.

2. TYPES OF MUTANTS

2.1. Plaque Morphology Mutants

Spontaneous mutants that exhibit larger or smaller plaques are occasionally observed during routine titrations of group A togaviruses (e.g., Marshall *et al.,* 1962; Quersin-Thiry, 1961; Bose *et al.,* 1970). At present, plaque morphology mutants have not proven to be useful in genetic studies. If an efficient system for the demonstration of recombination (see Section 3.2) can be devised, plaque-type mutants might usefully serve as a third marker in three-factor crosses involving two different temperature-sensitive mutants.

Persistently infected cultures probably represent a strongly selective environment that is markedly different from that of the usual lytic infection. Thus it is not surprising that mutants that produce altered plaques come to predominate under these conditions. Simizu and Takayama (1969) discovered two different large-plaque mutants of western equine encephalitis virus in a study of chronically infected mouse sarcoma cells. Schwöbel and Ahl (1972) noted that a persistent Sindbis virus infection of BHK cells selected a small plaque variant. Chronically infected *Aedes albopictus* cells yielded a small plaque mutant of Semliki Forest virus (Davey and Dalgarno, 1974).

Little is known of the physiology of the various plaque morphology mutants that have been isolated. In one case, the mutation affects the surface of the virion, presumably through changes in the amino acid sequences of one or another of the envelope glycoproteins, because the plaque mutants and the wild-type virus can be resolved by chromatography on calcium phosphage (Bose *et al.,* 1970). In another case, sensitivity to an inhibitor present in agar was responsible for the small plaques of a mutant (Schleupner *et al.,* 1969).

2.2. Host Range Mutants

Group A togaviruses characteristically have a broad host range. They multiply efficiently in a variety of avian, mammalian, and insect cell cultures (Pfefferkorn and Shapiro, 1974). Mutations that act to extend or restrict this host range have not been commonly sought. Symington and Schlesinger (1975) noted that their wild-type Sindbis virus grew poorly in a mouse plasmacytoma line. Serial passage in this line selected a stable mutant that grew with much greater efficiency than the wild type on a variety of cells derived from the mouse. This extended host range mutant retained its ability to replicate efficiently in chick cells.

I have commented above (Section 1) that the requirement that togaviruses multiply in both arthropod and vertebrate hosts may account for the relatively large amount of genetic information devoted to nonvirion proteins. If the virus does indeed have genes that need be expressed only in one host and not in the other, it should be possible to select mutants that grow in mosquito cells but not in vertebrate cells, and *vice versa*.

2.3. Mutants in Which the Stability of the Virion Is Altered

Group A togaviruses are readily inactivated by heat. The virion apparently contains two different thermosensitive targets. The inactivation of one predominates at physiological temperatures, while the other is more significant at temperatures above 41°C (Fleming, 1971). Burge and Pfefferkorn (1966a) selected their heat-resistant (HR) strain by repeatedly heating at 60°C and regrowing the survivors. The resulting HR strain was subsequently used as the wild type for the isolation of *ts* mutants (see Section 2.7). The HR strain has mutation(s) that affect only the thermal event that is significant above 41°C. At 37°C, the HR mutant is no more stable than the strain from which it was derived.

It might be profitable to cast the net wider in the selection of mutants with resistant virions. For example, Semliki Forest virus has been shown to be inactivated by urea and guanidine (Fleming, 1971), while Sindbis virus is susceptible to dithiothreitol (Carver and Seto, 1968). If they can exist, mutants resistant to these chemicals should be readily isolated and may be useful in the study of protein–protein interactions in the virion.

2.4. Mutants in Which the Morphology of the Virion Is Altered

Group A togavirions are approximately the same size, 45–75 nm in diameter (see Pfefferkorn and Shapiro, 1974). Most of the variation in reported diameters can probably be ascribed to differences in sample preparation for electron microscopy rather than true biological variation. One systematic study, however, suggests that the size of the virions can be altered by mutation. Tsilinsky *et al.* (1971) isolated clones of Venezuelan equine encephalitis virus that differed in diameter by as much as 20%. Furthermore, 5-fluorouracil mutagenesis of a strain characterized by small virions allowed the isolation of a mutant with reduced plaque size, greater thermostability, and larger virions. Brown and Gliedman (1973) noted even more dramatic changes in the diameter of Sindbis virions during continuous passage in mosquito cell culture. Two distinct smaller viral particles soon outnumbered the standard-sized virions. Although these smaller particles are antigenically related to Sindbis, their infectivity has not been established and they may be simply lethal errors in viral assembly. Brown and Gliedman (1973) suggest that these particles have smaller icosahedral nucleocapsids constructed from the same capsid protein but with a different triangulation number.

Most togaviruses in any given preparation have but a single nucleocapsid per virion, but a small fraction are occasionally observed to have more than one nucleocapsid within a common envelope (e.g., Bykovsky *et al.*, 1969; Higashi *et al.*, 1967; Tsilinsky, *et al.*, 1971). These abnormal virions presumably are the result of errors in assembly. This error, whatever it is, is greatly amplified in a γ-ray-induced, small plaque mutant western equine encephalitis virus isolated by Simizu *et al.* (1973). Fully half of the progeny of this mutant consist of rapidly sedimenting virions in which a single envelope encloses two or more nucleocapsids. The nature of the mutation causing this error in assembly is unknown.

2.5. Mutants with Reduced Virulence

Togavirus mutants with reduced virulence have been described in several laboratories (e.g., Bradish *et al.*, 1971; Bradish and Allner, 1972; Takayama, 1972; Rasmussen *et al.*, 1973; Brown and Officer, 1975). Most of these emerged after prolonged passage in culture and would be classed as vaccine strains. Since these vaccine strains are almost certainly multiple-step mutants, they are less attractive for genetic studies but may be useful in the analysis of viral pathogenesis.

2.6. Defective Interfering Mutants

Several laboratories have isolated defective interfering mutants from group A togaviruses (reviewed by Pfefferkorn and Shapiro, 1974).

Analogy with other better-studied systems suggests that these defective-interfering particles are likely to be lethal deletion mutants that have an intracellular growth advantage over the normal virion but are, in turn, dependent on coinfection with the normal virion to supply the deleted function. The principal obstacle to the use of these supposed deletion mutants in genetic studies is that, at present, there is no way to separate them from the normal virions that are required for their production.

2.7. Temperature-Sensitive Mutants

Temperature-sensitive (*ts*) mutants are selected for their inability to form plaques at a high (restrictive) temperature that permits plaque formation by the wild (*ts*$^+$) type. At a lower (permissive) temperature, both the *ts* mutant and the wild type grow and form plaques normally. Thus the *ts* mutants can be propagated at the permissive temperature and their defects studied at the restrictive temperature. Togaviruses are ideal for the isolation of *ts* mutants because their natural growth in both arthropods and vertebrates has selected for efficient replication over a broad range of temperature. All of the togavirus *ts* mutants that have come to my attention are listed in Table 1.

Temperature-sensitive (*ts*) mutants have proven to be the most useful class of mutants for all animal viruses. Their advantage lies in their

TABLE 1

Temperature-Sensitive Mutants of Group A Togaviruses

Virus	Reference	Number of mutants	Mutagens[a]
Sindbis	Burge and Pfefferkorn (1966*a*)	23	EMS, NA, NTG
Semliki Forest	Tan *et al.* (1969)	38	FU, HA, NTG
Western equine encephalitis	Simizu and Takayama (1971)	1	None[b]
Eastern equine encephalitis	Zebovitz and Brown (1970)	4	NA
Western equine encephalitis	Simizu and Takayama (1972)	2	NTG
Sindbis	Atkins *et al.* (1974*b*)	104	EMS, FU, HA, NA, NTG
Sindbis	Stollar *et al.* (1974)	1	None[b]
Semliki Forest	Keränen and Kääriäinen (1974)	16	NTG

[a] EMS, ethylmethanesulfonic acid; FU, 5-fluorouracil; HA, hydroxylamine; NA, nitrous acid; NTG, *N*-methyl-*N*′-nitro-*N*-nitrosoguanidine.
[b] Spontaneous mutants that appeared in chronically infected cultures.

relative ease of isolation and in their generality. Since a change in amino acid sequence can alter the temperature-dependent conformation of any protein, *ts* mutations should be possible in every cistron that has a protein product. In practice, this generalization can be tested only in microorganisms in which the genome can be thoroughly mapped. A detailed study of bacteriophage T4 (Epstein *et al.,* 1963) has shown a few cistrons identified through amber mutants for which no *ts* mutants were detected in a catalogue larger than is likely in most studies of animal viruses. Nonetheless, *ts* mutants of animal viruses should at least encompass most of the viral genome.

A review of the techniques for isolation of togavirus *ts* mutants (Pfefferkorn, 1969) requires only a few additions. Atkins *et al.* (1974*a*) avoided tedious blind selection by picking as potential *ts* mutants those plaques that failed to enlarge upon shift from the permissive to the restrictive temperature. Several additional mutagens should be considered by anyone seeking more mutants: fluorouracil and hydroxylamine (Tan *et al.,* 1969; Atkins *et al.,* 1974*a*), azacytidine (Halle, 1968), and various additional alkylating agents (Solyanik *et al.,* 1974).

Initial characterization of *ts* mutants should include both the back-mutation frequency and the degree of leakiness. The back-mutation frequency is measured by growing a stock of mutant virus and determining its plaque titer at both the restrictive and the permissive temperature. The ratio of these two values is the back-mutation frequency, which is a rough index of the back-mutation rate. The back-mutation rate, which is seldom if ever measured, is the probability that back-mutation will occur per genome replication. Although back-mutation rate is, in theory, a constant, back-mutation frequency of individual stocks of a given mutant will vary. It is often advantageous to select a stock that, by chance, has a particular low back-mutation frequency. Back-mutation frequencies for the larger catalogues vary from 5×10^{-3} to 1×10^{-7} (Burge and Pfefferkorn 1966*a*; Tan *et al.,* 1969; Atkins *et al.,* 1974*a*; Keränen and Kääriäinen, 1974). These values are probably lower than the natural rate, for all workers tend to discard as unusable a few mutants with excessively high reversion frequencies. Back mutation of *ts* mutants to *ts*$^+$ does not always restore the complete phenotype of the wild type. Several revertants of the same *ts* mutant varied in virion thermostability (Burge and Pfefferkorn, 1966*a*) and in plaque size (Pfefferkorn, unpublished observation). Since the selection of *ts* mutants involves the use of potent chemical mutagens, the possibility that some are double mutants should always be borne in mind. One *ts* mutant has been shown to have another temperature-inde-

pendent mutation (Keränen and Kääriäinen, 1974). The leakiness of a
ts mutant is measured by the production of *mutant* progeny in infections at the restrictive temperature. Leakiness can be expressed either
as the ratio of mutant virus production by a *ts* mutant at the restrictive
and at the permissive temperature or as the ratio of mutant virus
production by the mutant at the restrictive temperature and wild-type
virus production by the wild type at the restrictive temperature. In
either case, the values found are 10^{-3}–10^{-6}. Leakage by *ts* mutants is
generally the limiting factor in the detection of complementation.

3. INTERACTIONS OF TOGAVIRUS MUTANTS IN MIXED INFECTIONS

3.1. Phenotypic Mixing

Phenotypic mixing has been demonstrated to occur between
Sindbis virus and the closely related eastern and western equine encephalitis viruses (Burge and Pfefferkorn, 1966c). The Sindbis parent in
these experiments was a *ts* mutant, the virion of which was resistant to
heating at 60°C. The other viruses were wild type with respect to *ts*
lesions and their virions were thermolabile at 60°C. To demonstrate
phenotypic mixing, the progeny of a mixed infection at the permissive
temperature were heated to eliminate virions that were phenotypically
thermolabile. The survivors were then assayed by plaque formation at
the restrictive temperature to exclude the Sindbis *ts* genotype. The
mixed infections, but not the control single infections, yielded heat-stable virions that were genotypically eastern or western equine encephalitis virus. Thus the genomes of the equine encephalitis viruses must
occasionally have been enclosed in an envelope that contained enough
Sindbis virus glycoproteins to confer thermostability. The principal
value of this observation is that it demonstrates that genetically different togaviruses can simultaneously replicate in the same cell, a
necessary condition for both complementation and recombination.

Lagwinska *et al.* (1975) observed phenotypic mixing between
Sindbis virus and the structurally similar lactic dehydrogenase virus. In
contrast, Burge and Pfefferkorn (1966c) noted that Sindbis virus and a
morphologically distinct enveloped RNA virus, vesicular stomatitis
virus, failed to show any evidence of phenotypic mixing. This single
negative experiment should not be overinterpreted, since Burge and
Pfefferkorn (1966c) presented no evidence to show that a mixed infection was indeed established. Furthermore, other tests, such as neu-

tralization with specific antibody, might reveal phenotypic mixing that did not confer thermostability. Recent demonstrations of phenotypic mixing between phylogenetically unrelated viruses suggest that this phenomenon may be widespread among enveloped viruses.

3.2. Recombination

Genetic recombination, if and when it recurs, should be relatively easily detected, since many *ts* mutants of togaviruses (Table 1) with different defects and acceptably low back-mutation frequencies are available. To test for recombination, mixed infections are established at the permissive temperature and the progeny are titered at both the permissive and the restrictive temperature. Only true recombinants and revertants will make plaques at the restrictive temperature. Control single infections done in parallel with the genetic cross serve to measure the contribution of back mutants. Using this procedure with extensive catalogues of mutants, neither Burge and Pfefferkorn (1966*b*), nor Tan (1969), nor Atkins *et al.* (1974*a*) were able to detect recombination. Burge and Pfefferkorn (1966*b*) would have detected recombination had it occurred at a frequency of 10^{-4}. There is but one preliminary report of genetic recombination in togaviruses. Brawner and Sagik (1971) were able to demonstrate marker rescue between ultraviolet light-inactivated wild-type Sindbis virus and an unirradiated *ts* mutant. The resulting recombinant progeny were genetically stable and able to form plaques at the restrictive temperature. Brawner and Sagik (1971) ascribe their success to clumping the inoculum with $MgCl_2$ to promote multiple infection within a localized area of the same cell. The resulting proximity of the parental genomes was presumed to increase the probability of genetic interaction.

The observations of Brawner and Sagik (1971) are potentially most important. The successful mapping of the poliovirus genome described elsewhere in this volume is an example of what can be accomplished with RNA-containing animal viruses. The demonstration of recombination is such an important goal that additional methods to ensure a physically localized infection should be considered. A useful system might be to isolate *ts* mutants from the mutant of western equine encephalitis that Simizu *et al.* (1973) have shown to produce multiploid virions.

A mixed infection with two *ts* multiploid mutants should yield some multiploid particles with genomes bearing each *ts* mutation. Upon the next round of infection, the probability of recombination, provided that it is improved by proximity, should be significantly elevated. The problem of determining the genotype of the progeny in the face of the multiploid characteristic should be eliminated by extracting infectious RNA from the mixedly infected cells and using it to assay for wild-type recombinants.

3.3. Complementation

Complementation results in the production of *ts* mutant progeny virus by cells mixedly infected with two different *ts* mutants at the restrictive temperature. This virus production is measured as an increase over a control level that is the sum of the virus titers of parallel independent infections by the two mutants in question. If two mutants fail to complement, they may share the same defect, and are assigned to the same complementation group. If they do complement, the mutants are presumed to be defective in different functions, although the possibility of intracistronic complementation must be borne in mind (Fincham, 1966). The probability that all of the structural proteins of group A togavirus are produced by translation of the 26 S (interjacent) messenger RNA and cleavage of the resulting precursor (reviewed by Pfefferkorn and Shapiro, 1974) poses an additional problem in the interpretation of complementation assays. Any mutation that alters the conformation of the precursor protein may also affect the normal pattern of cleavage. In fact, as seen below (Sections 4.2 and 4.3), a common effect is inhibition of the normal cleavage process and accumulation of precursors in cells infected with *ts* mutants at the restrictive temperature. Since both the amino acid sequence at the cleavage site and the overall conformation of the precursor are determinants of cleavage, it is entirely possible that a mutation that affects the cleavage of one protein may actually be located in the amino acid sequence of another protein that is part of the same precursor. If, as is likely, small segments of the precursor are discarded and degraded during normal cleavage, mutations in these segments may also have profound effects. Under these circumstances, complementation may simply be too crude a tool to assign mutations to individual cistrons. Two alternative attacks are possible. First, a genetic map produced by measurement of recombination frequencies would show if, for example, mutations apparently affecting the capsid protein were really located in that protein. The difficulties involved in demonstration of recombination are noted in Section 3.2. A laborious but more reasonable approach might be to determine the amino acid sequence of each structural protein of the wild type and compare the results with those of selected mutants.

Complementation between *ts* mutants of Sindbis virus was first noted by Burge and Pfefferkorn (1966*b*). With few exceptions, the complementation was inefficient, generally representing a few percent of the wild-type growth under comparable conditions. In many cases, the yield was due to complementation so low that special procedures were required to disclose it. In particular, it was essential to rinse the monolayers several hours after mixed infection to remove virus that had been transiently adsorbed and had subsequently eluted back into the medium. Although only a small fraction of the inoculum was thus eluted, it was sufficient in many cases to obscure the low level of complementation.

Several parameters of togaviral complementation have been explored using *ts* mutants incapable (RNA$^-$) or capable (RNA$^+$) of viral RNA synthesis in infections at the restrictive temperature. In crosses of RNA$^+$ × RNA$^+$ mutants and RNA$^+$ × RNA$^-$ mutants, the complementation was roughly symmetrical; both genotypes were found in the progeny (Burge and Pfefferkorn, 1966*b*). The efficiency of complementation was not increased by multiplicities of infection greater than one RNA$^+$ parent per cell, presumably because this type of mutant is capable of genome replication. Conversely, complementation was increased by higher multiplicities of RNA$^-$ mutants (Burge and Pfefferkorn, 1966*b*; Pfefferkorn and Burge, 1967).

Representative results illustrating complementation between *ts* mutants of Sindbis virus are recorded in Table 2. These and other data (Burge and Pfefferkorn, 1966*b*; Pfefferkorn and Burge, 1967, 1968) allow several conclusions. Complementation is regularly observed when one parent is RNA$^+$ and the other is RNA$^-$. Within each of these two major classes of mutants, complementation allows recognition of three complementation groups.

Most RNA$^-$ mutants have been assigned to complementation group A despite the fact that some of them exhibit inefficient complementation with one another. The data from crosses within group A fall into no coherent pattern and are difficult to interpret. Intracistronic complementation (Fincham, 1966) may explain some or all of the positive results, but the possibility that misassigned members of as yet undesignated complementation groups may lurk in complementation group A cannot be ignored.

The only consistent exception to the rule that complementation between Sindbis virus mutants is inefficient involves an RNA$^-$ mutant,

TABLE 2

Complementation between *ts* Mutants of Sindbis Virus

Comple-mentation group	Mutant	Complementation level[a] in mixed infection with											
		*ts*21	*ts*19	*ts*17	*ts*4	*ts*24	*ts*11	*ts*6	*ts*2	*ts*5	*ts*10	*ts*23	*ts*20
A	*ts*21	—	0.2	0.1	0.1	1.5	17.6	200	43	27	24	ND[b]	ND
A	*ts*19		—	0.4	0.5	3.2	120	485	ND	16	19	43	12
A	*ts*17			—		4.5	30	393	25	31	17	19	23
A	*ts*4				—	0.36	9.0	127	19	ND	27	ND	8
A	*ts*24					—	4.2	364	22	29	18	16	5
A′	*ts*11						—	280	1.8	50	43	ND	12
B	*ts*6							—	62	93	64	68	21
C	*ts*2								—	1.0	36	27	5.2
C	*ts*5									—	345	61	8.0
D	*ts*10										—	0.7	16.7
D	*ts*23											—	8.5
E	*ts*20												—

[a] Since these data are from several independent experiments (Burge and Pfefferkorn, 1966b; Pfefferkorn and Burge, 1967; Pfefferkorn, unpublished observations), the viral titers are not strictly comparable and are not reported. The numbers recorded are relative values calculated as complementation levels as defined by Burge and Pfefferkorn (1966b). The complementation level is the ratio of the viral titer produced by a mixed infection of two *ts* mutants at the restrictive temperature to the sum of the viral titers produced in parallel single infection.
[b] Not done.

*ts*6. In crosses with other RNA⁻ mutants, *ts*6 allows an efficiency of complementation that represents 10–50% of the wild-type yield under comparable conditions. Pfefferkorn and Burge (1967) have thus assigned mutant *ts*6 to complementation group B, of which it is the sole representative. Complementation with *ts*6 is so extensive that it has been detected by biochemical as well as genetic techniques. Burge and Pfefferkorn (1967) reported that cultures supporting complementation synthesized actinomycin D-resistant (i.e., viral) [³H]uridine-labeled RNA that was qualitatively similar to the virus-specific RNA found in wild-type virus infected cells. Furthermore, the labeled RNA of one of the infecting virions could also be traced into an RNase-resistant form in cultures exhibiting complementation but not in control single infections. *Ts*6 paired with other RNA⁻ *ts* mutants complements so effeciently that continuous complementation can give rise to small plaques. Monolayers of chick embryo cells were infected with *ts*6 and *ts*4 each at a multiplicity of 10 PFU/cell. After 2 h at 40°C, the infected cells were dispersed with trypsin, diluted, and allowed to adsorb to fresh monolayer cultures that were then overlaid with agar medium and incubated at the restrictive temperature. Most of the infected cells yielded small (0.5–1.0 mm) plaques after 3 days' incubation. The progeny of isolated plaques were all of the *ts* phenotype and thus the plaques could have been formed only by several rounds of complementation (Pfefferkorn, unpublished observation).

Mutant *ts*11 is the sole representative of a third RNA⁻ complementation group called A′. Uncertainty as to the status of this mutant accounts for the ambiguity of its "prime" designation. It was originally assigned to an independent group (Burge and Pfefferkorn, 1966*b*), then demoted to the well-populated A group (Pfefferkorn and Burge, 1967), and finally reassigned to an independent complementation group. The status of mutant *ts*11 should still be regarded as unsettled.

The RNA⁺ *ts* mutants of Sindbis virus fall into three complementation groups: C, D, and E (Table 2). Here again, the complementation was inefficient but reproducible. It is gratifying that these assignments proved to be concordant with subsequently detected physiological defects (see Sections 4.2 and 4.3).

Although inefficient, complementation between *ts* mutants of Sindbis virus is a reproducible phenomenon. Both Atkins *et al.* (1974*a*) and Strauss (personal communication) have reported complementation using the same set of mutants. These successes stand in sharp contrast to the inability of Tan *et al.* (1969) to detect any significant complementation in studies of their catalogue of *ts* mutants of Semliki Forest virus. The first hint of a solution to this paradox comes from the important work of Atkins *et al.* (1974*a*), who were also unable to observe complementation in their very extensive catalogue of Sindbis virus mutants. The most significant difference between the two sets of Sindbis virus *ts* mutants, one of which exhibits complementation and one of which does not, is the wild-type strain from which they were derived. Burge and Pfefferkorn (1966*a*) used the HR strain, which they had previously selected for thermostability of the virion, while Atkins *et al.* (1974*a*) used the standard strain AR 339. It is likely that the HR strain has some genetic characteristic that permits complementation, while both the standard and Sindbis and Semliki Forest virus strains lack it. This characteristic may be related to the phenomenon of interference described below (Section 3.4).

Rettenmeir *et al.* (1975) have described a new procedure that allows selection of mutants that are dependent on complementation. A suitable modification of this procedure might allow selection of a complementing *ts* mutant of the AR 339 strain of Sindbis virus and thus allow a genetic attack on the control of complementation.

3.4. Interference

In this context, *interference* is defined as the inhibition of the growth of one virus in a given cell by some action of another infectious virus on that same cell. Interferon is presumably not involved in this phenomenon. Although interference is not a genetic interaction, it deserves consideration because it must be avoided in order to establish mixed infections that might allow phenotypic mixing, complementation, or genetic recombination. In general, when two group A togaviruses infect the same cell, the virus with a temporal or multiplicity advantage will produce most of the progeny (Zebovitz and Brown, 1968). This interference is more extensive than would be predicted on a simple kinetic model. That is, synthesis of the genome of the superinfecting virion is actually inhibited, perhaps as a consequence of competition for limited sites of replication or substrate (Zebovitz and Brown, 1968). Homologous interference was more extensively explored by Johnston *et al.* (1974) with the aid of *ts* mutants of Sindbis virus. They found that RNA^+ mutants efficiently interfered with the growth of wild-type virus at the restrictive temperature, while RNA^- mutants generally did not. However, viral RNA synthesis did not appear to be required, because one RNA^- mutant, *ts*6, also interfered with the replication of superinfecting wild-type virus at the restrictive temperature.

Interference is also seen in mixed infections of group A togaviruses and other unrelated viruses. For example, poliovirus effectively excludes Sindbis virus in mixed infections, possibly by inhibiting the initiation step of togaviral protein synthesis (Sreevalson and Rosemond-Hornbeak, 1974).

Conversely, preinfection with Sindbis virus blocks the replication of Newcastle disease virus, as evidenced by inhibition of hemadsorption. This phenomenon, intrinsic interference, has been explored through the use of *ts* mutants. Marcus and Zuckerbraun (1970) found that all RNA^+ mutants were capable of inducing intrinsic interference at the restrictive temperature while all RNA^- mutants, with one exception, were incapable. The exception, mutant *ts*11, proved to be variable in its activity, although serial tests in the same cell line yielded repeatable positive or negative results. Marcus and Zuckerbraun (1970) were forced to conclude that some lines of their green monkey kidney cells contained an activity, the alien A´ activity, that complemented only the defect in mutant *ts*11 (previously assigned to complementation group A´; see Section 3.3).

4. PHYSIOLOGICAL DEFECTS IN TEMPERATURE-SENSITIVE MUTANTS

4.1. Temperature-Sensitive Mutants with Defective or Altered Viral RNA Synthesis

Those *ts* mutants that induce little or no viral RNA synthesis in infections at the restrictive temperature are called RNA⁻, while those that induce substantial amounts of viral RNA are called RNA⁺ (Burge and Pfefferkorn, 1966a). Some authors designate as RNA± a third class of mutants that induce RNA synthetic capacities 1–10% of normal (Tan *et al.*, 1969; Atkins *et al.*, 1974a; Keränen and Kääriäinen, 1974). Assignment to these three categories can be made by titrating infectious RNA or by measuring incorporation of RNA precursors in the presence of actinomycin D. The results from these independent determinations are generally concordant (Burge and Pfefferkorn, 1966a). One mutant that synthesizes poorly infectious but grossly normal virion RNA has been described by Zebovitz and Brown (1970). It would be wise to examine the production of infectious RNA in all mutants classed as RNA± on the basis of [³H]uridine incorporation. Some may prove to be quite defective in the synthesis of infectious RNA and should then be regarded, functionally at least, as RNA⁻ mutants. On the other hand, a mutant able to make 10% of the wild-type level of infectious RNA at the restrictive temperature is likely to have some additional *ts* block that prevents plaque formation.

In each large series of *ts* mutants (Table 1), half or more are either RNA⁻ or RNA±. This distribution could reflect the participation of a large part of the viral genome in RNA synthesis. Alternatively, the method of selection might favor the isolation of mutants with a defect in RNA synthesis. For example, in cultures infected by an RNA⁺ mutant at the restrictive temperature, viral RNA replication in the initially infected cell allows additional opportunities for reversion to the wild type and thus production of a plaque. Consequently, only RNA⁺ mutants with very low back-mutation rates (back mutations per round of RNA replication) would have acceptable back-mutation frequencies. A final possible explanation for the preponderance of RNA⁻ is that structural proteins can tolerate more amino acid substitutions than can enzymatic proteins.

Although many RNA⁻ mutants have been isolated, very little is known of their defects. As noted above (Section 3.3), most RNA⁻ mutants of Sindbis virus have been assigned to complementation group

A. The highly efficient complementation of Sindbis mutant *ts*6 strongly suggests the existence of a second cistron involved in viral RNA synthesis. Complementation by mutant *ts*11, while not as impressive as that of *ts*6, probably defines a third complementation group that Burge and Pfefferkorn have designated A′. Nonetheless, it seems likely that the RNA⁻ mutants will be further classified by biochemical rather than genetic techniques. Unfortunately, the biochemical attack on these mutants has not yet yielded decisive data. Temperature-shift experiments in which infected cultures are incubated at the restrictive temperature for 4 h and then moved to the permissive temperature for an additional 4 h show that RNA⁻ mutants are, as might be expected, blocked in an early function (Tan *et al.*, 1969). Various RNA⁻ mutants differ in their response to a shift from the permissive to the restrictive temperature. Some mutants continue to produce virus and induce the formation of actinomycin D-resistant RNA, while in others both functions are rapidly compromised (Burge and Pfefferkorn, 1965, 1966*a*; Pfefferkorn and Burge, 1967; Tan *et al.*, 1969). This shiftup may serve to distinguish between those mutants that have defects in proteins required only in the early hours of infection and those mutants that have defects in proteins required throughout the infection. But an alternative explanation is at least equally likely. It supposes that all of the proteins that are affected by the various RNA⁻ mutations are actually required to maintain viral RNA synthesis throughout the infection. These mutant proteins differ, however, in that some, once synthesized at the permissive temperatures, are stable upon shift to the restrictive temperature, while others are denatured. If the latter suggestion is correct, it should be possible to detect the *in vitro* thermolability of some togaviral mutant RNA polymerases. Martin (1969) examined several RNA⁻ mutants of Semliki Forest virus and found only one that had induced a polymerase significantly more thermolabile than that of the wild type. Although that mutant (*ts*5) was the one that might have been expected, on the basis of temperature-shift experiments (Tan *et al.*, 1969), to have a labile polymerase, Martin (1969) concluded that the *in vitro* effect was not sufficiently great to explain the observed temperature sensitivity of the mutant. It should be noted that Martin's (1969) assay employed a relatively crude preparation that was capable only of synthesizing double-stranded RNA. The present availability of more active preparations that synthesize characteristic double- and single-stranded species of viral RNA (Sreevalsan and Yin, 1969; Michel and Gomatos, 1973) should make the *in vitro* approach more attractive for future studies.

An alternative to direct assay of viral RNA polymerases is to trace the conversion of labeled parental viral RNA to a double-stranded form in infected cells. The synthesis of togaviral RNA is undoubtedly similar to that of other plus-stranded RNA viruses. The initial step is synthesis of a minus strand that subsequently serves as a template for further production of plus-stranded RNA. Either the synthesis of the minus strand or the subsequent steps could be defective in an RNA$^-$ts mutant. Pfefferkorn et al. (1967) were able to trace the RNA of wild-type Sindbis virions into an RNase-resistant (presumably replicative) form during the first hour of infection. Unfortunately, both ts4 and ts6, representatives of complementation groups A and B, proved to be defective in this vital function at the restrictive temperature (Pfefferkorn et al., 1967; Pfefferkorn and Burge, 1968). Complementation groups A´ and B each are represented by but one Sindbis virus mutant. There is at present no direct biochemical evidence to suggest that these two mutants are different from one another or from the many other mutants of complementation group A. Rather indirect biological evidence (see Section 3.4), however, does serve to set these mutants apart. Of all the RNA$^-$ mutants tested, only ts6 was able to induce homologous interference at the restrictive temperature (Johnston et al., 1974). In a test for induction of intrinsic interference at the restrictive temperature, only mutant ts11 was able to respond to the presence of "alien A´" activity (Marcus and Zuckerbraun, 1970).

Cells infected by wild-type group A togaviruses contain two principal types of single-stranded RNA. The larger sediments at about 42 S and is presumably identical to the RNA found in virions. The smaller 26 S RNA is the polycistronic messenger RNA for the virion proteins. It represents about one-third of the base sequences of the virion RNA. A plausible mechanism for the synthesis of 26 S RNA has been presented (Simmons and Strauss, 1972b). The ratio of 42 S:26 S RNA in wild-type virus infected cells is affected by the temperature of incubation (Keränen and Kääriäinen, 1974) and by the strain of virus (compare data for Sindbis virus, Pfefferkorn and Burge, 1967; Western equine encephalitis virus, Sreevalsan and Lockart, 1966; Semliki Forest virus, Mécs et al., 1967). Since the controlled production of the 26 S RNA is presumably a function of the viral genome, it is not surprising that the ratio of 42 S:26 S RNA can be distorted by mutation. Such mutations need not be lethal, that is, allow no viral production at the restrictive temperature, but may simply result in less efficient viral growth. Thus alterations in this ratio may be the biochemical equivalent of a mutation affecting plaque size. The possibility exists that the substantial mutagenesis required for the isolation of *ts* mutants may also affect the ratio of viral single-stranded RNAs through the agency of a second mutation. Such seems to be the case in the Semliki Forest virus mutant *ts*1 studied by Keränen and Kääriäinen (1974). This mutant was selected for temperature sensitivity and shown to be RNA$^+$ and capable of nucleocapsid formation (see Sections 4.2 and 4.3). The ratio of 42 S:26 S RNA made in cells infected by this mutant was increased fivefold over the wild-type ratio, but this increase was *independent* of temperature and thus presumably not associated with the *ts* lesion. Atkins *et al.* (1974a) surveyed a broad spectrum of RNA$^+$ and RNA$^\pm$ *ts* mutants of Semliki Forest virus and found several with increased or decreased ratios. At present, there is no evidence that these distortions are temperature sensitive. Scheele and Pfefferkorn (1969) have described an RNA$^-$ mutant, *ts*24, in which the control of 26 S RNA synthesis may be temperature sensitive. In cells infected with this mutant, a shift to the restrictive temperature resulted in a preferential decline in 26 S RNA synthesis. However, this may just be another instance of a double mutation in which both the lesion affecting viral RNA synthesis and the one determining the 42 S:26 S RNA ratio are temperature sensitive.

One *ts* mutant of eastern equine encephalitis virus deserves special mention (Zebovitz and Brown, 1970). This mutant causes the synthesis of abnormally *large* amounts of all species of virus-specific RNA. However, the 42 S (virion) RNA extracted from the infected cells had only 2% of the specific infectivity of the comparable wild-type RNA. The biochemical basis for this observation remains unclear and, again, the mutation causing the synthesis of defective RNA may not be related to the *ts* defect of the mutant.

4.2. Temperature-Sensitive Mutants with an Apparent Defect in the Assembly of Nucleocapsids

Nucleocapsids of group A togaviruses, which sediment at about 140 S, are readily detected in cytoplasmic extracts of infected cells. Four laboratories have described *ts* mutants that are defective in nucleocapsid assembly at the restrictive temperature (Burge and Pfefferkorn, 1968; Yin and Lockart, 1968; Tan *et al.*, 1969; Keränen and Kääriäinen, 1974). Typical data that disclose such a defect are illustrated in Fig. 1.

Since the C protein is probably cleaved from the amino-terminal end of protein that is a precursor of all virion proteins, two classes of *ts*

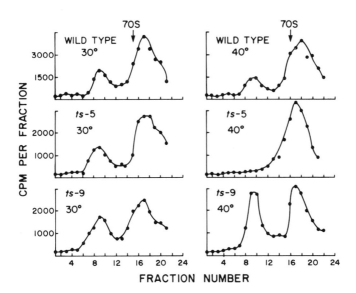

Fig. 1. Demonstration that Sindbis virus mutant *ts*5 is defective in the production of nucleocapsids at the restrictive temperature. Chick fibroblast cells were infected in the presence of actinomycin D, 1 μg/ml, and labeled with [³H]uridine from 2 to 6 h after infection. A cell-free extract was analyzed by centrifugation through a 15–30% glycerol gradient for 85 min at 39,000 rpm. Acid–precipitable radioactivity was measured. The 70 S marker is ferritin. Redrawn from Pfefferkorn and Burge (1968). Reproduced by permission of Academic Press.

mutants defective in nucleocapsid formation are possible. In the first, the cleavage proceeds normally but the resulting C protein is unable to assume a functional conformation at the restrictive temperature. In the second class of mutants, the cleavage is defective at the restrictive temperature and no protein product corresponding to the C protein is produced. Both classes of mutants have been observed. Keränen and Kääriäinen (1974) have described a *ts* mutant of Semliki Forest virus that is incapable of nucleocapsid assembly at the restrictive temperature. At this temperature, however, the 130,000 dalton precursor of the virion proteins is efficiently cleaved to yield a protein that is electrophoretically identical to the C protein but is apparently nonfunctional.

Burge and Pfefferkorn (1968) found that three *ts* mutants of Sindbis virus, all previously assigned to complementation group C, failed to produce nucleocapsids in cells infected at the restrictive temperature. Although these mutants were independently isolated and induced by three different mutagens (Burge and Pfefferkorn, 1966*a*), each appears to have the same defect. At the restrictive temperature, cells infected by these mutants accumulate a precursor protein of molecular mass approximately 130,000 daltons (Strauss *et al.,* 1969; Scheele and Pfefferkorn, 1970). The mutants of complementation group C are thus unable to cleave the precursor that ordinarily yields the structural proteins of the virion. Scheele and Pfefferkorn (1970) used a pulse of [³H]leucine to label the high molecular mass precursor accumulated in cells infected with mutant *ts*2 at the restrictive temperature. When the infected cells were subsequently shifted to the permissive temperature and incubated in unlabeled medium, the radioactively labeled 130,000 dalton precursor remained intact and was not cleaved into structural proteins. The stability of the mutant precursor protein once synthesized at the restrictive temperature was presumed to result from incorrect folding.

Remarkably enough, the phenotype of these mutants is exactly reproduced in an *in vitro* protein-synthesizing system. Messenger (26 S) RNA extracted from mutant-infected cells is translated into capsid protein at the permissive temperature and 130,000 dalton precursor protein at the restrictive temperature (Cancedda *et al.,* 1974; Simmons and Strauss, 1974). Several models will explain this observation: (1) An amino acid substitution might alter the conformation of the precursor in such a manner that it could not be recognized by cellular cleavage enzymes present in the protein-synthesizing extract. But accurate cleavage has not always been observed in extracts primed with other polycistronic viral messenger RNAs. (2) The mutation might result in a temperature-sensitive messenger RNA, blocking, at the restrictive temperature, the normal termination of translation at the end of the capsid protein. But mammalian and animal viral messengers are generally thought to lack signals for internal chain termination (Summers and Maizel, 1968; Jacobson and Baltimore, 1968). (3) A viral-coded protease might be synthesized during the *in vitro* incubation. Either the conformation of protease or the conformation of its specific cleavage site at the carboxy-terminal end of the C protein could be temperature sensitive. Actually, given the limited coding capacity of the 26 S RNA, the protease would have to be a part of the precursor protein and probably the C protein itself. It should be noted that there is no evidence for a viral-coded cleavage enzyme in any other system. Although objections can be posed to each of the above explanations, one of them is likely to be valid. I believe that the third should be given special consideration.

One RNA⁻ mutant *ts*11 has been shown in temperature shiftup experiments to induce the formation of a precursor protein of the same electrophoretic mobility as that which accumulates in cells infected by mutants of complementation group C (Waite, 1973). Mutant *ts*11 may thus be a double mutant with a defect in cleavage as well as RNA synthesis.

4.3. Temperature-Sensitive Mutants with Defects in Envelope Protein

The envelope proteins of group A togaviruses are first inserted into the plasma membrane of infected cells and then incorporated into virions as the nucleocapsid buds through the virus-modified membrane (reviewed by Pfefferkorn and Shapiro, 1974). Recent evidence from cross-linking studies (Garoff, 1974) suggests that the two large glyco-proteins of Semliki Forest virus are present in the viral envelope as E1–E2 dimers. The components of these dimers may act in concert to yield the biological activities of the virion surface, the hemagglutinin and the neutralizing antigen. Thus one should be cautious in assigning these activities to one protein or another. However, Pederson and Eddy (1974) have shown that only one of the envelope proteins of Venezuelan equine encephalitis virus is capable of inducing neutralizing hemaggluti-nation-inhibiting antibodies.

Only one test, hemadsorption, has been used to examine the func-tional-state envelope proteins in cells infected by *ts* mutants (Yin and Lockart, 1968; Burge and Pfefferkorn, 1968; Tan *et al.,* 1969). Typical results of a test for a mutant temperature sensitive in hemadsorption are presented in Fig. 2. Burge and Pfefferkorn (1968) used ^{5}Cr-labeled goose red cells to measure hemadsorption by cells infected by various RNA$^+$ mutants of Sindbis virus at the restrictive temperature. Of the three RNA$^+$ complementation groups, only group D, represented by *ts*10 and *ts*23, failed to exhibit hemadsorption. It seems likely that com-plementation group D defines a gene that determines an envelope pro-tein involved in hemadsorption. Support for this conclusion comes from the interesting observation that the hemagglutinating capacity of mutant *ts*23 is reversibly thermolabile (Yin, 1969). Preparations of this mutant grown at the permissive temperature fail to agglutinate goose red cells at the restrictive temperature but are fully functional upon cooling. Thus, within the virion, the envelope protein bearing the muta-tion of *ts*23 can assume two conformations of which only one is func-tional. The other representative of complementation group D, *ts*10, does not have a thermolabile hemagglutinin (Scheele and Pfefferkorn, 1970) and thus may represent a different mutation of the same protein. Another morphological consequence of the temperature-sensitive defect

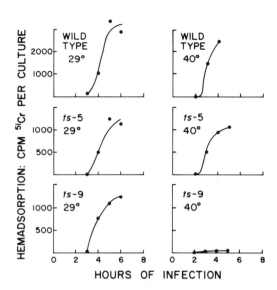

Fig. 2.   Demonstration that Sindbis virus mutant *ts*9 is defective in the induction of hemadsorption at the restrictive temperature. Infected chick fibroblast cells were washed and exposed to ⁵¹Cr-labeled goose red blood cells and washed again. The adsorbed radioactivity was measured. Redrawn from Pfefferkorn and Burge (1968). Reproduced by permission of Academic Press.

in mutants of complementation group D has been disclosed by electron microscopy. Brown and Smith (1975) noted that at the restrictive temperature the intracellular nucleocapsids of mutant *ts*23 did not become associated with the inner surface of the plasma membrane but remained randomly scattered in the cytoplasm. In contrast, the nucleocapsids of *ts*20 (complementation group E) were found attached to the inner surface of the plasma membrane. These observations suggest that mutation of *ts*23 affects not only hemadsorption but also the process by which nucleocapsids recognize a virus-modified patch of plasma membrane. This recognition is probably made through that portion of the envelope protein that extends through the lipid bilayer and into the cytoplasm (Garoff and Simons, 1974). No defect in capsid–membrane interaction was noted in an electron microscopic survey of cells infected by *ts* mutants of Semliki Forest virus (Tan, 1970).

One of the complementation groups characterized by induction of hemadsorption at the restrictive temperature has already been discussed (see Section 4.2). It is complementation group C, the members of which have a defect in assembly of nucleocapsids because the common precursor of all virion proteins cannot be cleaved in cells infected at the restrictive temperature. Since the envelope proteins are also locked up in this precursor, it is logical to ask how mutant virus-infected cells can exhibit hemadsorption at the restrictive temperature. The answer probably lies in the fact that the test for hemadsorption is very sensitive. I suspect that it will detect a few hundred molecules of viral hemagglutinin and rapidly rise to a maximum when the cell membrane contains the hemagglutinin equivalent of 10 or 20 virions. While the test for nucleocapsid formation (Fig. 1) is a reasonable measure of the amount of functional C protein produced, the test for hemadsorption is by no means a linear function of the amount of hemagglutinin in the membrane. A small amount of leakiness, i.e., normal cleavage, would yield a positive hemadsorption without detectable nucleocapsids. Leakiness of these mutants is probably also required for complementation.

The envelope proteins of group A togaviruses are produced from a precursor protein through a series of at least three proteolytic cleavages (reviewed by Pfefferkorn and Shapiro, 1974). In addition, the envelope proteins are further processed by glycosylation. There are several opportunities for mutation to interrupt this orderly process. The defect in cleavage of the 130,000 dalton precursor of all virion proteins that characterizes complementation group C has already been described. I know of no mutant defective in the second cleavage that produces the envelope protein E1 and the final precursor PE2. Two laboratories have reported temperature-sensitive defects in the cleavage of this final precursor to yield E2 and, at least in Semliki Forest virus, E3 (Simons et al., 1973; Jones et al., 1974). Jones et al. (1974) found that cells infected at the restrictive temperature by the sole representative of Sindbis complementation group E, ts20, accumulated the precursor PE2 in their membranes. In contrast to the 130,000 dalton precursor accumulated in cells infected by mutants of complementation group C, this smaller precursor, once labeled at the restrictive temperature, was cleaved after shift to the permissive temperature. Jones et al. (1974) suggest that cleavage of PE2 may take place during the budding of virions. Since mutant ts20 is positive in tests for hemadsorption at the restrictive temperature, its protein product is probably not the hemagglutinin.

4.4. Temperature-Sensitive Mutants and the Synthesis of Cellular Macromolecules

Group A togaviruses have two general effects on macromolecular metabolism of cells that they infect. The synthesis of cellular protein and RNA is inhibited, while the production of one particular protein, interferon, is stimulated. These effects of viral infection have been explored with the use of *ts* mutants of Sindbis and Semliki Forest viruses. The inhibitory effects appear to require viral RNA synthesis, for they are seen at the restrictive temperature only in cells infected by RNA$^+$ mutants (Tan *et al.*, 1969; Waite and Pfefferkorn, 1970). The situation with respect to interferon induction is more complex. There is general agreement that both wild type and *ts* mutants are efficient interferon inducers at the permissive temperature. At the restrictive temperature, RNA$^+$ and RNA$^-$ mutants have been reported to be both capable and incapable of inducing interferon (Lockart *et al.*, 1968; Lomniczi and Burke, 1970; Atkins *et al.*, 1974*b*).

Atkins *et al.* (1974*b*) provide the most coherent synthesis of these confusing data. They conclude that a threshold level of viral RNA synthesis is essential for the induction of interferon. Thus, in general, only RNA$^+$ mutants should be effective inducers at the restrictive temperature. The RNA$^+$ mutants may, however, fail if their RNA synthesis is partially compromised, particularly if the restrictive temperature is set too high. Atkins *et al.* (1974*b*) further suggest that induction of interferon by RNA$^-$ mutants at the restrictive temperature may be ascribed to the effect of back mutants or leakiness.

4.5. Virulence of *ts* Mutants

One of the long-range goals of animal virus genetics should be a fuller understanding of *in vivo* virulence and pathogenesis. Since virulence is likely to be determined by many (all?) of the viral genes, this is by no means a simple problem. Several investigators have begun the exploration of *in vivo* infections with *ts* mutants of group A togaviruses. Simizu and Takayama (1971, 1972) made an interesting comparison of two *ts* mutants of western equine encephalitis virus. One was a single-step mutant isolated after chemical mutagenesis, while the other appeared spontaneously after prolonged passage in a persistently infected culture. Both mutants were markedly less virulent in adult mice, but large inocula of either *in vivo* yielded neurovirulent revertants. However, only the neurovirulent revertant from the presumably single-step *ts* mutant also became *ts*$^+$. The *ts* mutant from the persistently infected culture presumably was thus a multiple-step mutant. That temperature sensitivity and neurovirulence were not covarient was confirmed by *in vitro* selection of a *ts*$^+$ revertant from the presumed multiple-step mutant and demonstration that it had not recovered the neurovirulent character of the original wild type.

Embryonated eggs are useful for the study of *in vivo* infections with *ts* mutants because their temperature can be rigorously controlled. Schluter *et al.* (1974) have begun an analysis of this potentially valuable system. They observed that *ts* mutants of Sindbis virus were generally avirulent at the restrictive temperature. At the permissive temperature and in temperature-shift experiments, the mutants were somewhat less virulent than the wild type, thus permitting a more detailed kinetic study of viral invasiveness. Schluter and Brown (1974) also noted that embryos infected with RNA$^+$ *ts* mutants at the restrictive temperature and then shifted after various intervals to the permissive temperature were protected from infection and death by as little as 2 h at the restrictive temperature. In contrast, embryos infected with RNA$^-$ mutants and incubated at the restrictive temperature for as long as 12 h were not protected against death upon shift to a lower temperature. This pattern parallels that observed *in vitro* by Pfefferkorn and Burge (1967), although it is by no means certain that the same mechanism is involved.

Although the data of Schluter and Brown (1974) only hint of the possibility that the *ts* mutants may cause a chronic or "slow" infection, I believe that all *ts* mutants should be handled with the care that would be exercised with a highly virulent group A togavirus such as eastern equine encephalitis virus.

ACKNOWLEDGMENTS

I am indebted to the following persons for preprints and helpful comments: A. Brown, D. T. Brown, L. Kääriäinen, S. I. T. Kennedy, M. J. Schlesinger, S. Schlesinger, K. Simons, and J. Strauss. The personal research reported in this chapter was supported by NIH Grant AI 08238.

5. REFERENCES

Atkins, G. J., Samuels, J., and Kennedy, S. I. T., 1974*a*, Isolation and preliminary characterization of temperature-sensitive mutants of Sindbis virus strain AR339, *J. Gen. Virol.* **25**:371.

Atkins, G. J., Johnston, M. D., Westmacott, L. M., and Burke, D. C., 1974*b*, Induction of interferon in chick cells by temperature-sensitive mutants of Sindbis virus, *J. Gen. Virol.* **25**:381.

Bose, H. R., Carl, G. Z., and Sagik, B. P., 1970, Separation of Sindbis virus plaque-type variants by calcium phosphate chromatography, *Arch. Ges. Virusforsch.* **29**:83.

Bradish, C. J., and Allner, K., 1972, The early responses of mice to respiratory or intraperitoneal infection by defined virulent and avirulent strains of Semliki Forest virus, *J. Gen. Virol.* **15**:205.

Bradish, C. J., Allner, K., and Maber, H. B., 1971, The virulence of original and derived strains of Semliki Forest virus for mice, guinea-pigs and rabbits, *J. Gen. Virol.* **12**:141.

Brawner, T. A., and Sagik, B. P., 1971, Rescue of ultraviolet-inactivated Sindbis virus, *Abst. Annu. Meet. Am. Soc. Microbiol.*, p. 218.

Brown, A., and Officer, J. E., 1975, An attenuated varient of Eastern encephalitis virus: Biological properties and protection induced in mice, *Arch. Ges. Virusforsch.* **47**:123.

Brown, D. T., and Gliedman, J. B., 1973, Morphological variants of Sindbis virus obtained from infected mosquito tissue culture cells, *J. Virol.* **12**:1534.

Brown, D. T., and Smith, J. F., 1975, Morphology of BHK-21 cells infected with Sindbis virus temperature-sensitive complementation groups D and E, *J. Virol.* **15**:1262.

Brown, D. T., Waite, M. R. F., and Pfefferkorn, E. R., 1972, Morphology and morphogenesis of Sindbis virus as seen with freeze-etching techniques, *J. Virol.* **10**:524.

Brown, F., Smale, C. J., and Horzinek, M. C., 1974, Lipid and protein organization in vesicular stomatitis and Sindbis viruses, *J. Virol.* **22**:455.

Burge, B. W., and Pfefferkorn, E. R., 1965, Conditional-lethal mutants of an animal virus: Identification of two cistrons, *Science* **148**:959.

Burge, B. W., and Pfefferkorn, E. R., 1966*a*, Isolation and characterization of conditional-lethal mutants of Sindbis virus, *Virology* **30**:204.

Burge, B. W., and Pfefferkorn, E. R., 1966*b*, Complementation between temperature-sensitive mutants of Sindbis virus, *Virology* **30**:214.

Burge, B. W., and Pfefferkorn, E. R., 1966*c*, Phenotypic mixing between group A arboviruses, *Nature (London)* **210**:1397.

Burge, B. W., and Pfefferkorn, E. R., 1967, Temperature-sensitive mutants of Sindbis virus: Biochemical correlates of complementation, *J. Virol.* **1**:956.

Burge, B. W., and Pfefferkorn, E. R., 1968, Functional defects of temperature-sensitive mutants of Sindbis virus, *J. Mol. Biol.* **35**:193.

Bykovsky, A. F., Yershov, F. I., and Zhdanov, V. M., 1969, Morphogenesis of Venezuelan equine encephalomyelitis virus, *J. Virol.* **4**:496.

Cancedda, R., and Schlesinger, M. J., 1974, Formation of Sindbis virus capsid protein in mammalian cell-free extracts programmed with viral messenger RNA, *Proc. Natl. Acad. Sci. USA* **71**:1843.

Cancedda, R., Swanson, R., and Schlesinger, M. J., 1974, Viral proteins formed in a cell-free rabbit reticulocyte system programmed with RNA from a temperature-sensitive mutant of Sindbis virus, *J. Virol.* **14**:664.

Carver, D. H., and Seto, D. S. Y., 1968, Viral inactivation by disulfide bond reducing agents, *J. Virol.* **2**:1482.

Davey, M. W., and Dalgarno, L., 1974, Semliki Forest virus replication in cultured *Aedes albopictus* cells: Studies on the establishment of persistence, *J. Gen. Virol.* **24**:453.

Epstein, R. H., Bolle, A., Steinberg, C. M., Kellenberger, E., Boy De La Tour, E., Chevalley, R., Edgar, R. S., Susman, M., Denhardt, G. H., and Lielausis, A., 1963, Physiological studies of conditional-lethal mutations of bacteriophage T4D, *Cold Spring Harbor Symp. Quant. Biol.* **28**:375.

Fincham, J. R. S., 1966, *Genetic Complementation*, Benjamin, New York.

Fleming, P., 1971*a*, Thermal inactivation of Semliki Forest virus, *J. Gen. Virol.* **13**:385.

Fleming, P., 1971*b*, Inactivation and reactivation of Semliki Forest virus by urea and guanidine hydrochloride, *J. Gen. Virol.* **13**:393.

Garoff, H., 1974, Cross-linking of the spike glycoproteins in Semliki Forest virus with dimethylsuberimidate, *Virology* **62**:385.

Garoff, H., and Simons, K., 1974, Location of the spike glycoproteins in the Semliki Forest virus membrane, *Proc. Natl. Acad. Sci. USA* **71**:3988.

Garoff, H., and Simons, K., 1975, Viral envelope composition: Proteins, in: *Cell Membranes and Viral Envelopes* (H. A. Blough and J. M. Tiffany, eds.), Academic Press, New York.

Garoff, H., Simons, K., and Renkonen, O., 1974, Isolation and characterization of the membrane proteins of Semliki Forest virus, *Virology* **61**:493.

Halle, S., 1968, 5-Azacytidine as a mutagen for arboviruses, *J. Virol.* **2**:1228.

Higashi, N., Matsumoto, A., Tabata, K., and Nagatomo, Y., 1967, Electron microscope study of development of Chikungunya virus in green monkey kidney stable (VERO) cells, *Virology* **33**:55.

Jacobson, M. F., and Baltimore, D., 1968, Polypeptide cleavages in the formation of poliovirus proteins, *Proc. Natl. Acad. Sci. USA* **61**:77.

Johnston, R. E., Wan, K., and Bose, H. R., 1974, Homologous interference induced by Sindbis virus, *J. Virol.* **14**:1076.

Jones, K. J., Waite, M. R. F., and Bose, H. R., 1974, Cleavage of a viral envelope precursor during the morphogenesis of Sindbis virus, *J. Virol.* **13**:809.

Keränen, S., and Kääriäinen, L., 1974, Isolation and basic characterization of temperature-sensitive mutants from Semliki Forest virus, *Acta Pathol. Microbiol. Scand. Sect. B* **82**:810.

Lagwinska, E., Stewart, C. C., Adles, C., and Schlesinger, S., 1975, Replication of lactic dehydrogenose virus and Sindbis virus in mouse peritoneal macrophages: Induction of interferon and phenotypic mixing, *Virology* **65**:204.

Lockart, R. Z., Jr., Bayliss, N. L., Toy, S. T., and Yin, F. H., 1968, Viral events necessary for the induction of interferon in chick embryo cells, *J. Virol.* **3**:962.

Lomniczi, B., and Burke, D. C., 1970, Interferon production by temperature-sensitive mutants of Semliki Forest virus, *J. Gen. Virol.* **8**:222.

Marcus, P. L., and Zuckerbraun, H. L., 1970, Viral polymerase proteins as antiviral agents (intrinsic interference), *Ann. N.Y. Acad. Sci.* **173**:185.

Marshall, I. D., Scrivani, R. P., and Reeves, W. C., 1962, Variation in the size of plaques produced in tissue culture by strains of Western equine encephalitis virus, *Am. J. Hyg.* **76**:216.

Martin, E. M., 1969, Studies on the RNA polymerase of some temperature-sensitive mutants of Semliki Forest virus, *Virology* **39**:107.

Mécs, E., Sonnabend, J. A., Martin, E. M., and Fantes, K. H., 1967, The effect of interferon on the synthesis of RNA in chick cells infected with Semliki Forest virus, *J. Gen. Virol.* **1**:25.

Michel, M. R., and Gomatos, P. J., 1973, Semliki Forest virus-specific RNAs synthesized *in vitro* by enzyme from infected BHK cells, *J. Virol.* **11**:900.

Pedersen, C. E., Jr., and Eddy, G. A., 1974, Separation, isolation, and immunological studies of the structural proteins of Venezuelan equine encephalomyelitis virus, *J. Virol.* **14**:740.

Pfefferkorn, E. R., 1969, Temperature-sensitive mutants of animal viruses: Isolation and preliminary characterization, in: *Fundamental Techniques in Virology* (K. Habel and N. P. Salzman, eds.), pp. 87–93, Academic Press, New York.

Pfefferkorn, E. R., and Burge, B. W., 1967, Genetics and biochemistry of arbovirus temperature-sensitive mutants, in: *The Molecular Biology of Viruses* (J. S. Colter and W. Paranchych, eds.), Academic Press, New York and London.

Pfefferkorn, E. R., and Burge, B. W., 1968, Morphogenic defects in the growth of *ts* mutants of Sindbis virus, *Perspect. Virol.* **6**:1.

Pfefferkorn, E. R., and Clifford, R. L., 1964, The origin of the protein of Sindbis virus, *Virology* **23**:217.

Pfefferkorn, E. R., and Shapiro, D., 1974, Reproduction of togaviruses, in: *Comprehensive Virology,* Vol. 2 (H. Fraenkel-Conrat and R. R. Wagner, eds.), pp. 171–230, Plenum Press, New York.

Pfefferkorn, E. R., Burge, B. W., and Coady, H. M., 1967, Intracellular conversion of the RNA of Sindbis virus to a double-stranded form, *Virology* **33**:239.

Quersin-Thiry, L., 1961, Nutritive requirements of a small plaque mutant of Western equine encephalitis virus, *Br. J. Exp. Pathol.* **42**:511.

Rasmussen, L. E., Armstrong, J. A., and Ho, M., 1973, Interference mediated by a variant of Sindbis virus. I. Isolation of an avirulent variant and *in vivo* interference, *J. Infect. Dis.* **128**:156.

Renkonen, O., Kääriäinen, L., Simons, K., and Gahmberg, C. G., 1971, The lipid class composition of Semliki Forest virus and of plasma membranes of the host cells, *Virology* **46**:318.

Rettenmeir, C. W., Dumont, R., and Baltimore, D., 1975, Screening procedure for complementation-dependent mutants of vesicular stomatitis virus, *J. Virol.* **15**:41.

Scheele, C. M., and Pfefferkorn, E. R., 1969, Inhibition of interjacent RNA (26S) synthesis in cells infected by Sindbis virus, *J. Virol.* **4**:117.

Scheele, C. M., and Pfefferkorn, E. R., 1970, Virus-specific proteins synthesized in cells infected with RNA^+ temperature-sensitive mutants of Sindbis virus, *J. Virol.* **5**:329.

Schleupner, C. J., Postic, B., Armstrong, J. A., Atchison, R. W., and Ho, M., 1969, Two variants of Sindbis virus which differ in interferon induction and serum clearance. II. Virological characterizations, *J. Infect. Dis.* **120**:348.

Schluter, B., and Brown, A., 1974, Pathogenesis of temperature-sensitive mutants of Sindbis virus in the embryonated egg. II. Control of the infectious process, *Infect. Immun.* **9**:76.

Schluter, B., Bellomy, B., and Brown, A., 1974, Pathogenesis of temperature-sensitive mutants of Sindbis virus in the embryonated egg. I. Characterization and kinetics of viral multiplication, *Infect. Immun.* **9**:68.

Schwöbel, W., and Ahl, R., 1972, Persistance of Sindbis virus in BHK-21 cell cultures, *Arch. Ges. Virusforsch.* **38**:1.

Simizu, B., and Takayama, N., 1969, Isolation of two plaque mutants of Western equine encephalitis virus differing in virulence for mice, *J. Virol.* **4**:799.

Simizu, B., and Takayama, N., 1971, Relationship between neurovirulence and temperature sensitivity of an attenuated Western equine encephalitis virus, *Arch. Ges. Virusforsch.* **34**:242.

Simizu, B., and Takayama, N., 1972, Virulence of a temperature-sensitive mutant of Western equine encephalitis virus, *Arch. Ges. Virusforsch.* **38**:328.

Simizu, B., Yamazaki, S., Suzuki, K., and Terasima, T., 1973, Gamma ray-induced small plaque mutants of Western equine encephalitis virus, *J. Virol.* **12**:1568.

Simmons, D. T., and Strauss, J. H., 1972a, Replication of Sindbis virus. I. Relative size and genetic content of 26 S and 49 S RNA, *J. Mol. Biol.* **71**:599.

Simmons, D. T., and Strauss, J. H., 1972b, Replication of Sindbis virus. II. Multiple forms of double-stranded RNA isolated from infected cells, *J. Mol. Biol.* **71**:615.

Simmons, D. T., and Strauss, J. H., 1974, Translation of Sindbis virus 26 S RNA and 49 S RNA in lysates of rabbit reticulocytes, *J. Mol. Biol.* **86**:397.

Simons, K., Keränen, S., and Kääriäinen, L., 1973, Identification of a precursor for one of the Semliki Forest virus membrane proteins, *FEBS Lett.* **29**:87.

Smith, A. E., Wheeler, T., Glanville, N., and Kääriäinen, L., 1974, Translation of Semliki-Forest virus 42-S RNA in a mouse cell-free system to give virus-coat proteins, *Eur. J. Biochem.* **49**:101.

Solyanik, R. G., Fedorov, Y. U. V., and Rapoport, I. A., 1974, The mutagenic effect of some alkylating compounds on eastern equine encephalomyelitis virus, *Sov. Genet.* **8**:412.

Sreevalsan, T., and Lockart, R. Z., Jr., 1966, Heterogeneous RNAs occuring during the replication of Western equine encephalomyelitis virus, *Proc. Natl. Acad. Sci. USA* **55**:974.

Sreevalsan, T., and Rosemond-Hornbeak, H., 1974, Inhibition of Sindbis virus in HeLa cells by poliovirus, *Antimicrob. Agents Chemother.* **5**:55.

Sreevalsan, T., and Yin, F. H., 1969, Sindbis virus-induced viral ribonucleic acid polymerase, *J. Virol.* **3**:599.

Stollar, V., Peleg, J., and Shenk, T. E., 1974, Temperature sensitivity of a Sindbis virus mutant isolated from persistently infected *Aedes aegypti* cell culture, *Intervirology* **2**:337.

Strauss, J. H., Jr., Burge, B. W., and Darnell, J. E., 1969, Sindbis virus infection of chick and hamster cells: Synthesis of virus-specific proteins, *Virology* **37**:367.

Summers, D. F., and Maizel, J. V., Jr., 1968, Evidence for large precursor proteins in poliovirus synthesis, *Proc. Natl. Acad. Sci. USA* **59**:966.

Symington, J., and Schlesinger, M. J., 1975, Isolation of a Sindbis virus varient by passage on mouse plasmacytoma cells, *J. Virol.* **15**:1037.

Takayama, N., 1972, Further characterization of an attenuated Western equine encephalitis virus: Search for *in vitro* markers. *Arch. Ges. Virusforsch.* **36**:363.

Tan, K. B., 1969, Studies with temperature-sensitive mutants of Semliki Forest virus, Ph.D. thesis, Australian National University, Canberra.

Tan, K. B., 1970, Electron microscopy of cells infected with Semliki Forest virus temperature-sensitive mutants: Correlation of ultrastructural and physiological observations, *J. Virol.* **5**:632.

Tan, K. B., Sambrook, J. F., and Bellett, A. J. D., 1969, Semliki Forest virus temperature-sensitive mutants: Isolation and characterization, *Virology* **38**:427.

Tsilinsky, Y. Y., Gutshin, B. V., Klimenko, S. M., and Lvov, D. K., 1971, Morphological pecularities of virions in clones and populaitons of Venezuelan equine encephalomyelitis virus, *Arch. Ges. Virusforsch.* **34**:301.

Utermann, G., and Simons, K., 1974, Studies on the amphipathic nature of the membrane proteins of Semliki Forest virus, *J. Mol. Biol.* **85**:569.

Waite, M. R. F., 1973, Protein synthesis directed by an RNA⁻ temperature-sensitive mutant of Sindbis virus, *J. Virol.* **11**:198.

Waite, M. R. F., and Pfefferkorn, E. R., 1970, Phospholipid synthesis in Sindbis virus infected cells, *J. Virol.* **6:**637.

Yin, F. H., 1969, Temperature-sensitive behavior of the hemagglutinin in a temperature-sensitive mutant virion of Sindbis, *J. Virol.* **4:**547.

Yin, F. H., and Lockart, R. Z., Jr., 1968, Maturation defects in temperature-sensitive mutants of Sindbis virus, *J. Virol.* **2:**728.

Zebovitz, E., and Brown, A., 1968, Interference among group A arboviruses, *J. Virol.* **2:**1283.

Zebovitz, E., and Brown, A., 1970, Altered viral ribonucleic acid synthesis by a temperature-sensitive mutant of Eastern equine encephalitis virus, *J. Mol. Biol.* **50:**185.

CHAPTER 6

Genetics of Rhabdoviruses

C. R. Pringle

Medical Research Council, Virology Unit
Institute of Virology
Glasgow G11 5JR, Scotland

1. INTRODUCTION: SOME RELEVANT BIOLOGICAL FEATURES OF RHABDOVIRUSES

The rhabdoviruses are enveloped bullet-shaped viruses infecting a wide range of organisms (for reviews, see Howatson, 1970; Knudsen, 1973; Wagner, 1975). The host may be a vertebrate (bird, fish, or mammal), an invertebrate (insect or arachnid), or a plant. Some rhabdoviruses, like Chandipura virus or vesicular stomatitis virus (VSV), have a wide host range and may be vector transmitted in nature. Indeed, although VSV is known because of the disease it produces in man and domestic animals, it is capable of multiplying in both its invertebrate vector and the vertebrate host, and it has been suggested that VSV is not primarily a virus of vertebrates (Tesh *et al.,* 1970). The plant rhabdovirus, lettuce necrotic yellows virus, can also multiply in its insect vector, and one rhabdovirus, sigma virus, is known only as a hereditary infection of the insect *Drosophila*. However, other rhabdoviruses, such as rabies virus, are restricted in their host range and no insect vector appears to be involved in their spread.

All animal rhabdoviruses are assumed to be negative-strand RNA viruses by analogy with VSV, where the deproteinized genome is not infectious *in vivo* and the complementary RNA isolated from polysomes of infected cells functions as a template for protein synthesis *in vitro* (Morrison *et al.,* 1974; Knipe *et al.,* 1975). The presence of an

RNA-dependent RNA polymerase. in the virion is necessary for transcription of messenger RNA in the infected cell. This transcription on the parental template is designated *primary transcription*. Operationally, it is synonymous with the viral RNA synthesis observed in infected cells in the presence of the inhibitor of protein synthesis cycloheximide. Replication occurs in the cytoplasm, since it has been shown that various animal rhabdoviruses can multiply efficiently in enucleate cells (Follett *et al.,* 1974, 1975). Plant rhabdoviruses such as lettuce necrotic yellows virus, which mature in the cytoplasm and possess a virion-associated RNA-dependent RNA polymerase, can be expected to have the same genetic properties as animal rhabdoviruses. However, other plant rhabdoviruses such as potato yellow dwarf virus have a nuclear phase in their development, and maturation appears to take place at the inner nuclear membrane (Macleod *et al.,* 1966). The nature and function of the genome of these viruses, therefore, may not have much in common with the concept of the rhabdovirus genome elaborated in this chapter, which is based on information from two or three animal viruses. Furthermore, not all animal rhabdoviruses may conform to this generalized pattern, since it has not yet been shown, for example, that rabies virus possesses a virion transcriptase (Bishop and Flamand, 1975*a*) or can multiply in enucleate cells (Wiktor and Koprowski, 1974). The rabies-related Mokola virus, however, was one of the rhabdoviruses shown to be competent in enucleate cells by Follett *et al.* (1975). Sokol and Koprowski (1975) have described variation in the pattern of *in vivo* phosphorylation of structural polypeptides of different rhabdoviruses and have suggested that the rhabdovirus group represents an evolutionary series running from the host-dependent nuclear plant viruses and rabies virus to fully independent cytoplasmic viruses like VSV.

VSV, generally regarded as the prototype of the rhabdovirus group, has been the subject of most genetic research because of the experimental convenience of its rapid growth cycle and ease of propagation in many types of cells. A limited amount of information is available concerning Chandipura virus, a human rhabdovirus isolated in India, which resembles VSV in many respects but is serologically unrelated. Genetic study of rabies virus, the most important pathogen in the rhabdovirus group, is under way and will assume increasing importance in the future in view of the persistence and in some instances expansion of rabies. By contrast, the genetic study of the CO_2 sensitivity induced in *Drosophila* by infection with sigma virus has a long history antedating identification of the infectious agent (see the reviews of L'Heritier, 1958; Seecof, 1968; Printz, 1973), and some aspects of sigma virus genetics fall outside the scope of this chapter. Variation in the biological properties of plant viruses during routine propagation has been recorded. One strain of potato yellow dwarf virus, for instance, which was transmitted experimentally from plant to plant over a long period, lost the ability to be transmitted by the leafhopper vector (Black, 1953). However, no detailed genetic study of plant viruses has been reported so far. Consequently, most of the content of this chapter will concern one or other of the serological types of VSV.

2. CODING CAPACITY OF THE GENOME OF RHABDOVIRUSES

The molecular weight of the nucleic acid component of VSV is about 4×10^6, while the total molecular weight of the polypeptides comprising the five structural proteins of VSV (the L, G, N, NS, and M proteins) is approximately 393×10^3 (Pringle and Wunner, 1975). Thus approximately 98% of the coding capacity of the genome is accounted for by the known structural components of the virion, and little remains for nonstructural proteins necessary for virus synthesis or additional structural components. However, a degree of uncertainty is introduced into this calculation by the inaccuracy inherent in the estimates of the molecular weight of the various polypeptides, particularly the L protein ($\sim 200 \times 10^3$). Nonetheless, the existence of six complementation groups of *ts* mutants of VSV suggests that there may be at least one virus-specified polypeptide in addition to the five structural components of the virion.

VSV is thus a remarkably simple genetic system since most of the gene products can be identified, and all the functions of the viral genome may reside in the five structural components of the virion and possibly one additional polypeptide. The large size of the virion (175 nm by 68 nm) and its unique bullet-shaped morphology make VSV an ideal model system for analysis of the nature and mode of biosynthesis of the negative-strand virus.

Differences in the molecular weights of the RNA of different VSV serotypes have been reported (Schaeffer and Soergel, 1972) which suggested that VSV New Jersey might have a greater coding capacity than VSV Indiana. This would have provided a rationale for the existence of an additional complementation group in VSV New Jersey, despite the greater genetic attention accorded VSV Indiana (Pringle and Wunner, 1975). These differences in molecular weight of the RNA would appear to be a strain characteristic only, because Wunner and Pringle (unpublished) were unable to distinguish the RNAs of the M strain of VSV New Jersey and the C strain of VSV Indiana by electrophoresis in polyacrylamide gel, although VSV Cocal RNA was different from both. The problem has been resolved in another way by the finding of the missing sixth complementation group of VSV Indiana by Rettenmier *et al.* (1975) using a screening procedure designed to eliminate commonly occurring mutants and increase the frequency of rarer types.

The molecular weight of the RNA of rabies virus and potato yellow dwarf has been estimated as 4.6×10^6 (Sokol *et al.*, 1969; Reeder *et al.*, 1972), which gives these viruses a slightly greater coding capacity than VSV. The additional structural protein in the membrane of these viruses may be a reflection of this increased coding capacity.

A feature of the genome RNA of the few rhabdoviruses which have been studied so far is the overall similarity of base composition and the near unity of their $G + C$ ratios (Knudsen, 1973). The latter is generally regarded as fortuitous since the RNA extracted from the virion is undoubtedly single stranded (Weber *et al.*, 1974). Remarkably, there is little sequence homology between the RNAs of different rhabdoviruses. Repik *et al.* (1974) showed that little or no exact sequence homology ($<10\%$) existed between the virion RNA of VSV Indiana, VSV New Jersey, VSV Cocal, Chandipura virus, Piry virus, and rabies virus. However, some limited inexact homology was observed between VSV Indiana and VSV Cocal, which are ranked as subtypes of the one serotype (Federer *et al.*, 1967), and to a lesser degree between different VSV serotypes, i.e., VSV New Jersey and VSV Cocal, or VSV Indiana and VSV New Jersey.

3.   RHABDOVIRUS MUTANTS

3.1.   Phenotypes

Table 1 illustrates the range of genetic variation which has been utilized experimentally in genetic studies of rhabdoviruses. The sigma virus phenotypes, with the exception of the *ts* mutants and possibly the rho/ultrarho defectives, represent natural variation observed between different strains. All other examples in Table 1 represent spontaneous or induced intrastrain variation.

The intrastrain mutants can be subdivided into two broad categories: mutants with specific phenotypes, and conditional lethal mutants where a common phenotype embraces many if not all indispensable functions of the genome. Examples of the former are the *tl* mutants of VSV Indiana where the phenotype is due to the thermosensitivity of the virion envelope (Závada, 1972*a*), or the Rif⁺ phenotype where the drug rifampin appears to inhibit directly the activity of the virus-specified transcriptase (Moreau, 1974). The conditional lethal mutants of rhabdoviruses are either temperature-sensitive (*ts*), host-restricted (*hr*), or temperature-dependent host range (*td*CE) mutants. The majority of the conditional lethal mutants of VSV appear to be "missense" mutations, and no supressor-sensitive "nonsense" mutations or frameshift mutations have been identified (Pringle, 1975), although the complementation-dependent (*cd*) mutants isolated by Rettenmier *et al.,* (1975) have not yet been characterized and could fall into any of these categories.

3.2. Spontaneous Mutants

Ts mutants dominate rhabdovirus genetics because of their general utility and simplicity of assay. *Ts* mutants of VSV, Chandipura virus, rabies virus, and sigma virus have been obtained with varying facility, generally by chemical mutagenesis. Different strains of VSV have different characteristic frequencies of spontaneous mutants, e.g., the frequency of spontaneous *ts* mutants in the Indiana C strain was 0.9% (Pringle, 1970*a,b*). On the other hand, Flamand (1969, 1970) was able to isolate 71 spontaneous *ts* mutants of VSV Indiana from a strain in which the frequency of mutants was 2.3%. This frequency was a stable characteristic of the strain during sequential passage at 30°C. Destabilization followed upshift to 39.5°C, and frequencies as high as 8% were observed during initial passages at this temperature. The effect was transitory and the original frequency was regained by the ninth transfer at 39.5°C. It was suggested that the initial high frequency at 39.5°C was a consequence of a higher frequency of miscoding by the virus-specified polymerase at high temperature, and restoration of the original frequency required selection of a polymerase which was more competent at high temperature (Flamand, 1973).

High frequencies of spontaneous *ts* mutants have also been obtained by culture of VSV Indiana in *Drosophila* cells maintained at 22°C (Mudd *et al.,* 1973). VSV produced a noncytocidal persistent infection of *Drosophila* cells, and by the ninth passage a considerable fraction of the virus yield had a *ts* phenotype. Characterization of individual clones showed that several phenotypic classes were present, one of which was predominant. Earlier, Printz (1970) had found that plaque

TABLE 1

Mutants and Variants of Rhabdoviruses

Virus	Serotype	Mutant designation	Phenotype	Mutagen[a]	Reference
VSV	Indiana	—	Plaque morphology	None, Sp.	Wagner et al. (1963)
	New Jersey	—	Plaque morphology	UV	Schechmeister et al. (1967)
	Indiana	L/s	Plaque morphology	None, Sp.	Wertz and Levine (1973)
	Indiana	ts	Temperature sensitive	5-FU, NA, EMS, P	Flamand (1969)
	Indiana	ts	Temperature sensitive	5-FU, 5-AzaC, EMS	Holloway et al. (1970)
	Indiana	ts	Temperature sensitive	5-FU, NA, NTG	Pringle (1970a,b)
	New Jersey	ts	Temperature sensitive	UV, NA	Rettenmier et al. (1975)
	New Jersey	ts	Temperature sensitive	5-FU	Pittman (1965)
	Cocal	ts	Temperature sensitive	5-FU	Pringle et al. (1971)
	Indiana	tl	Thermolabile	5-FU	Pringle and Wunner (1973)
	Indiana	hr	Host range (restricted in HeLa cells)	5-FU, NTG	Závada (1972b)
	New Jersey	hr	Host range (restricted in CE cells)	5-FU	Simpson and Obijeski (1974)
	Indiana	tdCE	Host range (conditionally restricted in CE cells)	5-FU	Pringle (unpublished)
					Pringle (unpublished)

Virus	Gene	Character	Selection	Reference
New Jersey	*td*CE	Host range (conditionally restricted in CE cells)	5-FU	Szilágyi and Pringle (1975)
Cocal	*td*CE	Host range (conditionally restricted in CE cells)	5-FU	Pringle (unpublished)
Indiana	Rif⁺	Rifampin sensitivity	None, Sp.	Moreau (1974)
Indiana	*cd*	Complementation dependent	NA, NTG	Rettenmier *et al.* (1975)
Chandipura	*ts*	Temperature sensitive	5-FU	Pringle and Wunner (1973)
	*td*CE	Host range (conditionally restricted in CE cells)	5-FU	Gadkari and Pringle (unpublished)
Rabies	*ts*	Temperature sensitive	5-FU	Clark and Koprowski (1971)
	—	Plaque size	None, Sp.	Kondo, cited by Matsumoto (1970)
Sigma	*ts*	Temperature sensitive	5-FU	Contamine (1973)
	Tr	Temperature resistance	None, Sp.	Ohanessian-Guillemain (1959)
	P⁺/P⁻	Host range	None, Sp.	Guillemain (1953)
	—	"Plaque size"	None, Sp.	Brun (1963)
	—	"Plaque type"	None, Sp.	Vigier (1966)
	rho	Replication defective	None, Sp.	Brun (1963)
	ultrarho	Replication defective	None, Sp.	Brun (1963)
	g⁺/g⁻	Germinal transmission	None, Sp.	Duhamel (1954)
	pr⁺/pr⁻	Egg invasiveness	None, Sp.	Duhamel (1954)
	V⁺/V⁻	Sperm invasiveness	None, Sp.	Goldstein (1949)

[a] Sp., spontaneous; 5-FU, 5-fluorouracil; 5-AzaC, 5-azacytidine; NA, nitrous acid; NTG, N-methyl-N'-nitro-N-nitrosoguanidine; EMS, ethylmethane sulfonate; P, proflavine; UV, ultraviolet light.

morphology variants accumulated when VSV was passed in *Drosophila* imagoes.

Clark and Wiktor (1974) reported that the frequency of spontaneous *ts* mutants of the rabies-related Lagos bat and Mokola viruses was probably higher than that of the CVS strain of "fixed" rabies virus when cultured in BHK-21 cells under comparable conditions. For instance, four of 32 clones of Lagos bat virus picked at random appeared to be temperature sensitive. Lagos bat and Mokola viruses also exhibited great phenotypic variability with regard to virulence in mice and plaque morphology in comparison with CVS rabies virus. Cloning did not eliminate this variability. The greater phenotypic stability of "fixed" rabies virus may be a reflection of its prolonged history in laboratory culture, whereas Lagos bat and Mokola viruses were isolated from the field relatively recently.

3.3. Induced Mutants

Nonetheless, the frequency of spontaneous mutants is low in most strains and it has usually been necessary to use chemical mutagens to isolate conditional lethal mutants in reasonable numbers. The mutagens favored have been the base analogues 5-fluorouracil (5-Fu) and 5-azacytidine (5-AzaC), the alkylating agent ethylmethane sulfonate (EMS), nitrous acid (NA), N-methyl-N'-nitro-N-nitrosoguanidine (NTG), proflavine (P), and ultraviolet light (UV) (Table 1). It has been general experience that 5-Fu is more effective than other mutagens for induction of *ts* mutants (Clark and Koprowski, 1971; Holloway *et al.*, 1970; Pringle, 1970*a,b*; Rettenmier *et al.*, 1975) and *hr* mutants (Simpson and Obijeski, 1974). The yield of *ts* mutants from VSV Indiana grown in BHK-21 cells was proportional to mutagen dose, rising from < 1.0% in the absence of mutagen to about 46% at 100 μg 5-Fu/ml (Pringle, 1970*a,b*). However, 5-Fu was not equally effective with all strains of VSV, although spontaneous mutant frequencies did not differ markedly (Pringle and Wunner, 1975; Pringle, 1975). For instance, an approximately threefold greater concentration of 5-Fu was needed to obtain the same proportion of *ts* mutants from VSV Cocal 39 as from VSV Indiana, or 25-fold more in the case of VSV New Jersey. The variation in the response of strains to 5-Fu can be interpreted as heritable differences in the fidelity of the VSV polymerase, which, being a virus-coded enzyme, is subject to modification by mutation of the viral genome (Pringle, 1975).

There was no evidence of any mutagen specificity, and indeed the induced *ts* mutants of VSV Indiana fell into the same complementation groups as spontaneous *ts* mutants, and in comparable proportions (Pringle and Wunner, 1975).

3.4. Techniques for Isolation of *ts* and *hr* Mutants

Random isolation of clones from unselected plaques and subsequent screening for *ts* or *hr* phenotypes is a straightforward and feasible method of obtaining mutants (Pringle, 1970a,b; Holloway *et al.*, 1970; Clark and Koprowski, 1971). An economical variation of this procedure was introduced by Flamand (1970) in which several isolates could be screened simultaneously on the same plate. Uninfected monolayers were overlaid with agar and marked off in sectors. Isolates were stabbed through the overlay onto the appropriate sectors of replicate plates, and then a second overlay was added to seal the perforations. One replicate was incubated at permissive temperature and the other at restrictive temperature. Rettenmier *et al.* (1975) further increased the capacity of the replicate plating technique by using cells embedded in agar instead of agar-overlaid monolayers.

Several selective or enrichment methods have been described. A temperature downshift regime successfully increased the yield of late mutants belonging to complementation group III from mutagenized VSV Indiana stock (Pringle and Duncan, 1971). Závada (1972b) used neutralizing antibody to select mutants affecting the G (spike) protein of VSV. Bishop (personal communication) has isolated *ts* mutants of a fish rhabdovirus directly from infected monolayers of fathead minnow cells by ringing plaques before temperature upshift and establishing clones from plaques whose diameter was not increased. Indicator monolayers containing a mixture of two cell types have been used to obtain *hr* mutants of VSV Indiana, VSV New Jersey, and VSV Cocal (Simpson and Obijeski, 1974; Pringle, in preparation). Recently, Rettenmier *et al.* (1975) devised a procedure which facilitated the recovery of *ts* mutants belonging to the rarer complementation groups (see Section 5.2). Monolayers were infected with a mutant of the most frequently occurring group—*ts*G11 of group I*—and simultaneously

---

* In this chapter, the nomenclature for mutants of VSV Indiana suggested by Cormack *et al.* (1973) will be followed. The number of the mutant is prefixed by the letters B (for Bratislava), G (for Glasgow), O (for Orsay), M (for Massachusetts), T (for Toronto), or W (for Winnipeg) to indicate the laboratory of origin. For clarity, the complementation group of the mutant will follow in parenthesis, e.g., *ts*G11 (group I) is *ts* mutant No. 11 of the Glasgow collection of mutants, classified in complementation group I.

with a low multiplicity of mutagenized virus. By incubation at restrictive temperature, only wild type and complementing *ts* mutants produced plaques; group I mutants were automatically eliminated. Subsequent screening of these plaques by replicate plating led to the discovery of a previously unknown complementation group—group VI. An additional by-product of this selection was the recognition of a new type of mutant—the *cd* phenotype. These mutants did not produce cytopathic effects at permissive or restrictive temperature, and were only detected by their ability to complement *ts*G11 at 39°C. The *cd* phenotype has not yet been characterized in detail.

3.5. Isolation of *tl* Mutants

Závada (1972*b*) devised a selective procedure for the isolation of thermolabile (*tl*) mutants, whose efficacy has been verified by independent experiment (Hallam and Pringle, unpublished observations). (The *tl* phenotype refers to the heat stability of virus *in vitro,* whereas the *ts* phenotype indicates the ability of the virus to grow in cells at high temperature. *tl* mutants may be simultaneously *ts,* and *vice versa,* depending on the nature of the mutational defect.) The VSV Indiana mutant *ts*O45 (complementation group V) is thermolabile *in vitro* and the mutational lesion is considered to involve the virion glycoprotein (G protein) which carries the neutralizing antigen (see Section 6.4). Závada reasoned, therefore, that thermolabile (*tl*) mutants might be obtained if VSV was grown at low temperature in the presence of neutralizing antibody, and he succeeded in isolating a *tl* mutant of VSV Indiana after three passages in the presence of VSV antiserum. This mutant (*tl*2) was thermolabile *in vitro* at 42°C. An enhancement of thermolability was obtained by growing *tl*2 in the presence of 5-fluorouracil for one cycle, followed by three passages in the presence of neutralizing antibody. Cloning of this material yielded a mutant (*tl*9) which was thermolabile *in vitro* at 42°C. A third mutant (*tl*17) was obtained by a reptition of this procedure of mutagenization and selection, which was thermolabile *in vitro* at 38°C. This mutant was presumably a multiple mutant carrying at least three independent mutations. It was neutralized less rapidly than the starting material, as predicted.

Závada and Závodská (1974) later showed that mutants *tl*2, *tl*9, and *tl*17 were also temperature sensitive *in vivo* and failed to complement group I *ts* mutants. It is likely that the group I *ts* phenotype was fortuitously associated with the *tl* phenotype, since group I mutants are the most frequent type of *ts* mutant (see Section 5.2). Mutants *tl*9 and *tl*17, in addition, failed to complement group V *ts* mutants. In this case, it is more likely that the group V *ts* mutation and the *tl* phenotypes are associated, but this has not been definitely established.

Thermolabile mutants, such as *tl*17, were valuable in improving limits of resolution in the detection of pseudotypes (see Section 8).

4. ABSENCE OF RECOMBINATION

Genetic recombination in RNA viruses with unsegmented genomes appears to be limited to the picornavirus group (see Subak-Sharpe and Pringle, 1975), and linear recombination maps have been described for both poliovirus, type 1 (Cooper *et al.,* 1971), and foot-and-mouth disease virus, type O (Lake *et al.,* 1975). On the other hand, wild-type recombinant clones isolated from crosses of *ts* mutants of several negative-strand viruses (Newcastle disease virus, Sendai virus, and respiratory syncytial virus) have failed to breed true, and the parental mutants have reappeared during subsequent cloning. This phenomenon has been attributed to the existence of polyploid particles containing multiple genomes carrying different complementing *ts* mutants (Simon, 1972). Thus the apparent recombination of negative-strand viruses is mediated by complementation, which involves the interaction of gene products rather than the genomes themselves.

In crosses of *ts* mutants of VSV, the frequencies of presumptive wild-type recombinants ranged from 0.2 to 2.3% and were ten- to a hundredfold higher than the frequency of wild-type virus in self-crosses (Pringle, 1970*a*). None of these recombinants, however, was genetically stable, and segregation was invariably observed during subsequent cloning (Pringle, 1970*b*; Wong *et al.,* 1971; Rettenmier *et al.,* 1975). As with other negative-strand viruses, the existence of multiploid particles heterozygous for complementing mutants best explains the phenomenon, since "recombinants" were never observed in circumstances where complementation could be excluded (e.g., crosses within the same complementation group or between strains of different serotype) (Pringle and Wunner, 1975). Nevertheless, the uniform bullet shape of the VSV virion makes the idea of multiploid particles less acceptable than in the case of the more pleomorphic para- and metamyxoviruses. It has never been clearly established that the complementing heterozygotes of VSV are really polyploid particles and not merely viral aggregates (Pringle, 1975). However, double-length particles have been observed at frequencies as high as 1% in some preparations (Prevec, personal communication), which gives credence to the existence of polyploid particles of VSV.

Stable multimutant clones have been isolated at low frequency in the progeny from tri- and quadriparental crosses of complementing *ts* mutants of VSV Indiana. These unusual clones did not have the characteristics of recombinants, since a *ts* marker not included in the cross sometimes appeared in the progeny. It was suggested that these multimutant clones were the products of an aberrant mutation-generating polymerase (Pringle and Wunner, 1975).

Ohanessian-Guillemain (1959, 1963) found no evidence of recombination in a cross of two strains of sigma virus which could be distinguished by five different marker characteristics. On the other hand, in an experiment in which *Drosophila* parents carrying different sigma viruses were crossed, nonparental types of sigma virus were generated. These apparent recombinant sigma viruses were unstable and underwent segregation for at least one marker. These segregating clones were interpreted as heterozygotes (partial diploids), although the complexity of the situation would allow other interpretations of the data.

Absence of genetic recombination is unpropitious for any theory of replication of the genome which requires ligation of independently replicated subgenomic units.

5. COMPLEMENTATION

5.1. General Characteristics

Genetic complementation has been an effective means of grouping the *ts* mutants of VSV, and of defining the functional subunits of the genome. Complementation is usually expressed as an index, which is the ratio of the yield obtained from the mixed infection at the restrictive temperature to the sum of the single-infection yields. Values greater than 1 indicate complementation, and a simple statistical test can be used to estimate the significance of the index (Pringle and Wunner, 1973). The efficiency of complementation, when measured as the ratio of the yield from mixedly infected cells incubated at the restrictive temperature to the yield obtained at permissive temperature, never exceeded 1%, and maximum complementation indices were obtained at fairly low multiplicity of infection ($\sim$5 PFU/cell) (Pringle, 1970*a*). Subsequent work has shown that complementation is very sensitive to T-particle-mediated homologous interference, however, and the presence of T particles may have influenced the outcome of these early experiments.

In general, *ts* mutants of VSV Indiana are not complemented by T particles (the formal equivalent of deletion mutants) isolated from wild-type or *ts* mutant stocks (see Section 7.1). The inability of T particles to participate in complementation may be related to their lack of *in vitro* transcriptase activity, which appears to be due to a defect of the template rather than an absence of enzyme (Emerson and Wagner, 1972). Mori and Howatson (1973), however, have described transcriptase-positive T particles, and recently Deutsch (1975) has reported that UV-irradiated wild-type T particles can rescue *ts* mutants in mixed infection at the nonpermissive temperature (see Section 7.1).

The progeny obtained by complementation was phenotypically *ts*, and the evidence suggested that both parental genotypes appeared in the progeny (Pringle, 1970*a*)—i.e., complementation was symmetrical—in contrast to polio virus where the complementation yield contained one parental type only (Cooper, 1965). Subsequently, the genotype of progeny clones was determined directly by complementation tests, and it was confirmed that both parental genotypes were present in the progeny (Pringle, unpublished). Cormack *et al.* (1973) have obtained similar results in mixed infections of *ts*W16B (group IV) and mutants from group I, II, or III. In each case, clones of both genotypes were present in the progeny, although the proportions were equal only in mixed infections involving *ts*W16B (group IV) and group 1 mutants.

Efficient complementation is not dependent on a particular host cell, because the homologies of *ts* mutants in the Glasgow, Orsay, Massachusetts, Toronto, and Winnipeg collections were established with little difficulty, although the mutants had been isolated and propagated in different cell systems (Flamand and Pringle, 1971; Cormack *et al.*, 1973; Stanners *et al.*, 1975; Rettenmier *et al.*, 1975). Furthermore, complementation occurs efficiently in enucleate cells (Pringle and Follett, unpublished data). It is noteworthy that RNA⁻ mutants belonging to complementation groups II and IV were not isolated in the screening procedure of Rettenmier *et al.* (see Table 2).

Complementation has yet to be reported for either the *hr, hr/ts, hr*CE, or *td*CE mutants of VSV, or for the *ts* mutants of rabies virus. In the case of the rabies mutants, there are technical problems to be overcome, but it is not clear whether this alone accounts for the lack of information for the others.

Deutsch (1975) has described rescue of group V *ts* mutants by UV-irradiated virus (wild type, mutant, or T particle). Rescue of the

TABLE 2

Classification of VSV Indiana *ts* Mutants into Complementation Groups

Reference	Origin	Selection	Cell	I	II	III	IV	V	VI	Multiple or unclassified	Total
Flamand (1970)	Spontaneous	None	CE	58	2	4	4	3	0	0	71
Holloway *et al.* (1970)	Induced	None	L	7	0	2	2	0	0	14	25
Pringle (1970*b*)	Induced	None	BHK	151	2	1	15	0	0	6	175
Pringle and Duncan (1971)	Induced	Temperature downshift	BHK	26	0	2	7	0	0	0	35
Rettenmier *et al.* (1975)	Induced	Complementation with *ts*G11 (I)	L	0	0	3	0	2	2	1	8
Total				242	4	12	28	5	2	21	314

Column group header: Complementation group (spanning I, II, III, IV, V, VI, Multiple or unclassified)

unirradiated mutant was dependent on the multiplicity of the UV-irradiated virus, and was unaffected by an inhibitor of protein synthesis. Triggering of maturation by a polypeptide contributed by the irradiated parent appeared to be the mechanism of rescue. Deutsch deduced from these observations that complementation can occur by reutilization of nondefective virion components, presumably in this case the G protein (see Section 6.4). However, it is unlikely that primary transcription would be completely inhibited by UV irradiation, and the rescuing virion could contribute mRNA for the synthesis of nondefective G protein.

5.2. Classification of *ts* Mutants into Complementation Groups

Table 2 summarizes the data from different laboratories for 314 *ts* mutants of VSV Indiana. The mutants could be classified into groups unequivocally, with a few exceptions, some of which were obviously multiple mutants. The Glasgow mutants fell into nonoverlapping groups; i.e., mutants in any one group were able to complement mutants in any other group, but failed to complement mutants in the same group (Pringle, 1970*a,b*). Similar results were obtained with the Orsay and Winnipeg mutants, with the exception that weak complementation was observed between certain mutants belonging to the same group—this was interpreted as evidence of intracistronic complementation (Flamand, 1970; Wong *et al.*, 1972).

The majority (84.6%) of the mutants fell into group I. Group IV mutants were the next most frequent (9.9%), and the other groups were relatively rare. Indeed, no group V mutants had been isolated in mammalian cells before Rettenmier *et al.* (1975) developed their screening procedure for the less frequent types of mutant, and group VI was unknown.

Almost identical results were obtained with the serologically related VSV Cocal (Table 3). VSV New Jersey, however, exhibited a different pattern. Six nonoverlapping groups were evident from the outset, and two groups (A and B) were almost equally frequent (Pringle *et al.,* 1971). The sample of Chandipura mutants was small, but the pattern resembled that of VSV Indiana and VSV Cocal, where a single group predominated.

5.3.   Interstrain Complementation

Complementation was unrestricted between mutants derived from different wildtype strains of VSV Indiana. No complementation could be detected between mutants of unrelated viruses, i.e., Chandipura virus and the VSV serotypes, nor between different serotypes in the VSV group, i.e., VSV Indiana or VSV Cocal and VSV New Jersey. Limited complementation, however, was observed between serologically related strains within the same serotype, i.e., VSV Indiana and VSV Cocal (Pringle and Wunner, 1973). Surprisingly, in view of the lack of specificity inherent in the pseudotype phenomenon (see Section 8), it appeared that the specificity of complementation followed serological relationships within the VSV group. Interference by T particles also showed a similar specificity. Later, Repik *et al.* (1974) showed that there was only limited exact-sequence homology between genomes of

TABLE 3

Classification of *ts* Mutants of Other VSV Serotypes and Chandipura Virus into Complementation Groups

Virus	VSV New Jersey[a]							VSV Cocal[b]					Chandipura[b]		
Group	A	B	C	D	E	F	Unclassified	α	β	γ	δ	Unclassified	ChI	ChII	Unclassified
Number	17	21	4	1	3	2	1	29	2	3	6	0	18	2	0
Total			49							40				20	

[a] Pringle *et al.* (1971).
[b] Pringle and Wunner (1973). Recently, an additional 22 *ts* mutants of Chandipura virus have been isolated and the number of complementation groups has increased to five (Gadkari and Pringle, in preparation).

rhabdoviruses such as VSV Indiana and VSV Cocal. These data suggest that complementation involves enzymatic processes rather than assembly functions; indeed, the assembly of viral components may be virtually automatic, and there is probably no information in the VSV genome devoted solely to control of assembly.

Nevertheless, the failure to observe complementation between VSV Indiana and VSV New Jersey may be due to heterotypic interference (Cooper, 1958), although Bowie and Pringle (unpublished data) have been unable to reproduce heterotypic interference under the conditions of simultaneous infection used in the complementation experiments. (On the other hand, determination of the antigenic type of progeny clones from mixed infections failed to show that individual cells could release both parental-type viruses, which tends to support the heterotypic interference explanation. These experiments were difficult to interpret because of a lack of proportionality between number of productively infected cells and multiplicity of infection.) Petric and Prevec (1970) have described an example of heterotypic interference which was mediated by the long T particle present in the Toronto HR strain of VSV Indiana. An identical long T particle present in the Indiana C strain, however, interfered only homotypically and could not have been responsible for the absence of complementation. Whatever the reason, it proved impossible to establish the homologies of the complementation groups of the different VSV serotypes by genetic criteria alone.

6. TEMPERATURE-SENSITIVE MUTANTS IN THE ANALYSIS OF GENOME FUNCTION

6.1. Phenotype and Complementation Group

Pringle and Duncan (1971) showed that mutants could be categorized as RNA negative (RNA^-) or RNA positive (RNA^+) by measurement of cumulative incorporation of [^{3}H]uridine into acid-insoluble material in the presence of actinomycin D. In general, Wunner and Pringle (1972a,b) found that virus-specified polypeptides could be detected in cells infected with RNA^+ mutants, but not in cells infected with RNA^- mutants; i.e., the intracellular RNA and polypeptide phenotypes were correlated.

Mutants classified in the same complementation group had a common phenotype, with certain exceptions. The exceptions were group II (VSV Indiana), group E (VSV New Jersey), and group δ (VSV Cocal), which included both RNA$^+$ and RNA$^-$ mutants. All the other groups appeared to contain mutants of one phenotype only (Table 4). Similar results were reported for the RNA phenotype of the Orsay mutants (Lafay, 1969) and the Winnipeg mutants (Wong *et al.*, 1972).

Knowing the group phenotypes, an attempt could be made to equate the VS.V Indiana and VSV Cocal groups. Group I and group α are probably homologous since they are the majority groups of RNA$^-$ mutants. Groups IV and group β are the minority RNA$^-$ groups, and group II and group δ contain mutants of both RNA$^-$ and RNA$^+$ phenotypes. Therefore, it is reasonable to equate these two groups. The remaining groups III and γ were assumed to be homologous on the basis of frequency and phenotype. Furthermore, group III complemented groups α, β, and δ of VSV Cocal, but not group γ (Pringle and Wunner, 1973). Subsequent detailed characterization of the phenotype of $ts\gamma1$ (see Section 6.4) indicated that the lesion involved the glycoprotein; therefore, group γ should be equated with group V rather than group III (Buller 1975; Buller and Wunner, in preparation). In the interstrain complementation experiments, group V complemented groups α and β, but not γ or δ, which does not conflict with this assignment.

Lesnaw and Reichmann (1975) examined the ability of representative mutants of the six complementation groups of VSV New Jersey to carry out primary transcription and amplification of RNA synthesis in BHK-21 cells at restrictive temperature. Mutants *ts* C1 and *ts* D1 from the RNA$^+$ complementation groups were able to amplify RNA synthesis, whereas the mutants *ts* A1, *ts* B1, *ts* E1, and *ts* F1 from the RNA$^-$ groups failed to amplify RNA synthesis. Mutants *ts* A1 and *ts* E1 could carry out primary transcription, however, and temperature-shift experiments suggested that these mutants were defective in replication. Mutants *ts* B1 and *ts* F1, on the other hand, were unable to carry out primary transcription and failed to synthesize any RNA.

TABLE 4

Phenotypic Characteristics of Complementation Groups

| Virus | Group phenotype | | | |
	RNA$^-$/protein$^-$	RNA$^+$/protein$^+$	Mixed	Undetermined
VSV Indiana	I, IV	III, V	II	VI
VSV Cocal	α, β	γ	δ	—
VSV New Jersey	A, B, F	C, D	E	—
Chandipura	ChI	ChII	—	—

Temperature-shift experiments with these mutants suggested that transcription and replication are functionally linked processes in VSV New Jersey.

On the basis of these findings Lesnaw and Reichmann suggested that groups A, B, and E of VSV New Jersey correspond to groups IV, I, and II, respectively, of VSV Indiana, and groups C and D correspond to groups III and V. The sixth VSV New Jersey group, group F, appeared to have no counterpart in VSV Indiana.

6.2. Phenotypic Characterization of the VSV Indiana Complementation Groups

A considerable amount of information has been accumulated concerning the phenotypes of mutants belonging to the VSV Indiana complementation groups (reviewed by Pringle, 1975). A synopsis of the data is presented in Table 5.

Inspection of Table 5 will show that there is more agreement than disagreement, and much of the latter is attributable to individuality of mutants within the groups. It should be noted here that the RNA phenotype in Table 4 refers only to the amplification of RNA synthesis which occurs as a result of virus replication; the RNA⁻ phenotype is not absolute, therefore, and many of these mutants carry out primary transcription *in vivo*. Viral RNA synthesis can be subdivided into three distinct phases: primary transcription (synthesis of mRNA from parental templates), secondary transcription (synthesis of mRNA from progeny templates), and replication (synthesis of complete plus and minus strands). The phenotypes of individual *ts* mutants of the RNA⁻ groups overlap these subdivisions, and the data strongly suggest that transcription and replication are interdependent processes. It has been concluded that replication occurs by modification of transcription, rather than by induction of an independent replicase, and that pleiotropic effects are common because of the role of the polymerase as a structural component of the virion (Bishop and Flamand, 1975*a,b*; Combard *et al.*, 1974; Huang, 1975; Perleman and Huang, 1973, 1974; Printz *et al.*, 1975; Unger and Reichmann, 1973; Pringle and Wunner, 1975).

Synthesis of 40 S replicative RNA was not inhibited when certain mutants of groups I and IV of VSV Indiana were transferred from permissive to restrictive temperature, although transcription of mRNA was greatly reduced. If protein synthesis was inhibited by addition of cycloheximide after temperature upshift of mutant *ts*G114 (group I), replicative RNA synthesis was abolished and transcription restored

(Perleman and Huang, 1973, 1974; Huang, 1975; Reichmann, personal communication). This finding supports the hypothesis that the viral transcriptase was modified by addition of another polypeptide to read off uninterrupted whole genome transcripts, which then became intermediates in replication. The absence of genetic recombination is circumstantial evidence in support of a hypothesis of replication via a complete 40 S complementary strand.

Three viral polypeptides can be assigned to cistrons (complementation groups) by consideration of the data in Table 5. One more polypeptide can be assigned if the New Jersey and Cocal mutants are considered in addition. These assignments are illustrated diagrammatically in Fig. 1. The gene order is arbitrary.

6.3. Polymerase Mutants

The *in vitro* activity of the virion transcriptase of thermolabile group I mutants was irreversibly inhibited at 39°C, suggesting that the transcriptase itself was inactivated at this temperature (Szilágyi and Pringle, 1972). These findings were confirmed by Hunt and Wagner (1974), who further established by elegant reconstitution experiments that the enzyme was defective rather than its template. Mutant and wild-type virions were dissociated into a sedimentable ribonucleoprotein complex (template) and a soluble (enzyme) fraction, which separately possessed no enzyme activity. *In vitro* enzyme activity was obtained at 39°C when wild-type enzyme and mutant template were combined, but not when mutant enzyme and wild-type template were combined. Since the L protein is the predominant component of the soluble fraction, these experiments strongly suggest that the L protein is the transcriptase itself, and that the L polypeptide is the product of the group I cistron. In fact, Hunt *et al.* (1976) have been able to confirm experimentally, using the reconstitution technique, that thermosensitivity of the L protein accounts for the defectiveness of the transcriptase of group I mutants. The *in vitro* transcriptase activities of three group I mutants (*ts* G13, *ts* G16, and *ts* G114) at 39°C were restored by purified L protein from wild-type virus. Soluble NS protein from wild-type virus did not restore activity, and NS protein from group I mutants displayed the wild-type phenotype in reconstitution assays. Furthermore, neither the L nor the NS proteins were capable of restoring the defective transcriptase of the template-defective mutant *ts* W16B of group IV. The prevalence of group I mutants (>80% of all *ts* mutants) may be a reflection of the size of the L polypeptide which accounts for half the coding capacity of the genome.

TABLE 5
Physiological Properties of the VSV Indiana Complementation Groups[a]

Property	Complementation group, VSV Indiana						Reference
	I	II	III	IV	V	VI	
Revertant frequency	Low or none[1] (< 10^{-7})	High[1,2]	High[1]	High in most stocks[1]	Moderate (~ 10^{-4})[1]	N.D.	1. Pringle (1970b; unpublished. 2. Flamand and Lafay (1973)
Heat stability of virion	Labile mutants frequent[1]; nucleocapsid defect[2]	Variable[3]	Stable[3,4]	Minor variations[3]	Thermolabile envelope[5]	N.D.	1. Szilágyi and Pringle (1972) 2. Buller (1975) 3. Pringle and Duncan (1971) 4. Wong et al. (1972) 5. Deutsch and Berkaloff (1971)
Time of action as defined by temperature shift	Early function, continuous requirement[1]; early function, gene product with long half-life[2]; variable[3]	Early function, stable gene product[1]	Late function[1,5]; maturation block, gene product irreversibly labile[6]	Early function, continuous requirement[1]; early function, stable gene product[5]	Late function[7]	N.D.	1. Pringle and Duncan (1971) 2. Flamand and Lafay (1973) 3. Martinet and Printz-Ané (1970) 4. Holloway et al. (1970) 5. Wong et al. (1972) 6. Lafay and Berkaloff (1969) 7. Deutsch and Berkaloff (1971)

						References
Stability of infectious centers (R.T.)	More labile than wild type[1]	Very labile[1]	As wild type	More labile than wild type[1]	As wild type	N.D.	1. Flamand and Lafay (1973)
Intracellular polypeptides at restrictive temperature (R.T.)	None[1,2]	None[1]; failure of glycosylation and insertion into the cell membrane[2]	All present[1]; M absent[2]; M atypical[3]	Traces[1,5]; L and N affected by shiftup[6]; L and N not affected by shiftup[7]	All present[1-5]	N.D.	1. Wunner and Pringle (1972a) 2. Printz and Wagner (1971) 3. Lafay (1971, 1974) 4. Buller (1975) 5. Printz et al. (1975) 6. Combard et al. (1974) 7. Perleman and Huang (1974)
Intracellular ribonucleoprotein at R.T.	None[1]	None[1,2]	Overproduction[1]	None[1]	As wild type	N.D.	1. Unger and Reichmann (1973) 2. Deutsch (1970) 3. Printz and Wagner (1971)
Transcriptase activity in vitro at R.T.	Frequently thermolabile[1-3,5]	As wild type[1]	As wild type[1]	As wild type[1,2]; thermolabile[4]	N.D.	N.D.	1. Szilágyi and Pringle (1972) 2. Printz-Ané et al. (1972) 3. Cormack et al. (1971) 4. Cairns et al. (1972) 5. Hunt et al. (1976)

(continued)

TABLE 5 (Continued)

Property	Complementation group, VSV Indiana						Reference
	I	II	III	IV	V	VI	
Primary transcription in vivo at R.T.	Yes, except very thermolabile mutants[1-5]	Yes[1-3]	Yes[1-3]	Yes[1-3]	Yes[1-3]	N.D.	1. Unger and Reichmann (1973) 2. Flamand and Bishop (1973) 3. Bishop and Flamand (1975a) 4. Printz-Ané et al. (1972) 5. Repik et al. (1976)
Secondary transcription and replication in vivo at R.T.	None[2-4]	Variable[1,3]	As wild type[1-3]	None[2,3]	As wild type[1-3]	N.D.	1. Flamand and Bishop (1973) 2. Flamand and Bishop (1974) 3. Unger and Reichmann (1973) 4. Repik et al. (1976)
Inhibition of host macromolecular synthesis	As wild type[1-3] None[4]	As wild type[3]	As wild type[1]; reduced inhibition of uridine uptake[3]	As wild type[1-4]	N.D.	N.D.	1. Holloway et al. (1970) 2. Genty and Berreur (1973) 3. Genty (1975) 4. McAllister and Wagner (1976)
Inferred defect	Transcriptase (L protein)	?	Matrix protein (M protein)	?	Glycoprotein spike (G protein)	?	

[a] N.D., no data; ?, unknown.

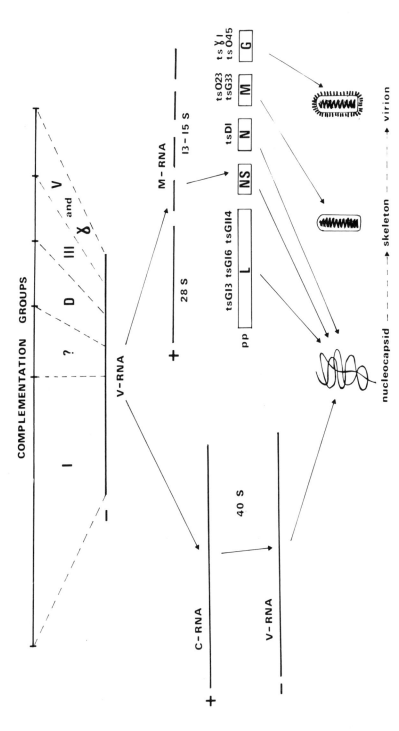

Fig. 1. Schematic representation of the biosynthesis of VSV and the relationship of viral gene and gene product. The order of the genes is arbitrary and no polarity is implied. Recently, Ball and White (1976) have determined the apparent target sizes for expression of the various virus genes in a cell-free system allowing coupled transcription and translation, and the probable gene order has been deduced as 5′-(L)-G-M-NS-N-3′. Abraham and Banerjee (1976) derived a similar gene order (5′-L-G-M/NS-N-3′) from studies of the polar effects of UV-irradiation on mRNA transcription.

Repik *et al.* (1976) have studied the ability of various *ts* mutants to synthesize intracellular viral complementary RNA at restrictive temperature. Synthesis of viral complementary RNA could always be detected by a sensitive hybridization procedure, except in the case of cells infected with the most highly thermosensitive group I mutant, *ts* G114. This result confirms that the *in vivo ts* phenotype of mutant *ts* G114 is accounted for by the thermosensitivity of the virion enzyme. It was also observed that the transcription defect of *ts* G114 could be complemented by wild-type VSV New Jersey, but not by Mokola virus (a rabies-related rhabdovirus). This complementation was inhibited by puromycin, which suggested that a VSV New Jersey gene product, presumably the transcriptase or a transcriptase component, was involved. This apparent interaction between VSV Indiana and VSV New Jersey gene products is interesting in view of the failure to detect complementation in genetic experiments (Section 5.3).

Ngan *et al.* (1974) and Cormack *et al.* (1975) obtained similar results and further established that the template was defective in group IV mutants, indicating that either the N or NS polypeptide is the site of the group IV mutational lesion. (It is possible, however, that RNA conformation may affect template activity.)

Other non-*ts* mutants are known to affect polymerase activity, notably the rifampin-sensitive mutant isolated by Moreau (1974). The transcriptase activity of some of the *hr/ts* mutants described by Simpson and Obijeski (1974) and Obijeski and Simpson (1974) was defective *in vitro* at permissive temperatures. The *td*CE mutants include mutants with defective *in vitro* transcriptase activity at restrictive temperatures (Szilágyi and Pringle, 1975). These mutants differ from the group I mutants in one important respect. *In vitro* transcriptase activity at 39°C was not irreversibly inhibited and activity could be restored instantaneously by downshift to 31°C, indicating that the function of the transcriptase was temperature sensitive. Reversion of the *td*CE phenotype to wild type was accompanied by restoration of normal transcriptase function at 31°C and 39°C.

6.4. Glycoprotein Mutants

The experiments of Závada, Lafay, and Buller implicated the group V cistron as the site of mutations involving the G protein. A more precise association has been described by Buller (1975) and Buller and Wunner (in preparation) for mutant $ts\gamma1$ of VSV Cocal. Normal glycosylation of polypeptide G was partially defective at 31°C and completely inhibited at 39°C. However, polypeptide G glycosylated at 31°C could become incorporated into virions at 39°C, suggesting that the mutational lesion involved the site or process of glycosylation rather than inducing a conformational change in the polypeptide itself. Reversion of the temperature-sensitive phenotype was accompanied by restoration of normal glycosylation.

6.5. A Nucleoprotein Mutant

Mutant tsD1, the only member of complementation group D of VSV New Jersey, has been shown to have a temperature-sensitive defect involving the N polypeptide (Wunner and Pringle, 1974). Mutant tsD1 is apparently a double mutant, since the electrophoretic mobility of both the G and the N polypeptides was abnormal in polyacrylamide gel. The molecular weight differences of G and N from wild type were 3500 and 1000, respectively. Isolation and characterization of revertants showed that only the N mobility difference was associated with the ts phenotype, however. Surprisingly, the mutant polypeptide phenotype was expressed at permissive temperature without any apparent effect on viability.

6.6. Matrix Protein Mutants

Lafay (1971, 1974) has shown that M protein synthesized in cells infected with tsO89 (group III) at 39°C was defective, because it did not become incorporated into virions following transfer to 31°C. Buller (1975) and Buller and Wunner (in preparation) have detected differences in the electrophoretic mobility of the M polypeptide of three different group III mutants (tsO23, tsG32, and tsG33) relative to wild-type M at 39°C using a gradient slab gel system of high resolution. Reversion of the ts phenotype was accompanied by changes in mobility of the M polypeptide, although the wild-type pattern was not always restored. Taken together, the results indicate that the M polypeptide is specified by the group III cistron.

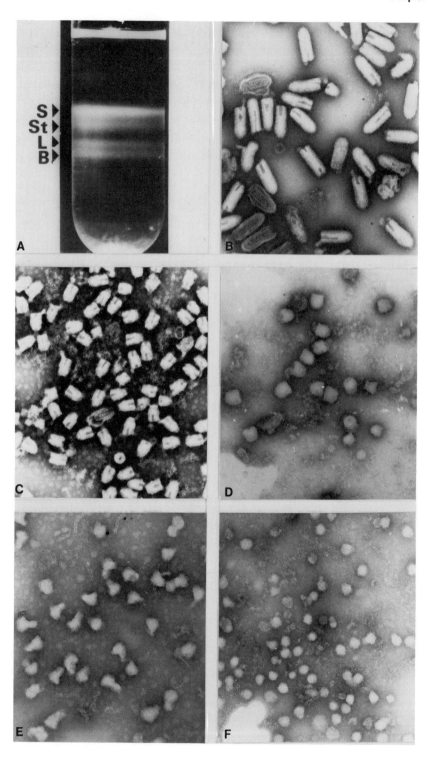

7. DEFECTIVENESS

7.1. T Particles and *ts* Mutants

Defective particles of rhabdoviruses are more easily studied than those of other viruses, because they can be distinguished morphologically from competent virions, and homogeneous preparations can be obtained by rate zonal centrifugation. The T particles of VSV are shorter than the virion and contain less RNA. The RNA is the negative strand, like the RNA of the complete genome; consequently, T particles can be regarded as *deletion mutants*. T particles contain all the virion structural proteins, but they lack transcriptase activity, and their genetic information remains unexpressed. T particles are not infectious and they can be replicated only in the presence of competent virions. They are distinguished biologically by their ability to interfere with multiplication of infectious VSV of the same serotype, probably by inhibiting replication rather than transcription or translation. The manifestation of interference is highly variable, however, and largely dependent on host cell type (Perrault and Holland, 1972). (For a general review, see Huang, 1973.)

Little is known about the genesis of T particles, other than that they accumulate during high-multiplicity passage. T particles of several morphological types with RNA contents ranging from 8% to 50% of the viral genome were found associated with particular *ts* mutants of VSV Indiana (Fig. 2). The various T particles were characteristic of individual mutants rather than complementation groups (Reichmann *et al.*, 1971). The T particle associated with wild-type VSV Indiana, designated the standard T particle (Fig. 2D), had a sedimentation coefficient of 330 S compared with the 610 S of the virion. A T particle of similar size but reduced structural stability was associated with *ts*G41 (group IV) (Fig. 2E). A long T particle approximately half the length of the virion and containing an RNA of 1×10^6 molecular weight (Fig.

Fig. 2.   The virion and four morphological types of T particles of VSV Indiana. (A) The separation of purified virion (B), long T (L), standard T (St), and short T (S) particles from a mixture by rate zonal centrifugation in a 15–45% sucrose gradient. (B) The virion (Glasgow wild type). (C) The long T particle associated with *ts*G11 (group I) and *ts*G22 (group II). The long T particle described by Petric and Prevec (1970) in the Toronto HR strain is indistinguishable. (D) The standard T particle from the Glasgow wild type. (E) A structurally unstable T particle associated with *ts*G41 (group IV). Fixation before negative staining produced a standard T (see Reichmann *et al.*, 1971). (F) The short T particle associated with mutants *ts*G31, *ts*G32, and *ts*G33 (all group III).

2C) was associated with *ts*G11 (group I) and *ts*G22 (group II). Finally, a very short T particle (Fig. 2F), spherical in shape and containing only one-twelfth of the genome, was associated with *ts*G31, *ts*G32, and *ts*G33 (all group III).

None of these types of T particles showed any genetic activity in complementation experiments with purified *ts* mutants, nor were wild-type T particles able to rescue *ts* mutants. The T-particle preparations had biological activity, however, since they all induced interference with infectious VSV of homologous serotype. Like wild-type T particles, they were less able to interfere with VSV of heterologous serotype. In this respect, they differ from a long T particle isolated from the Toronto HR wild-type strain by Petric and Prevec (1970). The HR long T particle had the unique property of interfering with heterotypic strains as efficiently as with homotypic strains. However, like other T particles it had no genetic activity in complementation experiments (Pringle and Prevec, unpublished data).

Deutsch (1975) has reported, however, that UV-irradiated wild-type T particles rescued mutant *ts*O45 (group V) under certain conditions. This complementation probably occurred as a result of reutilization of T-particle components (see Section 5.1). Unirradiated T particles were unable to rescue mutant *ts*O45 under the same conditions.

7.2. Physical Mapping of the Genome

The relationship of the genetic information present in the T particle to the complete viral genome has been deduced by annealing T-particle RNA with purified VSV messenger RNA. Leamnson and Reichmann (1974) concluded from such studies that the RNA fragment in the HR long T particle contained nucleotide sequences complementary to all messenger RNA species in the 13–18 S size class—the putative messages for the G, N, NS, and M polypeptides—and very few if any to the 30 S class—the putative message for the L protein. In contrast, the RNA of *ts*G11 long T particle (Reichmann, personal communication) and all the shorter T particles contained sequences predominantly or wholly complementary to the 30 S messenger RNA. Furthermore, the longer RNA fragments contained all the nucleotide sequences of the shorter species. A map locating the T-particle deletion fragments in the genome was prepared from this and other information (Fig. 3). One conclusion which can be drawn from this map is that if there is a common sequence in the genome responsible for interference,

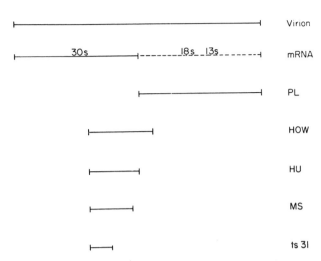

Fig. 3. Tentative map of T-particle RNA species on the viral genome. The RNA species are located in relation to the 30S and 13–18S mRNA domains. PL, Long T particle from the Toronto HR wild type; HOW, standard T particle from Toronto HR wild type; HU, standard T particle from the Massachusetts wild type; MS, standard T particle from the California wild type; *ts*31, short T particle from *ts*G31 (group III). Reproduced from the *Journal of Molecular Biology*.

it must be very short. Furthermore, the possible region of overlap between the HR long T and the other T-particle sequences is at opposite ends of the RNA fragments in relation to the 3′–5′ orientation.

The lack of genetic activity of the *ts*G11 long T and the short T particles can be attributed to absence of a complete viral cistron in these particles. This argument does not explain the inactivity of the HR long T particle, which should include at least one complete viral cistron. It seems probable, however, that the unique heterotypic interference induced by the HR long T is related in some way to its map position or possession of complete viral cistrons.

These observations have been extended by Schnitzlein and Reichmann (1976) recently and a revised map of T particle RNAs relative to viral cistronic regions proposed; the HR T particle remains unique in its possession of nucleotide sequences complementary to the 13–18S mRNAs. In addition, they concluded that the ability of the HR long T particle of VSV Indiana to interfere heterotypically with VSV New Jersey was not a function of the size of its RNA, since three other T particle RNAs of comparable size did not exhibit this property. Heterotypic interference appeared to be a property of nucleotide sequences originating from the 13–18S mRNA cistrons. The HR T particle RNA had no overlap of nucleotide sequence with other T particle RNAs; some apparent complementarity between the HOW T particle and the 13–18S RNA observed previously was due to impurities. The extent of a residual ability in other T particles to interfere heterotypically appeared to be host-cell dependent; greater residual heterotypic interference was observed in BHK-21 cells than in L cells.

A map of the VSV genome which has been derived independently by Prevec (1974) has much in common with the Leamnson and Reichmann map, and Stamminger and Lazzarini (1974) have derived a third map which attempts to define the 5′-3′ orientation. In this map, one of the 13 S cistrons is located to the left of the 30 S cistron, and the other three are to the right (the 5′ end).

These findings are provisional, and may have to be revised drastically in the light of the isolation of T particles (DI_{O11}) containing covalently linked negative- and plus-strand RNA which assumes a hairpin structure on deproteinization (Lazzarini et al., 1975), and the presence of separate molecules of negative- and plus-strand RNA in populations of long T particles of the HR strain of VSV (Roy et al., 1973). The principle of the mapping procedure has been established, however.

The DI_{O11} particles studied by Lazzarini et al. (1975) interfered with the replication of complete virus, like other T particles. It is not yet known whether the presence of nongenomic sequences affects the specificity of interference (see Section 7.1).

8. PHENOTYPIC MIXING AND PSEUDOTYPES

Phenotypic mixing was known to occur between related strains of enveloped viruses, and even between the related paramyxovirus and orthomyxovirus groups (Granoff and Hirst, 1954). More recently, it has been shown that rhabdoviruses can undergo phenotypic mixing with a wide range of enveloped viruses. Choppin and Compans (1970) showed that VSV genomes could be released from cells infected with the paramyxovirus SV5 within an envelope provided partially or entirely by SV5. Between 9% and 45% of the VSV plaque-forming virus possessed both SV5 and VSV antigens in their envelope. A further 0.6–1.2% of the yield was neutralized by SV5 antiserum, but not by VSV antiserum, suggesting that these particles were VSV (SV5) pseudotypes with the envelope provided entirely by the heterologous virus. It was subsequently confirmed by polyacrylamide gel electrophoresis of virion polypeptides that the pseudotype contained the core polypeptides of VSV and the envelope polypeptides of SV5 (McSharry *et al.*, 1971). The list of viruses able to undergo phenotypic mixing with VSV was later extended to include fowl plaque virus (Závada and Rosenbergová, 1972), avian and murine leukoviruses (Závada, 1972*a,b*), and herpes simplex virus (HSV) (Huang *et al.*, 1974). Finally, Bishop *et al.* (1975*c*) have obtained phenotypic mixing between different VSV serotypes, and even pseudotypes of VSV with heterologous viruses (personal communication), by the reassociation *in vitro* of spikeless particles and envelope components from different viruses.

Phenotypic mixing has not been detected between VSV and the arbovirus Sindbis virus (Burge and Pfefferkorn, 1966), which indicates that there are some constraints on the interaction of VSV nucleocapsids with heterologous viral envelope components.

Závada (1972*b*) showed that neutralization-resistant VSV particles released from cells chronically infected with avian myeloblastosis virus (AMV) or Moloney murine leukemia virus (MMLV) had the host range and interference specificity of the tumor virus, indicating that these particles were VSV (AMV) or VSV (MMLV) pseudotypes. Furthermore, VSV mutants *ts*O44 and *ts*O45 (group V), where the membrane glycoprotein is thought to be defective, were complemented (i.e., rescued by phenotypic mixing) in AMV-infected cells incubated at nonpermissive temperature. Mutants of complementation groups I, II, III, and IV were not complemented under the same conditions, which supports the view that the mutational lesion in these groups does not involve the viral glycoprotein. Love and Weiss (1974) showed that VSV could become phenotypically mixed with the envelope antigen of an endogenous avian leukovirus in cells positive for chick helper factor (*chf*), yielding the VSV (*chf*) pseudotype. This experiment disposed of the trivial explanation that pseudotypes are produced by some nonspecific mechanism such as extracellular clumping of virus particles. Boettiger *et al.* (1975) studied the efficiency of penetration of mammalian cells by pseudotypes of avian leukosis (ALV) and sarcoma (ASV) viruses. Only pseudotypes with the envelope of subgroup D viruses penetrated mammalian cells efficiently, confirming previous findings that the viral envelope plays a major role in determining whether avian leukoviruses can infect and transform mammalian cells. The efficiency of penetration of the VSV (ASV) pseudotype was a hundred- to a thousandfold higher than the efficiency of transformation; consequently, the expression of transforming genes is dependent on more than successful penetration of the mammalian cell. VSV (MLV) pseudotypes have been used in an analogous manner to show

that the host restriction of MLV controlled by the *Fv-1* locus—the N-
and B-cell tropism—acts after penetration of the genome into the host
cell (Huang *et al.,* 1973; Krontiris *et al.,* 1973). The types of particles
released from cells simultaneously infected with VSV and an oncornavirus, and their operational identification are summarized in Fig. 4
and Table 6.

The biological importance of the pseudotype phenomenon is
twofold. First, the reciprocal pseudotype where the tumor virus genome
is enclosed in a VSV coat potentially expands the host range of the
generally restricted tumor viruses (Weiss *et al.,* 1975). It should be
remembered, therefore, that there is a potential biohazard associated
with any pseudotype experiment. Second, VSV can be used as a probe
for detection of cryptic tumor viruses. This aspect of the phenomenon
has been exploited extensively by Závada and colleagues, who selected
ts and *tl* mutants to improve the discrimination of pseudotypes by
rendering the parental VSV thermolabile (Závada, 1972*b*; Závada and
Závodská, 1974). Release of VSV pseudotypes from cell lines derived
from a human mammary carcinoma (Závada *et al.,* 1972, 1974), a pro-
static carcinoma, a myeloma, and a sarcoma (Závada *et al.,* 1975) have
been reported. Although the origin of some of these cell lines is in
doubt, the principle of the technique has been demonstrated, nonetheless, and it may yet be successful in the search for cryptic human tumor
agents. A disadvantage is that VSV is probably partially restricted in

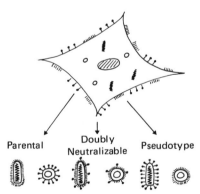

Fig. 4. Diagrammatic representation of the types of particles released from cells
simultaneously infected with VSV and an oncornavirus. VSV genomes are shown as
helices, oncornavirus genomes as *rings,* VSV glycoprotein as *spikes,* and oncornavirus
glycoprotein as *knobs.* Each viral genome may become enveloped during budding from
the cell membrane by its own glycoprotein (*parental* combination), by homologous and
heterologous glycoproteins (*doubly neutralizable*), or entirely by heterologous glycoprotein (*pseudotype*). The criteria for identification of these types of particles are summarized in Table 6.

TABLE 6

Synopsis of the Host Range and Neutralization Resistance of the Virus Particles Released from Cells Simultaneously Infected with an Avian Oncornavirus and VSV[a]

Type of particle			Host cell susceptible to homologous ALV			Host cell resistant to homologous ALV			Host cell chronically infected with homologous ALV		
Description	Core	Coat	No antibody	Anti-VSV	Anti-ALV	No antibody	Anti-VSV	Anti-ALV	No antibody	Anti-VSV	Anti-ALV
Parental	ALV	ALV	+	+	−	−	−	−	−	−	−
	VSV	VSV	+	−	+	+	−	+	+	−	+
Doubly neutraliz- able	ALV	ALV/VSV	+	−	−	−	−	−	−	−	−
	VSV	VSV/ALV	+	−	−	?	−	−	?	−	−
Full pseudotype	ALV	VSV	+	−	+	+	−	+	?	−	?
	VSV	ALV	+	+	−	−*	−	−	−	−	−

[a] Symbols: +, productive infection (ALV or VSV); −, no productive infection (ALV or VSV); ?, outcome not known, remains to be established. *, the same pattern is observed when VSV is grown in cells infected with murine oncornaviruses, except that the asterisked category would become a productive infection because restriction in murine cells does not act at the level of the surface receptor as it does in avian cells.

most human cells (Obijeski and Simpson, 1974). The human rhabdovirus, Chandipura virus, may be a more suitable probe than VSV in human cells, although preliminary experiments indicate that it produces pseudotypes with herpes simplex virus less efficiently than VSV (Hallam and Pringle, unpublished data).

Indeed, the occurrence of phenotypic mixing between VSV and both RNA and DNA viruses greatly extends the scope of VSV as a probe for cryptic oncogenic information. Surprisingly, phenotypic mixing between VSV and HSV is efficient, although the latter is thought to acquire its envelope during release from the nucleus; as much as 30% of the yield may be VSV (HSV) pseudotype. Experiments are now in progress using VSV and Chandipura virus as probes in an attempt to detect HSV gene expression in cell lines transformed by HSV.

9. HOST-CONTROLLED MODIFICATION

Phenotypic changes which are not heritable may appear as a result of growth of VSV in different hosts. This host-controlled modification is possible because the envelope of VSV may contain lipid and glycolipid of host origin in addition to viral glycoprotein (Cartwright and Brown, 1972). The carbohydrate moiety of the glycoprotein of VSV is another source of host-controlled modification, since the VSV genome does not have spare capacity to specify the number of glycosyltransferases necessary for synthesis of the appropriate oligosaccharides. Minor differences in the size and composition of the oligosaccharide chains of VSV grown in different cells have been detected (Burge and Huang, 1970; McSharry and Wagner, 1971; Etchison and Holland, 1974; Moyer and Summers, 1974). For example, Etchison and Holland found that fucose was present in VSV glycoprotein synthesized in BHK, HeLa, and MDCK cells, but was absent from VSV glycoprotein synthesized in mouse L929 cells.

Schloemer and Wagner (1975) have reported that the glycoprotein of VSV grown in cells of the mosquito *Aedes albopictus* was deficient in sialic acid, which correlated with an absence of sialic acid and sialyltransferase from these cells. Virons released from these cells had reduced hemagglutinating activity and low infectivity for mammalian cells. Since it was known that neuraminic acid residues were essential for efficient attachment of VSV to cells, Schloemer and Wagner suggest that lack of sialic acid is an important factor in the nonlytic nature of VSV infection of insect cells. In fact, sialylation *in vitro* of VSV virions released from mosquito cells produced a hundredfold increase in infectivity and hemagglutinating activity.

VSV grown in SV40-transformed hamster cells acquired the TSTA membrane antigen, which is invariably associated with SV40 virus transformation (Ansel, 1974). The virus-specified nature of TSTA is open to question in view of the very limited coding capacity of the SV40 genome. Ansel and Tournier (personal communication) suggest that the TSTA antigens may be a cellular glycolipid because trypsin treatment of VSV to produce naked spikeless particles did not remove the TSTA antigen. Phospholipase C treatment, on the other hand, did remove the TSTA antigen while leaving the spikes intact.

10. VIRULENCE AND PERSISTENT INFECTION

10.1. Role of T Particles

Huang and Baltimore (1970) suggested that defective particles might play a role in the pathogenesis of slow virus disease *in vivo*, and Doyle and Holland (1973) confirmed this by showing that large doses of T particles administered intracerebrally altered the pathogenesis of VSV in mice. T particles protected mice against low but fatal doses of VSV, and when large doses of VSV were injected a normally rapid fatal infection was converted to a slow progressive disease. T particles do not kill cultured cells (Marcus and Sekellick 1974), but they are important factors in the establishment of noncytocidal persistent infection in cultured cells. Holland and Villareal (1974) reported that carrier cultures could be regularly established by coinfection of BHK-21 cells with mutant tsG31 (group III) and its associated short T particle (see Fig. 2F). Carrier cultures established in this way could be maintained for many months by incubation under quasirestrictive conditions (37°C). The phenomenon was mutant specific, since carrier cultures could not be established from cells infected with mutants of other complementation groups or wild-type virus in the presence of their various homologous T particles. Cytopathic effect could be induced in these carrier cultures by transfer to 31°C, or by cocultivation with uninfected BHK-21 cells at 37°C. A long T particle was present in lysates from cells cocultivated at 37°C which was effective in inducing the carrier state with wild-type VSV. Thus specific T particles rather than temperature sensitivity per se were the determining factor in establishment of the carrier state. Wild-type particles produced in the presence of this long T particle had greatly reduced transcriptase activity.

Younger et al. (1976) also reported that noncytocidal persistent infection of mouse L cells at 37°C could be established only in the presence of a large excess of T particles. There was a rapid selection of spontaneous ts virus, until by the 63rd day of culture 100% of clones isolated from the persistent infection were ts at 39.5°C. Eight clones were examined and all exhibited an RNA⁻ phenotype and behaved as group I mutants in a complementation test. T particles were no longer detectable in these cultures by physical and biological tests. Futhermore, other persistent infections could be established in L cells at 37°C using low multiplicities of one of these group I clones (ts pi 364). In the light of these findings Younger et al. (1976) suggested that persistent infection at 37°C could be initiated either by an excess of T particles or by an appropriate ts mutant at low multiplicity. In fact, Younger and Quagliana (1976) demonstrated experimentally that some ts mutants of VSV Indiana may behave as conditionally defective interfering particles under certain conditions.

The existence of a proviral DNA form of VSV has been reported by Zhdanov (1975–1976), but evidence for involvement of proviral DNA in the maintenance of the persistent VSV infections described by Holland and Younger was lacking. Younger et al. (1976) proposed instead that persistent infection at 37°C was maintained by the rapid accumulation of *ts* virus, which both interfered with the replication of wild-type virus and could be rescued by wild-type virus. Younger and Quagliana (1976) provided support for this hypothesis by showing experimentally that the replication of *ts* virus was dominant over that of wild type virus in BHK-21 cells. Mutants belonging to complementation groups I, II, and IV all inhibited replication of wild-type virus in BHK-21 cells at permissive or restrictive temperatures. Mutant *ts* G41 was the most effective in this respect, the yield of wild-type virus being reduced one-thousandfold at 32°C. In the case of group I and II mutants (but not *ts* G41) there was a simultaneous enhancement (~15,000-fold) of the yield of the coinfecting mutant at restrictive temperature. These experiments suggest that wild-type revertants will not replace a *ts* mutant population selected during persistent infection at 37°C, even though this temperature is not optimal for replication of the mutants.

10.2.   *ts* Mutants and Neurotropism

Farmilo and Stanners (1972) have described a mutant of complementation group I of VSV Indiana, designated *ts*T1026, which under semipermissive conditions regularly established a persistent infection in L cells. Cell DNA synthesis and division continued despite the presence of viral glycoprotein in the plasma membrane and viral RNA in the cytoplasm. The rapid death of the host and the dissemination of virus throughout the body, which are characteristic of infection with wild-type VSV, were not observed when this mutant was injected into newborn hamsters. Instead, death was delayed and was preceded by neurological symptoms. At death, virus could be recovered from the brain only. Subsequent investigation established that neurotropism was not a special characteristic of *ts*T1026 or group I mutants in general, but rather an inevitable consequence of extended survival of the infected animal (Stanners and Goldberg, 1975). Any mutant which allowed survival beyond 3 days could be recovered in higher titer in the brain than in other organs (Fig. 5). These findings point to the existence of a resistance mechanism capable of clearing virus rapidly from peripheral organs but not from the CNS. The neurotropism of *ts* mutants of VSV in newborn hamsters was correlated with the reversion frequency or leakiness characteristic of individual mutants rather than complementation group (Table 7).

Inoculation of mutant *ts*T1026 into older animals produced long-term effects reminiscent of slow virus disease. Low doses of wild-type

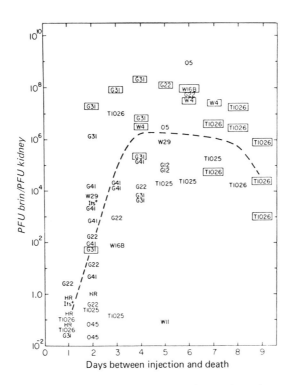

Fig. 5. Neurotropism of VSV Indiana *ts* mutants in newborn hamsters. Hamsters were injected subcutaneously with a range of doses of different mutants of VSV within 24 h after birth. The titer of virus recovered from homogenates of brain and kidney of dead or dying animals taken at the time indicated was determined by plaque assay on hamster embryo monolayers. The ratio of PFU in the brain to PFU in the kidney is presented for individual animals, except for those animals where no virus could be detected in the kidneys. The latter, shown within a box, represent the actual brain titer in PFU. The dashed line represents the approximate logarithmic average. Reproduced from the *Journal of General Virology.*

VSV in 20-day-old hamsters caused either early death or recovery and survival for the normal life span. High doses of *ts*T1026, on the other hand, produced few early deaths, but the life span of the survivors was shortened and neurological symptoms were common (Stanners *et al.,* 1975). Mutants such as *ts*T1026 may provide models for virus disease caused by persistent infection.

Rabinowitz, Dal Canto, and Johnson (1976) have made a study of the capacity of VSV to produce CNS infection in weanling mice. They found that certain *ts* mutants of VSV Indiana produced an altered pattern of disease after intracerebral inoculation, unlike the rapidly fatal encephalitis characteristic of wild-type virus. For example, after intracerebral inoculation of mutant *ts* G31 (group III), weanling Swiss

TABLE 7

Virulence of *ts* Mutants of Groups I, II, III, IV, and V of VSV Indiana in Hamsters[a]

Mutant[b]	Complementation group	Time to death of 50% of animals (days)	Phenotype of virus recovered[c]
ts+ (T)	—	1	Wild type, LP
ts+ (G)	—	1	Wild type, LP
*ts*G22	II	1.5	Wild type, LP + SP
*ts*O45	V	1.5	Wild type, LP + SP
*ts*T1025	I	1.5	Wild type, LP
*ts*G41	IV	2	Wild type, SP
*ts*G31	III	2.5	Wild type, LP + SP and *ts*
*ts*W4	I	2.5	Wild type, LP
*ts*W11	I	1–4	Wild type, LP
*ts*O5	I	4.5	Wild type, LP + SP
*ts*T1026	I	7.5	*ts*
*ts*G12	I	5–>400	*ts*
*ts*G11	I	>400	None
*ts*G13	I	>400	None
*ts*G114	I	>400	None

[a] Adapted from Stanners and Goldberg (1975). The mutants are listed in order of decreasing virulence.
[b] 10^3–10^4 PFU injected subcutaneously into 30 newborn (~ 24-hr-old) hamsters.
[c] Phenotype of virus recovered in organ homogenates at time of death. LP, large plaques; SP, small plaques.

mice developed hind-limb paralysis beginning 4–5 days after infection and persisting for 3–4 days until death of the animals. Wild-type infected mice, on the other hand, died within 2–3 days without obvious neurological signs. Subsequently, Dal Canto, Rabinowitz, and Johnson (1976) investigated the histopathological lesions in the brain and spinal cord of weanling Swiss mice infected with wild-type VSV and mutants *ts*G11, *ts*G22, *ts*G31, and *ts*G41. Mice infected intracerebrally with wild-type virus exhibited lesions consisting principally of occasional foci of perivascular mononuclear cell infiltration and rare foci of necrosis. In contrast mice infected intracerebrally with mutants *ts*G22 (group II) or *ts*G31 (group III) developed spongiform lesions limited to the grey matter of the spinal cord, beginning 4 days after inoculation. These lesions rapidly spread to involve the entire grey matter of the spinal cord within 5–7 days of infection. Vacuolar changes were restricted to neuronal processes and astrocytes. Progressive neurological illness was apparent by day 4 and the majority of mice died by day 7. Mice infected with *ts*G11 (group I) or *ts*G41 (group IV), on the other hand, remained well and were free of neurological lesions although both viruses multiplied to some extent in the CNS.

The lesions associated with *ts*G22 or *ts*G31 infection resembled the status spongiosus characteristic of the subacute viral spongiform encephalopathies (i.e., Creutzfeldt-Jakob disease, Kuru, scrapie, and transmissible mink encephalopathy), apart from the absence of astrocytosis and the presence of inflammation in VSV infection. Nevertheless, the experimental disease induced by the VSV Indiana mutants *ts*G22 and *ts*G31 provides a convenient system for further study of viral spongiform myelopathy and the nature of the host–virus relationship in the pathogenesis of virus infection.

10.3. *ts* Mutants as Vaccines

The virulence of wild-type VSV Indiana and *ts* mutants of groups I, II, and IV in 3 to 4-week-old mice has been studied by Wagner (1974). All the *ts* mutants were less virulent than wild type by the intracerebral or intranasal route. Neither wild type nor mutants were pathogenic by the intraperitoneal route. Intranasal vaccination with *ts* mutants produced a solid immunity to intranasal challenge with a lethal dose of wild-type virus within 3 days. A group IV mutant, *ts*G41, was the most effective in this respect. Possibly the ability of the Group IV mutant to carry out primary transcription enhanced its potential as an immunogen. Antibody could be detected in bronchial washings by 12 h, indicating that local immunity was established very rapidly after vaccination.

10.4. Pathogenesis of Rabies Virus *ts* Mutants in Mice

Two of the five *ts* mutants of rabies virus isolated by Clark and Koprowski (1971) have been characterized in detail. Mutant *ts*1 formed normal plaques, was more thermolabile than wild type, but exhibited normal pathogenicity for weanling mice apart from a slightly increased incubation period. Mutant *ts*2 formed minute plaques *in vitro* and induced an abnormal pathological response *in vivo*. The incidence of lethal infection of weanling mice was markedly reduced and the incubation period prolonged. A singular feature of *ts*2 infection was a very irregular dose–response relationship. Nevertheless, mice which survived infection, irrespective of the dose administered, were immune to challenge with wild-type virus. Other unusual features of *ts*2 infection of mice have been noticed and the mechanism of pathogenesis is being investigated in greater detail (Clark and Wiktor, personal communication).

10.5. Mechanism of Cell Killing

Vero cells infected with the transcriptase-defective mutant tsG114 (group I) were not killed, whereas cells infected with tsW10 (group IV)—an RNA$^-$ mutant with an active transcriptase—were killed (Marcus and Sekellick, 1975). It was concluded, therefore, that transcription of the viral genome was necessary for cell killing. Accumulation of transcripts *per se,* however, was not responsible for cell death. If tsG114-infected cells were incubated at 31°C in the presence of cycloheximide, transcripts accumulated; nevertheless, cell death did not ensue when the drug was removed and the cells were transferred to 40°C. This suggested that single-stranded mRNA molecules did not mediate cell killing. Transcription is necessary but not sufficient for cell death, and an event subsequent to transcription is required—possibly synthesis of double-stranded RNA, which is potentially cytotoxic even in very small amounts (Collins and Roberts, 1972).

11. SIGMA VIRUS AND GERMINAL TRANSMISSION

Sigma virus is prevalent in *Drosophila* in nature, and can be transmitted to other insects in the laboratory, but it does not infect vertebrate cells. It is transmitted predominantly via the female germ cells and is not associated with any disease (see reviews by L'Heritier, 1958; Seecof, 1968; Printz, 1973). VSV and related rhabdoviruses can be adapted to grow in *Drosophila* adults or cells in culture with minimal pathogenic effects, as can another vertebrate virus—Sindbis virus. VSV infection of *Drosophila* adults, however, induced the unique sensitivity to CO_2 which was characteristic of sigma virus infection, whereas Sindbis virus did not. The temporal expression of CO_2 sensitivity was complex and dependent on the VSV strain inoculated, probably as a consequence of the involvement of different ganglia (thoracic vs. abdominal) (Bussereau, 1973). Unlike sigma virus, even *Drosophila*-adapted VSV does not appear to be transmitted via the germ line.

Various host genes are known to influence the hereditary transmission of sigma virus in *Drosophila.* The best characterized is the semidominant refractory gene (*re*) located on the second chromosome (Ohanessian-Guillemain, 1963). Sigma virus multiplication is blocked in homozygous (*re/re*) flies. The *re* gene is expressed equally in the adult insect and in cell lines established from it (Richard-Molard, 1975). The mechanism of regulation of sigma virus multiplication by the *re* gene has not been elucidated.

Certain naturally occurring strains of sigma virus are not restricted by the *re* gene. These viruses are designated P^+, since they multiply in the homozygous *re/re* Paris strain of *Drosophila*. It has also been possible experimentally to select resistant variants of sigma virus by serial passage in semipermissive *re$^+$/re* flies (Gay, 1968). *Drosophila*-adapted VSV, however, is not restricted by the *re* gene.

Other variants of sigma virus are listed in Table 1. The rho variant is a maturation-defective sigma, which is transmitted hereditarily, restricted by the *re* gene, and renders flies immune to superinfection. Rho-carrying flies may yield small amounts of normal sigma virus late in life, possibly as a result of back mutation (Brun, 1963).

Rho-carrying strains sometimes yield ultrarho defectives. These ultrarho strains have never been observed to revert to rho or sigma and are interpreted as deletion mutants of rho. Flies carrying ultrarho are resistant to superinfection, but do not show the CO_2 sensitivity associated with sigma virus multiplication. (In general, CO_2 sensitivity is correlated with virus production and may be a consequence of modification of the cell membrane following insertion of viral protein.) Flies can be cured of ultrarho infection by the same procedures which eliminate sigma virus (Brun, 1963; Brun and Diatta, 1973). The hypothesis advanced to explain these observations is that the ultrarho genome can still replicate, but maturation of the virion is blocked. Although the physical nature of the genome has not been determined directly, there is no evidence that the hereditary transmission of sigma, rho, or ultrarho is analogous to lysogeny. Richard-Molard (1973) found that primary cultures of cells from ultrarho flies exhibited superinfection immunity initially but gradually lost this property on subsequent passage. This instability suggested that the virus was not maintained in an integrated state in the host cell genome.

Virus transmission is influenced by the viral genome. Viruses of genome g^- did not invade the germ line and germinal transmission was absent, in contrast to the normal g^+ sigma. Virus of genotype V^- were excluded from the sperm, whereas V^+ viruses were not. Finally, the pr^- genotype controlled invasiveness of the female germ cells.

Temperature-sensitive (*Ts*) and temperature-resistant (*Tr*) strains of sigma have been described, but more recently a significant advance in sigma genetics has been made by the isolation of *ts* mutants from a cloned strain of sigma virus after mutagenization with 5-fluorouracil (Contamine, 1973). Three *ts* mutants were identified among 148 clones isolated from four mutagen-exposed flies, whereas no *ts* mutants were found among 89 clones isolated from two untreated flies. Two of the mutants have been characterized. Hereditary transmission of mutant *ts*9 was unaffected at the restrictive temperature, although CO_2 sensitivity was inhibited. This mutant appears to be defective in a maturation function, and at the restrictive temperature it behaves phenotypically like the rho/ultrarho variants isolated by Brun. Mutant *ts*4, on the other hand, appeared to be defective in a replicative function, since hereditary transmission at restrictive temperature was blocked. These observations add support to the hypothesis that sigma virus is maintained in *Drosophila* in a carrier state rather than by integration into the genome of the host cell.

12. FUTURE PROSPECTS

Of immediate concern will be the assignment of functions to complementation groups II, IV, and VI of VSV Indiana, followed by a comparative analysis of the structure and function of the genome of other serotypes of VSV. The availability of better methods for assay of rabies virus *in vitro* will undoubtedly stimulate research into the genetic properties of this important animal and human pathogen and its increasing number of relatives. Similarly, a need for live virus vaccines is likely to stimulate genetic investigation of the recently discovered rhabdoviruses of fish, some of which are becoming economically important as pathogens in fish farming.

The wide variation in the host range of different members of the rhabdovirus group points to the existence of host controls of virus multiplication. Investigation of these controls by means of host-restricted mutants is likely to be another trend in rhabdovirus genetics.

ACKNOWLEDGMENTS

I am indebted to the many colleagues who provided information and papers prior to publication; to Bill Wunner, who read the manuscript; and to Eddie Follett, who provided the electron micrographs for Fig. 2.

13. REFERENCES

Abraham, G., and Banerjee, A. K., 1976, Sequential transcription of the genes of vesicular stomatitis virus, *Proc. Natl. Acad. Sci. USA* **73**:1504.

Ansel, S., 1974, Incorporation de l'antigène tumoral de transplantation specifique du SV40 (TSTA-SV40) dans le virus de la stomatite vesiculaire cultivée en cellule de hamsters transfermée par le SV40, *Int. J. Cancer* **13**:773.

Ball, L. A., and White, C. N., 1976, Order of transcription of genes of vesicular stomatitis virus, *Proc. Natl. Acad. Sci. USA* **73**:442.

Bishop, D. H. L., and Flamand, A., 1975a, Transcription processes of animal RNA virus, in: *Control Processes in Virus Multiplication* (D. C. Burke and W. C. Russell, eds.), pp. 95–151, Cambridge University Press, Cambridge.

Bishop, D. H. L., and Flamand, A., 1975b, The transcription of VSV and its mutants *in vivo* and *in vitro*, in: *Negative Strand Viruses*, Vol. 1 (B. W. J. Mahy and R. D. Barry, eds.), pp. 327–352, Academic Press, New York.

Bishop, D. H. L., Repik, P., Obijeski, J. F., Moore, N. F., and Wagner, R. R., 1975c, Restitution of infectivity to spikeless vesicular stomatitis virus by solubilized viral components, *J. Virol.* **16**:75.

Black, L. M., 1953, Loss of vector transmissibility by viruses normally insect transmitted, *Phytopathology* **43**:466.

Boettiger, D., Love, D. N., and Weiss, R. A., 1975, Virus envelope markers in mammalian tropism of avian RNA tumor viruses, *J. Virol.* **15**:108.

Brun, G., 1963, Etude d'une association du virus et de son hôte la Drosophile: l'état stabilisée, These Biol. Exp., Orsay.

Brun, G., and Diatta, F., 1973, Guérison germinale de femelles de drosophile stabilisées pour le virus sigma, a la suite d'un traitement par la température ou par l'éthylméthane-sulfonate, *Ann. Microbiol. (Inst. Pasteur)* **124A**:421.

Buller, R. M. L., 1975, Biological and biochemical characterization of vesicular stomatitis virus and temperature-sensitive maturation mutants, Ph.D. thesis, University of Glasgow.

Burge, B. W., and Huang, A. S., 1970, Comparison of membrane protein glycopeptides of Sindbis virus and vesicular stomatitis virus, *J. Virol.* **6**:176.

Burge, B. W., and Pfefferkorn, E. R., 1966, Phenotypic mixing between group A arboviruses, *Nature (London)* **210**:1397.

Bussereau, F., 1973, Étude du symptome de la sensibilité au CO_2 product par le virus de la stomatite vésiculaire chez *Drosophila melanogaster*. III. Souches de differentes serotypes, *Ann. Microbiol. (Inst. Pasteur)* **124A**:535.

Cairns, J. E., Holloway, A. F., and Cormack, D. Y., 1972, Temperature-sensitive mutants of vesicular stomatitis virus: *In vitro* studies of virion-associated polymerase, *J. Virol.* **10**:1130.

Cartwright, B., and Brown, F., 1972, Glycolipid nature of the complement-fixing host cell antigen of vesicular stomatitis virus, *J. Gen. Virol.* **15**:243.

Choppin, P. W., and Compans, R. W., 1970, Phenotypic mixing of envelope proteins of the parainfluenza virus SVS and vesicular stomatitis virus, *J. Virol.* **5**:609.

Clark, H. F., and Koprowski, H., 1971, Isolation of temperature-sensitive conditional lethal mutants of "fixed" rabies virus, *J. Virol.* **7**:295.

Clark, H. F., and Wiktor, T. J., 1974, Plasticity of phenotypic characters of rabies-related viruses: Spontaneous variation in plaque morphology, virulence, and temperature-sensitivity characters of serially propagated Lagos bat and Mokola viruses, *J. Infect. Dis.* **130**:608.

Collins, F. D., and Roberts, W. K., 1972, Mechanism of mengo virus-induced cell injury in L cells: Use of inhibitors of protein synthesis to dissociate virus-specific events, *J. Virol.* **101**:969.

Combard, A., Martinet, C., Printz-Ané, C., Friedmann, A., and Printz, P., 1974, Transcription and replication of vesicular stomatitis virus: Effects of temperature-sensitive mutations in complementation group IV, *J. Virol.* **13**:922.

Contamine, D., 1973, Étude de mutants thermosensibles du virus sigma, *Mol. Gen. Genet.* **124**:233.

Cooper, P. D., 1958, Homotypic non-exclusion by vesicular stomatitis virus in chick cell culture, *J. Gen. Microbiol.* **19**:350.

Cooper, P. D., 1965, Rescue of one phenotype in mixed infections with heat-defective mutants of type 1 poliovirus, *Virology* **25**:431.

Cooper, P. D., Geissler, E., Scotti, P. D., and Tannock, G. A., 1971, Further characterisation of the genetic map of poliovirus temperature-sensitive mutants, in: *Strategy of the Viral Genome* (G. E. W. Wolstenholme and M. O'Connor, eds.), pp. 75–100, Churchill Livingstone, Edinburgh.

Cormack, D. V., Holloway, A. F., Wong, P. K. Y., and Cairns, J. E., 1971, Temperature-sensitive mutants of vesicular stomatitis virus. II. Evidence of defective polymerase, *Virology* **45**:824.

Cormack, D. V., Holloway, A. F., and Pringle, C. R., 1973, Temperature-sensitive mutants of vesicular stomatitis virus; homology and nomenclature, *J. Gen. Virol.* **19**:295.

Cormack, D. V., Holloway, A. F., and Ngan, J. S. C., 1975, RNA polymerase defects in temperature-sensitive mutants of vesicular stomatitis virus, in *Negative Strand Viruses*, Vol. 1 (B. W. J. Mahy and R. D. Barry, eds.), pp. 361–366, Academic Press, New York.

Dal Canto, M. C., Rabinowitz, S. G., and Johnson, T. C., 1976, Status spongiosus resulting from intracerebral infection of mice with temperature-sensitive mutants of vesicular stomatitis virus, *Br. J. Exp. Path.* **57**:321.

Deutsch, V., 1970, Mise en évidence d'une accumulation de nucléocapsides infectieuses du virus de la stomatite vésiculaire (VSV) dans le cytoplasme des fibroblastes de poulet, *C. R. Acad. Sci. Paris* **271**:273.

Deutsch, V., 1975, Nongenetic complementation of group V temperature-sensitive mutants of vesicular stomatitis virus by UV-irradiated virus, *J. Virol.* **15**:798.

Deutsch, V., and Berkaloff, A., 1971, Analyse d'un mutant thermolabile du virus de la stomatite vésiculaire (VSV), *Ann. Inst. Pasteur* **121**:101.

Doyle, M., and Holland, J. J., 1973, Prophylaxis and immunisation in mice by use of virus-free defective T particles to protect against intracerebral infection by vesicular stomatitis virus, *Proc. Natl. Acad. Sci. USA* **71**:2956.

Duhamel, C., 1954, Étude de la sensibilité héréditaire à l'anhydride carbonique chez la Drosophile: Description de quelques variants du virus, *C. R. Acad. Sci. Paris* **239**:1157.

Emerson, S. U., and Wagner, R. R., 1972, Dissociation and reconstitution of the transcriptase and template activities of vesicular stomatitis B and T virions, *J. Virol.* **10**:297.

Etchison, J. J., and Holland, J. J., 1974, Carbohydrate composition of the membrane glycoprotein of vesicular stomatitis virus grown in four mammalian cell lines, *Proc. Natl. Acad. Sci. USA* **71**:4011.

Farmilo, A. J., and Stanners, C. P., 1972, Mutant of vesicular stomatitis virus which allows deoxyribonucleic acid synthesis and division in cells synthesizing viral ribonucleic acid, *J. Virol.* **10**:605.

Federer, K. E., Burrows, R., and Brooksby, J. B., 1967, Vesicular stomatitis virus— The relationship between some strains of the Indiana serotype, *Res. Vet. Sci.* **8**:103.

Flamand, A., 1969, Etude des mutants thermosensibles du virus de la stomatite vésiculaire: Mise au point d'un test de complémentation, *C. R. Acad. Sci. Paris* **268**:2305.

Flamand, A., 1970, Etude génétique du virus de la stomatite vésiculaire: Classement de mutants thermosensibles spontanés en groupes de complémentation, *J. Gen. Virol.* **8**:187.

Flamand, A., 1973, Genetical behaviour of vesicular stomatitis virus during successive passages at high and low temperatures, *Mutat. Res.* **17**:177.

Flamand, A., and Bishop, D. H. L., 1973, Primary *in vivo* transcription of vesicular stomatitis virus and temperature-sensitive mutants of five vesicular stomatitis virus complementation groups, *J. Virol.* **12**:1238.

Flamand, A., and Bishop, D. H. L., 1974, *In vivo* synthesis of RNA by vesicular stomatitis virus and its mutants, *J. Mol. Biol.* **87**:31.

Flamand, A., and Lafay, F., 1973, Etude des mutants thermosensibles du virus de la stomatite vesiculaire appartenant au groupe de complementation II, *Ann. Microbiol. (Inst. Pasteur)* **124A**:261.

Flamand, A., and Pringle, C. R., 1971. The homologies of spontaneous and induced temperature-sensitive mutants of vesicular stomatitis virus isolated in chick embryo and BHK-21 cells, *J. Gen. Virol.* **11**:81.

Follett, E. A. C., Pringle, C. R., Wunner, W. H., and Skehel, J. J., 1974, Virus replication in enucleate cells: Vesicular stomatitis virus and influenza virus, *J. Virol.* **13**:394.

Follett, E. A. C., Pringle, C. R., and Pennington, T. H., 1975, Virus development in enucleate cells: Echovirus, poliovirus, pseudorabies virus, reovirus, respiratory syncytial virus and Semliki Forest virus, *J. Gen. Virol.* **26**:183.

Gay, P., 1968, Adaptation d'une population virale à se multiplier chez un hôte refractaire, *Ann. Genet.* **11**:98.

Genty, N., 1975, Analysis of uridine incorporation in chicken embryo cells infected by vesicular stomatitis virus and its temperature-sensitive mutants: Uridine transport, *J. Virol.* **15**:8.

Genty, N., and Berreur, P., 1973, Métabolisme des acides ribonucléiques et des protéines de cellules d'embryon de poulet infectées par le virus de la stomatite vésiculaire: Etude des effects de mutants thermosensibles, *Ann. Microbiol. (Inst. Pasteur)* **124A**:133.

Goldstein, L., 1949, Contribution à l'étude de la sensibilité héréditaire au gaz carbonique chez la Drosophile: Mise en evidence d'une forme nouvelle du genoide, *Bull. Biol. France Belg.* **83**:177.

Granoff, A., and Hirst, G. K., 1954, Experimental production of combination forms of virus. IV. Mixed influenza A–Newcastle disease virus infections, *Proc. Soc. Exp. Biol. Med.* **86**:84.

Guillemain, A., 1953, Découverte et localization d'une gène empêchant le multiplication du virus de la sensibilité héréditaire au CO_2 chez D.M., *C. R. Acad. Sci. Paris* **236**:1085.

Holland, J. J., and Villareal, L. P., 1974, Persistent noncytocidal vesicular stomatitis virus infections mediated by defective T particles that suppress virion transcriptase, *Proc. Natl. Acad. Sci. USA* **71**:2956.

Holloway, A. F., Wong, P. K. Y., and Cormack, D. V., 1970, Isolation and characterisation of temperature-sensitive mutants of vesicular stomatitis virus, *Virology* **42**:917.

Howatson, A. F., 1970, Vesicular stomatitis and related viruses, *Adv. Virus Res.* **16**:195.

Huang, A. S., 1973, Defective interfering viruses, *Annu. Rev. Microbiol.* **27**:101.

Huang, A. S., 1975, Ribonucleic acid synthesis of vesicular stomatitis virus, in: *Negative Strand Viruses*, Vol. 1 (B. W. J. Mahy and R. D. Barry, eds.), pp. 353–360, Academic Press, New York.

Huang, A. S., and Baltimore, D., 1970, Defective viral particles and viral disease processes, *Nature (London)* **226**:325.

Huang, A. S., Besmer, P., Chu, C., and Baltimore, D., 1973, Growth of pseudotypes of vesicular stomatitis virus with N-tropic murine leukaemia virus coats in cells resistant to N-tropic viruses, *J. Virol.* **12**:659.

Huang, A. S., Palma, E. L., Hewlett, N., and Roizman, B., 1974, Pseudotype formation between enveloped RNA and DNA viruses, *Nature (London)* **252**:743.

Hunt, D. M., and Wagner, R. R., 1974, Location of the transcription defect in group I temperature-sensitive mutants of vesicular stomatitis virus, *J. Virol.* **13**:28.

Hunt, D. M., Emerson, S. U., and Wagner, R. R., 1976, RNA⁻ temperature-sensitive mutants of vesicular stomatitis virus: L protein thermosensitivity accounts for transcriptase restriction of group I mutants, *J. Virol* **18**:596.

Knipe, D., Rose, J. K., and Lodish, H. F., 1975, Translation of individual species of vesicular stomatitis viral mRNA, *J. Virol.* **15**:1004.

Knudsen, D. L., 1973, Rhabdoviruses, *J. Gen. Virol. (Symp. Suppl.)* **20**:105.

Krontiris, T. G., Soeiro, R., and Fields, B. N., 1973, Host restriction of Friend leukemia virus, role of the viral outer coat, *Proc. Natl. Acad. Sci. USA* **70**:2549.

Lafay, F., 1969, Étude des mutants thermosensibles du virus de la stomatite vésiculaire (VSV): Classification de quelques mutants d'après des critères de fonctionnment, *C. R. Acad. Sci. Paris* **268**:2385.

Lafay, F., 1971, Étude des fonctions du virus de la stomatite vésiculaire altérées par une mutation thermosensible: Mise en evidence de la protéine structurale affectée par la mutation *ts*23, *J. Gen. Virol.* **13**:449.

Lafay, F., 1974, Envelope proteins of vesicular stomatitis virus: Effect of temperature-sensitive mutation in complementation groups III and V, *J. Virol.* **14**:1220.

Lafay, F., and Berkaloff, A., 1969, Étude des mutants thermosensibles du virus de la stomatite vésiculaire (VSV): Mutants de maturation, *C. R. Acad. Sci. Paris* **269**:1031.

Lake, J. R., Priston, R. A. J., and Slade, W. R., 1975, A genetic recombination map of foot-and-mouth disease virus. *J. Gen. Virol.* **27**:355.

Lazzarini, R. A., Weber, G. H., Johnson, L. D. and Stamminger, G. W., 1975, Covalently linked message and anti-message (genomic) RNA from a defective vesicular stomatitis virus particle, *J. Mol. Biol.* **97**:289.

Leamnson, R. N., and Reichmann, M. E., 1974, The RNA of defective vesicular stomatitis virus particles in relation to viral cistrons, *J. Mol. Biol.* **85**:551.

Lesnaw, J. A., and Reichmann, M. E., 1975, RNA synthesis by temperature-sensitive mutants of vesicular stomatitis virus, New Jersey serotype, *Virology* **63**:492.

L'Heritier, P., 1958, The hereditary virus of *Drosophila, Adv. Virus Res.* **5**:276.

Love, D. N., and Weiss, R. A., 1974, Pseudotypes of vesicular stomatitis virus determined by exogenous and endogenous avian RNA tumour viruses, *Virology* **57**:271.

Macleod, R., Black, L. M., and Moyer, F. H., 1966, The fine structure and intracellular localization of potato yellow dwarf virus, *Virology* **29**:540.

Marcus, P. I., and Sekellick, M. I., 1974, Cell killing by viruses. I. Comparison of cell killing, plaque-forming, and defective-interfering particles of vesicular stomatitis virus, *Virology* **57**:321.

Marcus, P. I., and Sekellick, M. I., 1975, Cell killing by viruses. II. Cell killing by vesicular stomatitis virus: A requirement for virion-derived transcription, *Virology* **63**:176.

Martinet, C., and Printz-Ané, C., 1970, Analyse de la synthèse de l'ARN viral du virus de la stomatite vésiculaire (VSV) utilisation de mutants thermosensibles, *Ann. Inst. Pasteur* **119**:411.

Matsumoto, S., 1970, Rabies virus, *Adv. Virus Res.* **16**:257.

McAllister, P. E., and Wagner, R. R., 1976, Differential inhibition of host protein synthesis in L cells infected with RNA⁻ temperature-sensitive mutants of vesicular stomatitis virus, *J. Virol.* **18**:550.

McSharry, J. J., and Wagner, R. R., 1971, Carbohydrate composition of vesicular stomatitis virus, *J. Virol.* **7**:412.

McSharry, J. J., Compans, R. W., and Choppin, P. W., 1971, Proteins of vesicular stomatitis virus and of phenotypically mixed vesicular stomatitis virus–simian virus 5 virions, *J. Virol.* **8**:722.

Moreau, M.-C., 1974, Inhibition of a vesicular stomatitis virus mutant by rifampin, *J. Virol.* **14**:517.

Mori, H. and Howatson, A. F., 1973, *In vitro* transcriptase activity of vesicular stomatitis virus B and T particles: Analysis of product, *Intervirology* **1**:168.

Morrison, T., Stampfer, M., Baltimore, D., and Lodish, H. F., 1974, Translation of vesicular stomatitis virus messenger RNA by extracts from mammalian and plant cells, *J. Virol.* **13**:62.

Moyer, S. A., and Summers, D. F., 1974, Vesicular stomatitis virus envelope glycoprotein alterations induced by host cell transformations, *Cell* **2**:63.

Mudd, J. A., Leavitt, R. W., Kingsbury, D. T., and Holland, J. J., 1973, Natural selection of mutants of vesicular stomatitis virus by cultured cells of *Drosophila melanogaster, J. Gen. Virol.* **20**:341.

Ngan, J. S. C., Holloway, A. F., and Cormack, D. V., 1974, Temperature-sensitive mutants of vesicular stomatitis virus: Comparison of the *in vitro* RNA polymerase defects of group I and group IV mutants, *J. Virol.* **14**:765.

Obijeski, J. F., and Simpson, R. W., 1974, Conditional lethal mutants of vesicular stomatitis virus. II. Synthesis of virus-specific polypeptides in nonpermissive cells infected with "RNA⁻" host-restricted mutants, *Virology* **57**:369.

Ohanessian-Guillemain, A., 1959, Étude génétique du virus héréditaire de la Drosophile (σ); mutations et recombinaison génétique, *Ann. Genet.* **1**:59.

Ohanessian-Guillemain, A., 1963, Étude de facteurs génétique controlant les relations du virus σ et la Drosophile son hôte, *Ann. Genet.* **5**:1.

Perleman, S. M., and Huang, A. S., 1973, RNA synthesis of vesicular stomatitis virus. V. Interactions between transcription and replication, *J. Virol.* **12**:1395.

Perleman, S. M., and Huang, A. S., 1974, Virus-specific RNA specified by the group I and IV temperature-sensitive mutants of vesicular stomatitis virus, *Intervirology* **2**:312.

Perrault, J., and Holland, J. J., 1972, Variability of vesicular stomatitis virus auto-interference with different host cells and virus serotypes, *Virology* **50**:148.

Petric, M., and Prevec, L., 1970, Vesicular stomatitis virus—A new interfering particle, intracellular structures, and virus-specific RNA, *Virology* **41**:615.

Pittman, D., 1965, Temperature-sensitive mutants of a rod-shaped RNA animal virus, *Genetics* **52**:468.

Prevec, L., 1974, Physiological properties of vesicular stomatitis virus and some related rhabdoviruses, in: *Viruses, Evolution and Cancer*, pp. 677–697, Academic Press, New York.

Pringle, C. R., 1970*a*, The induction and genetic characterisation of conditional lethal mutants of vesicular stomatitis virus, in: *The Biology of Large RNA Viruses*, (R. D. Barry and B. W. J. Mahy, eds.), pp. 567–582, Academic Press, New York.

Pringle, C. R., 1970*b*, Genetic characteristics of conditional lethal mutants of vesicular stomatitis virus induced by 5-fluorouracil, 5-azacytidine and ethylmethane sulfonate, *J. Virol.* **5**:559.

Pringle, C. R., 1975, Conditional lethal mutants of vesicular stomatitis virus, *Curr. Top. Microbiol. Immunol.* **69**:85.

Pringle, C. R., and Duncan, I. B., 1971, Preliminary physiological characterisation of temperature-sensitive mutants of vesicular stomatitis virus, *J. Virol.* **8**:56.

Pringle, C. R., and Wunner, W. H., 1973, Genetic and physiological properties of temperature-sensitive mutants of Cocal virus, *J. Gen. Virol.* **12**:677.

Pringle, C. R., and Wunner, W. H., 1975, A comparative study of the structure and function of the VSV genome, in: *Negative Strand Viruses*, Vol. 2 (B. W. J. Mahy and R. D. Barry, eds.), pp. 707–724, Academic Press, New York.

Pringle, C. R., Duncan, I. B., and Stevenson, M., 1971, Isolation and characterisation of temperature-sensitive mutants of vesicular stomatitis virus, New Jersey serotype, *J. Virol.* **8**:836.

Printz, P., 1970, Adaptation du virus de la stomatite vésiculaire a *Drosophila melanogaster*, *Ann. Inst. Pasteur* **119**:510.

Printz, P., 1973, Relationship of sigma virus to vesicular stomatitis virus, *Adv. Virus. Res.* **18**:143.

Printz, P., and Wagner, R. R., 1971, Temperature-sensitive mutants of vesicular stomatitis virus: Synthesis of virus-specific proteins, *J. Virol.* **7**:651.

Printz, P., Combard, A., Printz, C., and Martinet, C., 1975, The use of temperature-sensitive mutants of vesicular stomatitis virus for studying transcription and replication, in: *Negative Strand Viruses*, Vol. 1, (B. W. J. Mahy and R. D. Barry eds.), pp. 367–378, Academic Press, New York.

Printz-Ané, C., Combard, A., and Martinet, C., 1972, Study of the transcription and the replication of vesicular stomatitis virus by using temperature-sensitive mutants, *J. Virol.* **10**:889.

Rabinowitz, S. G., Dal Canto, M. C., and Johnson, T. C., 1976, Comparison of central nervous system disease produced by wild-type and temperature-senstitive mutants of vesicular stomatitis virus, *Infect. Immun.* **13**:1242.

Reeder, G. S., Knudsen, D. L., and Macleod, R., 1972, The ribonucleic acid of potato yellow dwarf virus, *Virology* **50**:301.

Reichmann, M. E., Pringle, C. R., and Follett, E. A. C., 1971, Defective particles in

BHK cells infected with temperature-sensitive mutants of vesicular stomatitis virus, *J. Virol.* **8**:154.

Repik, P., Flamand, A., Clark, H. F., Obijeski, J. F., Roy, P., and Bishop, D. H. L., 1974, Detection of homologous RNA sequences among six rhabdovirus genomes, *J. Virol.* **13**:250.

Repik, P., Flamand, A., and Bishop, D. H. L., 1976, Synthesis of RNA by mutants of vesicular stomatitis virus (Indiana serotype) and the ability of wild type VSV New Jersey to complement the VSV Indiana *ts* G114 transcription defect, *J. Virol.* **20**:157.

Rettenmier, C. W., Dumont, R., and Baltimore, D., 1975, Screening procedure for complementation dependent mutants of vesicular stomatitis virus, *J. Virol.* **15**:41.

Richard-Molard, C., 1973, Étude de la multiplication du virus sigma dans plusieurs cultures primaires et dans une lignée continue de cellules de Drosophile issues d'embryous perpétuant un virus sigma defectif, *C. R. Acad. Sci. Paris* **277**:121.

Richard-Molard, C., 1975, Isolement de lignées cellulaires de *Drosophila melanogaster* de différents genotypes et étude de la multiplication de deux variants du rhabdovirus sigma dans ses lignées, *Arch. Ges. Virusforsch.* **47**:139.

Roy, P., Repik, P., Hefti, E., and Bishop, D. H. L., 1973, Complementary RNA species isolated from vesicular stomatitis (HR strain) defective virions, *J. Virol.* **11**:915.

Schaeffer, F. L., and Soergel, M. G., 1972, Molecular weight estimates of vesicular stomatitis virus ribonucleic acids from virions, defective particles, and infected cells, *Arch. Ges. Virusforsch,* **39**:203.

Schechmeister, I. L., Streckfuss, J., and St. John, R., 1967, Comparative pathogenicity of vesicular stomatitis virus and its plaque type mutants, *Arch. Ges. Virusforsch* **21**:127.

Schloemer, R. H., and Wagner, R. R., 1975, Mosquito cells infected with vesicular stomatitis virus yield unsialylated virions of low infectivity, *J. Virol.* **15**:1029.

Schnitzlein, W. M., and Reichmann, M. E., 1976, The size and the cistronic order of defective vesicular stomatitis virus particle RNAs in relation to homotypic and heterotypic interference, *J. Mol. Biol.* **101**:307.

Seecof, R., 1968, The sigma virus infection of *Drosophila melanogaster, Curr. Top. Microbiol. Immunol.* **42**:59.

Simon, E. H., 1972, The distribution and significance of multiploid virus particles, *Prog. Med. Virol.* **14**:36.

Simpson, R. W., and Obijeski, J. F., 1974, Conditional lethal mutants of vesicular stomatitis virus. I. Phenotypic characterisation of single and double mutants exhibiting host restriction and temperature sensitivity, *Virology* **57**:357.

Sokol, F., and Koprowski, H., 1975, Structure–function relationships and mode of replication of animal rhabdoviruses, *Proc. Natl. Acad. Sci. USA* **72**:933.

Sokol, F., Schlumberger, H. D., Wiktor, T. J., Koprowski, H., and Hummeler, K., 1969, Biochemical and biophysical studies on the nucleocapsid and the RNA of rabies virus, *Virology* **38**:651.

Stamminger, G., and Lazzarini, R. A., 1974, Analysis of the RNA of defective VSV particles, *Cell* **3**:85.

Stanners, C. P., and Goldberg, V. J., 1975, The mechanism of neurotropism of vesicular stomatitis virus in newborn hamsters. I. Studies with temperature-sensitive mutants, *J. Gen. Virol.* **29**:281.

Stanners, C. P., Farmilo, A. J., and Goldberg, V. J., 1975, Effects *in vitro* and *in vivo* of a mutant of vesicular stomatitis virus with attenuated cytopathogenicity, in: *Negative Strand Viruses,* Vol. 2 (B. W. J. Mahy and R. D. Barry, eds.), pp. 785–798, Academic Press, New York.

Subak-Sharpe, J. H., and Pringle, C. R., 1975, Viral information controlling DNA and RNA animal virus replication, in: *Control Processes in Virus Multiplication* (D. C. Burke and W. C. Russell, eds.), pp. 363–403, Cambridge University Press, Cambridge.

Szilágyi, J. F., and Pringle, C. R., 1972, Effect of temperature-sensitive mutations on the virion-associated RNA transcriptase of vesicular stomatitis virus, *J. Mol. Biol.* **71**:281.

Szilágyi, J. F., and Pringle, C. R., 1975, Virion transcriptase activity differences in host range mutants of vesicular stomatitis virus, *J. Virol.* **16:** 927.

Tesh, R. B., Peralta, P. H., and Johnson, K. M., 1970, Ecologic studies of VSV, *Am. J. Epidemiol.* **91**:216.

Unger, J. T., and Reichmann, M. E., 1973, RNA synthesis in temperature-sensitive mutants of vesicular stomatitis virus, *J. Virol.* **12**:570.

Vigier, P., 1966, Contribution à l'étude de l'mutabilité génétique du virus σ de la Drosophile, *Ann. Genet.* **9**:5.

Wagner, R. R., 1974, Pathogenicity and immunogenicity for mice of temperature-sensitive mutants of vesicular stomatitis virus, *Infect. Immun.* **10**:309.

Wagner, R. R., 1975, Reproduction of rhabdoviruses, in: *Comprehensive Virology,* Vol. 4 (H. Fraenkel-Conrat and R. R. Wagner, eds.), pp. 1–93, Plenum Press, New York.

Wagner, R. R., Levy, A. H., Snyder, R. M., Raycliff, G. A., and Hyatt, D. F., 1963, Biologic properties of two plaque variants of vesicular stomatitis virus (Indiana serotype), *J. Immunol.* **91**:112.

Weber, G. H., Dahlberg, J. E., Cottler Fox, M., and Heine, U., 1974, Electron microscopy of single-stranded RNA from vesicular stomatitis virus, *Virology* **62**:284.

Weiss, R. A., Boettiger, D., and Love, D. N., 1975, Phenotypic mixing between vesicular stomatitis virus and avian RNA tumor viruses. *Cold Spring Harbor Symp. Quant. Biol.* **39**:913.

Wertz, G. W., and Levine, M., 1973, RNA synthesis of vesicular stomatitis virus and a small plaque mutant: effects of cycloheximide, *J. Virol.* **12**:253.

Wiktor, T. J., and Koprowski, H., 1974, Rhabdovirus replication in enucleated host cell, *J. Virol.* **14**:300.

Wong, P. K. Y., Holloway, A. F., and Cormack, D. V., 1971, Search for recombination between temperature-sensitive mutants of vesicular stomatitis virus, *J. Gen. Virol.* **13**:477.

Wong, P. K. Y., Holloway, A. F., and Cormack, D. V., 1972, Characterisation of three complementation groups of vesicular stomatitis virus, *Virology* **50**:829.

Wunner, W. H., and Pringle, C. R., 1972*a,* Protein synthesis in BHK-21 cells infected with vesicular stomatitis virus. I. *Ts* mutants of the Indiana serotype, *Virology* **48**:104.

Wunner, W. H., and Pringle, C. R., 1972*b,* Protein synthesis in BHK-21 cells infected with vesicular stomatitis virus. II. *Ts* mutants of the New Jersey serotype, *Virology* **50**:250.

Wunner, W. H., and Pringle, C. R., 1974, A temperature-sensitive mutant of vesicular stomatitis virus with two abnormal virion proteins, *J. Gen. Virol.* **23**:97.

Younger, J. S., Dubovi, E. J., Quagliana, D. O., Kelly, M., and Preble, O. T., 1976, Role of temperature-sensitive mutants in persistent infections initiated with vesicular stomatitis virus, *J. Virol.* **19**:90.

Younger, J. S., and Quagliana, D. O., 1976, Temperature-sensitive mutants of vesicular stomatitis virus are conditionally defective particles that interfere with and are rescued by wild-type virus, *J. Virol.* **19**:102.

Závada, J., 1972a, Pseudotypes of vesicular stomatitis virus with the coat of murine leukemia and of avian myeloblastosis viruses, *J. Gen. Virol.* **15**:183.

Závada, J., 1972b, Vesicular stomatitis virus pseudotype particles with the coat of avian myeloblastosis virus, *Nature (London) New Biol.* **240**:122.

Závada, J., and Rosenbergová, M., 1972, Phenotypic mixing of vesicular stomatitis virus with fowl plaque virus, *Acta Virol.* **16**:103.

Závada, J., and Závodská, 1974, Complementation and phenotypic stabilisation of vesicular stomatitis virus temperature-sensitive mutants by avian myeloblastosis virus, *Intervirology* **2**:25.

Závada, J., Závadová, Z., Maliř, A., and Kočent, A., 1972, VSV pseudotype produced in cell line derived from human mammary carcinoma, *Nature (London) New Biol.* **240**:124.

Závada, J., Závadová, Z., Widemaier, R., Bubeník, J., Indrová, M., and Altaner, C., 1974, A transmissible antigen detected in two cell lines derived from human tumours, *J. Gen. Virol.* **24**:327.

Závada, J., Bubeník, J., Widmaier, R., and Závadová, Z., 1975, Phenotypically mixed vesicular stomatitis virus particles produced in human tumor cell lines, *Cold Spring Harbor Symp. Quant. Biol.* **39**:907.

Zhdanov, V. M., 1975–76. Integration of genomes of infectious RNA viruses, *Intervirology* **6**:129.

CHAPTER 7

Genetics of Reoviruses

Rise K. Cross

The Rockefeller University
New York, New York 10021

and

Bernard N. Fields

Department of Microbiology and Molecular Genetics
Harvard Medical School
Boston, Massachusetts 02115

1. INTRODUCTION: STRUCTURE AND REPLICATION OF REOVIRUSES AS THEY RELATE TO GENETICS

One of the most striking features of the reoviruses is the unusual nature of their genetic material. The genome of reovirus consists of ten unique segments of double-stranded (ds) RNA which are packaged within a double-shelled capsid composed of protein subunits (Bellamy *et al.*, 1967; Shatkin *et al.*, 1968; Watanabe *et al.*, 1968) (Fig. 1). Each of these dsRNA fragments falls into one of three size classes: there are three large (L), three medium (M), and four small (S) molecules with molecular weights of about 2.7, 1.4, and 0.7×10^6, respectively; the total genome equivalent molecular weight is about 15×10^6. Although the exact topology of the ten segments within the double-shelled capsid is unknown and even less information is available regarding the mechanism which ensures their encapsidation, several lines of evidence attest to their structural as well as functional discreteness (Joklik, 1974). The plus strand of all of the dsRNA segments has quite recently been found to contain an unusual blocked, methylated 5′-terminal structure with the

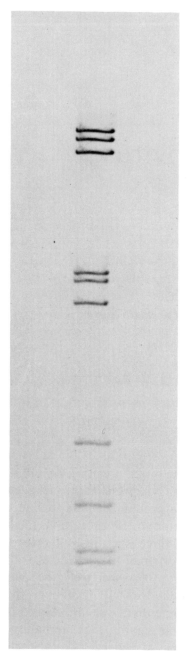

Fig. 1. Autoradiogram of double-stranded RNA from virions of reovirus type 3 wild type separated by gel electrophoresis. Note three large species, three middle-sized species, and four small species. The largest RNA species are at the top, the smallest at the bottom of the gel shown. From R. Cross (unpublished data).

sequence m⁷G(5′)ppp(5′)G^mpCp ... (Furuichi *et al.,* 1975). Each segment of genome RNA serves as a template for the synthesis of a monocistronic messenger RNA molecule which is translated into a unique polypeptide species (McDowell *et al.,* 1972; Both *et al.,* 1975).

Although a detailed account of the replication of reoviruses will not be presented here, the reader is referred to the comprehensive review on the subject by Joklik (1974). A brief description of the multiplication cycle follows: Shortly after entry by phagocytosis into a permissive cell, reoviruses are converted to subviral particles by lysosomal enzymes (Silverstein and Dales, 1968). This process, involving only a partial uncoating of the reovirus genome, is sufficient to activate the core-associated viral transcriptase (Silverstein *et al.,* 1972), which then transcribes each of the ten segments of the dsRNA genome into single-stranded (ss) RNA molecules (Shatkin *et al.,* 1968; Watanabe *et al.,* 1968). A major portion of each of the ten species of ssRNA are associated with polysomes and serve as messenger RNA molecules (Bellamy and Joklik, 1967). In addition, they function as templates for the synthesis of complementary strands to form progeny (ds) RNA (Schonberg *et al.,* 1971). The enzyme responsible for this activity, often referred to as a "replicase," is associated with particulate structures containing newly synthesized viral ssRNA and polypeptides (Sakuma and Watanabe, 1971). Completed dsRNA molecules within progeny subviral particles also serve as templates for further ssRNA synthesis before final assembly of these particles into fully mature virions.

Several aspects of the replicative cycle are especially critical to an understanding of the genetics of reovirus. Genetic information is transferred from parent to progeny via single-stranded RNA intermediates. Transcription of ssRNA is fully conservative (Skehel and Joklik, 1969). Viral ssRNA plus (+) strands (so designated because they have the same polarity as viral mRNA) are synthesized from only one strand of each of the ten segments of dsRNA. Synthesis of the complementary minus (−) strand occurs sequentially and asynchronously (Schonberg *et al.,* 1971). Minus strands which are never found free in the cytoplasm are copied from preformed plus-stranded transcripts to yield dsRNA molecules (Acs *et al.,* 1971).

It is likely that the assortment of RNA molecules occurs at the level of single-stranded RNA. At no time in the replication cycle does dsRNA exist in a free or naked form. Parental genomes remain within subviral particles throughout the cycle. The synthesis of progeny dsRNA molecules occurs within particulate structures that contain all ten ssRNA molecules (Zweerink *et al.*, 1972). Completed progeny dsRNA remain associated within these structures.

Because of the unique mode of replication and structure of its genome, reovirus offers one of the most novel animal viral genetic systems. The organization of the viral genomes into discrete genomic subunits that are in certain respects analogous to chromosomes affords an excellent opportunity for the study of genetic interactions, as well as the development of insight into general features of transcription and translation in mammalian cells. As with most genetic studies of animal viruses, conditional lethal, temperature-sensitive (*ts*) mutants form the basis of genetic analysis of reovirus. This chapter will, therefore, address itself largely to a review of data relating to the genetic and biochemical characterization of *ts* mutants of reovirus type 3, one of the three serotypes of mammalian reoviruses. The focus of this presentation will be directed to (1) discussion of the different mechanisms involved in viral gene interactions, (2) the physiological basis of mutant behavior as it is related to gene function, and (3) the impact of the viral genome on the host.

2. GENETIC INTERACTIONS

2.1. Conditional Lethal Temperature-Sensitive Mutants

Two laboratories have successfully isolated conditional lethal, temperature-sensitive (*ts*) mutants of the Dearing strain of reovirus type 3.

Ikegami and Gomatos (1968) reported the isolation of six *ts* mutants. Two of these arose spontaneously, and four appeared after exposure to mutagens: two were induced by treatment with nitrous acid, and two after growth of the virus in the presence of 5′-fluorouracil. In contrast to the wild-type virus which multiplied optimally at 37°C, the optimal growth temperature of the *ts* mutants was 30–33°C; 37°C was nonpermissive. On the basis of differential thermosensitivity at 52°C, the ratio of infectivity to hemagglutinating activity, and responses to shift in temperature, these six mutants have been classified into two groups. One group (*ts*26a and *ts*44b) possessed less hemagglutinating activity per infectious unit and was more heat labile than the other group (*ts*53a, *ts*90b, *ts*133a). Mutants *ts*44b and *ts*53a differed in their behavior in temperature-shift experiments: after incubation at the nonpermissive temperature and shiftup to the restrictive temperature, viral synthesis continued in cells infected with *ts*44b but ceased in those cells infected with *ts*53a. Additional *ts* mutants were subsequently isolated, five after exposure of the virus to hydroxylamine and three after exposure to nitrous acid (Ikegami and Gomatos, 1972). The temperature sensitivity of the 14 *ts* mutants isolated in this laboratory is believed to be due to marked inhibition of both cellular and viral protein synthesis late in infection (Section 3.4). Classification of these mutants by genetic analysis has not yet been reported.

Fields and Joklik (1969) isolated approximately 60 *ts* mutants after treatment of the Dearing strain with chemical mutagens and selection by a plaque enlargement method. Viral stocks were mutagenized with either nitrous acid or *N*-methyl-*N'*-nitro-*N*-nitrosoguanidine or permitted to replicate in the presence of proflavin. Surviving virus was plated at the permissive temperature (31°C); after appearance of plaques, the plates were shifted to the nonpermissive temperature (39°C). Nonenlarging plaques were harvested as presumptive *ts* mutants. Although *ts* mutants are intrinsically "leaky," a large number of stable mutants possessed a sufficiently wide difference in the efficiency of plating at 31°C and 39°C to be useful. These have been classified into seven groups (A–G) on the basis of their ability to yield wild-type (*ts*⁺) recombinant virus in the progeny of pairwise crosses at the permissive temperature (Section 2.2) (Fields and Joklik, 1969; Cross and Fields, 1972). Extensive biochemical and genetic analyses of these *ts* mutants have been carried out. These studies are reviewed below. Prototype strains and other frequently studied mutants, as well as their classification into genetic groups, are presented in Table 1. The relationship of the *ts* mutants of Ikegami and Gomatos to those of Fields and Joklik has not yet been established.

2.2. Two-Factor Crosses

Because of the segmented nature of the reovirus genome, wild-type (*ts*⁺) progeny from cells infected with two different *ts* mutants might be generated either by intramolecular recombination or by reassortment of RNA segments. Intramolecular recombination would be expected to occur at a very low frequency in view of the small size of the individual molecules of viral RNA. On the other hand, if each of the segments behave as independently reassorting genetic units, high-frequency recombination would be expected for markers lying on different genome segments, and no recombinants would occur between markers

TABLE 1

Selected *ts* Mutants of Reovirus Type 3

Class	*ts* strain	Mutagen[a]	EOP 39°C/31°C[b]
A	201[c]	PRO	0.10
	234	NTG	0.06
	270	PRO	0.02
	279	PRO	0.25
	290	PRO	0.0002
	340	NA	0.001
	438	NTG	0.025
	470	NTG	0.3
	474	NTG	0.008
B	271	PRO	0.005
	352[c]	NA	0.0025
	405	NA	0.001
C	447	NTG	0.0004
D	357[c]	NA	0.02
	585	NTG	0.006
E	320[c]	NA	0.3
F	556[c]	NTG	0.02
G	453[c]	NTG	0.0002

[a] NA, nitrous acid; PRO, proflavine; NTG, N-methyl-N'-nitro-N-nitrosoguanidine.
[b] (Number of plaques at 39°C/number of plaques at 31°C).
[c] Standard prototype strain.

residing on identical genome segments (unless intramolecular recombinants could occur). The results of two-factor genetic crosses should reflect the manner in which genetic material is exchanged.

To perform two-factor (*ts* × *ts*) genetic crosses with reovirus *ts* mutants, cells are simultaneously infected with mutant pairs or with each mutant alone at the permissive temperature; after a period of 24–30 h, the virus yields are titered at both the permissive and nonpermissive temperatures (Fields and Joklik, 1969). The percentage of ts^+ "recombinants" for any two mutants A and B can be determined by the following formula:

$$\% \text{ recombinants} = \frac{\text{yield }(A \times B)^{39°C} - \text{yield }(A)^{39°C} - \text{yield }(B)^{39°C}}{\text{yield }(A \times B)^{31°C}} \times \frac{100}{1}$$

Since reciprocal double-mutant recombinants are not scored, the theoretical frequency of recombination is assumed to be twice the calculated percentage of ts^+ recombinants.

The results of this type of analysis strongly indicated reassortment between pieces of viral RNA rather than intramolecular recombination (Fields and Joklik, 1969). The frequency of ts^+ recombinants from all pairwise crosses was found to be either high (values ranging from 3% to 50%) or zero (Fields and Joklik, 1969) (Table 2). Pairs of mutants that did not form recombinants were placed in the same genetic group and presumed to carry a mutation either on the same genome segment or on segments for which exchange is forbidden. Conversely, mutants that did recombine presumably carried mutations on different segments that could be exchanged. Five recombination groups (A–E) were initially defined in this manner (Fields and Joklik, 1969), and two additional groups (F and G) have been subsequently identified in a similar fashion (Cross and Fields, 1972). It should be possible to define three additional groups by two-factor crosses since the genome of reovirus consists of a set of ten unique dsRNA segments.

A statistical analysis of recombination frequencies resulting from two-factor crosses with ts mutants of groups A–E was undertaken to detect possible linkage between pairs of ts markers on different genome segments (Fields, 1973). The recombination frequencies in these studies were observed to range from 5.2% to 15.8%. The differences in frequencies between crosses were, for the most part, not statistically significant (on the basis of Student's t test), suggesting that they could

TABLE 2

Presence and Absence of Genetic Recombination between Several ts Mutants at the Permissive Temperature (31°C)^a

Virus strain used in infection	Yield at 24 h (PFU/ml) 39°C	Yield at 24 h (PFU/ml) 31°C	Efficiency of plating 39°C/31°C	Presumed wild-type recombinants (% of 31°C titer)
Wild type	3×10^7	3×10^7		
ts201	3×10^4	1×10^8	3×10^{-4}	—
ts352	1×10^3	1×10^8	1×10^{-5}	—
ts447	2×10^3	5×10^7	4×10^{-5}	—
ts234	1×10^3	2×10^8	5×10^{-6}	—
ts201 $\times$ ts352	7×10^6	1×10^8	7×10^{-2}	7
ts201 $\times$ ts447	3×10^6	3×10^7	1×10^{-1}	10
ts201 $\times$ ts234	2×10^4	3×10^8	7×10^{-5}	0
ts352 $\times$ ts447	2×10^7	1×10^8	2×10^{-1}	20
ts352 $\times$ ts234	3×10^6	1×10^8	3×10^{-2}	3
ts447 $\times$ ts234	3×10^6	4×10^7	8×10^{-2}	8

^{a} From Fields and Joklik (1969).

have arisen by chance. The few frequencies that appeared statistically different involve a "leaky" mutant (ts320) and therefore are potentially artifactual. It has been concluded that there is no linkage between ts markers.

The "all-or-none" nature of recombination (in which the percentage of recombinants is either high or zero) and the lack of statistical differences in recombination frequencies suggest that ts^+ recombinants are generated by a mechanism of reassortment of segments of viral RNA. Recombination frequencies, however, rarely approach a level of 50% as might be expected if there were completely random reassortment of unlinked RNA. This might be partly artifactual. Growth of stock ts^+ reovirus at 31°C has been found to change the efficiency of plating (39°C/31°C) from 0.5–1.0 to 0.15–0.5 (Fields, unpublished data). Since all reovirus mutants are also grown at 31°C, this falsely lowers the true plating efficiency at 39°C and thus decreases the overall calculated percentage of recombinants. Differences in the growth rate of some of the mutants at 31°C (Section 4.1.1) and slight variations in the multiplicity of infection (see below) might also explain the less than random level of reassortment. These studies were limited by the lack of a stable, independent plaque morphology, host range, or biochemical marker so that three-factor crosses that would unambiguously resolve the question of linkage might be performed (Section 2.3).

The fact that two-factor crosses suggest a nonlinkage (or "reassortment") between ts markers does not provide insight into the precise mechanism of how this may occur. Although there is no direct evidence, the biology of the virus demands that the reassortment of ts markers on different genome segments must occur among single-stranded RNA molecules. While both parental and progeny dsRNA genomes remain packaged within a subviral particle throughout the replicative cycle of reovirus, individual ssRNA transcripts of each segment are extruded from these structures into the cytoplasm, where they are capable of genetic interaction. The mechanism by which these ssRNA molecules are eventually arranged into sets of ten unique molecules has not yet been identified. However, RNA–RNA or RNA–protein interactions are likely to play an important role.

The term "genetic reassortment" has been applied to the high-frequency recombination that results from the exchange of physically discrete units of viral RNA (Fenner, 1974). This type of recombination is also characteristic of influenza viruses, which, like the reoviruses, contain a segmented RNA genome (Pons and Hirst, 1969; Duesberg and Robinson, 1967). Although the genome of influenza virus is single-stranded RNA, while that of reovirus is double-stranded RNA, the fact that reassortment in the latter probably proceeds at the level of ssRNA suggests obvious similarities. Recombination in animal viruses was first demonstrated with influenza virus, utilizing naturally occurring strains that differed from each other in a variety of properties (for a review, see Kilbourne, 1963). High-frequency recombination led Hirst (1962) to postulate that the influenza viral genome was fragmented, and that recombination between strains might occur by random reassortment of subgenomic fragments of both parental types.

While certain features of the genetics of reovirus are similar to that of influenza, others differ. The effects of length of incubation and multiplicity of infection (MOI) on recombination frequencies have been investigated with both viruses. As with influenza, kinetic experiments indicate that maximal recombination frequencies following infection with pairs of reovirus *ts* mutants are observed early (between 6 h and 12 h postinfection at 31°C), and do not significantly increase later when maximal virus yields are obtained (Fields, 1971; Spandidos and Graham, 1976*a*). Those observations suggest that recombination occurs early in the growth cycle and that there is a single cycle of mating. A similar interpretation has been suggested for influenza virus (Mackenzie, 1970). The results of studies of the effect of input multiplicity of infection (MOI) on the percentage of reovirus ts^+ recombinants (Fields, 1971) are shown in Table 3. The maximal percentage of recombinants with input multiplicities of 1 and 0.1 PFU/cell paralleled the decrease in the theoretical number of cells doubly infected. Unlike influenza virus, these data suggest that although reovirus stocks contain a high proportion of non-plaque-forming particles (50–150 particles/PFU), they are not a source of recombinants (Simpson and Hirst, 1968; Mackenzie, 1970; Sugiura *et al.*, 1972; Hirst, 1973; Hirst and Pons, 1973). The total particle/PFU ratio may simply reflect the efficiency with which any particular particle initiates productive infection. Alternatively, since non-plaque-forming reovirus particles may comprise a population of defective virions (Section 2.7), these findings are consistent with the recent comments of Spandidos and Graham (1976*a*) that a defective virion lacking the L1 segment of genome RNA does not form recombinants with *ts* mutants of reovirus (Section 2.7). By contrast, Hirst (1973) has reported that it is possible to generate influenza ts^+ recombinants by a one-hit process involving mixed aggregate particles, or by a two-hit process in which noninfectious particles are the principal source of recombinants. In reovirus, complementation by mixed aggregate

TABLE 3
Effect of Varying Input Multiplicity on Percentage of Recombinants

		Experiment A ts447					Experiment B ts447					Experiment C ts201		
		MOI[a]					MOI					MOI		
		<0.1	1	10			1	10	100			1	10	100
	0.1	0.1	0.15	0.5		1	1.7	1.7	0.7		1	1.8	0.7	0.1
ts352	1	0.2	1.0	2.5	ts352	10	0.8	4.5	4.2	ts352	10	4.0	7.0	1.0
MOI	10	0.1	1.0	3.0		100	<0.1	0.35	4.3		100	2.5	1.8	3.0

Theoretical percentage of cells mixedly infected using the formula $(1 - e^{-M_A})(1 - e^{-M_B})100$, where M_A and M_B were the input multiplicities of the infecting viruses.

		MOI (A)			
		0.1	1	10	100
	0.1	1	6.3	10	10
	1	—	40	63.2	63.2
MOI (B)	10	—	—	100	100
	100	—	—	—	100

[a] MOI refers to multiplicity of infections (plaque-forming units/cell). Number refers to the percentage of recombinants as described in Table 2. From Fields (1971).

particles is also not a significant mechanism for generating the ts^+ phenotype (Fields, 1971, 1973) (Section 2.5).

Although genetic reassortment is most often simply referred to as "recombination," true intramolecular recombination has never been demonstrated in reovirus. In view of the size of each segment of RNA (the molecular weight of the largest species of ssRNA is less than 1.5×10^6), it would be extremely difficult to detect intramolecular recombinants against the background levels of spontaneous revertants. The only probable example of this type of recombination among RNA-containing animal viruses has been described by Cooper (1968) for poliovirus. The frequency of ts^+ recombinants from pairwise crosses between ts mutants in this system is generally < 1%. The single-stranded genome of poliovirus is about 2.6×10^6 daltons (Granboulan and Girard, 1969). While it is possible to postulate a mechanism in which poliovirus recombinants might be generated (by a copy-choice mechanism involving loosely associated dsRNA replication intermediates and utilizing the viral replicase enzyme), the mode of replication of reovirus makes it difficult to envision how intramolecular recombination between reovirus ssRNA plus-strands could occur. No host cell or viral enzymes capable of breaking and rejoining pieces of ssRNA are currently known.

2.3. Three-Factor Crosses

Three-factor genetic crosses lend even stronger support to the concept that viral RNA segments are undergoing "reassortment" during viral replication. The aberrant electrophoretic behavior of the $\mu 1$ and $\mu 2$ polypeptides of certain ts mutants has offered an independent, genetically stable, non-temperature-sensitive marker for such crosses (Section 3.4).

Three-factor crosses between the group D ($ts357$) mutant and group B ($ts352$) or C ($ts447$) mutants have been performed (Cross, 1975; Cross and Fields, 1976c). The group D mutant ($ts357$) was selected for these studies because it induces the synthesis of aberrant $\mu 1/\mu 2$ polypeptides (designated μ^{--}) that are easily distinguished from the wild type (μ^+) polypeptides by their more rapid electrophoretic migration (Fig. 2). Groups B and C represent two of the three groups of mutants that exhibit a normal μ^+ polypeptide pattern. The third group (E) is very "leaky," and technically difficult to use in genetic experiments. Three-factor crosses between these mutants are of the following genotypes:

i. $[tsD^-\ tsB^+\ \mu^{--}] \times [tsD^+\ tsB^-\ \mu^+]$
ii. $[tsD^-\ tsC^+\ \mu^{--}] \times [tsD^+\ tsC^-\ \mu^+]$

Ts^+ recombinants were selected from among the progeny of these crosses and were subsequently analyzed for the unselected μ marker. It might be expected that if the ts and μ markers reside on different, unlinked genome segments that are randomly reassorted, the unselected μ marker should segregate independently of the ts markers, and there should be an equal chance for ts^+ recombinants to express the μ^+ or μ^{--} phenotypes. If, on the other hand, any of these markers are linked, then the ts^+ recombinants will be predominantly or exclusively μ^+ or μ^{--}.

Although only limited numbers of recombinant clones have been analyzed, the μ phenotypes were found to segregate independently of either ts marker in both crosses (i and ii above). Approximately 50% of the ts^+ recombinants express the μ^+ phenotype, while the remainder are μ^{--}. Extensive study of progeny of numerous recombinant $ts^+\mu^+$ and

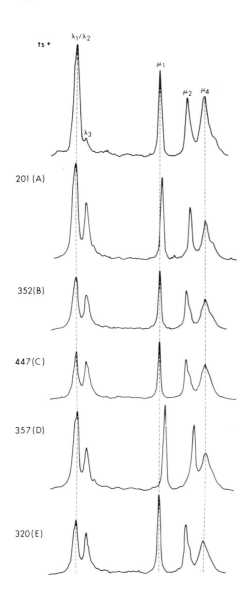

Fig. 2. Densitometer tracing of autoradiogram of large-sized (λ) and medium-sized (μ) cytoplasmic polypeptides induced by ts mutant groups A–E, separated by gel electrophoresis. Note the aberrant $\mu 1/\mu 2$ migration induced by 201 (A) and 357 (D). From Cross and Fields (1976b).

$ts^+\mu^{--}$ clones has indicated that the μ phenotype, once acquired, is inherited in a stable manner (Fig. 3).

Recloning of ts strains containing the μ^+ or μ^{--} phenotype indicates that the mutation rate of μ^+ to μ^{--} or μ^{--} to μ^+ is not sufficiently high to account for these results. In addition, no $ts^+\mu^+$ recombinants were detected in a $ts\mathrm{D}^- \times ts\mathrm{G}^-$ cross (where both mutants are μ^{--}), strongly suggesting that the μ^+ phenotype of the ts^+ recombinants generated in $ts\mathrm{D}^- \times ts\mathrm{B}^-$ or $ts\mathrm{D}^- \times ts\mathrm{C}^-$ crosses did not arise by back mutation of μ^{--} to μ^+. It has been concluded, therefore, that the equal distribution of the μ^+ and μ^{--} phenotypes among ts^+ recombinants reflects genetic reassortment and not mutation.

Evidence that about half of the ts^+ recombinants generated by a $tsD^- \times tsB^-$ or $tsD^- \times tsC^-$ cross are $ts^+\mu^{--}$, and all of the recombinants generated by a $tsD^- \times tsG^-$ are $ts^+\mu^{--}$, further established the independence of the μ and ts loci, since generation of the ts^+ phenotype by recombination (or by reversion, Section 3.7) does not simultaneously restore the wild-type μ^+ phenotype. These findings preclude the possibility that the aberrant μ^{--} phenotype results from a pleiotropic effect of either group G or group D ts mutations.

Since neither the μ^{--} phenotype of the group D mutant nor the μ^+ phenotype of groups B and C was favored in $tsD^- \times tsB^-$ and $tsD^- \times tsC^-$ crosses, the determinant of the phenotype appears not to be linked to either the tsD, tsC, or tsB gene. Therefore, independent segregation of the μ marker among ts^+ recombinants in two three-factor genetic crosses strongly favors a mechanism of recombination in which recombinants are generated by a random assortment of unlinked RNA segments from a common pool. Because parental double-stranded RNA molecules are never fully uncoated (Silverstein *et al.*, 1970; Chang and Zweerink, 1971) and progeny dsRNA molecules are synthesized in virion core-like structures (Acs *et al.*, 1971; Zweerink *et al.*, 1972), reassortment must occur between single-stranded RNA molecules. Thus these data imply that any linkage between these ssRNA molecules, through either RNA or protein interactions, must be

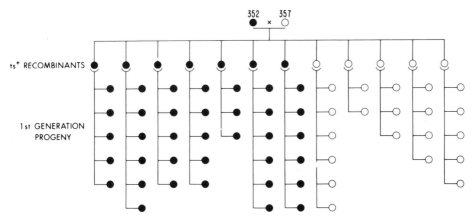

Fig. 3. Summary of the μ phenotypes of progeny of ts^+ recombinant clones from mixed infection with group D ($ts357$) and group B ($ts352$); μ^+ phenotypes are represented by ●; μ^{--} phenotypes are represented by ○. From Cross and Fields (1967c).

extremely weak or occur after reassortment has taken place. Additional crosses are being carried out to further substantiate these results.

In contrast to the observation that the μ^{--} and μ^+ phenotypes segregate equally among ts^+ recombinants derived from mixed infection with groups D and B or C, all of the ts^+ recombinants derived from a cross between groups D and A exhibit the μ^{--} phenotype of the group D mutant $ts357$ (Cross and Fields, 1976c). The group A mutants induce an aberrant $\mu1/\mu2$ polypeptide, designated as μ^-, that migrates slightly slower than the μ^{--} polypeptide (Fig. 2). This result suggests that the μ determinant and the tsA gene are linked, since the ts^+ recombinants acquire both the tsA$^+$ gene and μ^{--} marker from the tsD$^-$ parent. The μ^- phenotype would, of necessity, be excluded with the tsA$^-$ gene. The fact that ts^+ recombinants are generated by reassortment of RNA segments would imply that the tsA gene and the determinant of the μ phenotype lie on the same genome segment, and affect, therefore, the same gene product (Section 3.7.2). Further crosses between the group A mutants and other groups are necessary to confirm this hypothesis. The fact that upon reversion of the group A mutant ($ts201$) to ts^+, expression of the μ phenotype is often affected (a significant number of revertants are μ^{--} or μ^+) supports the data obtained from studies of genetic crosses (Section 3.7.2b).

2.4. Complementation

Standard complementation tests between ts mutants of reovirus require simultaneous infection of L cells with pairs of ts mutants or with each mutant alone, and, after removal of unadsorbed virus, incubation at the nonpermissive temperature for about 24 h. The yield of virus is titered at 31°C and 39°C, and the complementation index for any two strains A and B is calculated according to the formula

$$\frac{\text{yield } (A \times B)^{31°C} - \text{yield } (A \times B)^{39°C}}{\text{yield } (A)^{31°C} + \text{yield } (B)^{31°C}}$$

Early studies by Fields and Joklik (1969) suggested that complementation occurs between ts mutants, but that it is inefficient and difficult to measure. Complementation indices ranging from 2 to approximately 10 (on the borderline of significance) have been recorded (Fields and Joklik, 1969; Spandidos and Graham, 1975b). Since complementation indices were low, there had been no systematic attempt to correlate these indices with classification into groups by genetic recombination.

Ito and Joklik (1972*a*) have applied an approach to the study of complementation between mutant strains that involves determination of the ability of mutants to synthesize viral RNA at 39°C following mixed infection. When pairs of RNA⁻ mutants of different recombination groups (C, D, or E) are used to coinfect cells, a small but significant increase in virus-specific RNA, larger than that following infection with each mutant alone, is observed. They have interpreted this enhanced RNA synthesis as evidence of complementation. Although this method appears to be useful in classifying *ts* mutants and is consistent with reassortment data, it is important to confirm that complementation has actually taken place by progeny testing. Since reassortment occurs at both 39°C and 31°C, the yield of virus from mixed infection at 39°C contains a considerable yield of *ts⁺* virions (Fields, unpublished data). It is possible, therefore, that the enhanced RNA synthesis that follows mixed infection reflects genetic reassortment rather than complementation. The fact that reassortment of gene segments occurs early and is so efficient in reovirus-infected cells, even at 39°C, is a possible reason for the difficulty in detecting complementation in this system.

Spandidos and Graham (1975*b*) have recently devised an alternative method for studying complementation. They have utilized a plaque assay on cell monolayers mixedly infected with defective reovirions lacking the L1 segment (Section 2.7) and prototype *ts* mutants. An increase in the number of plaques on plates mixedly infected at 39°C over controls infected with the defective virus or each *ts* mutant alone is indicative of a significant degree of complementation. Complementation, not recombination, is believed to be measured by this method because there is no detectable recombination between defective virions and any of the *ts* mutants. Mutants of groups A, B, D, F, and G are complemented by the defectives, while groups C and E are not. Analysis of the virus progeny by density gradient centrifugation to detect reciprocal complementation has demonstrated that mutants of all groups except C complement the defective reovirions. On the basis of these experiments, it was concluded that the *ts* lesion in the C mutant is in a *trans*-acting function that resides in the L1 genome segment, and that only the group E mutation is in a *cis*-acting function (Spandidos and Graham, 1975*a,b*). In addition to experiments using *ts* mutants derived from reovirus type 3, wild-type reovirus type 1 can complement L1 type 3 defectives that are deletion mutants (Spandidos and Graham, 1975*b*).

Subsequently, Spandidos and Graham (1976*b*) developed an infectious center assay to measure recombination and complementation.

The mutants fell into complementation groups corresponding to the previously defined recombination groups.

2.5. Nongenetic Variables

Plaques that appear on assay plates at the nonpermissive temperature following mixed infection at permissive temperature with *ts* mutants of certain viruses (Newcastle disease virus, Dahlberg and Simon, 1969*a,b*; Hirst, 1962; influenza, Hirst and Pons, 1973; RNA tumor viruses, Weiss *et al.,* 1973; vesicular stomatitis virus, Pringle and Duncan, 1971) have often been shown to be produced by aggregates of complementing *ts* mutants or by heteropolyploids. Several experiments have been performed to prove that the plaques appearing at 39°C following mixed infection with reovirus mutants are due to the generation of "true" ts^+ recombinants (Fields, 1973).

The contribution of virus aggregates to plaque formation was examined by studying the effect of ultrasonic vibration and filtration on the yield of virus from mixed infection and on an artificial mixture of mutants (Fields, 1973) (Table 4). While some clumps are present after mixed infection with group B and C mutants, sonication or filtration (conditions known to disrupt or eliminate aggregated virus) reduce their contribution to plaque formation equally. This finding suggests that the remaining level of recombinants (6%) is not the result of aggregates of complementing mutants. Artificial mixtures of mutants of groups B and C also yield plaques on assay plates at the nonpermissive temperature. Sonication, however, decreases their level to 3.3% of that

TABLE 4
Effect of Sonication and Filtration on Plaquing of Mixed Yield and Mixture of two *ts* Mutants[a]

Sample	Treatment	PFU/ml 31°C	PFU/ml 39°C	Percentage of recombinants $\dfrac{\text{PFU/ml } 39°C}{\text{PFU/ml } 31°C} \times 100$
(A) Mixed yield	(1) None	8.0×10^7	1.4×10^7	20
(ts352 × ts447)	(2) Sonic vibration	1.1×10^9	7.0×10^7	6
	(3) Filtered	3.2×10^7	2.0×10^6	6
(B) Artificial mixture	(1) None	1.9×10^9	3.5×10^5	0.2
(ts352 + ts447)	(2) Sonic vibration	1.2×10^9	2.7×10^5	0.2
	(3) Filtered	6.0×10^8	2.0×10^4	0.03

[a] From Fields (1973).

produced by mixed infection at 31°C, and filtration further reduces their contribution another tenfold. The residual numbers of plaques may result from aggregation of complementing *ts* mutants. However, at the very high concentrations used in these reconstruction experiments, they probably reflect mixed infection of cells on the assay plate. In any event, their contribution to the recombination frequency is negligible.

Because there is no evidence of polyploid particles of reovirus, complementing heterozygotes are also unlikely to be a complicating factor. Presumptive ts^+ recombinants have been found to have a high efficiency of plating (between 30% and 100%) similar to that of the wild-type strain (Fields, 1971). In the absence of recombination, the number of plaques appearing at the nonpermissive temperature cannot exceed the level of heterozygosity. The high efficiency of plating, therefore, strongly suggests that heterozygotes, which at best are negligible in reovirus populations (as are aggregates of complementing *ts* mutants), are not major factors in contributing to formation of plaques at 39°C. Furthermore, studies on density-banded, radiolabeled virus from a mixed infection at 31°C have indicated that the efficiency of plating is virtually identical in virus of all densities and the specific infectivity (PFU/cpm) constant, whether measured at 31°C or 39°C. Likewise, purification of input virus by density banding has no effect on recombination frequencies when compared with unpurified viral suspensions. These data lend additional, independent proof that hetero-polyploids are not present. However, density gradient centrifugation would not resolve particles with duplication of a single genomic segment, leaving open the possibility of partially diploid heterozygotes.

In addition, virtually all of the ts^+ recombinant clones resulting from mixed infection at 31°C with the group D mutant *ts*357 (which exhibits a μ^{--} polypeptide phenotype) and either the group B or C mutants (which possess the μ^+ phenotype) (Section 2.3) were found to express either the μ^{--} or μ^+ phenotype, but not both. A small proportion of mixed $ts^+\mu^+/\mu^{--}$ clones were also detected, but these are not stable and segregate immediately into genetically stable $ts^+\mu^+$ or $ts^+\mu^{--}$ phenotype upon recloning. Thus the gene segment responsible for the μ^+ or μ^- phenotype appears to be present in only one copy in most ts^+ recombinant clones, suggesting that stable heterozygotes are not a problem in reovirus genetics.

2.6. Multiplicity Reactivation

Following exposure of suspensions of reovirus to moderate doses of ultraviolet light, virus titers decrease in an exponential fashion

(McClain and Spendlove, 1966). However, with high-titer preparations of virus and larger doses of ultraviolet light, multiplicity reactivation (MR) may occur. All three serotypes of mammalian reovirus exhibit MR, and are also capable of interacting in mixed infection with high efficiency to yield infectious virus. Although indirect, these observations suggested that reovirus could, in fact, undergo genetic recombination.

MR is probably achieved by reassortment between undamaged genome segments rather than intramolecular recombination within damaged segments. The fact that the three serotypes readily undergo MR suggests that a similar type of reassortment may occur in heterologous infections with different reovirus serotypes. Considering the ubiquitous nature of reoviruses, reassortment between various types might, in fact, provide a source of antigenic variation. Recently, efficient reassortment between temperature-sensitive mutants of reovirus type 3 and reovirus types 1 and 2 has been demonstrated (Ramig *et al.*, 1977*b*; Sharpe *et al.*, 1977). However, mouse L cells infected with type 3 reovirus and the avian reovirus did not interact to allow synthesis of avian virus (Spandidos and Graham, 1976*c*). This result suggests that the mammalian reoviruses may be genetically isolated from the avian reoviruses.

2.7. Deletion Mutants

As is characteristic of many other animal viruses, serial passage of reovirus results in the accumulation of defective particles. These were first demonstrated by Nonoyama *et al.* (1970), who observed that two populations of core particles resulted after treatment of stock virus with chymotrypsin. Heavy (H) cores ($\sigma = 1.43$ g/cm^3) were derived from complete, infectious virions; light (L) cores ($\sigma = 1.415$ g/cm^3) were obtained from defective virions. The L cores were morphologically indistinguishable from H cores and possessed an active transcriptase, but lacked the largest (L1) segment of genome dsRNA. Defective virions were not infectious and required coinfection with complete virions for propagation: they could be virtually eliminated from stocks by passages at multiplicities of less than 1. Since defective virions lack a segment of genome RNA, they are essentially deletion mutants and as such offer considerable potential for the study of the genetics of reovirus.

Serial passage of freshly cloned virus results in the accumulation of defective particles with the L1 deletion by the seventh to eighth passage (Nonoyama and Graham, 1970; Schuerch *et al.*, 1974). Schuerch *et al.* (1974) have noted that newly cloned stocks of two mutants, group C *ts*447 and group F *ts*556, when passaged at the permissive temperature, yield defective particles much sooner than the wild-type strain. Passage of *ts*447 gives rise immediately to an equal number of nondefective and defective particles devoid of segment L3; particles that lack L1 (as in the case of the wild-type strain) form on prolonged passage. When *ts*556 is passaged as few as three times, particles that lack either L3 or both L1 and L3 are formed in approximately equal proportions. All of these defective particles contain a normal polypeptide complement and possess full transcriptase activity. Further investigation of these mutants should provide insight into the little-understood mechanism that ensures the encapsidation of a set of ten unique pieces of RNA into progeny virions.

It has not been possible until recently to separate defective particles from infectious virions: defective virions could be demonstrated only in viral populations after treatment with chymotrypsin, as described above. Spandidos and Graham (1975*a*), however, have succeeded in obtaining an almost pure population of defective virions that lack the L1 segment. This was accomplished by growth of defective virions in the presence of the group E mutant. This mutant complements the missing L1 function in *trans* at 39°C but does not itself replicate, since the *ts* defect appears to be in a *cis*-acting function. These defective virions have subsequently been used as deletion mutants in complementation studies with various *ts* mutants to define mutant lesions (Sections 2.4 and 3.7.4). Using defective reovirus lacking the L1 segment in recombination experiments, Spandidos and Graham (1976*a*) have found that no recombination was detectable when the defective virus was crossed with the different classes of *ts* mutants. The significance of this result is unclear.

3. GENE FUNCTION

3.1. Phenotype of Genetic Groups

Seven groups of *ts* mutants have been defined on the basis of two-factor genetic crosses. Each of these falls into three general types with respect to their phenotype at the nonpermissive temperature: (1) Group A and F mutants are rapidly uncoated, synthesize viral RNA and polypeptides as efficiently as the wild type, and assemble noninfectious particles that are morphologically similar to wild type. (2) Group B and

TABLE 5

Properties of *ts* Mutant Groups

Group (prototype)	Percent synthesized dsRNA	Percent synthesized ssRNA	Percent synthesized Protein	Morphogenesis	Cell killing	Aberrant ds RNA hybrid	Aberrant proteins
A (*ts*201)	100	100	100	Full virion	Like wild	L_2	μ_2^-
B (*ts*352)	25–50	25–50	25	Corelike	Minor	—	—
C (*ts*447)	~ 0.1	~ 5	5–10	Outer capsid shell	Minor	—	—
D (*ts*357)	~ 0.1	~ 5	10–20	Mixed capsid shell	Intermediate	M_2	μ_2^{--}
E (*ts*320)	~ 1	~ 5	5–10	Uncertain	Intermediate	S_3	—
F (*ts*556)	50–100	50–100	50–100	Full virion	Like wild	—	μ_2^-
G (*ts*453)	15–25	20	25	Corelike	Like wild	—	μ_2^{--}

G mutants initiate the synthesis of viral ssRNA and dsRNA in a delayed fashion with a significantly reduced yield of both species of RNA as well as viral polypeptides. In addition, the group G mutant transcribes less ssRNA *in vitro* than wild type. Subviral particles accumulate that are "corelike" in composition, i.e., lack the outer coat proteins. (3) Group C, D, and E mutants are RNA⁻ and synthesize only small amounts of ssRNA and virtually no dsRNA. Polypeptide synthesis is also greatly diminished. *In vitro* transcriptase activity is, however, comparable to that of the wild-type strain. Empty particles resembling "top component" accumulate.

Further details will be described below and are summarized in Table 5.

3.2. Transcription

The ability of representative *ts* mutants to transcribe viral ssRNA *in vitro* and in infected cells has been examined. Mutants from groups A–F were found not to differ significantly from the wild-type strain in their capacity to transcribe viral ssRNA *in vitro* at both the permissive (31°C) and nonpermissive (39°C) temperatures as well as at 50°C (Cross and Fields, 1972; Ito and Joklik, 1972*a*). The group G mutant, however, was found to synthesize less ssRNA *in vitro* than mutants of all other groups at all three temperatures (Cross and Fields, 1972). The reaction products and heat stability of the core-associated transcriptase of this mutant were comparable to those of the wild-type strain and mutants of other groups. It appears that although the group G mutant possesses a defective core-associated transcriptase, it is not clear that this defect is responsible for its temperature sensitivity.

None of the mutants isolated by Ikegami and Gomatos possesses a *ts* defect in the core-associated viral transcriptase. The assay conditions for *in vitro* RNA synthesis, kinetics of synthesis, reaction products, and heat stability at 52°C of the transcriptase of viral cores derived by treatment of mutant virions with chymotrypsin are identical to those of wild-type virus (Ikegami and Gomatos, 1972).

Reovirus-specific ssRNA synthesis in infected cells has been divided into early RNA, transcribed from parental subviral particles, and late RNA, transcribed from immature progeny virus particles (Joklik, 1974). The kinetics of appearance of viral-specific RNA in cells infected at 39°C with each of the mutant groups A–G has been studied using actinomycin D to selectively inhibit host cell RNA synthesis (Fields and Joklik, 1969; Cross and Fields, 1972). The quantity of RNA induced by mutants of groups A and F is comparable to or exceeds that of the wild type, consisting of early and late RNA. The peak of RNA synthesis occurs somewhat earlier than in the wild virus; more rapid uncoating and activation of the viral transcriptase are a reasonable explanation for this phenomenon. Mutants of groups B and G synthesize less than one-third the quantity of RNA induced by wild type, and exhibit a greater lag period before the appearance of RNA. This RNA is presumably a mixture of early RNA and reduced amounts of late RNA. Negligible quantities of RNA are induced by mutants of groups C, D, and E. Since progeny dsRNA-containing virus particles are not formed in cells infected with any of these groups of mutants, this RNA is exclusively early.

Analysis of the individual viral ssRNA transcripts has been carried out by hybridization of radiolabeled plus-strand ssRNA from cells infected with each mutant with minus-strand RNA from wild-type virions, followed by electrophoresis on polyacrylamide gels (Ito and Joklik, 1972a; Cross and Fields, 1972). Mutants of each group induce the synthesis of all ten species of viral ssRNA at the nonpermissive temperature. The relative quantities of each RNA species are similar to those of wild type. A minor but significant retardation in the electrophoretic mobility of certain species of heterologous dsRNA molecules consisting of mutant plus-strands and wild-type minus-strands has been demonstrated (Ito and Joklik, 1972b; Schuerch and Joklik, 1973). The significance of this observation in assignment of the *ts* mutation to genome segment is discussed in Section 3.7.

The group C, D, and E mutants synthesize between 1% and 5% as much ssRNA as the wild type (Ito and Joklik, 1972a). The diminished capacity of mutants of groups C, D, and E to transcribe viral ssRNA in infected cells (although equally competent as the ts^+ strain *in vitro*) is undoubtedly related to their inability to synthesize progeny dsRNA (Section 3.3). Exposure to high concentrations of drugs such as cycloheximide and actinomycin D, that also inhibit the replication of progeny dsRNA, similarly results in a substantial reduction in ssRNA (Watanabe *et al.*, 1968; Silverstein *et al.*, 1974). Presumably this low level of ssRNA is transcribed from the parental genome of partially uncoated input virus, and, by definition, is "early" RNA.

Watanabe *et al.* (1968) have reported that when protein synthesis is arrested by cycloheximide and dsRNA synthesis is consequently blocked, only four species of "early" RNA (l1, m3, s3, and s4) are transcribed. Yet the mutants of groups C, D, and E that synthesize virtually no progeny dsRNA transcribe all ten species of ssRNA. Whether the four "early" species are an artifact of treatment with cycloheximide, reflecting merely those species synthesized in greatest quantity (and more likely detected) at a time when RNA synthesis is low (Joklik, 1974), or are the result of repression of late RNA by a preexisting host cell repressor that requires *de novo* synthesis of protein to reverse its effect (Millward and Graham, 1974) remains to be determined. Recent studies in Graham's laboratory lend further credence to the idea of a cellular repressor. Using either defective reovirus lacking the L1 segment or the C (*ts*447) mutant, Spandidos *et al.* (1976) showed a temporal control over transcription similar to that for wild type virions. The same four segments are also transcribed in nonpermissive infection of L cells infected with avian reovirus (Spandidos and Graham 1976c). When L cells are co-infected with the avian reovirus and type 3, all ten segments of the avian genome are transcribed. There is currently no indication as to the nature, or mechanism of action, of the putative cellular repressor.

3.3. Replication

Mutants of groups A, B, F, and G synthesize all ten species of viral dsRNA in cells infected at the nonpermissive temperature, although somewhat reduced quantities are produced by groups B and G (Cross and Fields, 1972). The relative proportion and size of each of these dsRNA molecules are identical to those of wild type (Cross and Fields, 1972).

The most striking feature of three groups of mutants (C, D, and E) is their inability to replicate viral dsRNA at the nonpermissive temperature (Ito and Joklik, 1972a; Cross and Fields, 1972). Group C (ts447) and D (ts585) mutants synthesize no detectable dsRNA. Another group D mutant (ts357) makes about 15% of the normal quantities, but this probably reflects the leakiness of this mutant. The group E mutant synthesizes less than 1.0% of that of wild type.

An examination of dsRNA synthesis following temperature shift from 31°C to 39°C revealed differences between the C, D, and E mutants (Ito and Joklik, 1972a). Following shiftup, dsRNA synthesis ceases abruptly in cells infected with mutants of groups C and D, while in those cells infected with the group E mutant it continues at an undiminished rate once dsRNA synthesis has commenced. The ts lesion of the group E mutant appears to reside in a very early function that is confined to the first hour of replication. It is for this reason that it is necessary to adsorb this mutant at 4°C, or inoculate it at MOI < 5 in order to examine its ts characteristics at the nonpermissive temperature.

The failure of mutants of groups C, D, and E to replicate dsRNA results in a substantial reduction in viral ssRNA (Section 3.2). This observation is consistent with other data indicating that the bulk of ssRNA synthesized in virus-infected cells (late RNA) is transcribed from the completed progeny dsRNA of immature virus particles (Kudo and Graham, 1965; Shatkin and Rada, 1967).

Further characterization of the group C mutant (ts447) suggests that the mutant polypeptide is a structural component of the complexes within which progeny dsRNA are replicated (Matsuhisa and Joklik, 1974). These dsRNA-synthesizing structures (DSRSS) do not develop at 39°C in cells infected with ts447, but, once formed at 31°C, are able to synthesize dsRNA in vitro at 39°C. The ts447 DSRSS produced at 31°C are more heat labile than those of the wild-type strain. Because core polypeptides are components of DSRSS (Zweerink et al., 1972, Zweerink, 1974), this phenomenon is consistent with independent evidence reported by Matsuhisa and Joklik (1974) that suggests that one of the two innermost core polypeptides, $\lambda 1$ or $\sigma 2$ of ts447, is probably defective (Section 3.5). Such a defect might prevent the formation of the inner core structure and replication of viral RNA. Viral "factories" within cells infected at the nonpermissive temperature with the group C and D mutants accumulate "empty" particles (Section 3.5). This suggests that under nonpermissive conditions, core polypeptides are incapable of proper assembly.

3.4. Translation

Protein synthesis by host cells does not decrease for several hours following infection with reovirus (Zweerink and Joklik, 1970). At 39°C, the background of cellular protein synthesis remains quite high in contrast to that observed at 31°C. The technique of immunological precipitation was employed by Fields *et al.* (1972) in order to detect viral-specific polypeptides against an appreciable background of host-cell protein synthesis at the elevated temperature. By using antiserum against whole virus to selectively precipitate reovirus-specific polypeptides from infected cell extracts, viral polypeptides can be detected in cells infected with wild type or with *ts* mutants of groups A–E at both 31°C and 39°C. The quantity of radiolabeled protein precipitated by antiviral antiserum at 39°C is roughly proportional to the total ssRNA transcribed in cells similarly infected (Section 3.2). While 16% and 10% of the acid-precipitable radiolabel in cytoplasmic lysates is recovered from cells infected with the wild type and the group A mutant, respectively, less than 3% is detected in cells infected with mutants of groups B, C, D, and E. Analysis of polypeptide species by polyacrylamide gel electrophoresis suggests that each of the mutants synthesizes all of the major capsid proteins, and none has a demonstrable defect in the cleavage of polypeptide $\mu 1$ to $\mu 2$.

High-resolution discontinuous gel electrophoresis has recently been used to examine the virus-specified polypeptides synthesized in reovirus-infected cells (Both *et al.*, 1975; Cross and Fields, 1976*a*). Additional polypeptides that presumably correspond to the ten primary gene products have been identified by this procedure (Fig. 4). Analysis of the polypeptides synthesized by the mutants at 39°C confirms and extends earlier data (Cross and Fields, 1976*b*). The same viral-specific species synthesized in cells infected with wild type are synthesized in those infected with mutants of groups A–G at the nonpermissive temperature. Mutants of each group are capable of carrying out the synthesis of all of the viral structural polypeptides, as well as the two major nonstructural species. This is entirely consistent with the observation that all ten species of mRNA are transcribed in mutant-infected cells under nonpermissive conditions (Cross and Fields, 1972; Ito and Joklik, 1972*a*), and with the demonstration of viral antigens and structures in nonpermissively infected cells by immunofluorescence and electron microscopy (Fields *et al.*, 1971). The failure to detect mature viral particles in cells infected with some of the mutants (B, C, D, G) at the nonpermissive temperature, even though the appropriate polypeptides are synthesized,

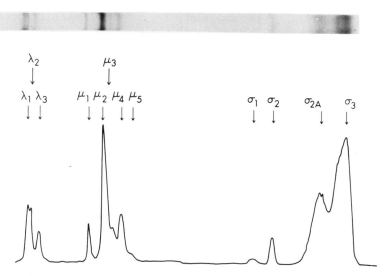

Fig. 4. Densitometer tracing of autoradiogram of viral polypeptides immunologically precipitated from cells infected with reovirus type 3 wild type separated by gel electrophoresis. Note three large species, four (or five) middle-sized species, and four small species. μ_4 and σ_{2A} are nonstructural polypeptides.

suggests a posttranslational defect in either processing or assembly of viral polypeptides. It is unlikely, however, that a failure to cleave properly is involved, because it has been conclusively demonstrated that the ability to yield the $\mu2$ cleavage product is not impaired at the elevated temperature. It is likely that the synthesized polypeptides are unable to assume a functional configuration at the nonpermissive temperature, thereby hindering the normal assembly process and resulting in the accumulation of particles whose completion is blocked (Section 3.5).

All of the polypeptides, except $\mu1$ and $\mu2$ from groups A, D, F, and G, synthesized by the mutant strains at the nonpermissive temperature exhibit the same electrophoretic mobility on polyacrylamide gels as the respective wild-type species (Fig. 2). The migration of the $\mu1$ polypeptide and the $\mu2$ cleavage product of five group A mutants and of the group F mutant is faster than that of the polypeptides of wild type. The behavior of the group D mutant $ts357$ and the group G mutant $\mu1$ and $\mu2$ species on polyacrylamide gels is likewise aberrant; however, the $\mu1$ and $\mu2$ polypeptides of these mutants migrate even more rapidly than those of groups A and F. The other group D mutant $ts585$ synthesizes wild-type $\mu1/\mu2$ polypeptides. The wild-type $\mu1/\mu2$ polypeptides have been designated μ^+ while the aberrant polypeptides of groups A and F and groups D and G have been designated as μ^- and

μ^{--}, respectively. The expression of μ^- and μ^{--} phenotypes is not temperature dependent. Synthesis of the $\mu1$ and $\mu2$ polypeptides of these four mutants at the permissive temperature does not restore the electrophoretic behavior to that of the wild type. The aberrant species are present not only in cytoplasmic extracts of permissively infected cells but also in mature, infectious virions (Cross and Fields 1976b).

It is likely that the mutation that results in the aberrant $\mu1$ (and $\mu2$) polypeptide products resides on a medium-sized RNA segment. Data obtained from *in vitro* protein-synthesizing systems have demonstrated conclusively that the λ, μ, and σ classes of reovirus polypeptides are translated from the mRNA transcripts of the large (L), medium (M), and small (S) size classes of dsRNA, respectively (Graziadei and Lengyel, 1972; Both *et al.*, 1975). It has not yet been ascertained precisely which species of RNA within a size class codes for a particular polypeptide. The mutation affecting the $\mu1$ polypeptide could therefore lie on any of the three medium-sized (M) genome segments. The fact that the $\mu1$ and $\mu2$ polypeptides are simultaneously affected lends additional proof to the precursor–product relationship of those polypeptides deduced from pulse-chase experiments by Zweerink and Joklik (1970). It also indicated that the mutation responsible for the aberrant migration occurs in a region of RNA coding for the conserved portion of the $\mu1$ polypeptide.

Whether or not the faster migration of the mutant $\mu1$ and $\mu2$ polypeptides actually indicates that these species are smaller than the corresponding species of wild type has not yet been determined. A reduction in molecular weight of the aberrant polypeptide could result from a deletion in genome RNA. This is unlikely, since no differences have been detected in the molecular weight of any dsRNA species (Ito and Joklik, 1972b; Cross and Fields, 1972; Schuerch and Joklik, 1973). A reduction in molecular weight might also arise from a nonsense mutation in a medium RNA segment that results in premature chain termination during translation. The difference in molecular mass (based on the distance migrated) between the wild-type and mutant proteins is of the order of 1000–3000 daltons (Ramig, unpublished observation). This could correspond to a difference of about 10–30 amino acids. It is also entirely conceivable that, since the $\mu2$ polypeptide is a phosphoprotein (Krystal *et al.*, 1975), a missense mutation in a critical location in a medium RNA segment might affect the conformation of the polypeptide and, in this way, affect the availability of particular residues for phosphorylation. Alternatively, a missense mutation might directly change one of the many serines (or possibly threonines) to another amino acid that cannot be phosphorylated. In either case, the difference in electrophoretic behavior of the μ^+, μ^-, and μ^{--} species may be due to variability in the phosphorylation of these polypeptides that could alter electrophoretic mobility. It is also possible that a missense mutation might alter the electrophoretic mobility of the μ polypeptide, without having any effect on a secondary modification of this type.

The common occurrence of altered $\mu 1$ and $\mu 2$ polypeptides suggests that one of the medium-sized RNA segments may contain a mutational "hot spot" and/or that such mutations are not excluded by selective pressures. They are both good possibilities because $\mu 2$ is a major outer structural polypeptide in which minor changes might be tolerated. Differences between serotypes of blue tongue virus, another dsRNA-containing virus, appear to be associated primarily with variations in the two major proteins of the outer coat (DeVilliers, 1974). However, examination of the cytoplasmic polypeptides induced by reovirus serotypes 1, 2, and 3 revealed different electrophoretic mobilities following electrophoresis in SDS-polyacrylamide gels in almost every capsid protein (Ramig *et al.*, 1977*a*). Thus, it appears that changes in every viral polypeptide can be tolerated.

The preceding discussion has assumed that the aberrant μ phenotype is the result of a mutation in one of the medium (M) RNA segments. However, it is also conceivable that alteration of a μ polypeptide species might result from the pleiotropic effect of a mutation in another gene. Thus it might be postulated that the association of the $\mu 2$ polypeptide with the defective product of another gene may affect its proper folding and subsequent phosphorylation, and so result in an aberrant migration. If this is in fact the cause, a temperature-sensitive defect in any of a number of different polypeptides might affect the migration and phosphorylation(?) of the μ polypeptides, and explain the frequent occurrence of an aberrant species in four of seven groups of *ts* mutants. Genetic studies of revertants to the *ts*$^+$ phenotype argue against the possibility that the aberrant μ phenotype of the group D and G mutant strains is the result of a pleiotropic effect of mutations to temperature sensitivity (Section 3.7.2).

On the basis of studies of the sequential digestion of virions with chymotrypsin (Section 3.7.2), Ito and Joklik (1972*c*) have suggested that both group D mutants possess an altered structural $\mu 2$ polypeptide. The relationship of this observation to the aberrant migration of the *ts*357 (D) $\mu 1$ and $\mu 2$ polypeptides is not known. While the $\mu 2$ polypeptides of the group D mutant *ts*357 exhibit a novel digestion

product and an aberrant electrophoretic behavior, no unique intermediate was derived from digestion of the D mutant ts585, although the
kinetics of digestion was slower than that of the ts^+, and no difference
in the migration of the μ2 species of this mutant from ts^+ was noted.

Ikegami and Gomatos (1972) have studied host and viral protein
synthesis in cells infected at the nonpermissive temperature with ts
mutants isolated in their laboratory. A marked inhibition of both viral
and cellular protein synthesis was found to occur late in infection with
all 14 of the mutants. Preexisting host polyribosomes were disrupted
and only viral-specific polyribosomes were detected. It has been suggested that newly synthesized host mRNA molecules do not form a
stable association with ribosomes during viral infection. Virus-coded
factors involved in stable binding of mRNA to ribosomes preferentially
recognize viral-specific mRNA and exclude host mRNA. Although viral
mRNA is associated with polysomes in mutant-infected cells, subsequent translation is inhibited at the nonpermissive temperature. It has
been suggested that additional factors that may also be virus coded are
required for the synthesis of virus-specified polypeptides, and that the ts
mutants are temperature-sensitive in these factors, but not in those that
affect the binding of host mRNA to ribosomes. None of these
hypothetical factors has yet been identified.

3.5. Assembly

The accumulation of viral antigen in mutant-infected cells has
been studied using the technique of indirect immunofluorescence
(Fields et $al.$, 1971). While the distribution of viral antigen as indicated
by cytoplasmic fluorescence is identical in cells infected at 31°C, reproducible differences are observed at 39°C. Large coalescent cytoplasmic
masses characteristic of wild-type infection appear in cells infected with
mutants of groups A and F. Intermediate-size cytoplasmic masses form
in cells infected with the group D mutant, and discrete, small cytoplasmic masses of uniform size are induced by mutants of groups B, C,
and G. Variable results are obtained with the "leaky" group E mutant.

Electron microscopy has revealed the intracytoplasmic distribution
and ultrastructural morphology of viral cytoplasmic inclusions or "factories" induced by representative mutants in infected cells (Fields et $al.$,
1971). The size and distribution of these correspond well with the patterns of fluorescent antigen described above. The structures observed
within "factories" in cells infected at 31°C with each of the mutants

are identical with those of wild type; full, mature, double-shelled particles, occasionally arranged in crystalline arrays also containing empty capsids, are apparent. In contrast, there are striking differences in the ultrastructure of the virus particles which accumulate in "factories" at 39°C in cells infected with the various mutants.

Cells infected with mutants of groups A and F are capable of assembling particles at 39°C that resemble those of the wild type morphologically, but are not infectious [Fig. 5(1)]. All ten segments of newly synthesized dsRNA are packaged within a double-shelled capsid (Cross, unpublished observation), although the final stages in the morphogenetic pathway are either incomplete and/or aberrant. It is possible that a defective polypeptide present in either the core or the outer layer interferes with necessary conformational changes, or that there is a deficiency of certain polypeptides in these particles. The fact that mutants of groups A and F synthesize normal amounts of viral RNA and protein but not oligo(A) (Section 3.6) is consistent with their classification as late mutants.

Cells infected with mutants of groups B and G accumulate "corelike" particles (particles lacking a normal outer capsid shell) [Fig. 5(2)] that are occasionally detected in cells infected with the wild-type strain, and are probably intermediates in viral morphogenesis (see below). These mutants are blocked in an earlier stage of assembly than the group A and F mutants. Either an aberrant outer capsid polypeptide cannot bind to viral cores, or completion of the outer shell is blocked by a defective core polypeptide. Particles that are basically corelike in composition are capable of replicating dsRNA and transcribing ssRNA *in vitro* (Sakuma and Watanabe, 1971; Zweerink *et al.,* 1972; Zweerink, 1974). It is not surprising, therefore, that these mutants are able to synthesize both dsRNA and ssRNA, although in somewhat diminished quantities.

To explore the possibility that "corelike" particles are intermediates in viral morphogenesis, Morgan and Zweerink (1974) isolated progeny subviral particles from cells infected at 39°C with wild type and mutants of groups B and G. These subviral particles, which sediment at 400 S in sucrose gradients, closely resemble reovirus cores prepared by digestion of virions with chymotrypsin. Like cores, they have a buoyant density in CsCl of 1.44 g/cm^3, are about 50 nm in diameter, and are capable of synthesizing ssRNA. They also are composed primarily of the four core polypeptides ($\lambda1$, $\lambda2$, $\mu1$, $\sigma2$) and contain all ten segments of dsRNA. However, their surface is slightly different. Polypeptide $\lambda2$ is present in reduced amounts, and small and variable

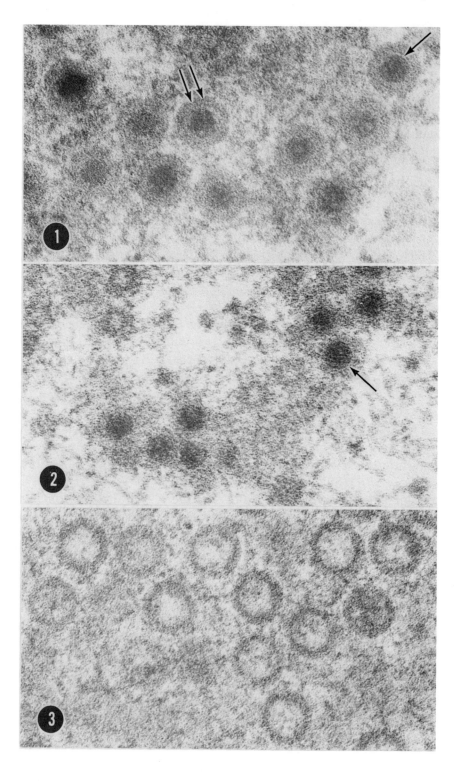

quantities of the outer capsid ($\mu2$ and $\sigma3$) and noncapsid ($\mu0$) polypeptides are also present. Cells infected with wild-type virus at 39°C accumulate both virions and 400 S particles; the latter are not observed at 31°C. Only 400 S particles accumulate at 39°C in cells infected with the group B and G mutants: this is consistent with the results of electron microscopic studies demonstrating the presence of corelike particles in cells infected with these mutants. The appearance of 400 S corelike particles early in replication, before the formation of progeny reovirions, suggests that these may function as intermediates in viral morphogenesis. Unfortunately, pulse-chase conditions combined with temperature-shift experiments (39°C → 31°C) that might have proven this hypothesis conclusively are hampered by the large pools of viral ssRNA and polypeptides in reovirus-infected cells.

The mutants isolated by Ikegami and Gomatos (1968, 1972) are similar to the group B and G mutants; they accumulate viral cores but not mature virus under restrictive conditions (Ikegami and Gomatos, 1972). Although the number of viral cores present in cells infected with mutant virus is initially equivalent to that in the wild strain, the synthesis of viral cores in all mutant-infected cells is inhibited late in infection. Viral cores isolated from cells infected either with mutants or wild type have a buoyant density of about 1.43 g/cm^3 and are capable of synthesizing viral ssRNA *in vitro*.

Ultrastructural studies of cells infected with group C and D mutants reveal the presence of empty, thin-shelled particles resembling outer viral capsids (group C) (Fig. 5-3), or a heterogeneous mixture of empty single- and double-shelled capsid particles (group D) (Fields *et al.*, 1971). Although these structures have been termed "empty," a close examination reveals that the majority contain electron-dense material similar to that described by Silverstein *et al.* (1974) within particles that accumulate in wild-type infected cells in the presence of high concentrations of actinomycin D. Whether these structures contain viral ssRNA or are devoid of nucleic acid has not yet been determined. The appearance of "empty" capsids in these two mutant groups is consistent with the observation that replication of progeny dsRNA does not occur. These structures are presumably by-products of the ineffectual assembly of immature virion precursor particles

Fig. 5. (1) Group A mutant: Each virion displays an electron-dense RNA core surrounded by inner (single arrow) and outer (double arrow) protein shells. Surrounding the virions are 5-nm kinky filaments. ×200,000. (2) Group B mutant: Note that each particle lacks the normal outer protein shell. The inner shell is present (single arrow). ×200,000. (3) Group C mutant: These particles consist of outer capsid material. ×200,000. Modified from Fields *et al.* (1971).

within which dsRNA is replicated. The group C and D mutants are therefore arrested at an even earlier stage of morphogenesis than mutants of group A, F, B, or G. Analysis of these products may help elucidate the morphogenetic pathway of reovirions.

Additional studies have been done to determine the nature of the particles formed in cells infected with the group C mutant *ts*447 (Matsuhisa and Joklik, 1974). In contrast to wild type, *ts*447 forms two types of empty or top component particles at 33°C; these are H and L particles with buoyant densities of 1.31 and 1.30 g/cm³, respectively. The polypeptide composition and morphology of the H top component particles are indistinguishable from those of wild type. While the wild-type and *ts*447 H particles possess all seven structural polypeptides, L component particles contain all of those in the outer shell ($\mu2$, $\sigma1$, $\sigma3$) and two of those in the inner shell ($\lambda2$, $\mu1$), but lack polypeptides $\lambda1$ and $\sigma2$. The last two polypeptides are located on the innermost surface of the core (Martin *et al.,* 1973). Furthermore, while the capsids of wild-type or H particles are thick and consist of a double shell, L particle capsids are only about half as thick and appear to possess only a single outer shell. In this respect, they resemble the structures observed by electron microscopy in cells infected with *ts*447 at 39°C (Fields *et al.,* 1971, Fig. 5-3). This finding of a heterogeneous population of top component, consisting of H and L particles, may reflect the intermediate temperature (33°C) at which these studies were performed. It is difficult, however, to analyze the thin-walled structures synthesized at 39°C because of the small quantities produced at this temperature (Fields, unpublished data). Analysis of the *ts*447 L top component particles as well as the *ts*447 dsRNA-synthesizing structures (Section 3.3) led Matsuhisa and Joklik (1974) to suggest that the lesion of *ts*447 affects either core polypeptide $\lambda1$ or $\sigma2$, resulting in a failure to replicate dsRNA at the restrictive temperature.

The defect in viral assembly in cells infected with the group E mutant has been difficult to analyze because of the "leaky" nature of the single mutant within this group. However, the E group is believed to have a defect in a very early function (Ito and Joklik, 1972*a*).

3.6. Oligonucleotides

The small single-stranded oligoadenylates, oligo(A), present within the inner capsid of reovirions represent an interesting class of molecules whose function is poorly understood. Each virion contains about 850 copies of these molecules, which vary in chain length from 2 to 20 adenylate residues (Nichols *et al.*, 1972). An oligo(A)-synthesizing activity has recently been detected in purified virions, in infectious subviral particles derived by limited chymotrypsin digestion (Stoltzfus *et al.*, 1974), and in a particulate fraction derived from infected cells (Silverstein *et al.*, 1974). It has been suggested that the oligo(A) polymerase is an alternative activity of the virion ssRNA transcriptase (Nichols *et al.*, 1972; Joklik, 1973).

In an attempt to clarify the role of oligo(A) in the viral replicative cycle, *ts* mutants that are blocked at various stages of replication at the nonpermissive temperature were examined for their ability to synthesize oligo(A) (Johnson *et al.*, 1976). While all of the mutants were found to make oligo(A) at 31°C, none of the mutants carried out this synthesis at 39°C. It is not surprising that mutants which fail to replicate dsRNA (groups C, D, and E) or which accumulate subviral particles lacking an outer shell (groups B and G) are deficient in synthesis of oligo(A). Oligo(A) is formed within immature virions after completion of dsRNA synthesis (Silverstein *et al.*, 1974). It has been hypothesized that the core-associated ssRNA transcriptase within nascent particles is converted to an oligo(A) polymerase as a result of a regulatory effect by outer shell proteins during a late step in viral morphogenesis (Nichols *et al.*, 1972; Silverstein *et al.*, 1974; Stoltzfus *et al.*, 1974). The fact that cells infected with mutants of groups A and F, which synthesize normal quantities of both dsRNA and ssRNA and assemble particles that are morphologically indistinguishable from mature virions, do not synthesize any detectable quantities of oligo(A) is somewhat unexpected. The group A and F particles that accumulate at 39°C are not, however, infectious. While it is unlikely that an absence of oligo(A) accounts for lack of infectivity (Carter *et al.*, 1974), failure to synthesize oligo(A) suggests that the final stage of viral assembly in these mutants is defective. Mutants of groups A and F both possess an aberrant $\mu2$ polypeptide which is a major outer capsid species (Cross and Fields, 1976*b*); the group A mutants also contain a mutation in genome segment L2 that codes for one of the core polypeptides (Ito and Joklik, 1972*b*; Schuerch and Joklik, 1973). It is possible, therefore, that the inability of either of these polypeptide species to achieve a proper configuration within the maturing virion prevents the triggering of synthesis of oligo(A). A possible reason might be that the aberrant $\mu2$ polypeptide cannot exert a regulatory effect on the core-associated transcriptase, thereby converting it to an oligo(A) polymerase. Alternatively, a defective core polypeptide may not respond normally. The results of these studies therefore corroborate others, indicating that oligo(A) synthesis is a late event that coincides with final stages in the assembly of mature, infectious virions, but they reveal little about the function of oligo(A).

3.7. Specific Gene Lesions

A variety of methods have been used in an attempt to gain insight into the specific segment of the genome on which the *ts* mutation of each of the different groups resides. These have included biochemical and ultrastructural as well as genetic approaches. Although preliminary data have suggested a meaningful pattern, the different approaches have, in some instances, produced disparate answers. The purpose of this part of the discussion is to describe the various approaches as well as their potential difficulties and limitations.

3.7.1. Analysis of Hybrid dsRNA Molecules

Ito and Joklik (1972*b*) observed that certain species of heterologous dsRNA molecules composed of mutant (+) RNA strands and wild-type (−) RNA strands migrate slightly more slowly when electrophoresed in polyacrylamide gels than homologous hybrids in which both strands are either mutant or wild type, or than "reverse" hybrids composed of mutant (−) strands and wild-type (+) strands. The extent of hybrid retardation is greatly enhanced in gels that contain reagents (urea or formamide) which reduce hydrogen bond formation, suggesting that this effect is related to some feature of secondary structure. It was postulated that mutation of a base at a critical site results in mismatching and the formation of looped structures upon hybridization, which are retarded in electrophoretic mobility.

Detailed analysis of 35 available *ts* mutants has revealed several anomalous electrophoretic migration patterns (Ito and Joklik, 1972*b*; Schuerch and Joklik, 1973). Half of the group A mutants (13/26) yield retarded L2 hybrids, one of which also exhibits a retarded S3 species, and another a retarded "reverse" M1 species. Two of the three spontaneous non-temperature-sensitive revertants derived from a group A mutant (*ts*340) with an anomalous L2 RNA hybrid do not yield retarded hybrids. One of the group D mutants (*ts*357) yields both retarded L1 and M2 hybrids; the group E mutant (*ts*320) yields retarded L2 and S3 hybrids. A non-temperature-sensitive revertant of the group E mutant still possesses a retarded L2 hybrid, but exhibits a normally migrating S3 species. Aberrant migration is observed *in vitro* and *in vivo* when the mutant (+) RNA is synthesized at the permissive or at the nonpermissive temperature; this indicates that it is an intrinsic property of mutant RNA. No mutants in groups B, C, F, and G exhibit alteration in the electrophoretic migration of molecules of hybrid RNA.

Schuerch and Joklik (1973) have concluded on the basis of these observations that hybrid retardation appears to be mutant group specific. In those instances in which two retarded hybrids are detected, only one presumably represents the temperature-sensitive lesion, because reversion frequencies are not unusually low. Thus the mutations that lead to temperature sensitivity of groups A and E are proposed to reside in genome RNA segments L2 and S3, respectively, and the temperature-sensitive lesion of group D in the M2 genome segment, which is believed to be linked to an alteration in the polypeptide for which it codes (Section 3.7.2a).

3.7.2. Analysis of Variant Viral Polypeptides

3.7.2a. Group D Mutant Polypeptides

Controlled digestion of group D virions to cores by chymotrypsin has suggested that mutants of this group have an altered structural $\mu2$ polypeptide (Ito and Joklik, 1972c). While the principal derivative of the $\mu2$ polypeptide of ts^+ and groups C and E virus is a component "D," in the case of group D mutant $ts357$ a component denoted "D′" that is significantly smaller has been detected. This novel intermediate is not derived from digestion of the $\mu2$ polypeptide of the group D mutant $ts585$, but the kinetics of its digestion is slower than that of ts^+.

Because group D mutants appear to possess abnormal $\mu2$ polypeptides, and one of the mutants ($ts357$) also yields a retarded M2 hybrid dsRNA molecule (Section 3.7.1), it has been concluded that the group D-specific mutation to temperature sensitivity is in the M2 genome segment (which was presumed to code for $\mu2$). However, in light of recent observations (Section 3.7.2b) indicating that other mutant groups (A, F, and G), in addition to group D mutant $ts357$, possess aberrant $\mu2$ polypeptides (although they do not yield retarded M2 hybrid dsRNA species), it is no longer clear that this is a defect specific for group D. Thus, although the correlation of a retarded hybrid to an altered gene product is consistent, it may not necessarily constitute proof that hybrid retardation, as suggested by Schuerch and Joklik (1973), signifies a group-specific *ts* mutation.

3.7.2b.   Analysis of $\mu 1/\mu 2$ Polypeptides

Four of the groups of mutants (A, D-*ts*357, F, and G) synthesize $\mu 1$ and $\mu 2$ polypeptides that behave aberrantly on polyacrylamide gels; i.e., the $\mu 1$ polypeptide and its cleavage product $\mu 2$ migrate faster than the respective wild-type polypeptides (Section 3.4). The $\mu 1/\mu 2$ polypeptides of the group A and F mutants have been designated as μ^-, those of group D (*ts*357) and group G, that migrate slightly more rapidly than the group A and F species, have been designated as μ^{--}, and the wild-type polypeptides are μ^+ (Fig. 2) (Cross and Fields, 1976*b*).

The observation that four of the seven *ts* mutant groups exhibit the μ^- or μ^{--} phenotype is not inconsistent with their classification into separate genetic groups. These were defined by the ability of *ts* mutant pairs to yield *ts*$^+$ recombinants among the progeny of mixed infections at the permissive temperature. The mutation resulting in the μ^{--} phenotype of the group D mutant *ts*357 and the group G mutant *ts*453 is distinct from the mutation to temperature sensitivity; numerous spontaneous revertants of these mutants to *ts*$^+$ phenotype still exhibit aberrant μ^{--} polypeptides. Furthermore, it is unlikely that both mutations are responsible for the temperature-sensitive phenotype since the frequency of revertants is not unusually low, as would be expected for double mutants. Revertants of the group F mutant *ts*556 have not been examined. However, in striking contrast to *ts*$^+$ revertants of groups D and G, that retain the μ phenotype of the mutant strain from which they are derived, the spontaneous revertants of the group A mutant *ts*201 display a variety of phenotypes (Fig. 6). Some of the A revertants retain the μ^- phenotype of the group A mutant (Fig. 6D), while a significant number of revertants exhibit a μ^{--} (Fig. 6C) or μ^+ (Fig. 6B) phenotype similar to that of the group D or G mutants and wild type, respectively (Cross and Fields, 1976*c*).

One putative revertant clone of group A mutant *ts*201 retained the μ^- phenotype (clone 101, Fig. 6D) and was analyzed for the possibility that it was not a true revertant but rather a "pseudorevertant" containing a second suppressor mutation (Ramig *et al.*, 1977*c*). Backcrossing clone 101 with wild type yielded progeny of two types. One progeny type had a wild type efficiency of plating. The other had a temperature-

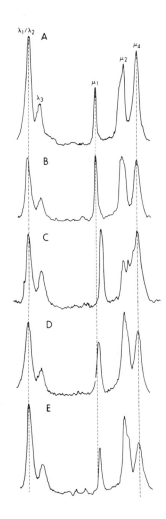

Fig. 6. Densitometer tracing of autoradiogram of large-sized (λ) and medium-sized (μ) cytoplasmic polypeptides of wild type, $ts201$, and three ts^+ revertants derived from $ts201$A. (A) Wild type, (B) clone 108, (C) clone 107, (D) clone 101, and (E) $ts201$A. From Cross and Fields (1976c).

sensitive phenotype. The ts progeny clones were shown to contain the tsA lesion. These results indicate that the ts lesion of clone 101 was suppressed by an extragenic mutation. The mechanism of this suppression is not yet understood.

The fact that many revertants of the group A mutant ($ts201$) are associated with changes in the μ^{--} or μ^+ suggests that the mutations leading to temperature sensitivity and to the μ^- phenotype may alter the identical polypeptide. The result of preliminary three-factor genetic crosses in which the tsA$^-$ and μ^- mutations appear to be linked also supports this conclusion (Section 2.3). It is particularly appealing to speculate that both the tsA mutation and the determinant of the μ

phenotype reside on a medium-sized (M) genome segment that codes for the $\mu 1/\mu 2$ polypeptides. A mutation that restores a functional tsA$^+$ polypeptide might affect the electrophoretic behavior of the $\mu 1/\mu 2$ polypeptide by introducing a nonsense or missense mutation at a critical site (Section 3.4). It is especially interesting in this regard that the prototype tsA mutant (ts201) used in these studies was originally obtained by proflavin mutagenesis. This mutagen is known to induce frameshift mutations which revert spontaneously and at high frequencies in T4, bacteria, and yeast (for review, see Roth, 1974). There are precedents, especially in the T4 lysosome gene, in which the addition or deletion of nucleic acid base pairs (i.e., frameshift mutations) does, in fact, result in a functional polypeptide species that differs in size from the original species. It will be necessary to examine (1) other proflavin-induced group A mutants, (2) proflavin-induced mutants of other groups, and (3) group A mutants induced by other mutagens to establish whether the unique behavior of group A (ts201) revertants is a result of the induction of ts201 by proflavin, and/or is related to the fact that the tsA mutation is located on the same gene segment that codes for the $\mu 1/\mu 2$ polypeptide. The observation that group A ts mutations might reside on a gene segment in which mutations are extremely frequent or easily tolerated might explain the fact that most of the ts mutants that have been isolated fall into this group. Also consistent with this possibility is the finding that group A mutants are more heat labile than those of groups B, C, D, and E (Fields, unpublished data); this suggests that they possess a ts structural protein (Fenner, 1974). This defective polypeptide may be one of the major outer capsid polypeptides ($\mu 2$ or $\sigma 3$) since viral cores produced by treatment of group A virions with chymotrypsin are not particularly heat labile (Section 3.2).

These analyses have favored the hypothesis that the determinant of the μ phenotype (and also the tsA mutation) is situated on a medium-sized genome RNA segment. However, it is possible that a mutation on another gene segment may have a pleiotropic effect on the $\mu 1/\mu 2$ polypeptide (Section 3.7.2a). Schuerch and Joklik (1973) have concluded that the mutation that causes temperature sensitivity of the group A mutants is in genome segment L2 (Section 3.7.1). This conclusion was based on the observation that 50% of the group A mutants yield retarded L2 hybrids composed of mutant (+) strand and ts^+ (−) strand, and that two out of three revertants of the group A mutant ts340 do not yield retarded L2 hybrids. Additional biochemical studies to determine the molecular basis of the aberrant migration $\mu 1/\mu 2$

polypeptides should reveal more about the nature of the *ts*A mutation. It must also be emphasized that Ito and Joklik (1972*c*) have suggested that the group D mutants possess a *ts* lesion in the M2 segment of RNA (which is presumed to code for the $\mu 1$ polypeptide) on the basis of studies on retardation of hybrid dsRNA (Section 3.7.1) as well as the effect of chymotrypsin on the $\mu 2$ polypeptide (Section 3.7.2a).

3.7.3. Analysis of Aberrant Viral Particles

Group B and G mutant-infected cells accumulate corelike particles (Fields *et al.,* 1971), which have been isolated and characterized (Morgan and Zweerink, 1974). Group C mutant-infected cells accumulate particles resembling empty thin-walled outer capsids (Fields *et al.,* 1971), and an aberrant top component particle has been described (Matsuhisa and Joklik, 1974). While the corelike structures contain reduced amounts of the $\lambda 2$ core polypeptide as well as variable amounts of all outer capsid polypeptides, precluding any insight into a specific protein defect, the aberrant top component particles lack only two polypeptides, $\lambda 1$ and $\sigma 2$. Thus it has been suggested that an inner peptide (Fields *et al.,* 1971) or $\lambda 1$ or $\sigma 2$ (core polypeptides) (Matsuhisa and Joklik, 1974) might be the mutant gene product(s) of group C. However, whether the absent polypeptide of an assembled viral structure is the aberrant gene product of a temperature-sensitive mutation is unclear. It is possible that a primary defect that affects the folding or function of one protein may indirectly result in the improper packaging or assembly of another protein located adjacent to the mutant polypeptide.

3.7.4. Deletion Mutants

Deletion mutants have been used in studies of the genetics of bacteriophage for the purpose of mapping single-site mutations (Benzer, 1961). Because reovirus deletion mutants lack entire genome segments (Section 2.7), they are a potentially useful tool in the assignment of each group-specific *ts* mutation to individual genome segments. The major obstacle to this approach is the fact that pure populations of different deletion mutants are difficult to separate from (1) infectious virions on whose replication they depend and (2) other deletion mutants that are often generated simultaneously. Although recombination between deletion and *ts* mutants does not occur at detectable levels (the reason for which is presently unclear), complementation tests between pairs of deletion and *ts* mutants are feasible (Spandidos and Graham, 1975*a,b*). Spandidos and Graham (1975*a*) have succeeded in obtaining a relatively pure preparation of L1 deletion mutants and have used them to allocate the *ts* lesion of the group C mutant to the L1 genome segment (Section 2.4). This is the only mutant that neither complements defective virions that lack the L1 segment nor is complemented by them.

3.7.5. Three-Factor Crosses

The known biochemical defects (dsRNA, polypeptides) (Sections 3.7.1 and 3.7.2) provide additional genetic markers for defining linkage of a *ts* mutation to a specific gene product. A three-factor cross using such markers has been described in Section 2.3. The results of the cross involving *ts*201 (A) and *ts*357 (D) suggested linkage of the μ^- phenotype to the *ts*A gene. Since many additional studies of this type need to be performed before final conclusions can be made, this must be considered a tentative conclusion. Ramig *et al.* (1977*a*) have found that the genome RNAs and polypeptides of the three reovirus serotypes could be distinguished following analysis by polyacrylamide gel electrophoresis. Analysis of recombinants between serotypes and mutants has allowed the tentative construction of a map correlating the temperature sensitive lesion with a physical segment (Ramig *et al.*, 1977*b*, Sharpe *et al.*, 1977). Four mutants have been mapped in this manner: *ts*C corresponds to S2 RNA; *ts*D to L1 RNA; *ts*E to S3 RNA; *ts*G to S4 RNA. These results disagree with some previous assignments (*ts*C and *ts*D; see Spandidos and Graham, 1975*b*; Ito and Joklik, 1972*b,c*); confirm others (*ts*C and *ts*E; see Matsuhuhisa and Joklik, 1974; Ito and Joklik, 1972*b*); and add a new assignment (*ts*G).

The current status of information concerning potential gene lesions and the methods used to generate them is presented in Table 6. The differences in results indicate discrepancies based on the varieties of approaches discussed in this section, and will undoubtedly be clarified over the next few years. Since little is known about the actual function of each of the reovirus polypeptides in the viral replication cycle, knowledge of the mutated RNA gene segment and corresponding altered gene product, together with extensive data regarding the physiological defects of each mutant group, should provide invaluable

TABLE 6

Current Status of Data Concerning Gene Lesions

Gene segment	Polypeptide	*ts* mutants[b]
L1	λ2[a]	C,[4] D[1,6]
L2	λ1	A,[1] C[3]
L3	λ3	
M1	μ3	
M2	μ1/μ2	D,[1,2] A,[2,5]
M3	μ4(μ0)[a]	
S1	σ1	
S2	σ2	C[3,6]
S3	σ2A[a]	E[1,6]
S4	σ3[a]	G[6]

[a] Gene product assignment based on cycloheximide experiments [four RNA species L1, M3, S3, and S4 and four polypeptides λ2, μ4(μ0), σ2A, and σ3] (Spandidos and Graham, 1975b; Cross and Fields, 1976a).
[b] Method: [1] Hybrid dsRNA method (Ito and Joklik, 1972b; Schuerch and Joklik, 1973). [2] Polypeptide analysis (Ito and Joklik, 1972c; Cross and Fields, 1976b). [3] Particle analysis (Matsuhisa and Joklik, 1974). [4] Deletion mutant complementation (Spandidos and Graham, 1975b). [5] Three-factor cross—aberrant polypeptides (Cross and Fields, 1976c). [6] Serotype genetic cross—RNA segregation (Ramig et al., 1977b).

information regarding the functional aspects of the reovirus gene products.

4. EFFECT ON HOST

4.1. Virus–Cell Interaction

4.1.1. Cytopathic Effect

The seven groups of *ts* mutants differ in their ability to induce cell destruction or cytopathic effect (CPE). Thirty to forty hours after infection at 31°C, extensive damage and lysis are apparent in cells infected with wild type and mutants of all groups except the C and G mutants. There is a delay in the development of CPE in cells infected with the group C mutant. The replicative cycle of this mutant is also delayed, but viral titers equivalent to the wild-type strain are ultimately reached. A premature cytopathic effect (20–30 h after infection) is observed in cells infected with the group G mutant and is associated with a slightly more rapid growth and lower yields of virus.

Two patterns of CPE develop at 39°C. The group A and F mutants rapidly induce extensive CPE similar to that produced by wild type. Fifteen hours after infection, 90–95% of the cells lyse; only cellular debris and nuclei are observed after 24 h. In contrast, a marked reduction in CPE is apparent in cells infected with mutants of groups B, C, D, and E. Twenty-four hours after infection, fewer than 20% of the cells lyse and the majority of the cells exclude the dye, trypan blue (Fields, unpublished data). Despite the fact that at least 90% contain viral antigen, as demonstrated by immunofluorescence, for as long as 7 days after infection, most of the cells remain viable. However, it has not been possible to establish persistently infected cell lines with these mutants at multiplicities of infection of 5–10 PFU/cell. In general, mutant groups A and F, which accumulate a large amount of viral-specific products and assemble noninfectious virions, cause major degrees of cytopathogenicity, while mutant groups B, C, D, and E, which are blocked earlier in replication, are less cytopathogenic.

4.1.2. Microtubules

Electron microscopic examination of the cytological changes that accompany viral infection under nonpermissive conditions has revealed differences in the effect of various mutants on cellular microtubules (Fields *et al.*, 1971). A characteristic feature of reovirus replication is the presence of microtubules coated with newly formed virus-specific proteins within viral factories (Dales, 1963). Coated microtubules are present in cells infected with mutants of groups A, C, D, and F. In contrast, there is a marked reduction in the number of coated micro-tubules in cells infected with group B and G mutants. This has also been confirmed *in vivo* with mutants of groups B and C (Raine and Fields, 1974). Coated microtubules are rarely observed in neurons of animals infected with the group B mutant, while large numbers of these structures are present after infection with the group C mutant.

The common feature of the mutants associated with normal coating of microtubules is the presence of either fully assembled virions (A, F) or empty capsids (C, D, E) in viral inclusions. The B and G mutants, which do not coat microtubules, induce the synthesis of partially assembled subviral particles ("cores") lacking a distinct outer coat. The coincidence of a lack of proper assembly of the outer virus capsid with an inability to stimulate the coating of microtubules suggests that assembly of the outer polypeptide species is the crucial event in this process. It should be noted that although the group B and G mutants assemble particles lacking the outer capsid polypeptides, these polypeptides are synthesized (Section 3.4). In these instances, failure to coat microtubules is not related to the absence of appropriate viral polypeptides.

4.1.3. Interferon

Reovirus is a potent inducer of interferon (Long and Burke, 1971; Oie and Loh, 1971). To gain insight into the mechanism involved in the induction of interferon, Lai and Joklik (1973) have examined the ability of *ts* mutants of six of the seven genetic groups to produce this substance in mouse L fibroblasts. These groups of mutants are blocked at various stages of viral replication under restrictive conditions; this offers an excellent opportunity to explore which viral function(s) is essential for induction of interferon. The results of these studies indicate that while at 31°C each of the mutants induces a quantity of interferon approximately equal to that induced by wild type, all induce markedly reduced amounts (only 1–17% as much) at 38.5°C. There is no correlation between the yield of interferon and the ability of the mutants to synthesize viral dsRNA, ssRNA, and proteins. Mutants that synthesize almost as much viral RNA and protein as wild type do not induce greater quantities of interferon than do those that synthesize negligible amounts of these species. The concentration of interferon induced appears in general to be only proportional to the yield of infectious virus. These observations indicate, therefore, that the induction process is initiated by a very late event in the replication of reovirus, or by the presence of mature progeny virions. In contrast, the mechanism by which UV-irradiated virus induces interferon is clearly different from that which occurs during a productive infection. The interferon-inducing capacity of wild type is decreased by ultraviolet irradiation, but not nearly so dramatically as is the reduction in infectivity (Long and Burke, 1971; Lai and Joklik, 1973). The ability of the group C mutant *ts*447 to induce interferon at 39°C, a temperature at which it is a poor inducer, is enhanced over thirtyfold after ultraviolet irradiation. However, negligible quantities of viral RNA (or infectious virus) are made under these conditions. It has been suggested that there may be a relation between the cytopathogenicity of UV-inactivated virus and stimulation of interferon; *ts*447 becomes quite cytopathic at 39°C only after irradiation.

Reovirus is also quite sensitive to the action of interferon (Wiebe and Joklik, 1975). Recent studies have been directed to define the stage in replication of reovirus that is inhibited by interferon (Wiebe and Joklik, 1975). The group C mutant (*ts*447), which is incapable at 39°C of synthesizing progeny dsRNA and late mRNA, was used in order to study the effects of interferon on early viral mRNA transcription and translation. The results of these studies indicate that, although transcription of early mRNA is only slightly sensitive to interferon (about 20% inhibition in cells treated with 75 PRD_{50}/ml), the translation of early mRNA, particularly the species that codes for polypeptide $\lambda 1$, is inhibited much more intensely (about 72% at 75 PRD_{50}/ml for the most sensitive species). Late viral functions such as the formation of progeny dsRNA, the transcription of late mRNA, and the formation of infectious virus are also suppressed (about 80%) after treatment of wild-type-infected cells with interferon. Because the $\lambda 1$ polypeptide is a component of the dsRNA replication complexes, on whose formation the expression of these late viral functions depends, it has been argued that the primary target for inhibition of replication of reovirus in interferon-treated cells is the translation of early mRNA and specifically the species that codes for the $\lambda 1$ polypeptide.

4.2. Role in Disease

The availability of well-defined viral mutants provides a tool for determination of the contribution of individual viral genes and gene products to the ultimate impact of the virus on the production of specific disease syndromes. Such an approach has been used in the study of the effect of wild type and two groups of *ts* mutants (B and C) on the central nervous system of young rats (Fields, 1972; Raine and Fields, 1974). Inoculation of the parental *ts*$^+$ strain into brains of newborn or suckling rodents causes an acute, highly lethal encephalitis; under appropriate conditions, almost 100% of the animals die. The site of viral replication and primary destruction is the neural cells. The pathology of infected brains is characterized by extensive necrosis and hemorrhage throughout the cerebral tissue (Margolis *et al.,* 1971; Raine and Fields, 1973; Raine and Fields, 1974).

Mutants of groups B and C are strikingly attenuated in their ability to produce acute encephalitis. A smaller percentage of animals (25–50%) die or develop acute illness. The pathoanatomical changes are similar to those induced by the parent strain. Survivors of group C infections exhibit no long-term residua. However, the animals that survive infection with group B mutants develop, after several weeks, an illness characterized by a reduced rate of growth and a "humped" posture. Examination of their brains reveals degeneration of cerebral tissue and hydrocephalus *ex vacuo.*

Ts mutants persist for 6–8 weeks in brain tissue of animals infected with both B and C mutants; however, virus cannot be isolated either directly or by cocultivation after that time. There is no evidence that the *ts* mutant strain has reverted to *ts⁺ in vivo.* The kinetics and levels of neutralizing antibody reached are the same in animals infected with either group of mutants (Raine and Fields, 1974; Fields, unpublished data).

These observations suggest that specific *ts* mutant lesions are associated with altered pathological properties. Particularly striking is the ability of the group B mutant to cause chronic neurological disease instead of the clinically apparent, acute, necrotizing encephalitis characteristic of wild-type infection. The group B mutant is blocked at a stage in assembly that results in the accumulation of corelike structures that lack a major portion of the outer coat (Fields *et al.,* 1971; Morgan and Zweerink, 1974). Fields (1972) has speculated that the *ts* defect of this mutant may play a specific role in establishing viral persistence and a chronic neurological syndrome. A parallel has been drawn between the inability of the group B mutant to assemble its outer coat and the inefficient assembly of the outer coat of the measleslike virus associated with the chronic neurological illness and viral persistence characteristic of subacute sclerosing panencephalitis (Fields, 1972). Whether specific mutations in outer coat proteins are, in fact, factors related to the altered pathological changes produced by group B reovirus mutants and the agents of SSPE remains an intriguing possibility.

Ikegami and Gomatos (1968) have carried out similar experiments with *ts* mutants, and have examined the production of disease in newborn hamsters. Wild type is highly neurovirulent at very low doses, while, as in the similar studies of Fields and Raine, all of the mutants are considerably attenuated. Ultrastructural examination of brain tissue was not performed and long-term effects were not studied; the experiments were terminated after 3 weeks.

Spandidos and Graham (1976*d*) utilizing a subcantaneous route of inoculation, confirmed that both the B and C mutants induce acute encephalitis in only a small percentage of infected rats. Defective virus lacking the L1 segment of the viral genome was recovered from brains both during the acute and chronic phase. In addition, defective virus exerted a protective effect when inoculated intracerebrally with the wild type virus. These authors have suggested that these defective viruses may play a major role in determining the course of this neurotropic infection.

ACKNOWLEDGMENTS

The authors wish to thank Dr. A. Graham, Dr. A. Shatkin, Dr. S. Silverstein, and Dr. H. Zweerink for making available preprints of unpublished data. The authors wish to thank particularly Dr. W. K. Joklik, in whose laboratory these studies were initiated and whose continued encouragement helped make this work possible.

Research by the authors was supported by Research Grant AI-10326 from the National Institutes of Health.

5. REFERENCES

Acs, G., Klett, H., Schonberg, M., Christman, J. K., Levin, D. H., and Silverstein, S. C., 1971, Mechanisms of reovirus double-stranded ribonucleic acid synthesis *in vivo* and *in vitro*, *J. Virol.* **8**:684.

Bellamy, A. R., and Joklik, W. K., 1967, Studies on reovirus RNA. II. Characterization of reovirus messenger RNA and the genome RNA segments from which it is transcribed, *J. Mol. Biol.* **29**:19.

Bellamy, A. R., Shapiro, L., August, J. T., and Joklik, W. K., 1967, Studies on reovirus RNA. I. Characterization of reovirus genome RNA, *J. Mol. Biol.* **29**:1.

Benzer, S., 1961, On the topography of the genetic fine structure, *Proc. Natl. Acad. Sci. USA* **47**:403.

Both, G. W., Lavi, S., and Shatkin, A. J., 1975, Synthesis of all the gene products of the reovirus genome *in vivo* and *in vitro*, *Cell* **4**:173.

Carter, C., Stoltzfus, C. M., Banerjee, A. K., and Shatkin, A. J., 1974, Origin of reovirus oligo(A), *J. Virol.* **13**:1331.

Chang, C.-T., and Zweerink, H. J., 1971, Fate of parental reovirus in infected cells, *Virology* **46**:544.

Cooper, P. D., 1968, A genetic map of poliovirus temperature-sensitive mutants, *Virology* **35**:584.

Cross, R. K., 1975, Characterization of temperature-sensitive mutants of reovirus type 3, Ph.D. Thesis, Albert Einstein College of Medicine.

Cross, R. K., and Fields, B. N., 1972, Temperature-sensitive mutants of reovirus type 3: Studies on the synthesis of viral RNA, *Virology* **50**:799.

Cross, R. K., and Fields, B. N., 1976a, Studies on reovirus specific polypeptides: Analysis using discontinuous gel electrophoresis, *J. Virol.* **19**:162.

Cross, R. K., and Fields, B. N., 1976b, Temperature-sensitive mutants of reovirus type 3: Evidence for aberrant μ1 and μ2 polypeptides species, *J. Virol.* **19**:174.

Cross, R. K., and Fields, B. N., 1976c, Use of an aberrant polypeptide as a marker in three-factor crosses: Further evidence for independent reassortment as the mechanism of recombination between temperature-sensitive mutants of reovirus type 3, *Virology* **74**:345.

Dahlberg, J. E., and Simon, E. H., 1969*a*, Recombination in Newcastle disease virus (NDV): The problem of complementing heterozygotes, *Virology* **38**:490.

Dahlberg, J. E., and Simon, E. H., 1969*b*, Physical and genetic studies of Newcastle disease virus: Evidence for multiploid particles, *Virology* **38**:666.

Dales, S., 1963, Association between the spindle apparatus and reovirus, *Proc. Natl. Acad. Sci. USA* **50**:268.

DeVilliers, E. H., 1974, Comparison of the capsid polypeptides of various bluetongue virus serotypes, *Intervirology* **3**:47.

Duesberg, P. H., and Robinson, W. S., 1967, On the structure of and replication of influenza virus, *J. Mol. Biol.* **25**:383.

Fenner, F., 1974, Virus genetics, in: *The Biology of Animal Viruses* (F. Fenner, B. R. McAuslan, C. A. Mims, K. J. Sambrook, and D. O. White, eds.), pp. 274–318, Academic Press, New York.

Fields, B. N., 1971, Temperature-sensitive mutants of reovirus type 3: Features of genetic recombination, *Virology* **46**:142.

Fields, B. N., 1972, Genetic manipulation of reovirus—A model for modification of disease? *N. Engl. J. Med.* **287**:1026.

Fields, B. N., 1973, Genetic reassortment with reovirus mutants, in: *Virus Research* (F. Fox, ed.), p. 461, Academic Press, New York.

Fields, B. N., and Joklik, W. K., 1969, Isolation and preliminary genetic and biochemical characterization of temperature-sensitive mutants of reovirus, *Virology* **37**:335.

Fields, B. N., Raine, C. S., and Baum, S. G., 1971, Temperature-sensitive mutants of reovirus type 3: Defects in virus maturation as studied by immunofluorescence and electron microscopy, *Virology* **43**:569.

Fields, B. N., Laskov, R., and Scharff, M. D., 1972, Temperature-sensitive mutants of reovirus type 3: Studies on the synthesis of viral peptides, *Virology* **50**:209.

Furuichi, Y., Muthukrishnan, S., and Shatkin, A. J., 1975, 5′-terminal m⁷G(5′)ppp(5′)G^mp *in vivo*: Identification in reovirus genome RNA, *Proc. Natl. Acad. Sci. USA* **72**:742.

Granboulan, N., and Girard, M., 1969, Molecular weight of poliovirus ribonucleic acid, *J. Virol.* **4**:475.

Graziadei, W. D., and Lengyel, P., 1972, Translation of *in vitro* synthesized reovirus messenger RNAs into proteins of the size of reovirus capsid proteins in a mouse L-cell extract, *Biochem. Biophys. Res. Commun.* **46**:1816.

Hirst, G. K., 1962, Genetic recombination with Newcastle disease virus, polioviruses, and influenza, *Cold Spring Harbor Symp. Quant. Biol.* **27**:303.

Hirst, G. K., 1973, Mechanism of influenza recombination. I. Factors influencing recombination rates between temperature sensitive mutants of strain WSN and the classification of mutants into complementation-recombination groups, *Virology* **55**:81.

Hirst, G. K., and Pons, M. W., 1973, Mechanism of influenza virus recombination. II. Virus aggregation and its effect on plaque formation by so-called noninfectious virus, *Virology* **56**:620.

Ikegami, N., and Gomatos, P. J., 1968, Temperature-sensitive conditional-lethal mutants of reovirus 3. I. Isolation and characterization, *Virology* **36**:447.

Ikegami, N., and Gomatos, P. J., 1972, Inhibition of host and viral protein syntheses during infection at the nonpermissive temperature with ts mutants of reovirus 3, *Virology* **47**:306.

Ito, Y., and Joklik, W. J., 1972*a*, Temperature-sensitive mutants of reovirus. I. Patterns of gene expression by mutants of groups C, D, and E, *Virology* **50**:189.

Ito, Y., and Joklik, W. K., 1972*b*, Temperature-sensitive mutants of reovirus. II. Anomalous electrophoretic migration behavior of certain molecules composed of mutant plus strands and wild type minus strands, *Virology* **50**:202.

Ito, Y., and Joklik, W. K., 1972*c*, Temperature-sensitive mutants of reovirus. III. Evidence that mutants of group D ("RNA-negative") are structural polypeptide mutants, *Virology* **50**:282.

Johnson, R. B., Soeiro, R., and Fields, B. N., 1976, The synthesis of A-rich RNA by temperature-sensitive mutants of reovirus, *Virology* **73**:173.

Joklik, W. K., 1973, Reovirus: A virus with a segmented double-stranded RNA genome, in: *Viral Replication and Cancer* (J. L. Melnick, S. Ochoa, and J. Oró, eds.), pp. 123–153, Editorial Labor, S.A., Barcelona.

Joklik, W. K., 1974, Reproduction of reoviridae, in: *Comprehensive Virology,* Vol. 2 (H. Frankel-Conrat and R. R. Wagner, eds.), Plenum Press, New York.

Kilbourne, E. D., 1963, Influenza virus genetics, *Prog. Med. Virol.* **5**:79.

Krystal, G., Winn, P., Millward, S., and Sakuma, S., 1975, Evidence for phosphoproteins in reovirus, *Virology* **64**:505.

Kudo, H., and Graham, A. F., 1965, Synthesis of reovirus ribonucleic acid in L cells, *J. Bacteriol.* **90**:936.

Lai, M.-H. T., and Joklik, W. K., 1973, The induction of interferon by temperature-sensitive mutants of reovirus, UV-irradiated reovirus, and subviral reovirus particles, *Virology* **51**:191.

Long, W. F., and Burke, D. C., 1971, A comparison of interferon induction by reovirus RNA and synthetic double-stranded polynucleotides, *J. Gen. Virol.* **12**:1.

Mackenzie, J. S., 1970, Isolation of temperature-sensitive mutants and the construction of a preliminary genetic map for influenza virus, *J. Gen. Virol.* **6**:63.

Margolis, G., Kilham, L., and Gomatos, N., 1971, Reovirus type III encephalitis: Observations of virus-cell interactions in neural tissues. I. Light microscopy studies, *Lab. Invest.* **24**:91.

Martin, S. A., Pett, D. M., and Zweerink, H. J., 1973, Studies on the topography of reovirus and bluetongue virus capsid polypeptides, *J. Virol.* **12**:194.

Matsuhisa, T., and Joklik, W. K., 1974, Temperature-sensitive mutants of reovirus. V. Studies on the nature of the temperature-sensitive lesion of the C group mutant ts447, *Virology* **60**:380.

McClain, M. E., and Spendlove, R. S., 1966, Multiplicity reactivation of reovirus particles after exposure to ultraviolet light, *J. Bacteriol.* **92**:1422.

McDowell, M. J., Joklik, W. K., Villa-Komaroff, L., and Lodish, H. F., 1972, Translation of reovirus messenger RNAs synthesized *in vitro* into reovirus polypeptides by several mammalian cell-free extracts, *Proc. Natl. Acad. Sci. USA* **69**:2649.

Millward, S., and Graham, A. F., 1974, Reovirus: Early events in the infected cell and structure of the double-stranded RNA genome, in: *Viruses, Evolution, and Cancer* (M. Kurstak and W. Maramarosch, eds.), p. 651, Academic Press, New York.

Morgan, E. M., and Zweerink, H. J., 1974, Reovirus morphogenesis: Core-like particles in cells infected at 39° with wild type and temperature-sensitive mutants of groups B and G, *Virology* **59**:556.

Nichols, J. L., Bellamy, A. R., and Joklik, W. K., 1972, Identification of the nucleotide sequences of the oligonucleotides present in reovirions, *Virology* **49**:562.

Nonoyama, M., and Graham, A. F., 1970, Appearance of defective virions in clones of reovirus, *J. Virol.* **6**:693.

Nonoyama, M., Watanabe, Y., and Graham, A. F., 1970, Defective virions of reovirus, *J. Virol.* **6**:226.

Oie, H. K., and Loh, P. C., 1971, Reovirus type 2: Induction of viral resistance and interferon production in fathead minnow cells, *Proc. Soc. Exp. Biol. Med.* **136**: 369.

Pons, M. W., and Hirst, G. W., 1969, The single- and double-stranded RNAs and the proteins of incomplete influenza virus, *Virology* **38**:68.

Pringle, C. R., and Duncan, I. B., 1971, Preliminary physiological characterization of temperature-sensitive mutants of vesicular stomatitis virus, *J. Virol.* **8**:56.

Raine, C. S., and Fields, B. N., 1973, Reovirus type III encephalitis—A virologic and ultrastructural study, *J. Neuropathol. Exp. Neurol.* **32**:19.

Raine, C. S., and Fields, B. N., 1974, Neurotropic virus–host relationship alterations due to variation in viral genome as studied by electron microscope, *Am. J. Pathol.* **75**:119.

Ramig, R. F., Cross, R. K., and Fields, B. N., 1977*a*, Genome RNAs and polypeptides of reovirus serotypes 1, 2, and 3, *J. Virol.* (in press).

Ramig, R. F., Sharpe, A., Mustoe, T., and Fields, B. N., 1977*b*, A genetic map of reovirus. II. Assignment of temperature-sensitive lesions to genome segments, submitted for publication.

Ramig, R. F., White R. M., and Fields, B. N., 1977*c*, Suppression of the temperature-sensitive phenotype of a mutant of reovirus type 3, *Science* **195**:406.

Roth, J. R., 1974, Frameshift mutations. *Annu. Rev. Genet.* **8**:319.

Sakuma, S., and Watanabe, Y., 1971, Unilateral synthesis of reovirus double-stranded ribonucleic acid by a cell-free replicase system, *J. Virol.* **8**:190.

Schonberg, M., Silverstein, S. C., Levin, D. H., and Acs, G., 1971, Asynchronous synthesis of the complementary strands of the reovirus genome, *Proc. Natl. Acad. Sci. USA* **68**:505.

Schuerch, A. R., and Joklik, W. K., 1973, Temperature-sensitive mutants of reovirus. IV. Evidence that anomalous electrophoretic migration behavior of certain double-stranded RNA hybrid species is mutant group-specific, *Virology* **56**:218.

Schuerch, A. R., Matsuhisa, T., and Joklik, W. K., 1974, Temperature-sensitive mutants of reovirus. VI. Mutant *ts*447 and *ts*556 particles that lack either one or two genome segments, *Intervirology* **3**:36.

Sharpe, A. S., Ramig., R. F., Mustoe, T. A., and Fields, B. N., 1977, A genetic map of reovirus. I. correlation of genome RNA's between serotypes 1, 2, and 3, submitted for publication.

Shatkin, A. J., and Rada, B., 1967, Reovirus-directed ribonucleic acid synthesis in infected L cells, *J. Virol.* **1**:24.

Shatkin, A. J., Sipe, J. D., and Loh, P., 1968, Separation of ten reovirus segments by polyacrylamide gel electrophoresis, *J. Virol.* **2**:986.

Silverstein, S. C., and Dales, S., 1968, The penetration of reovirus RNA and initiation of its genetic function in L-strain fibroblasts, *J. Cell Biol.* **36**:197.

Silverstein, S. C., Schonberg, M., Levin, D. H., and Acs, G., 1970, The reovirus replicative cycle: Conservation of parental RNA and protein, *Proc. Natl. Acad. Sci. USA* **67**:275.

Silverstein, S. C., Astell, C., Levin, D. H., Schonberg, M., and Acs, G., 1972, The mechanisms of reovirus uncoating and gene activation *in vivo, Virology* **47**:797.

Silverstein, S. C., Astell, C., Christman, J., Klett, H., and Acs, G., 1974, Synthesis of reovirus oligoadenylic acid *in vivo* and *in vitro, J. Virol.* **13**:740.

Simpson, R. W., and Hirst, G. K., 1968, Temperature-sensitive mutants of influenza A virus: Isolation of mutants and preliminary observations on genetic recombination and complementation, *Virology* **35**:41.

Skehel, J. J., and Joklik, W. K., 1969, Studies on the *in vitro* transcription of reovirus RNA catalyzed by reovirus cores, *Virology* **39**:822.

Spandidos, D. A., and Graham, A. F., 1975a, Complementation of defective reovirus by *ts* mutants, *J. Virol.* **15**:954.

Spandidos, D. A., and Graham, A. F., 1975b, Complementation between temperature-sensitive and deletion mutants of reovirus, *J. Virol.* **16**:1444.

Spandidos, D. A., and Graham, A. F., 1976a, Recombination between temperature-sensitive and deletion mutants of reovirus, *J. Virol.* **18**:117.

Spandidos, D. A., and Graham, A. F., 1976b. Infectious center assay for complementation and recombination between mutants of reovirus, *J. Virol.* **18**:1151.

Spandidos, D. A., and Graham, A. F., 1976c, Nonpermissive infection of L cells by an avian reovirus: Restricted transcription of the viral genome, *J. Virol.* **19**:977.

Spandidos, D. A., and Graham, A. F., 1976d, Generation of defective virus after infection of newborn rats with reovirus, *J. Virol.* **20**:234.

Spandidos, D. A., Krystal, G., and Graham, A. F., 1976, Regulated transcription of the genomes of defective virions and temperature-sensitive mutants of reovirus, *J. Virol.* **18**:7.

Stoltzfus, C. M., Morgan, M., Banerjee, A. K., and Shatkin, A. J., 1974, Poly(A) polymerase activity in reovirus, *J. Virol.* **13**:1338.

Sugiura, A., Tobita, K., and Kilbourne, E. D., 1972, Isolation and preliminary characterization of temperature-sensitive mutants of influenza virus, *J. Virol.* **10**:639.

Watanabe, Y., and Graham, A. F., 1967, Structural units of reovirus ribonucleic acid and their possible functional significance, *J. Virol.* **1**:665.

Watanabe, Y., Millward, S., and Graham, A. F., 1968, Regulation of transcription of the reovirus genome, *J. Mol. Biol.* **36**:107.

Weiss, R. A., Mason, W. S., and Vogt, P. K., 1973, Genetic recombinants and heterozygotes derived from endogenous and exogenous avian RNA tumor viruses, *Virology* **52**:535.

Wiebe, M. E., and Joklik, W. K., 1975, The mechanism of inhibition of reovirus replication by interferon, *Virology* **66**:229.

Zweerink, H. J., 1974, Multiple forms of SS → DS RNA polymerases activity in reovirus-infected cells, *Nature (London)* **247**:313.

Zweerink, H. J., and Joklik, W. K., 1970, Studies on intracellular synthesis of reovirus-specified proteins, *Virology* **41**:501.

Zweerink, H. J., Ito, Y., and Matsuhisa, T., 1972, Synthesis of reovirus double-stranded RNA within virus-like particles, *Virology* **50**:349.

CHAPTER 8

Genetics of RNA Tumor Viruses

Peter K. Vogt

Department of Microbiology
University of Southern California School of Medicine
Los Angeles, California 90033

1. INTRODUCTION

1.1. Scope of This Chapter

The genetic analysis of RNA tumor viruses has two main objectives: (1) to provide an understanding of virus replication and (2) to explain virus-induced transformation of the host cell. Virus replication results from a complex interaction of viral and cellular genomes. Viral genetics, however, considers only the virus side of this interaction; the numerous and specific cellular functions which are required for the synthesis of infectious virus will have to be defined by a genetic analysis of the host cell. In virus-induced transformation, viral genetic information presumably interferes with the genetic regulatory apparatus of the host cell, and here again it is important to realize that focusing on the viral information will reveal only part of a very complex interaction between two organisms. Despite these obvious limitations, the viral genome is at the moment that partner in this interaction which is more amenable to experimental study and offers realistic opportunities for an increase of our insight into virus replication and cellular transformation.

This review will deal with the structure and organization of the viral genome, the physiology of conditional and nonconditional viral mutants, genetic and nongenetic interactions affecting viral phenotypes, and the beginnings of a genetic map of avian sarcoma viruses. Genetic transmission of RNA tumor viruses from one host generation to the next will not be considered, and, as practically nothing is known about the genetics of type B viruses, these viruses will not be dealt with. The material reviewed here has been obtained only with type C viruses, which make up the vast majority of RNA tumor viruses. The terms "type C virus" and "RNA tumor virus" will therefore be used interchangeably in the course of this review. For reasons of familiarity, these vernacular names are preferred to the latinized term "Oncovirinae" (a subfamily within the family of Retroviridae), which was recently approved for RNA tumor viruses by the International Committee on Taxonomy of Viruses. In the past 3 years, several excellent review articles dealing with genetic aspects of RNA tumor viruses have appeared; they have been extensively consulted throughout the writing of this chapter and are highly recommended (Tooze, 1973; Wyke, 1974, 1975).

1.2. A Synopsis of RNA Tumor Virus Infection

RNA tumor viruses are enveloped, spherical viruses of approximately 100 nm diameter. They consist of RNA (about 2%), protein (about 65%), lipids (about 30%), and carbohydrates (about 3%). The virion polypeptides are specified by the high molecular weight RNA of the virus; low molecular weight virion RNA, carbohydrates, and lipids are products of the cell. The lipids of the viral envelope are derived from the plasma membrane, but there are some quantitative differences in lipid composition between plasma membrane and envelope (Rao *et al.,* 1966; Quigley *et al.,* 1972). Virion carbohydrates are mainly components of glycolipids and of glycoproteins. The virion contains six to seven structural proteins ranging in molecular weight from approximately 10,000 to 80,000. These proteins are individually referred to by "gp" (for glycoprotein) or "p" (for protein), followed by the first two digits of the five-digit molecular weight. For murine leukemia viruses, this list reads gp69/71, p15E, p30, p15, p12, and p10; for avian sarcoma and leukosis viruses, it reads gp85, gp37, p27, p19, p15, p12, and p10 (Ikeda *et al.,* 1975; Bolognesi, 1974). The glycoproteins protrude as spikes and knobs from the membranous viral envelope; they react with type- and subgroup-specific neutralizing antibody, mediate specific viral interference, and in some RNA tumor viruses control the host range. The envelope surrounds a probably icosahedral core shell composed mainly or exclusively of the largest and most abundant internal viral protein (p30 in the murine and p27 in the avian RNA tumor viruses). The core shell in turn encloses a nucleocapsid which appears to have helical symmetry and contains the virion RNA plus one structural protein (p10 in the murine and p12 in the avian viruses). The location and function of the other virion proteins are not definitely known, but some are phosphorylated (Pal and Roy-Burman, 1975; Pal *et al.*, 1975).

RNA tumor viruses appear to enter susceptible cells by viropexis, by fusion of the viral envelope with the plasma membrane, or by localized dissolution of viral and cellular membranes; there is no agreement on this point (Miyamoto and Gilden, 1971; Dales and Hanafusa, 1972; see also Morgan and Rose, 1968). Entry of virus into host cell requires a specific interaction between viral envelope glycoprotein and cell surface receptor (Piraino, 1967; Crittenden, 1968).

After entry of the virus into the cell, the virion RNA-dependent DNA polymerase becomes activated (Temin and Mizutani, 1970; Baltimore, 1970). Whether this step of infection requires the removal of internal nonglycosylated virion proteins besides the viral envelope is not known. The virion DNA polymearase transcribes the high molecular weight virion RNA first into single- and then into double-stranded DNA (Temin and Baltimore, 1972; Bishop and Varmus, 1975). Viral DNA is synthesized in the cytoplasm during the first few hours after infection, circularizes, then appears to migrate to the nucleus, and becomes integrated into cellular DNA (Hatanaka *et al.*, 1971; Varmus *et al.*, 1973a,b, 1974, 1975a; Lovinger *et al.*, 1974, 1975b; Gianni and Weinberg, 1975; Gianni *et al.*, 1975; Takano and Hatanaka, 1975). There is also some evidence for parental RNA entering the nucleus, but whether this RNA participates in the events which lead to integration is not clear (Dales and Hanafusa, 1972; Sveda *et al.*, 1974; Leis *et al.*, 1975). It appears that integration of the viral genome into cellular DNA is a prerequisite for transformation and for virus production. If integration is prevented by the presence of ethidium bromide during the initial phases of infection, virus synthesis and transformation are also inhibited (Guntaka *et al.*, 1975; see also Roa and Bose, 1974). However, this inhibition has not been seen by all investigators (Richert and Hare, 1972; Bader 1973). Ethidium bromide has no effect on virus synthesis after integration has taken place. Despite these intriguing observations, the possibility that some provirus remains unintegrated and can function in a free state has not been definitely ruled out.

Viral RNA is synthesized from integrated DNA provirus by cellular RNA polymerase II as judged by the sensitivity of this reaction to α-amanitin (Rymo *et al.,* 1974; Weissmann *et al.,* 1975; Dinowitz, 1975). The initiation of viral RNA synthesis shows a requirement for mitosis (Humphries and Temin, 1972, 1974). Newly produced viral RNA is found associated with polyribosomes as messenger RNA and also becomes incorporated into progeny virus. Both messenger and virion RNA have the same plus polarity. There is circumstantial evidence that virion RNA and messenger RNA constitute separate pools (Levin and Rosenak, 1976). Most viral messenger RNA is 35 S in size, but some is smaller (Leong *et al.,* 1972; Tsuchida *et al.,* 1972; Fan and Baltimore, 1973; Schincariol and Joklik, 1973; Shanmugam *et al.,* 1974; Gielkens *et al.,* 1974). Because much of the messenger RNA is large enough to encompass the whole genome, all primary translational products may be polyproteins from which functional viral proteins are derived by proteolytic cleavage, analogous to protein synthesis in poliovirus and other picornaviruses (Jacobson and Baltimore, 1968; Butterworth and Rueckert, 1972; Butterworth, 1973). However, so far only the internal nonglycosylated viral proteins have definitely been shown to come from a polyprotein precursor of about 80,000 molecular weight, although much larger viral polyproteins have been observed (Vogt and Eisenman, 1973; Eisenman *et al.,* 1975; Naso *et al.,* 1975; van Zaane *et al.,* 1975; Vogt *et al.,* 1975). RNA sarcoma viruses also appear to code for a nonvirion transforming protein besides structural proteins and RNA-dependent DNA polymerase. The existence of such a protein can be inferred from temperature-sensitive (*ts*) mutants which replicate but do not transform cells under nonpermissive conditions (Martin, 1970). Transformation of cells infected by such mutants occurs upon shift to permissive conditions but is inhibited in the presence of cycloheximide, suggesting a requirement for new protein synthesis (Kawai and Hanafusa, 1971; Biquard and Vigier, 1972; Bader, 1972). RNA tumor virus transformed cells also have been reported to contain a tumor-specific cell surface antigen (Kurth and Bauer, 1972*a,b*; Meyers *et al.,* 1972; Rohrschneider *et al.,* 1975). Whether this surface antigen is a viral gene product and whether it is related to the transforming protein are still open questions.

Virus release takes place by budding from the plasma membrane. Newly budded virus undergoes a process of extracellular maturation. Thin sections viewed with the electron microscope suggest a transition from particles with an electron-lucent to an electron-dense core (Dalton, 1962). This morphological change is paralleled by alterations in the virion RNA. In young particles, this RNA occurs in the form of 35 S components which are not or only weakly linked to each other; in mature particles, the hydrogen bonding between the 35 S components has become more extensive, resulting in a stable 70 S complex (Cheung *et al.*, 1972; Canaani *et al.*, 1973; Stoltzfus and Snyder, 1975).

2. BASIC PROPERTIES OF THE VIRUS GENOME

2.1. The Virion Contains Cellular and Viral RNA

The genome of RNA tumor viruses is in all probability the high molecular weight single-stranded RNA which can be extracted from virions with SDS and phenol and which sediments at about 60–70 S (Robinson *et al.*, 1965). Contained in the virion are also other RNA species of lower molecular weight sedimenting at 7, 5, and 4 S, respectively (Bishop *et al.*, 1970*a,b*; Faras *et al.*, 1973). Although none of these low molecular weight RNA species codes for viral products, at least some may be essential to the structure and function of the viral genome, and therefore they will be briefly considered at this point. The 7, 5, and 4 S RNA species of RNA tumor viruses are components of the host cells, as are occasional 18 S and 28 S ribosomal RNAs found in some virus preparations (Bishop and Varmus, 1975). The 7 S RNA is found in polyribosomal structures of uninfected cells (Erikson *et al.*, 1973; Walker *et al.*, 1974). The 5 S RNA is a part of the large subunit of normal ribosomes (Faras *et al.*, 1973). The 4 S RNA recovered from RNA tumor viruses represents a selected population of cellular tRNA species (Bonar *et al.*, 1967; Trávníček, 1968; Erikson, 1969; Bishop *et al.*, 1970*a*; Erikson and Erikson, 1970; Waters *et al.*, 1975), and can be divided into 4 S RNA species hydrogen-bonded to the 60–70 S virion RNA and 4 S RNA free inside the virus particle (Erikson and Erikson, 1971). Among those 4 S RNA species bound to the 60–70 S RNA is one which serves as a primer for RNA-dependent DNA synthesis *in vitro* (Canaani and Duesberg, 1972). Its structure has been determined; it is identical to a cellular tryptophan transfer RNA species and shows specific binding affinity to RNA-dependent DNA polymerase (Faras *et al.*, 1974; Dahlberg *et al.*, 1974, 1975; Panet *et al.*, 1975*b*). This 4 S RNA species is the only low molecular weight RNA species in the virion for which a function is known. It is attached to 30–40 S RNA by base pairing and is located near the 5′ end of the molecule (Taylor and

Illmensee, 1975; Faras, 1975). Recent studies indicate that it is the 3′ end of the primer molecule which binds to virion RNA (Eiden *et al.*, 1976). There is about one primer molecule per 30–40 S RNA (Taylor *et al.*, 1975).

2.2. The Molecular Weight of the 60–70 S RNA Is About 6–8 × 10⁶

The molecular weight of the 60–70 S RNA is only approximately known. Using Spirin's formula, Robinson *et al.* (1965) obtained a value of 9.6 × 10⁶ from an $S_{20,w}$ = 64 for the genome of Rous sarcoma virus (RSV). In the light of more recent data, this value may be too high. A lower molecular weight, 6.1 × 10⁶, was obtained by electron microscopy (Mangel *et al.*, 1974; Delius *et al.*, 1975). Bellamy *et al.* (1974) arrived at a molecular weight of between 3.8 and 4.8 × 10⁶ for the 60–70 S RNA of ASV, using an experimentally determined molecular weight of the whole virion as basis for their calculations. As pointed out by these authors, this value for the molecular weight of the 60–70 S RNA assumes that all virions contain about the same amount of RNA and that there is no substantial fraction of virus particles with little or no RNA. If this assumption is incorrect, the molecular weight of the 60–70 S RNA could be considerably higher than the upper limit of 4.8 × 10⁶ given by Bellamy *et al.* (1974). In a recent study, RNA of the Schmidt-Ruppin strain of RSV was measured by sedimentation and by gel electrophoresis and found to have a molecular weight of 7.6 × 10⁶ (King, 1976). Riggin *et al.* (1975) have determined the molecular weight of Moloney murine leukemia virus (MuLV) 60–70 S RNA by sedimentation equilibrium centrifugation. They obtained a value of 7.2 × 10⁶, in good agreement with the figure of 6.9 × 10⁶ published by King (1976). The molecular weight of the 60–70 S RNA has also been measured by electron microscopy for the feline endogenous RNA tumor virus RD114 and was found to be 5.7 × 10⁶ (Kung *et al.*, 1975a). It is probably safe to say that the molecular weight of the 60–70 S RNA is between 5 and 8 × 10⁶. Differences would be expected to exist between different RNA tumor viruses according to the amounts of genetic information which they carry. Some of these differences have been documented (Duesberg and Vogt, 1970; Duesberg *et al.*, 1975a).

2.3. The 60–70 S Complex Consists of Two 35 S RNA Molecules

Upon heating or treatment with DMSO, the sedimentation constant of the 60–70 S RNA is reduced to about 30–40 S (Duesberg,

1968; Montagnier *et al.,* 1969; Erikson, 1969). At the same time, the electrophoretic mobility of the RNA increases. These observations suggest that the processes of heating or treatment with DMSO, both of which disrupt hydrogen bonds, dissociate the 60–70 S RNA into several smaller molecules which presumably are held together by base pairing. The molecular weight of these components of the 60–70 S complex has been estimated from the sedimentation behavior and by electrophoresis in formamide-containing polyacrylamide gels (Duesberg and Vogt, 1973*a*; Maisel *et al.,* 1973). For the 30–40 S RNA derived from a nondefective avian sarcoma virus, the estimated molecular weight is between 2.4 and 3.4 $\times$ 10^6. A more definitive measurement obtained from a combination of sedimentation coefficients and retardation coefficients in gel electrophoresis gives a value of 3.3 $\times$ 10^6 (King, 1976). For a transformation-defective (*td*) avian tumor virus, a deletion mutant of avian sarcoma virus which is able to replicate in single infection but does not induce sarcomas in animals or foci of transformed fibroblasts in tissue culture, the value is 2.2–2.9 $\times$ 10^6. The dissociated RNA of the defective Kirsten murine sarcoma virus (MSV) migrates in formamide-containing gels as a molecule of 2.3 $\times$ 10^6 molecular weight; Kirsten MuLV shows a value of 2.5 $\times$ 10^6. Sedimentation equilibrium centrifugation of the 35 S RNA of Moloney MuLV has given a value of 3.4 $\times$ 10^6 (Riggin *et al.,* 1975). King (1976) obtained a molecular weight of 2.8 $\times$ 10^6 for this RNA species. Based on these molecular weight estimates, the number of 30–40 S RNA molecules per 60–70 S complex is probably two. Electron microscopy, to be discussed below, also suggests that there are only two 30–40 S molecules per 60–70 S complex.

The 3$'$ end of the 30–40 S RNA consists of poly(A), about 200 residues in length (Lai and Duesberg, 1972; Wang and Duesberg, 1974; Quade *et al.,* 1974*b*). Poly(A) is found on most 30–40 S molecules derived from a given virus preparation, and where it is absent it appears to have been lost secondarily as a result of nuclease action (King and Wells, 1976). There are no major differences between poly(A)-containing and poly(A)-lacking 30–40 S RNA molecules, as both show identical nucleotide fingerprint patterns (Wang and Duesberg, 1974; Quade *et al.,* 1974*b*; Rho and Green, 1974). The function of poly(A) in the 30–40 S RNA is not known. Complementary poly(U) has not been found in RNA tumor viruses. At the 5$'$ terminal, the 30–40 S RNA of Rous sarcoma virus carries 7-methylguanosine in 5$'$ linkage with the penultimate nucleotide which is methylated in the 2$'$-*O*-ribose position (Keith and Fraenkel-Conrat, 1975; Furuichi *et al.,* 1975). The significance of this end group which is found in various messenger RNAs is not known.

2.4.   The Genome of RNA Tumor Viruses Appears to Be Diploid

The 30–40 S RNA isolated from cloned virus has a uniform sedimentation constant, migrates as a single peak in polyacrylamide gels, and appears to contain poly(A) at the majority of the 3′ ends. This physical and chemical homogeneity of the 30–40 S RNA from a given RNA tumor virus raises the possibility that the 30–40 S molecules comprising a 60–70 S complex are identical. The 60–70 S complex would then represent a polyploid genome consisting of probably two unit genomes (Vogt, 1973). If, on the other hand, the 60–70 S complex were made up of genetically different 30–40 S RNAs, then the genome of RNA tumor viruses would be haploid, consisting of two genetically specialized 30–40 S segments. The two genome models, polyploid vs. haploid, make different predictions about the genetic complexity of RNA tumor viruses: If the 60–70 S RNA represents a polyploid genome, then its complexity is equal to that of a 30–40 S RNA; if the genome is haploid and segmented, its complexity would correspond to that of a 60–70 S RNA. Determinations of genome complexity have been made, and on balance the results favor a polyploid structure.

Three independent techniques were used to measure genetic complexity of RNA tumor viruses: (1) oligonucleotide fingerprinting, (2) size measurements of infectious DNA, and (3) RNA-DNA hybridization. In the first technique, the RNA was labeled with ^{32}P, digested exhaustively with RNase T_1, and fingerprinted by electrophoresis and chromatography or by two-dimensional gel electrophoresis (Billeter *et al.*, 1974; Quade *et al.*, 1974a; Beemon *et al.*, 1974, 1976; Weissmann *et al.*, 1975; Duesberg *et al.*, 1975b; Ostertag *et al.*, 1975). Oligonucleotides large enough to occur statistically only once in the 60–70 S complex were isolated, and the radioactivity in each oligonucleotide, the total RNA, and the molecular weight of the oligonucleotides were determined. The complexity of the RNA could then be computed according to the following formula:

$$\frac{cpm_{RNA}}{cpm_{olig}} = \frac{MW_{RNA}}{MW_{olig}}$$

where the molecular weight of the RNA refers to that of unique sequences. The four laboratories that have used this approach agree that the complexity of the RNA tumor virus genome corresponds to an RNA of about 3×10^6 molecular weight in unique sequences.

Infectious viral DNA has been obtained from RNA tumor virus-infected cells, indicating that the entire viral genome is present in the form of a provirus (Hill and Hillova, 1972; Karpas and Milstein, 1973). The smallest size of such DNA which is still infectious, showing single-hit kinetics of infection, has a molecular weight of about 6×10^6, corresponding in complexity to the 30–40 S RNA (Montagnier and Vigier, 1972; Hill and Hillova, 1974; Cooper and Temin, 1974, 1975; Levy et al., 1974; Hill et al., 1975; Smotkin et al., 1975).

With RNA-DNA hybridization, conflicting data have been obtained both in support of a highly complex and thus haploid genome of 10^7 molecular weight (Taylor et al., 1974; Fan and Paskind, 1974) and in support of the less complex and therefore polyploid genome (Baluda et al., 1975). These discrepancies probably result from the choice of different molecular weight standards for the RNA, and different hybridization conditions, both of which have a considerable influence on the results of complexity measurements. The conflict between the reported figures cannot be resolved on the basis of hybridization data alone. However, viewed in the context of results obtained by other techniques, the RNA-DNA hybridizations suggesting a lower complexity for the RNA tumor virus genome are probably the correct ones.

A relatively small genome size is also indirectly suggested by the UV resistance and hence small target size of RNA tumor viruses (Rubin and Temin, 1959; Latarjet and Chamaillard, 1962; Levinson and Rubin, 1966; Goldé and Latarjet, 1966). However, the nature of UV damage to RNA tumor viruses is still not understood (Owada et al., 1976), nor is there a simple and experimentally confirmed relationship between radiation target size and genome size in RNA tumor viruses (Friis, 1971). Therefore, the argument relating UV resistance to genome complexity must be considered with reservation.

2.5. The 35 S RNAs of an RNA Tumor Virus Contain the Same Sequences in Fixed Order

The low complexity of the viral RNA still allows several variant models of a polyploid genome, as pointed out by Billeter et al. (1974) and Weissmann et al. (1975): (1) the unit genomes of a virus contain identical genes but the gene order is permuted in different 35 S molecules, (2) the 35 S unit genome comprising of 60–70 S complex contains the same genes in fixed order, and (3) the two 35 S molecules making up a 60–70 S complex contain different genes, but two copies of each, so that the total complexity is still equivalent to that of one 35 S RNA molecule having unique sequences.

Recent studies have shown model (2) to be the correct one (Wang and Duesberg, 1974; Wang et al., 1975; Coffin and Billeter, 1976). In these studies, 35 S RNA was randomly fragmented with dilute alkali, and molecules with intact 3′ ends were then isolated by virtue of the fact that the poly(A) at the 3′ position binds to Millipore filters, to poly(U)-Sepharose, or to oligo(dT)-cellulose. The poly(A)-containing population of RNAs was then fractionated according to size, and individual fractions were fingerprinted. The complexity of such fingerprints was found to be a function of fragment size, with the largest fragments yielding the most complex fingerprints, equivalent to intact 35 S RNA. This observation rules out extensive permutation of the gene order and argues in favor of a fixed linear sequence in RNA tumor viruses. More convincing data on this point are supplied by electron microscopy and will be discussed below.

2.6. The 60–70 S RNA Is an Inverted Dimer of 35 S RNAs Linked at the 5′ Ends

Several laboratories have studied the high molecular weight RNA of RNA tumor viruses using modifications of the spreading technique introduced by Kleinschmidt (1968). The results of these electron microscopic investigations confirm and extend the structure and organization of the viral genome as determined by physical and chemical techniques. The 60–70 S complex of avian sarcoma virus has been visualized after reaction with protein of gene 32 from phage T4. This protein binds to and extends single-stranded nucleic acids. Prepared in this fashion, the 60–70 S RNA appears as a complex, largely single-stranded network with a length corresponding to a molecular weight of 6.1×10^6 to 7.2×10^6 (Mangel et al., 1974; Delius et al., 1975; Weissmann et al., 1975). If the RNA is first dissociated by heating or if it is prepared for electron microscopy in formamide and urea or in glyoxal, then stretched-out molecules representing the 30–40 S RNA components are seen (Mangel et al., 1974; Kung et al., 1974, 1975a,b; Delius et al., 1975; Chi and Bassel, 1975; Jacobson and Bromley, 1975a,b). The molecular weight of the 30–40 S RNA as estimated from length measurements is from

2.8×10^6 to 4.0×10^6 for avian sarcoma virus. The 30–40 S RNA of transformation-defective (*td*) deletion mutants of RSV was found to be about 10% shorter than the 30–40 S RNA of the nondefective parental sarcoma virus. Generally lower values for the molecular weight of the 30–40 S RNA have been reported by Weber *et al.* (1975). The same group of workers presented data supporting nonrandom degradation during the preparation of 30–40 S RNA (Heine *et al.*, 1975). This degradation generates distinct size classes of subgenomic fragments and may reflect the existence of preferred sites for nuclease action. Nonrandom size distributions of degraded 30–40 S RNA are also sometimes seen in polyacrylamide gels (Duesberg *et al.*, 1970).

Older electron microscopic studies have described stretched-out nucleic acid molecules of avian RNA tumor viruses with a maximal length corresponding to a molecular weight of 1.0×10^7 (Granboulan *et al.*, 1966; Kakefunda and Bader, 1969). These preparations were obtained under nondenaturing conditions under which single-stranded RNA, including the 60–70 S complex of RNA tumor viruses, shows a highly tangled and convoluted contour. The stretched-out molecules in these preparations are therefore more likely DNA, possibly of cellular origin, and not RNA. Nuclease digestion of such electron microscope mounts supports this interpretation (Delius *et al.*, 1975; Weber *et al.*, 1975).

More detailed information on the structure of the RNA tumor virus genome has come from investigations of the endogenous cat virus RD114 (Kung *et al.*, 1974, 1975a,b). Undenatured high molecular weight RNA of the virus has a sedimentation constant of 52 S. This composite molecule can be dissociated into two half molecules. The separation requires more strongly denaturing conditions than are needed to obtain the 30–40 S RNA of other RNA tumor viruses: 80°C in urea-formamide or methyl mercuric hydroxide and glyoxal at room temperature. Because the 52 S RNA of RD114 is stable under moderately denaturing conditions, it is possible to study its extended form in the electron microscope. Its length corresponds to a molecular weight of 5.8×10^6. The 52 S molecule shows a central Y-shaped structure and two loops located symmetrically to the center. Dissociation of the 52 S complex leads to half-length molecules with a molecular weight of about 2.8×10^6. In such half molecules obtained by heating in formamide urea and rapid cooling on ice, another secondary branchlike structure can be seen at a fixed position. The location of the poly(A) in RD114 RNA has been determined by annealing to poly(dT), which is itself linked to SV40 circular DNA (3.6×10^6 molecular weight). Using this readily observed marker, poly(A) is seen at both ends of the 52 S molecule (Bender and Davidson, 1976). These data are compatible with the view that the 52 S RNA of RD114 is not a tandem dimer with the genomes oriented in the same $3' \rightarrow 5'$ direction, but an inverted dimer, consisting of two identical half molecules which are linked by a Y-shaped structure involving base pairing at or near their $5'$ ends. The position of characteristic secondary structures at the same fixed locations in both half molecules argues against a genome consisting of different 30–40 S components in which individual genes are repeated two to three times, and supports a fixed nonpermuted sequence which is the same in all half molecules. This general structure appears to be of common occurrence at least among mammalian RNA tumor viruses (Davidson, 1975, personal communication; Bender and Davidson, 1976; Kung *et al.*, 1976).

2.7. Summary and Conclusions

The physical, chemical, and electron microscopic data on the RNA tumor virus genome are consistent with, but do not definitely prove, the following model: The genome is a single-stranded, linear RNA which, depending on virus strain, sediments at 50–70 S and has a molecular weight of about $6–8 \times 10^6$. This RNA consists of two identical half molecules which can be dissociated and which then sediment at about 30–40 S. They have a molecular weight of about 3×10^6. Each of the half molecules contains the entire genetic information of the virus, with the viral genes arranged in a fixed, nonpermuted sequence. In the 60–70 S complex, these unit genomes are held together at their $5'$ ends by a base-paired structure. The virion RNA is thus a symmetrically arranged dimer, comprising a diploid genome. Although this RNA, as extracted from the virus, is linear, its structure *in situ* may involve linkage of $3'$ to $5'$ ends.

As one looks at the reproductive cycle of RNA tumor viruses and the structure of the genome, three processes stand out as of potential significance for genetics: (1) Reverse transcription creates an opportunity for genetic exchange between the two unit genomes of the same 70 S complex. (2) Integration of viral DNA into cellular DNA and transcription of progeny viral RNA from this provirus may lead to the inclusion of cellular sequences into the viral genome. (3) Polycistronic transcription and translation could affect the operational definition of genetic elements by complementation tests. A genetic lesion anywhere in a precursor polypeptide may interfere with processing. All functional proteins derived from this precursor will then be affected and register as belonging to one cistron. On the other hand, a genetic lesion may not block processing, but the cleavage product carrying the lesion could show impaired function. In this event, the cleavage product would appear in a cistron separate from the other proteins derived from the same precursor.

3. NONCONDITIONAL MUTANTS AND MARKERS

The analysis of gene functions, of gene regulation, and of gene order requires mutants. In the past few years, many new conditional and nonconditional mutants of RNA tumor viruses have been isolated and characterized, and together with the natural genetic markers they provide ample material for genetic investigations. In this survey, the nonconditional mutants and natural markers will be described first. These data will then be used in a discussion of genetic and nongenetic interactions of RNA tumor viruses, which will be followed by a review of temperature-sensitive mutants.

In a perhaps oversimplified view of the RNA tumor virus genome, four principal genetic functions can be listed. These functions, which can be provisionally regarded as products of viral genes, are (1) the nonglycosylated structural proteins of the virion, (2) the RNA-dependent DNA polymerase, (3) the envelope glycoprotein(s), and (4) the transforming protein. These functions have been termed, somewhat noneuphoniously, *gag* for "group-specific antigen," *pol* for "polymerase," *env* for "envelope," and *onc* for "oncogenicity" (Baltimore, 1975). Since experimental evidence for a specific cell-transforming viral gene is restricted to sarcoma viruses, this function has been called more recently *src* for "sarcoma induction" (Wang *et al., 1976a*). The viral genome has also been broadly divided into functions concerned exclusively with the synthesis of infectious progeny virus (R functions), those which are needed only for transformation of the cell (T functions), and those which are coordinately required for both virus synthesis and transformation to occur (C functions). The R functions include *gag* and *env,* i.e., structural proteins. The T function is equivalent to *src* or *onc,* and the only known C function is *pol.* This division of the genome into three functional areas T(*onc/src*), R(*gag* + *env*), and C(*pol*) serves as a useful initial orientation and will be followed in the discussion of mutants.

3.1. Defective Viruses

3.1.1. Replication-Defective Avian Sarcoma Viruses with a Deletion Affecting *env*

RNA tumor viruses which carry a mutation affecting a replicative (R) function, and therefore fail to produce infectious progeny virus, are called "replication defectives" (*rd*) (Table 1). Two well-known *rd* viruses with a deletion in an R function are the Bryan high-titer strain of RSV (BH RSV) and the *NY*8 variant of the Schmidt-Ruppin RSV of subgroup A (SR RSV-A). Both have very similar defects. In single infection with these viruses, the host cell becomes transformed, but infectious sarcoma virus is not produced (Temin, 1962, 1963; Hanafusa *et al.,* 1963; Kawai and Hanafusa, 1973). Such transformed cells do not adsorb virus-neutralizing antibody and do not elicit the production of a neutralizing antibody when injected into chickens, indicating absence of viral surface glycoprotein from the transformed cells. If the nonproductively transformed cells are superinfected by an avian leukosis virus, the glycoprotein of the leukosis virus can be used for the maturation of infectious but still genetically defective sarcoma virus. The superinfected cells release both sarcoma and leukosis virus (Hanafusa *et al.,* 1964*a*). The genetically defective sarcoma virus carrying the envelope glycoprotein of the leukosis virus helper is called a "pseudotype" (Rubin, 1965). There is no genetic exchange between sarcoma and helper virus such that the *env* function of the leukosis virus is combined with the *src* function of the defective virus to produce a nondefective sarcoma recombinant, although recombination in other markers appears to occur (Hanafusa and Hanafusa, 1968). More will

TABLE 1

Properties of Replication-Defective (*rd*) Avian Sarcoma Virus with a Deletion in *env* [RSV(−), NY8]

Solitary infection with *rd* pseudotype:
    Oncogenic transformation of the cell. Production of noninfectious virions. Noninfectious virions lack envelope glycoproteins and 10–20% of the genomic RNA.
Noninfectious virions fused into cells:
    Cellular transformation and synthesis of noninfectious progeny.
Double infection with *rd* sarcoma and leukosis helper virus:
    Oncogenic transformation of the cell. Production of infectious sarcoma and leukosis virus. Sarcoma virus is a pseudotype, with glycoprotein specified by leukosis virus. No recombination yielding nondefective sarcoma virus.

be said about the action of helper viruses in the sections on phenotypic mixing and on recombination.

Through its glycoprotein, the helper leukosis virus controls virus-specific surface properties of the sarcoma pseudotype: thus antigenicity, host range, and sensitivity to viral interference are identical to those of the helper virus (Hanafusa et al., 1964a; Vogt, 1965; Hanafusa, 1965; Hanafusa and Hanafusa, 1966; Kawai and Hanafusa, 1973). The glycoprotein defect in the sarcoma virus can also be complemented by endogenous helper viruses or helper factors. Chicken cells which express endogenous helper activity for BH RSV or NY8 are called "chicken helper factor positive" (chf+). They synthesize env product of the endogenous virus which can be incorporated into BH RSV or NY8 to yield infectious pseudotypes BH RSV(chf) or NY8(chf). (Vogt, 1967a; Weiss, 1967, 1969a,b; T. Hanafusa et al., 1970b; H. Hanafusa et al., 1970, 1973; Halpern et al., 1975). Despite the absence of viral glycoproteins in helper factor-negative cells (chf−) transformed by the defective BH RSV or SR RSV-A, such cells do produce viral particles, but these particles are noninfectious (Dougherty and Di Stephano, 1965; Courington and Vogt, 1967; Robinson, 1967; Hanafusa and Hanafusa, 1968; T. Hanafusa et al., 1970a; Kawai and Hanafusa, 1973). In the case of BH RSV, these particles are referred to as RSV(−); with rd mutants of SR RSV-A, they are called NY8 particles (Weiss, 1972; Kawai and Hanafusa, 1973). The noninfectious RSV(−) and NY8 particles can be purified and have been shown to lack envelope glycoproteins, but contain all nonglycosylated structural proteins. In NY8, no carbohydrate label can be found in virion proteins (Kawai and Hanafusa, 1973), although in RSV(−) there may be small amounts of anomalous glycoprotein (Scheele and Hanafusa, 1971; Halpern et al., 1976). The absence of glycoprotein clearly prevents entry of the RSV(−) or NY8 particles into the host cell, since if these noninfectious particles are fused into cells with inactivated Sendai virus they are able to transform the cell and to direct the synthesis of noninfectious progeny particles (T. Hanafusa et al., 1970a; Kawai and Hanafusa, 1973). Since the virion glycoproteins form spikes and knobs visible with the electron microscope on the surface of infectious virus (Bolognesi et al., 1972), it would be expected that RSV(−) and NY8 lack these envelope structures. Recent studies have confirmed this expectation (De Giuli et al., 1975; Ogura and Friis, 1975). The RNA of the RSV(−) and NY8 particles has also been purified and compared to the RNA of nondefective sarcoma viruses in gel electrophoresis and by oligonucleotide fingerprint analysis (Duesberg et al., 1975a). The 35 S RNAs obtained from these rd sarcoma viruses are smaller than those of nondefective sarcoma viruses. In the case of $NY8$, the difference is 0.75×10^6 daltons, or 21% of the genome of SR RSV-A. RSV($-$), for which no congenic nondefective virus is available and which can only be compared to other nondefective RNA sarcoma viruses, contains 35 S RNA which is shorter by about 10% or 0.35×10^6 daltons than that of most nondefective avian sarcoma viruses. These data suggest that RSV($-$) and $NY8$ represent deletion mutants. This conclusion is supported by oligonucleotide fingerprint patterns of $NY8$ and its progenitor SR RSV-A. All RNase T_1-resistant large oligonucleotides identifiable in $NY8$ are also present in SR RSV-A. In addition, SR RSV-A has six oligonucleotides which are missing from $NY8$. These six oligonucleotides may be derived from the *env* gene.

3.1.2. The Defects in Other *rd* Avian Sarcoma Viruses Are Only Partially Known

A fairly large number of *rd* avian sarcoma viruses unrelated to RSV($-$) or to $NY8$ have been described in the literature. Most workers agree that mutagenization by UV or γ-rays or by chemicals induces or selects for such defectives in stocks of nondefective sarcoma viruses (Goldé, 1970; Toyoshima *et al.*, 1970; Kawai and Yamamoto, 1970; Weiss *et al.*, 1973). There is only one discordant series of experiments in which sarcoma virus survivors of mutagenization were invariably also producers of infectious progeny. This puzzling observation led to the hypothesis that R functions are required for oncogenic transformation (Graf and Bauer, 1970; Graf *et al.*, 1971). Although there are now enough examples of *rd* deletion mutants to make this hypothesis untenable, a satisfactory explanation for the results of Graf and coworkers has never been proposed, nor is the selection or induction of *rd* viruses by mutagens understood.

Most of the *rd* sarcoma viruses other than RSV($-$) or $NY8$ have not been studied extensively, and often very little is known about the nature of the defect. But in a few cases it is clear that the defects are distinct from those described for RSV($-$) or $NY8$. In Table 2 the characteristics of *rd* sarcoma viruses including the *env*$-$ deletion mutants RSV($-$) and $NY8$ are listed. Type 3 appears to be noncomplementable by leukosis virus, a situation for which there is no simple explanation in view of the current doctrine that leukosis viruses contain all genes necessary for the replication of avian sarcoma viruses. The *rd* virus referred to as "type 6" in the table has been studied in some detail

TABLE 2
Types of Replication-Defective Avian Sarcoma Virus

Type	Induces interference with leukosis virus of same glycoprotein subgroup	Directs synthesis of noninfectious virions	Is complemented by exogenous leukosis virus of different glycoprotein subgroup	Is complemented by endogenous leukosis virus	Recombines with leukosis virus in the defective function	Defective function	Example or reference
1	No	Yes	Yes	Yes	No	*env*	RSV(−), NY8 Hanafusa and Hanafusa (1968), Kawai and Hanafusa (1973)
2	No	Yes	Yes	No for *pol* Yes for *env*	Yes for *pol* No for *env*	*pol* and *env*	RSVα(−), NY8α Reference same as for type 1
3	No	NT	No	No	No	Unknown	Weiss (1973), Vogt *et al.* (1977)
4	NT[a]	Yes	NT	No	NT	Unknown, not *pol*	Kawai and Hanafusa (1973)
5	NT	NT	Yes	No	Yes	Unknown	Weiss (1973)
6	Yes	Few	Yes	NT	Yes	Probably *gag*	Vogt *et al.* (1977), Kawai and Yamamoto (1970)

[a] Not tested.

(Vogt *et al.*, 1977). Cells transformed by this agent (*LA*7365) produce very small amounts of virus particles with a 70 S RNA, but virtually no infectious virus is made. The size of the virion RNA indicates that no major genetic deletion has taken place. The "nonproducer" cells can complement and be complemented by RSV(−) and are resistant to superinfection by viruses of the same subgroup. Both facts indicate that viral glycoproteins are synthesized by this *rd* sarcoma virus. Complementation can also be obtained by superinfection with a leukosis virus of another glycoprotein subgroup. Unlike RSV(−) or *NY*8 pseudotypes, *LA*7365 rescued by either leukosis virus or RSV(−) contains nondefective sarcoma virus, suggesting that recombination with the helper virus has taken place and has led to a substitution of the defective marker in *LA*7365 by the corresponding wild-type gene. *LA*7365 is not complemented by conditional mutants affected in the internal nonglycosylated proteins and therefore may have a defect in one of these proteins. This nonconditional *rd* sarcoma virus may represent a point mutation, or at most a very small deletion, because upon prolonged passage cells infected with this virus start to release infectious virus spontaneously, suggesting that it mutates back to *wt*. Furthermore, the defective virus recombines with helper virus to yield nondefective sarcoma recombinants, an ability not seen with larger deletion mutants.

From the fragmentary information compiled in Table 2, it is clear that more work is needed on *rd* sarcoma viruses. Point mutations would yield useful information on various viral R genes, and deletions would offer much needed material for biochemical mapping experiments which hold great promise (Wang *et al.*, 1975).

3.1.3. Avian Sarcoma Viruses with a Defect in *pol*

In preparations of envelope-defective RSV(−) and of *NY*8, genetic variants with an additional defect in the polymerase can be found. These are termed RSVα(−) and *NY*8α, respectively, and in all properties relevant to the defect these viruses are alike. The defect in the polymerase cannot be complemented in cells which show partial expression of endogenous leukosis virus and which are positive for internal group-specific virion antigens (*gag*$^+$ or *gs*$^+$) and for envelope glycoprotein (*chf*$^+$ or *env*$^+$) (Hanafusa and Hanafusa, 1968; Kawai and Hanafusa, 1973). Thus *chf*$^+$ cells are used routinely to isolate RSVα(−) and *NY*8α and to differentiate these variants from RSV(−) and *NY*8, which are complemented in chf^+ cells (Hanafusa and Hanafusa, 1971; Kawai and Hanafusa, 1973). Cells infected and transformed by RSVα(−) or $NY8α$ elaborate noninfectious virions, but these particles cannot transform if fused into cells by inactivated Sendai virus (T. Hanafusa et al., 1970a). They lack reverse transcriptase activity and are also free of proteins which cross-react immunologically with reverse transcriptase (Hanafusa and Hanafusa, 1971; Hanafusa et al., 1972; Nowinski et al., 1972; Panet et al., 1975a). The inability of RSVα(−) and of $NY8α$ particles to transform after fusion into cells with inactivated Sendai virus reflects the coordinate nature of their defect: reverse transcriptase is required for both transformation and virus replication. Infectious sarcoma virus can be rescued by helper virus from cells infected and transformed by the defective RSVα(−) or $NY8α$, and this virus appears to be a pseudotype not only with respect to the envelope glycoproteins but also in the reverse transcriptase. However, unlike pseudotype formation with RSV(−) or $NY8$, which never leads to the genetic repair of the env defect, a significant proportion of the pseudotypes formed between RSVα(−) or $NY8α$ and avian leukosis helper virus acquire the genetic information for polymerase but retain the env lesion; i.e., these viruses become RSV(−) and $NY8$, respectively. This repair of the pol defect is probably the result of recombination with the helper virus (Hanafusa and Hanafusa, 1968; Kawai and Hanafusa, 1973). Do RSVα(−) and $NY8α$ have a deletion in the pol gene? The absence of reverse transcriptase and of cross-reacting material from the noninfectious RSVα(−) and $NY8α$ particles suggests that this is the case. Also in accord with the possibility of deletion in pol is the fact that neither RSVα(−) nor $NY8α$ shows spontaneous reversion to wt (Kawai and Hanafusa, 1973; Hanafusa, 1975, personal communication). However, biochemical evidence suggests that this putative deletion in pol is quite small. The RNA of $NY8α$ has been studied by fingerprint analysis of the major RNase T_1-resistant oligonucleotides and was found not to lack additional oligonucleotides as compared to $NY8$ (Duesberg, 1975, personal communication). The RNA of $NY8α$ is also not detectably smaller in size than that of $NY8$. If the major portion of the gene coding for the reverse transcriptase (molecular weight 60,000) was deleted, this would certainly be reflected in the fingerprint patterns and in the size of the RNA.

A possibly different defect in the polymerase gene of RSV(−) was described by Robinson and Robinson (1971). In this variant of BH RSV, RNA-dependent DNA polymerase activity was found missing, but a DNA-dependent activity could be detected in the noninfectious particles. Since the two enzyme activities could be physically separated, which cannot be done for virion reverse transcriptase, it is questionable whether the DNA-dependent polymerase activity in the noninfectious particles represented the viral enzyme rather than cellular contamination. If the DNA-dependent enzyme is cellular, the defective virus described by Robinson and Robinson could be the same as RSVα(−).

So far the polymerase defect seen in RSVα(−) and *NY8α* has been found only in the association with a deletion in *env*. Whether this association of the *env* deletion with a polymerase defect is fortuitous or has some significance is not known. The *pol* gene has not yet been mapped unambiguously, but a likely position for it is adjacent to *env*.

3.1.4. Transforming Viruses Which Fail to Produce Infectious Progeny Occur Also in Various Strains of Avian Leukosis

The study of viral defectiveness depends on rigorous cloning procedures. Helper-independent focus assays for transformation must be available to generate clones of cells infected and transformed by single particles of a defective virus. This condition is generally fulfilled in the case of sarcoma viruses; however, for many leukemia and leukosis viruses, transformation assays *in vitro* have not yet been developed. Exceptions among the avian leukosis viruses are avian myeloblastosis virus, which transforms yolk sac and bone marrow cultures under conditions of solitary infection, avian myelocytosis virus MC29, which causes foci of transformed cells in chicken embryo fibroblasts, and avian erythroblastosis virus strain R, which also transforms fibroblasts (Beaudreau *et al.,* 1960; Baluda and Goetz, 1961; Moscovici, 1967; Langlois and Beard, 1967; Ishizaki and Shimizu, 1970). These leukosis viruses which cause transformation *in vitro* have been tested for defectiveness. Stocks of all three viruses contain, besides the transforming agent, nontransforming, independently replicating associated viruses. These can be separated from the transforming component (Moscovici and Vogt, 1968; Ishizaki and Shimizu, 1970; Langlois *et al.,* 1971), and they could serve as helper viruses for *rd* leukosis.

If single foci of chicken macrophages transformed by avian myeloblastosis virus are isolated and tested, many fail to release virus which can again transform macrophages or cause myeloblastosis in the chicken (Moscovici and Zanetti, 1970; Moscovici *et al.,* 1975; Moscovici, 1975). The nonproducing cells can be grown into mass cultures, and macrophage-transforming virus can be rescued by superinfection with avian leukosis viruses. The transformed nonproducing cells, being derived from primitive macrophages, also show the selective suscepti- bility of the chicken macrophage to the glycoprotein subgroups of avian tumor viruses. Since chicken macrophages are susceptible only to subgroups B and C (Gazzolo *et al.*, 1974, 1975), leukosis viruses of these two subgroups are also the most efficient helper virus for defec- tive avian myeloblastosis. Subgroup A leukosis viruses, on the other hand, cannot rescue myeloblastosis virus from nonproducer clones, because macrophages are not susceptible to viruses of this subgroup. Subgroup D viruses behave irregularly in that they do complement defective avian myeloblastosis in nonproducing clones, although they do not replicate by themselves in macrophages (Moscovici, 1975). The nature of the replication defect in avian myeloblastosis virus has not been determined, nor is it known whether all leukemogenic virus in avian myeloblastosis stock preparations is replication defective or whether some can transform and synthesize infectious progeny in solitary infection. The defect in avian myeloblastosis virus may involve only structural proteins but could also include the DNA polymerase. No particles corresponding to RSV($-$) or *NY*8 have been described, but some of the avian myeloblastosis nonproducer lines release a myeloblastosis-associated helper virus (MAV-2 of subgroup B) without also producing the macrophage-transforming myeloblastosis virus itself. Therefore, at least two types of defective avian myeloblastosis virus exist: one cannot be rescued by myeloblastosis-associated helper virus, the other can be efficiently complemented. Complementation of defective avian myeloblastosis virus by endogenous avian leukosis virus appears to be very inefficient if it occurs at all, as judged by the high frequency of nonproducer clones in macrophage cultures derived from chicken embryos with constitutive expression of the endogenous viral genes *gag* and *env*. Transformed cells which do not release infectious virus have also been obtained from single neoplastic foci induced by avian leukosis virus MC29 in chicken embryo fibroblast cultures (Ishizaki *et al.*, 1971). Infectious MC29 can be rescued from these nonproducing cells by superinfection with helper leukosis viruses which do not transform fibroblasts. Helper viruses belonging to any of the four envelope subgroups A–D are effective. The other subgroups E–G have not been tested but would probably work as well, if the cells are susceptible to the helper virus. The defect in MC29 is only partially known. Nonproducing cells are free of viral glycoprotein and contain only very low levels of group-specific internal virion proteins, suggesting that the synthesis of several structural proteins is affected. It is therefore expected that noninfectious virions are not elaborated by MC29 nonproducer cells. Complementation of defective MC29 with endogenous virus does not appear to take place or may be very inefficient. The data on this point are incomplete.

3.1.5. Transformation-Defective Avian Sarcoma Viruses Have a Deletion in the *src* Region

The term "transformation defective" (*td*) is commonly used to designate nonconditional mutants of helper-independent sarcoma virus which are no longer able to transform fibroblast cultures or to induce sarcomas in the animal, but still synthesize infectious progeny virus in single infection. Defectiveness in transformation in this context refers specifically to the sarcoma-producing capacity of the virus (the *src* gene). Those *td* agents which have been tested still induce leukosis in the animal host and thus are not completely nononcogenic (Biggs *et al.,* 1973; Purchase, Weiss, and Vogt, 1974, unpublished observations). However, the conclusion that *td* viruses contain specific leukemogenic genes is not justified from the available data, because it is not known whether *td* viruses undergo some genetic change, such as acquisition of oncogenic information from the host cell, before they act as leukemogens. In the experiments of Biggs and associates, two *td* viruses derived from the Schmidt-Ruppin strain of RSV were used; one had a deletion amounting to about 15% of the parental genome, and in the other the deletion was smaller (Stone *et al.,* 1975). It is perhaps significant that a very low incidence of sarcomas was associated with infection by the virus having the smaller deletion but not with infection by *td* virus which had the more common size deletion of 15%.

Td viruses have been found in many nondefective avian sarcoma virus preparations. If the sarcoma virus has not been cloned recently, *td* viruses occur usually in excess of the sarcoma virus (Dougherty and Rausmussen, 1964; Hanafusa and Hanafusa, 1966; Duff and Vogt, 1969). However, *td* viruses are found even in cloned stocks of helper-independent avian sarcoma viruses, albeit in lower concentrations than the sarcoma-producing component (Vogt, 1971a; Kawai *et al.,* 1972). *Td* viruses are spontaneous segregants derived exclusively from nondefective sarcoma virus. They are not extraneous contaminants of the sarcoma virus stocks, nor are most of them recombinants between the sarcoma and endogenous leukosis viruses, although such recombination may occur (Weiss *et al.*, 1973). There are three lines of evidence which support the statement that *td* viruses arise directly from nondefective sarcoma virus: (1) *Td* viruses have the same envelope properties as the sarcoma viruses with which they are associated. These include specific antigens revealed in neutralization and fluorescent antibody straining, host range in various avian cell types, sensitivity to viral interference, and response of virus-cell adsorption to the presence of polycations (Hanafusa and Hanafusa, 1966; Duff and Vogt, 1969; Toyoshima *et al.*, 1970; Vogt, 1971*a*; Graf *et al.*, 1971). (2) The incidence of *td* viruses is not detectably higher if the sarcoma virus is grown in cells which express endogenous leukosis virus (Vogt, 1971*a*). (3) The RNA fingerprint pattern of large RNase T_1-resistant oligonucleotides obtained with the 30–40 S RNA of *td* viruses is contained in the pattern of the parental sarcoma virus. There are no new oligonucleotides in the *td* virus as compared to the sarcoma virus, as would be expected if *td* viruses arose by recombination with endogenous leukosis viruses. However, there are some (from one to three) oligonucleotides of the sarcoma virus, probably representing sarcomagenic information, which are missing in the *td* virus (Lai *et al.*, 1973; Duesberg *et al.*, 1975*a,b*). These fingerprint analyses of viral RNA which always show the loss of specific oligonucleotides in *td* mutants as compared to the sarcoma virus parent demonstrate that *td* viruses are deletions. In accord with these results is the observation that the RNA of *td* viruses is smaller than that of the sarcoma virus by about 15%, the respective molecular weights being about 3.0 and 3.5 × 10^6 (Duesberg and Vogt, 1970, 1973*b*). This difference in the size of the RNA is a property of the virus and is not caused by the growth of sarcoma and *td* viruses in transformed and normal fibroblasts, respectively. *Ts* mutants of sarcoma virus which fail to transform at the nonpermissive temperature but still replicate have the larger RNA characteristic of nondefective sarcoma viruses, even if grown under nonpermissive conditions in phenotypically normal cells, and *td* viruses propagated in chemically transformed cells retain the smaller RNA (Martin and Duesberg, 1972; Lai, 1975, personal communication). That *td* viruses are the result of a deletion is further indicated by genetic experiments. *Td* viruses fail to complement a large number of nonidentical sarcoma virus point mutations which are *ts* for maintenance of transformation. *Td* viruses also cannot form *wt* recombinants with such *ts* mutants (Bernstein *et al.*, 1976). These results suggest that the defect in *td* viruses overlaps all of the *ts* mutants. There are no reports of carefully controlled experiments showing the reversion of a *td* virus to a nondefective sarcoma virus, and such reversions would not be expected from deletion mutants, unless the *td* viruses can obtain the *src* gene by recombination with the host cell.

Td viruses segregate spontaneously from nondefective sarcoma viruses, probably in the process of virus replication either during reverse transcription or during synthesis of viral RNA from provirus. The observations of Hillova *et al.* (1974) favor the former possibility. These authors found no evidence for segregation of *td* viruses in permissive cells transfected with sarcoma viral DNA prepared from RSV-transformed mammalian cells. Such DNA is presumably free of *td* genomes, while transfection with DNA from virus-producing chicken cultures which probably includes *td* genomes also leads to the appearance of *td* viruses in the recipient cultures. However, even in chicken cell cultures transfected with DNA from mammalian Rous sarcoma cells, *td* deletions should appear eventually as the virus goes through several cycles of replication.

The levels of *td* viruses in sarcoma virus preparations appear to be increased after mutagenesis (Goldé, 1970; Toyoshima *et al.*, 1970; Graf *et al.*, 1971). Whether the defectives are induced by the mutagen or are merely selected for is not clear. At least for UV irradiation, the balance of available evidence is in favor of selection. For BH RSV, which in comparison to nondefective avian sarcoma viruses lacks about as much RNA as most *td* deletions, a smaller UV target size has been reported (Friis, 1971). If the rate of UV inactivation is also slower with *td* viruses as compared to nondefective sarcoma viruses, selection could account for the prevalence of *td* viruses in irradiated stocks. Recent work, however, has shown that there is no partial inactivation of the RNA tumor virus genome by UV; i.e., the *src* gene and possibly other markers as well cannot be rescued from UV-inactivated virus (Owada *et al.*, 1976; Bister *et al.*, 1977). Yet such partial inactivation of the genome would have to be postulated if UV were to generate rather than select *td* viruses.

Stocks of nondefective avian sarcoma viruses usually contain *td* virus in excess over sarcoma virus, unless there is a selection for viral progeny produced by transformed cells (Duesberg and Vogt, in preparation). There are five possible explanations for the prevalence of *td* viruses in conventionally grown sarcoma virus stocks: (1) Mutation from sarcoma to *td* virus is not reversible, leading to an accumulation of *td* deletions. (2) *Td* viruses have a faster growth rate than sarcoma viruses. (3) *Td* viruses are more heat stable than sarcoma viruses, so that the virus titers representing equilibrium between synthesis and inactivation are higher for *td* viruses. (4) The rates of virus production by transformed cells may be lower than those by nontransformed cells. (5) Sarcoma virus-transformed cells may have a shorter life span than normal fibroblasts. In mixed cultures of the two cell types, fibroblastic elements often prevail, with a concomitant preponderance of *td* viruses. Explanation (1) is definitely applicable and accounts for the known facts. Whether the other explanations play an additional role, must be decided by further experimentation.

3.1.6. Replication and Coordinately Defective Mammalian Sarcoma Viruses Often Have Deletions Encompassing Several Genes

Genetic defectiveness in replicative and coordinate functions and the ensuing dependence on helper viruses for the production of infectious progeny are more common among mammalian than among avian sarcoma viruses. In fact, all presently known mammalian sarcoma viruses—the four strains of murine sarcoma virus (Moloney, Kirsten, Harvey, and probably Finkel-Biskis-Jinkins), the two strains of feline sarcoma (Gardner and Snyder-Theilen), and simian sarcoma virus—are unable to produce infectious progeny virus in the absence of a helper virus (Hartley and Rowe, 1966; Huebner *et al.*, 1966; Aaronson and Weaver, 1971; Harvey and East, 1971; Sarma *et al.*, 1971; Levy *et al.*, 1973; Scolnick and Parks, 1973; Aaronson, 1973; Henderson *et al.*, 1974; Chan *et al.*, 1974). An exception to this general rule has been reported by Ball *et al.* (1973*b*) and by Lo and Ball (1974), who described a variant of the Moloney MSV which appeared to be helper independent and to contain a genome which is larger than that of defective MSV and of the MuLV helper virus. However, independent confirmation of these important data has not been forthcoming. Recent studies by Maisel (1975, personal communication) have failed to provide evidence for a nondefective MSV in the variant described by Ball *et al.* (1973*b*). While these preparations clearly contained a large excess of MSV over MuLV, the MSV was found to be replication defective, and the size of the virion RNA did not differ from that of known *rd* preparations of Moloney MSV.

The first observations on the defectiveness of MSV were made by Hartley and Rowe (1966), and from their data it appeared that murine sarcoma virus required a leukemia virus helper for transformation as well as replication of infectious progeny, because focus formation in mouse embryo fibroblast cultures followed two-hit kinetics and could become converted to single-hit by adding an excess of leukemia helper virus to the cultures. Therefore, focus formation itself appeared to be helper dependent. However, it was soon found that the two-hit kinetics for focus formation of MSV in mouse embryo fibroblast cultures was a peculiarity of the tissue culture system which required virus spread to neighboring cells for the development of foci. Cell culture systems in which a focus could arise by multiplication of the initially transformed cell without recruitment of neighboring cells clearly showed that transformation by MSV was helper independent (Parkman *et al.*, 1970; Aaronson and Rowe, 1970; Aaronson *et al.*, 1970; Levy, 1971). Susceptible cells which are infected by MSV in the absence of a helper become transformed but do not release infectious sarcoma virus progeny. Superinfection of these nonproducing cells with MuLV results in the production of both helper and sarcoma virus (Huebner *et al.*, 1966). Kinetic studies of this rescue process have shown that progeny of defective and of helper leukemia virus appear simultaneously and that a late function of the leukemia viruses is needed for the rescue (Peebles *et al.*, 1971; Rowe, 1971).

Various degrees of defectiveness have been found among mammalian sarcoma viruses. In the murine sarcoma viruses there are two principal levels of defectiveness. Nonproducing cells infected and transformed by the first type of defective virus do not release noninfectious particles and do not produce virus structural proteins (Huebner *et al.*, 1966; Aaronson and Rowe, 1970; Aaronson and Weaver, 1971; Levy, 1971). Nonproducer cells infected and transformed by the second, less defective type of MSV (also referred to as S^+L^- for "sarcoma positive, leukemia negative," or S^+H^- for "sarcoma positive, helper negative") produce internal nonglycosylated virion proteins and release noninfectious viral particles (Bassin *et al.*, 1971*a*; Gazdar *et al.*, 1973). The S^+L^- particles are noninfectious even if fused into cells with inactivated Sendai virus, probably because of a defect in an early function. This early viral function may be the virion RNA-dependent DNA polymerase; in S^+L^- particles, only very low levels of this essential viral enzyme have been found (Peebles *et al.*, 1972), and the similar S^+H^- particles described by Gazdar *et al.* (1973) also have a polymerase defect. The data on both types of defective MSV (those producing and those not producing virions) thus suggest defects in coordinate functions (e.g., the polymerase) as well as in purely replicative functions (e.g., virion structural proteins). The noninfectious S^+L^- and S^+H^- particles are also physically different from infectious MSV and MuLV. S^+H^- particles can be distinguished from infectious murine type C particles in thin sections with the electron microscope; they lack the electron-dense core characteristic of complete MSV (Hall *et al.*, 1974). S^+L^- particles seem to have a preponderance of low molecular weight RNA; most of the larger RNA species sediment at 28 and 18 S but have been reported to carry virus-specific sequences and are thus at least not entirely ribosomal (Phillips *et al.*, 1973). The two levels of defectiveness found in MSV are stable through repeated clonings, indicating that they are genetically determined (Aaronson *et al.*, 1972). These two types of defective MSV appear to be the main ones and are most extensively studied, but they are not the only ones. Recently, a new type of defective virus has been identified in the Kirsten strain of MSV (Bilello *et al.*, 1974). Rat cells infected and transformed by this agent do not contain the major structural protein p30 of the murine type C viruses, nor do they release noninfectious particles, but they synthesize viral glycoprotein, gp71. Whether this type of defect is genetically stable and whether it can be complemented by other types of defective murine sarcoma virus is not yet known. Still another type of MSV appears to be defective in both transformation and replication functions (T^-R^-) (Ball *et al.*, 1973*a*). Cells infected by this virus are not transformed morphologically and do not release noninfectious virus particles, but upon superinfection with MuLV they become transformed and release infectious sarcoma and leukemia virus. Whether the absence of morphological transformation in these cells reflects a genetic defect of the virus or whether it represents an uncommon response of the host cell is not known. In some cell lines infected with S^+L^- particles, the same observation of leukemia virus-dependent transformation has also been made, yet there is no evidence that S^+L^- particles have a genetic defect in their transforming function (Bassin *et al.*, 1970).

Nonproducer cells transformed by feline sarcoma viruses appear to be free of structural viral proteins and do not produce noninfectious sarcoma virions (Henderson *et al.*, 1974). No further information on the nature and the extent of the defect in feline sarcoma viruses is available at this time.

Several different levels of defectiveness have also been seen in simian sarcoma virus and are listed in Table 3 (Scolnick and Parks, 1973; Aaronson *et al.*, 1975). Some nonproducing transformed cell clones synthesize neither structural proteins nor noninfectious virions. Others synthesize one or several of the internal nonglycosylated virion proteins, and in certain clones small amounts of noninfectious particles have been detected as well. Whether these particles could transform if fused into cells with inactivated Sendai virus has not been determined.

TABLE 3
Levels of Defectiveness in Simian Sarcoma Virus

Type of nonproducing cell	Production of			
	p12	p30	gp70	Virions
I[a]	−	−	−	−
II[a]	+	−	−	−
III[a]	+	+	−	−
IV[a]	+	+	−	+
V[b]	+	+	NT[c]	+

[a] Data from Aaronson *et al.* (1975).
[b] Data from Scolnick and Parks (1973).
[c] Not tested.

Because the number of different nonproducing clones isolated so far from simian sarcoma virus-transformed cells is small, the list in Table 3 is probably not complete, and additional types of defective simian sarcoma virus may be found in the future. There is evidence that in the simian virus the various levels of viral defectiveness are genetically stable, as they are in murine sarcoma virus (Scolnick and Parks, 1973; Aaronson *et al.*, 1975).

Rescue of defective sarcoma virus from nonproducing cell lines transformed by any mammalian sarcoma virus can be accomplished by superinfection with a wide spectrum of type C leukemia viruses (Huebner *et al.*, 1966; Klement *et al.*, 1969, 1971; Aaronson and Rowe, 1970; Sarma *et al.*, 1970; Aaronson and Weaver, 1971; Levy, 1971; Scolnick *et al.*, 1972a: Peebles *et al.*, 1973; Aaronson, 1973; Henderson *et al.*, 1974; Levy, 1977; Weiss and Wong, 1977). There seems to be no virus-controlled and virus-specific restriction in helper activity: in principle, all mammalian and even some avian type C viruses can act as helper viruses for all mammalian sarcoma viruses. The only limitations are set by the cell, which must be susceptible to infection by the helper virus for rescue to take place. While leukemia viruses can act as helpers to sarcoma viruses, complementation between different defective sarcoma viruses (murine and simian) has not been observed, suggesting that they have overlapping defects (Scolnick and Parks, 1973).

In all instances which have been studied, the rescued sarcoma virus is a pseudotype; i.e., it carries virion proteins coded for by the helper virus, and thus its antigenic specificity is at least in part determined by the helper (Huebner *et al.*, 1966). There is no evidence for recombination between helper and defective sarcoma virus in those markers for which the sarcoma virus is defective. Recombination may occur, however, in other markers (Aaronson *et al.*, 1972, 1975; Scolnick and Parks, 1973). The defective mammalian sarcoma viruses appear to be deletion mutants which have lost coding capacity for some essential proteins. The 30–40 S RNA of MSV contains a component which is smaller than the RNA of murine leukemia virus, and this component is thought to represent the fibroblast-transforming information of the defective sarcoma virus plus sequences coding for some but not all replicative functions such as structural proteins (Maisel *et al.*, 1973; Tsuchida *et al.*, 1974). The larger component of the 30–40 S RNA obtained from MSV pseudotypes probably represents the RNA of the MuLV helper virus. Cross-hybridization data using the 70 S virion RNAs and their respective DNA transcripts of (1) Kirsten MuLV and (2) a mixture of Kirsten MSV and MuLV can be interpreted as showing that some MuLV sequences are quantitatively reduced in the sarcoma leukemia virus mixture (Stephenson and Aaronson, 1971). Similar conclusions were also reached by Roy-Burman and Klement (1975), who used viral RNA and DNA from normal and infected rat cells in their hybridization studies. Additional suggestive evidence for deletions in murine, feline, and simian sarcoma viruses is provided by the experiments of Scolnick and co-workers. The RNA of various nonproducing lines infected by the different mammalian sarcoma viruses was hybridized to DNA transcripts of leukemia viruses. Transcripts were derived from the same leukemia virus that also acted as a helper in the pseudotype preparation from which the nonproducer line was originally derived. Only part of the DNA transcripts entered hybrids. Assuming that all sequences of the defective sarcoma virus genome are represented in the cellular RNA preparation—a likely supposition because of the size of this viral RNA—this result suggests that some helper virus sequences presumably needed for synthesis of infectious virus are absent from the sarcoma viral genome (Benveniste and Scolnick, 1973; Scolnick *et al.*, 1973, 1974; Scolnick and Parks, 1974). The fact that nonproducing sarcoma cells, despite a lack of virus structural proteins, contain RNA which does hybridize to helper viral DNA suggests that the defective sarcoma virus genomes have coding capacity for some virion proteins and that the corresponding RNA is transcribed in the nonproducer cells. Why the sequences coding for virion proteins are not translated in nonproducer cells is not clear. It could be that the defective sarcoma viruses, besides being deletion mutants, also are regulatory mutants in the synthesis of structural proteins and possibly of the polymerase.

With the Moloney strain of MSV, Scolnick *et al.* (1975*b*) have also compared the RNA obtained from two nonproducer lines with different defects, one synthesizing the internal structural protein p30 (p30$^+$), the other one lacking it (p30$^-$). The surprising result of this study was that the deletions represented by these two types of nonproducing cells are only partially overlapping and that the p30$^-$ line which was expected to carry a larger deletion completely encompassing that of the p30$^+$ line had retained sequences not present in the p30$^+$ line. It will now be of interest to determine what viral proteins besides p30 are present in these two nonproducing cell lines. The observation on nonoverlapping deletion in p30$^+$ and p30$^-$ cell lines may also suggest that, especially in polycistronic systems, there is not necessarily a correlation between the size of a genetic deletion and the size of deleted proteins. A small genetic deletion could affect several viral proteins.

Further support in favor of the suggestion that mammalian sarcoma viruses are deletion mutants can be adduced from the inability of the *rd* sarcoma viruses to form a nondefective sarcoma virus by genetic crossover. As will be discussed in greater detail in the section on recombination, deletions could prevent crossover between the appropriate genes.

3.1.7. Replication-Defective Murine Leukemia Viruses Are Also Helper Dependent

The general rule that defectiveness in replication can be best studied if there is a focal assay for transformation applies also to murine leukemia viruses. There are two strains of MuLV for which such assays are available and which have been shown to contain transforming particles unable to produce infectious progeny without the aid of a helper virus: Friend leukemia virus and Abelson leukemia virus.

Friend leukemia virus is a mixture of two agents which differ in their pathogenic effects: a spleen focus-forming virus responsible for the erythroleukemic Friend disease and the lymphoid leukemia virus which induces only lymphoid neoplasms. The lymphoid leukemia virus can be obtained free of the spleen focus-forming virus, but the reverse seems not possible, indicating some dependence of the spleen focus-forming virus on the lymphoid leukemia agent for replication (Dawson *et al.*, 1968; Rowson and Parr, 1970; Steeves *et al.*, 1971). A nonproducing cell line from a Friend virus-induced reticulum cell sarcoma has been isolated, and Friend virus can be rescued from this line by superinfection with murine lymphoid or myeloid leukemia virus in tissue culture or in the animal (Fieldsteel *et al.*, 1969, 1971). The spleen focus-forming virus produced under these conditions and probably all spleen focus-forming components of the Friend murine leukemia virus are pseudotypes. Studies with antibody neutralization indicate that the helper virus in this system controls virion surface antigens, probably the glycoproteins (Eckner and Steeves, 1971, 1972). Whether the helper virus controls other virion proteins and thus other properties of the spleen focus-forming virus is not clear. Eckner and Steeves (1971) and Eckner (1973) have reported that the titration of spleen focus-forming virus which has an N-tropic helper follows two-hit kinetics in the resistant BALB C mouse (see discussion of murine leukemia virus host range in Section 3.2.2). Yet spleen focus formation in susceptible NIH Swiss mice shows single-hit kinetics. Thus there is no evidence that the helper is needed for the growth of a spleen focus, e.g., through infection and recruitment of neighboring cells. The behavior of the spleen focus-forming virus in the restrictive host can therefore be best explained by assuming that the helper virus contributes to the pseudotype some virion proteins other than envelope components which are functional early in infection and which are subject to restriction by the *Fv-1* locus. Recently, conditions have been worked out under which Friend leukemia virus induces the formation of erythroid colonies of mouse bone marrow cells in tissue culture. This *in vitro* assay of the spleen focus-forming virus should lead to a further elucidation of the defect in Friend leukemia virus (Clarke *et al.*, 1975).

The second MuLV which induces focal transformation is the Abelson strain. This virus causes lymphosarcomas and B-cell-derived lymphoblastic leukemia in mice (Abelson and Rabstein, 1970). It produces foci of altered cells in murine fibroblast cultures and can also transform hematopoietic cells *in vitro* (Sklar *et al.*, 1974; Scher and Siegler, 1975; Rosenberg *et al.*, 1975). From a focus of transformed fibroblasts, a nonproducing cell line has been isolated, and from this cell line Abelson MuLV can be rescued by superinfection with Moloney MuLV. Moloney MuLV also appears to be the natural helper of Abelson MuLV. The nature and extent of the replication defect in Abelson MuLV are not known.

3.1.8. *td* Mutants of MSV

The limited experience with nondefective MSV indicates that *td* deletions occur there as they do in stocks of nondefective avian sarcoma virus; as a matter of fact, segregation rates of *td* from sarcoma viruses appear much higher than in avian sarcoma virus strains (Ball *et al.*, 1973*b*). *Td* deletions derived from defective MSV have not been studied, because the double deletion in T and R functions would make it difficult to assay for such agents, if indeed the residual viral genome can be expressed at all. Exceptions are the nonconditional mutations in the *src* gene of Kirsten MSV which have been described by Greenberger *et al.* (1974*a*). These mutants were isolated from nonproducing MSV-infected cell lines mutagenized with mitomycin C. They can be rescued by pseudotype formation with MuLV from the nonproducer cells which have reverted to normal properties. The rescued mutants, identifiable as sarcoma-derived by hybridization, cannot transform new cells, although as pseudotypes they are infectious. The mutants do not complement each other and are therefore probably located in the same cistron. Since they show genetic reversion to *wt*, they are not deletions but probably point mutations.

3.2. Host Range Variants

The various RNA tumor viruses capable of infecting a single vertebrate species show differences in host range; each has a spectrum of cells which it can readily infect and others from which it is excluded or in which it is restricted. Both viral host range and cellular susceptibility or resistance are genetically determined. With avian leukosis or sarcoma viruses, the difference in plating efficiency between susceptible and resistant cells is usually very large, at least 10^3, often more than 10^6 (for review, see Tooze, 1973). Such efficient restriction has proved extremely valuable in the genetic selection for and against certain host range variants, and has been a component of most genetic crosses carried out with avian leukosis and sarcoma viruses. Therefore, the host range variants of these viruses, commonly referred to as "subgroups," constitute important genetic markers. Feline sarcoma and leukemia viruses appear to be subject to similar host range control, but this system has not yet been applied to genetic problems (Tooze, 1973). Host range control of ecotropic murine type C viruses (i.e., murine type C viruses capable of infecting primarily mouse cells) is quantitatively more moderate than that of the avian system and less suitable for genetic selection (Lilly and Pincus, 1973). However, the xenotropic murine type C viruses (i.e., those excluded from mouse cells but capable of infecting cells of several other species) show again similarities to the avian system of host range control (Besmer and Baltimore, 1975, personal communication). Little is known about the control of host range in the recently discovered amphotropic murine type C viruses which combine the host range of eco- and xenotropic viruses (Bryant and Klement, 1976; Hartley and Rowe, 1976; Rasheed *et al.,* 1976).

3.2.1. A Specific Interaction between Envelope Glycoprotein and Cellular Receptor Controls the Host Range of Avian Sarcoma and Leukosis Viruses

Avian leukosis and sarcoma viruses have been classified into seven different subgroups A–G (Vogt and Ishizaki, 1965; Duff and Vogt, 1969; T. Hanafusa *et al.,* 1970*b*; Hanafusa and Hanafusa, 1973; Fujita *et al.,* 1974). Subgroups A–E represent chicken viruses; F and G have been isolated from pheasants. Recent studies suggest that additional subgroups may be found in other galliform birds (Chen and Vogt, in press), but whether these new pheasant viruses qualify as subgroups of the avian (i.e., chicken) leukosis and sarcoma group remains to be seen. T. Hanafusa *et al.* (1976) have found that the viruses presently assigned to subgroup G (isolated from the pheasant genus *Chrysolophus*) show profound differences from the avian leukosis and sarcoma viruses in all structural proteins. There is no antigenic cross-reaction of internal, nonglycosylated virion proteins between G viruses and avian leukosis and sarcoma viruses and no nucleic acid homology. Since the groups (= species) of type C viruses are defined by the presence of shared antigens on the major virion core protein (p27 or p30), the G viruses will probably have to be accorded the status of a separate avian tumor virus group.

The subgroups of avian leukosis and sarcoma viruses are defined by various properties of the viral envelope—antigenicity, sensitivity to interference, and host range, the last being the most practical one. Table 4 summarizes the host range of the avian sarcoma and leukosis virus subgroups in various genetic types of chicken cells which show specific resistance against one or several of these viral subgroups. In the abbreviations for fibroblast phenotypes, C stands for "chicken," the bar (/) signifies "resistant to" and is followed by the subgroup that is

TABLE 4

Host Range of Avian Sarcoma and Leukosis Virus Subgroups in Different Genetic Types of Chicken Fibroblasts[a]

Fibroblast phenotype	Avian tumor virus subgroup						
	A	B	C	D	E	F	G
C/O	S	S	S	S	S	S	S
C/A	R	S	S	S	S	S	S
C/BE	S	R	S	SR	R	S	S
C/C	S	S	R	S	S	S	S
C/E	S	S	S	S	R	S	S

[a] Abbreviations: R, resistant; S, susceptible; SR; intermediate. See also footnote Table 5.

excluded from the particular cell. In Table 5, the same data are compiled for several other avian species. It is obvious from these tables that there exist cell types suitable for the selection for or against any of the seven host range subgroups of the avian sarcoma and leukosis viruses. The resistance in chicken fibroblasts does not interfere with efficient adsorption of the virus to the cell but does block penetration (Piraino, 1967; Crittenden, 1968). Viral host range is specified by the viral envelope glycoprotein(s) and is thus a function of the *env* gene. If the glycoprotein is changed by phenotypic mixing, e.g., in the formation of pseudotypes with the *env*⁻ deletion mutant RSV (−) or *NY*8, the host range is altered accordingly (Hanafusa, 1965; Vogt, 1965; Hanafusa and Hanafusa, 1966; Crittenden, 1968; Kawai and Hanafusa, 1973). However, pseudotypes of RSV(−) or *NY*8 may contain other helper-coded proteins besides the glycoprotein, and therefore they do not provide compelling proof for the exclusive role of the glycoprotein component in determining host range. Additional evidence comes from studies with pseudotypes of vesicular stomatitis virus, which have incorporated avian tumor virus glycoproteins in their envelope and which follow the host range pattern of the corresponding avian sarcoma and leukosis virus subgroup (Love and Weiss, 1974; Boettiger *et al.*, 1975). That penetration of virus into the cell is the site of restriction can also be shown by circumventing this step of infection. If an avian sarcoma or leukosis virus is fused into a genetically resistant cell with inactivated Sendai or Newcastle disease virus, the resistance block is bypassed and successful infection is established (Robinson *et al.*, 1967; Weiss, 1969*a*; T. Hanafusa *et al.*, 1970*a*). The cellular genetic control of resistance and susceptibility to avian sarcoma and leukosis virus subgroups is exerted through three autosomal loci termed *tva, tvb,* and *tvc,* which affect the cellular response to viruses of subgroups A, B, and C, respectively. *Tvb* also influences the response to subgroups D and E. In each of these loci, susceptibility is dominant over resistance, suggesting that they code for cellular receptors which may specifically mediate penetration for each of the subgroups (Crittenden *et al.,* 1963, 1964, 1967; Payne and Biggs, 1964, 1970; Rubin, 1965). The loci controlling resistance and susceptibility to host range subgroups A and C, *tva* and *tvc,* are linked to each other, but neither is linked to the locus for subgroup B, *tvb* (Payne and Pani, 1971). Resistance to subgroup B in the chicken but not in other avian species always carries with it a

TABLE 5

Resistance and Susceptibility of Embryonic Fibroblasts from Various Avian Species to Focus Formation by Avian Sarcoma Viruses[a]

Avian species	Avian sarcoma virus subgroup						
	A	B	C	D	E	F	G
Guinea fowl	S	S	S	S	S	NT	NT
Golden pheasant	S	R/S	S	R/S	S	S	S
Ghighi pheasant	S	R	S	S	S	NT	NT
Swinhoe pheasant	S	R	S	S	R	S	S
Silver pheasant	S	R	S	R	R	S	S
Ringnecked pheasant	S	R	SR	R	S	S	S
Green pheasant	S	R	SR	R	S	S	S
Mongolian pheasant	S	R	S	R	S	NT	NT
Reeve's pheasant	S	R	S	R	R	NT	NT
Japanese quail	S	R	SR	SR	S	S	S
Chinese quail	R	R	R	R	R	S	S
Bobwhite quail	R	R	R	SR	R	NT	NT
Turkey	S	R	S	SR	S	NT	NT
Chukar	S	R	R	R	R/S	NT	NT
Peking duck	R	R	S	R	R	S	R
Moscovy duck	R	R	S	R	R	NT	NT
Goose	R	R	S	R	R	R	R
Parakeet	R	R	R	R	R	NT	NT
Pigeon	R	R	R	SR	NT	NT	NT

[a] Abbreviations: R, efficiency of plating (EOP) $< 10^{-3}$ compared to C/O chicken cells; S, EOP $> 10^{-1}$; SR, EOP $< 10^{-1}$, $> 10^{-3}$; R/S, segregation for R and S; NT, not tested.

strong resistance to subgroup E (Vogt, 1970; Crittenden *et al.*, 1973; Crittenden and Motta, 1975). Cellular response to subgroup E is also influenced by an epistatic inhibitor gene, which induces a dominant resistance and appears to be associated with expression of endogenous leukosis virus group-specific antigen, and of chicken helper factor (*chf*), which indicates presence of subgroup E *env* product in the cell (Payne *et al.*, 1971; Crittenden *et al.*, 1973). A complete account of this situation has been given in several recent reviews (Payne *et al.*, 1973; Payne, 1972; Crittenden, 1975). Genetic resistance to subgroup B also reduces the susceptibility to subgroup D to a varying degree, usually not more than a hundredfold. The specific resistance locus for subgroup D in the chicken has not been identified; rather, the *tvb* locus appears to act pleiotropically to include response to this host range variant (Pani, 1975). While the inheritance of resistance and susceptibility to avian sarcoma and leukosis viruses in the chicken has been fairly well studied, virtually nothing is known about the genetic control of susceptibility in other avian species. Specific genetic loci controlling resistance and susceptibility to subgroups F and G have not been identified.

An epigenetic restriction of cellular susceptibility to avian sarcoma and leukosis virus subgroups has recently been described in chicken macrophages derived from C/O embryos. Contrary to expectation, these hematopoietic cells are not susceptible to all subgroups but only to B and C (Gazzolo *et al.*, 1974, 1975). The control of host range appears to be again at the penetration stage, with the viral envelope glycoprotein playing a decisive role. These observations suggest that macrophages lack cell surface receptors for subgroups A, D, E, F, and G despite the presence of appropriate genetic information in the cell.

3.2.2. The *Fv-1* Locus of the Mouse Controls an Early Postpenetration Function of Murine Leukemia Viruses

Murine ecotropic leukemia viruses are subject to a number of genetically determined and complex host restrictions which have been admirably reviewed by Lilly and Pincus (1973). The best studied of these genetic systems is controlled by the *Fv-1* locus of the mouse. *Fv* stands for "Friend virus," because originally this locus was discovered by its effect on Friend virus disease (Lilly, 1967), but its two alleles, *Fv-1^n* and *Fv-1^b*, control infection by murine leukemia viruses generally and allow a division of these viruses into three major host range categories, N-tropic, B-tropic, and NB-tropic (Hartley *et al.*, 1970; Pincus *et al.,* 1971*a,b*). N-Tropic viruses grow well in mouse cells which are homozygous for the $Fv-1^n$ allele, but are restricted by a factor of about 10^2 in cells which are homozygous for the $Fv-1^b$ allele. B-Tropic viruses show the reciprocal behavior—optimal growth in $Fv-1^{bb}$ cells and restriction in cells of $Fv-1^{nn}$ constitution. NB viruses grow well in both cell types. Mouse cells which are of the heterozygote $Fv-1^{nb}$ constitution are resistant to B- and N-tropic viruses. Thus in this system resistance is dominant over susceptibility, a fact which argues against the possibility that resistance is caused by the lack of a cellular receptor. Rather, it appears that resistance reflects the presence of some virus inhibitory protein coded for by the $Fv-1$ locus. In keeping with this suggestion is the observation that N- and B-tropism is not controlled by the virion envelope glycoprotein, and therefore probably does not involve virus entry into the cell as a critical step in $Fv-1$ restriction. Pseudotypes of vesicular stomatitis virus carrying the glycoprotein of MuLV in their envelope enter and replicate well in cells homozygous or heterozygous for the *n* or *b* allele of $Fv-1$ regardless of whether the glycoprotein was derived from N- or B-tropic leukemia virus (Krontiris *et al.,* 1973; Huang *et al.,* 1973). Therefore, it appears likely that the target of $Fv-1$ restriction is some internal virion component.

A recent study suggests that the restriction controlled by the $Fv-1$ locus extends also to focus formation induced by murine sarcoma virus under conditions where recruitment of neighboring cells is not required for the development of the focus. Under these conditions, restriction cannot be explained by its effect on the helper-dependent spread of the sarcoma virus (Bassin *et al.,* 1975). A similar interpretation can be applied to the more complex results of Yoshikura (1973*b*), who studied the effect of N- and B-tropic helper viruses on focus formation in $Fv-1$ permissive and restrictive cells under conditions requiring virus spread. These observations are in accord with the hypothesis that $Fv-1$ restriction, although acting after penetration, intervenes before integration and is directed against a virion component which, in the case of MSV pseudotypes, is derived from the helper leukemia virus. A different conclusion concerning the time point of $Fv-1$ restriction was reached by Sveda *et al.* (1974), who followed the fate of ^{32}P-labeled RNA of N- and B-tropic viruses in permissive and in restrictive cells. Since no difference was found in the extent to which labeled RNA became associated with host DNA, Sveda and co-workers proposed that $Fv-1$-controlled restriction occurred after integration. The data of Jolicoeur and Baltimore (1976) are compatible with either hypothesis; the amount of viral RNA was found reduced seventy- to a hundredfold in the cytoplasm and in the nucleus of resistant cells, which could be explained by an *Fv-1*-controlled restriction acting on the transcription of provirus or on an event prior to transcription. It could also mean that virus-specific RNA is rapidly degraded in resistant cells.

Fv-1-controlled resistance can also be transferred to virus-susceptible cells by treatment with cell-free extracts from resistant cells. The active substance in the extracts appears to be an RNA (Tennant *et al.*, 1974*b*).

An indication of the mechanism by which *Fv-1* restriction acts is provided by the titration patterns of restricted virus in resistant cells. This has been found to follow multiple-hit kinetics, and the implication of this observation is that virions must interact with each other in the nonpermissive cell to establish infection (Yoshikura, 1973*a*; Tennant *et al.*, 1974*a*; Declève *et al.*, 1975; Pincus *et al.*, 1975). It is not known whether the interacting particles are of the same or of different kinds. The two-hit titration patterns have recently been called into question in a study demonstrating clear single-hit titration kinetics in the restrictive cell (Jolicoeur and Baltimore, 1975). A resolution of these conflicting data is not available at this time; it will be of great importance for the understanding of *Fv-1* restriction.

The host range determinants of murine xenotropic leukemia viruses have been studied only recently (Levy, 1973). This work and that of Besmer and Baltimore (1975, personal communication) suggest that the viral surface controls the host range of xenotropic MuLV and suggests that the cellular counterpart of this control is a surface receptor which mediates penetration of the virus in the cell.

The third host range category of MuLV is referred to as "amphotropic," because these viruses combine host range characteristics of N-tropic and of xenotropic MuLV (Bryant and Klement, 1976; Hartley and Rowe, 1976; Rasheed *et al.*, 1976). Amphotropic MuLV has been isolated from feral mouse populations. After cloning, these isolates do not show interference or cross-neutralization with eco- or xenotropic MuLV; unlike xenotropic MuLV, they cannot infect duck or Japanese quail cells. The roles of envelope and internal virion components in determining amphotropic host range have not yet been defined.

3.3. Transformation Markers

Besides *td* mutants in which the ability to form foci in fibroblasts is completely lost, there exist qualitative modulations of transforming activity which are determined by the viral genome. Among the avian sarcoma viruses, two types of qualitative transformation markers have been recognized: the morphology of the individual transformed cell and the spatial relationships of transformed cells in a focus (Temin, 1960, 1961; Purchase and Okazaki, 1964; Vogt, 1967c; Yoshii and Vogt, 1970). These markers represent mutants in the *src* gene and are useful in analyzing genetic and nongenetic interactions between viruses. The virus-controlled shape of embryonic fibroblasts transformed by avian sarcoma viruses may be either round or fusiform, and foci composed of either round or fusiform cells can be easily distinguished in the same culture. However, attention to physiological conditions is necessary, as viruses inducing foci of the round cell type can occasionally produce fusiform foci, e.g., temperature-sensitive mutants at intermediate temperature (Martin, 1971), or *wt* virus plated on fibroblasts of the Japanese quail (Moscovici and Jimenez, 1971, unpublished observation). Toyoshima and co-workers recently observed the appearance of fusiform transformation markers in round clones of avian sarcoma virus B77 after passage in cultures of Japanese quail (Toyoshima *et al.,* 1975). Whether this drift from round to fusiform transformation represents a selection of spontaneous or preexisting virus mutants or a host-induced modification of *src* is not known. There is some evidence that fusiform transformation occupies an intermediate position between the normal and the rounded transformed cell type (Martin, 1971). Some parameters of transformation—for example, caseinolytic activity—seen with rounded transformed cells are not or only faintly expressed in fusiform cells (Balduzzi and Murphy, 1975).

Spatial arrangements of transformed cells differ with the strain of avian sarcoma virus (Bryan high titer, Schmidt-Ruppin, Prague, Harris, Carr-Zilber), and foci may be either compact or diffuse, monolayered or multilayered. Both cell morphology and focus architecture have been used as genetic markers of avian sarcoma viruses (Temin, 1961; Friis *et al.,* 1971; Kawai and Hanafusa, 1973). The ability to tell one kind of focus from another extends to avian leukosis viruses which can transform fibroblasts, and here too qualitative transformation markers have potential for genetic studies. Avian leukosis virus MC29 and erythroblastosis virus strain R both induce foci in chick embryo fibroblasts. These foci are distinguishable from those caused by avian sarcoma virus, and thus focus morphology could serve as a marker in crosses between these leukosis and avian sarcoma viruses (Langlois and Beard, 1967; Ishizaki and Shimizu, 1970). Different focus morphologies are also observed with various strains of murine sarcoma virus (Levy *et al.,* 1973). Through the use of murine xenotropic leukemia virus as helpers for RSV(−) and murine sarcoma virus, common host cell systems for murine and avian focus-forming viruses have now become available (Levy, 1975, 1977; Weiss and Wong, 1977). Foci induced by murine sarcoma viruses are distinct in their architecture from those of avian sarcoma viruses in cultures of the same host cell, a fact which should aid further studies on the interactions between these agents (Levy, 1975, personal communication).

4. INTERACTIONS BETWEEN RNA TUMOR VIRUSES

In a discussion of mutants and markers, the logical progression after presenting the data on nonconditional mutants would be to turn to conditional ones. However, while nonconditional mutants and markers of RNA tumor viruses can be covered adequately without going into the details and mechanisms of genetic and nongenetic interactions between viruses, a survey of conditional mutants involves recombination and complementation to a greater extent. Therefore, the basic aspects of these viral interactions will be considered at this point, relying heavily on the specific examples provided by the nonconditional mutants, but also including some material taken from conditional mutants. This section will then serve both as an application of the mutant data discussed so far and as an introduction to the investigations with conditional mutants.

4.1. Complementation and Phenotypic Mixing

"Complementation" is the general term for a nongenetic interaction between two viruses with mutations in different cistrons. If these viruses infect the same cells, they may utilize each other's gene products, and thus the infection becomes phenotypically *wt*. A genetic exchange is not a requirement for complementation, and the progeny of this mixed infection retain their mutant character. Phenotypic mixing can be regarded as a special case of complementation in which the functional gene products supplied to each other by the complementing viruses are proteins of the virion. The phenotypically mixed particles are recognized by specific properties of virion proteins, including control of host range, antigenicity, response to viral interference, and rate of heat inactivation.

4.1.1.   *Rd* Deletion Mutants Are Propagated as Pseudotypes, but Phenotypic Mixing Occurs Also between Nondefective RNA Tumor Viruses

Practically all examples of complementation between RNA tumor viruses involve phenotypic mixing, because most viral gene products are components of the virion. The classical case of phenotypic mixing between RNA tumor viruses is that of BH RSV, an *rd* deletion mutant which is complemented in the envelope function by avian leukosis helper virus (Hanafusa *et al.,* 1963). Phenotypic mixing includes not only structural components of the virion but the RNA-dependent DNA polymerase as well. In the *pol⁻* mutants $NY8\alpha$ and $RSV\alpha(-)$, the helper virus presumably supplies the polymerase besides the envelope glycoprotein (Hanafusa and Hanafusa, 1971; Kawai and Hanafusa, 1973). Analogous situations in which helper viruses supply various virion components are found in all other *rd* deletion mutants of RNA tumor viruses. In the murine sarcoma viruses several genes for structural proteins appear to be deleted, and in pseudotypes of MSV there is therefore an extensive phenotypic contribution of the helper virus. In all cases where genetic deletions cause the complete lack of a certain virion component, the degree of phenotypic mixing is of necessity extreme, as all of the missing components in such pseudotypes need to be supplied by the helper virus.

Phenotypic mixing also occurs between nondeleted virion components; for instance, the envelope glycoproteins of avian leukosis viruses become mixed if different viruses replicate in the same cell, and the same is true of nondefective sarcoma viruses (Vogt, 1967*b*). An open question in this context is whether there exist mosaic virions which carry the glycoproteins (or other virion components) of two or more parental viruses or whether all phenotypic mixing is really phenotypic *masking* with glycoproteins or other virion proteins of one virus enclosing the genome of another. Some evidence has been presented in favor of mosaics, but more work is needed to settle the question (Vogt, 1967*b*). Complementation by phenotypic mixing is also observed with *ts* mutants. Examples will be discussed in greater detail in a later section of this chapter. At this point, one instance will suffice: *LA*334, a *ts* mutant of avian sarcoma virus B77 has a late defect in virus production. This defect can be complemented by avian leukosis virus and by RSV(−) (Owada and Toyoshima, 1973; Hunter and Vogt, 1976). The complementation is probably due to phenotypic mixing involving an internal nonglycosylated virion protein.

4.1.2. Phenotypic Mixing Sometimes Combines Components of Unrelated Virions

Phenotypic mixing occurs rather indiscriminately between RNA tumor viruses. This is especially evident among mammalian leukemia viruses, all of which can act as helpers for the diverse replication-defective mammalian sarcoma viruses. A rare exception described in the literature is the porcine type C virus, which could not rescue Kirsten MSV from a nonproducer cell line (Todaro *et al.*, 1974). However, it is not known whether this absence of phenotypic mixing between Kirsten MSV and porcine type C virus is a property of the virus combination or of the cell system. Pseudotype formation has even been demonstrated to occur between xenotropic murine leukemia viruses (xMuLV) and replication-defective avian sarcoma viruses (Levy, 1977; Weiss, and Wong, 1977). Because xMuLV can infect duck cells and Japanese quail cells, it is possible to use it as helper virus in RSV(−)-transformed lines of these host species (Levy, 1975). The pseudotypes from this coinfection show the envelope properties, chiefly the host range of xMuLV, and can infect and transform a large number of different mammalian cells but not murine cells. The reciprocal pseudotypes between murine sarcoma virus and avian leukosis virus have also been created by an infection of duck cells with MSV (xMuLV) followed by superinfection with a subgroup C avian leukosis virus which is capable of growing in these cells. Progeny can replicate in chicken fibroblasts, but for unknown reasons fails to transform these cells. Phenotypic mixing has also been demonstrated between avian sarcoma virus, ecotropic murine leukemia virus, feline leukemia virus, and a primate leukemia virus (Levy, 1977; Weiss and Wong, 1977).

In the light of these observations, the apparent absence of phenotypic mixing between avian leukosis and sarcoma viruses on the one side and reticuloendotheliosis virus on the other is very puzzling (Halpern *et al.*, 1973). In the past, this lack of interaction has been explained by the absence of nucleic acid homology and antigenic cross-reaction between avian leukosis and sarcoma viruses and reticuloendotheliosis viruses (Halpern *et al.*, 1973; Maldonado and Bose, 1973; Mizutani and Temin, 1973; Kang and Temin, 1973; Moelling *et al.*, 1975), but since xMuLV also lacks relatedness to avian sarcoma and leukosis viruses this argument is no longer satisfactory, and a reinvestigation of possible interactions between REV and avian leukosis and sarcoma viruses is indicated.

An even wider distance between viral groups spans pseudotypes of vesicular stomatitis virus which contain the genome of this virus but carry envelope determinants of RNA tumor viruses (Závada, 1972). These pseudotypes have been extremely valuable in the analysis of host range determinants for RNA tumor viruses. It has been mentioned above that VSV pseudotypes carrying envelope markers of either N- or B-tropic MuLV are not restricted by the *Fv-1* locus, indicating that the envelope components are of no consequence in N- or B-tropic host range (Huang *et al.*, 1973; Krontiris *et al.*, 1973). Weiss and co-workers have made imaginative use of VSV pseudotypes equipped with avian sarcoma and leukosis virus glycoproteins in studies of avian tumor virus antigenicity and host range (Love and Weiss, 1974; Boettiger *et al.*, 1975; Weiss *et al.*, 1975). Their data demonstrate the dominant influence of the glycoprotein on the host range of avian leukosis and sarcoma viruses. This effect of the glycoprotein extends also to mammalian cells which can be infected by VSV pseudotypes only if they carry the avian glycoproteins of subgroups C or D, thus reflecting the host range of the avian sarcoma virus subgroups. These studies further demonstrate that, despite efficient penetration, avian sarcoma viruses have a reduced ability to transform mammalian cells. Boettiger (1974, 1975) and Varmus *et al.* (1973a,b, 1975a,b) have also shown that after infection with avian sarcoma viruses a substantial proportion of mammalian cells remain phenotypically normal but contain DNA provirus and yield infectious avian sarcoma virus after fusion with chicken cells. These observations suggest that there exists a second, postpenetration block in the transformation of mammalian cells by avian sarcoma viruses.

4.2. Recombination between RNA Tumor Viruses

Genetic recombination is common between RNA tumor viruses. It was first demonstrated in double infection with an avian sarcoma virus and an avian leukosis virus of different envelope-controlled host ranges (Vogt, 1971b; Kawai and Hanafusa, 1972b). The recombinants arising in these double infections unite in genetically stable form, the transforming ability (*src*) of the sarcoma virus with the envelope host range (*env*) of the leukosis virus. It can be shown that this combination of viral markers is not caused by continuous phenotypic mixing, because the recombinant properties persist through serial clonings of the virus in the absence of excess parental leukosis virus. The frequency of recombinants in mixed yields is surprisingly high, ranging from 10% to 40%.

4.2.1.   Recombination Occurs between Any Marker of Related RNA Tumor Viruses and Can Include Endogenous Viral Genes

All genetic markers of avian RNA tumor viruses can probably participate in recombination. Thus avian sarcoma viruses which are *ts* for the maintenance of transformation or nonconditional avian sarcoma virus mutants showing fusiform morphology of the transformed cell have been recombined into different envelope subgroups by cocultivation with an avian leukosis virus of the appropriate envelope specificity (Kawai *et al.,* 1972; Wyke, 1973*b*; Vogt, 1974, unpublished observation; Bernstein *et al.,* 1976). *Ts* avian sarcoma viruses with a mutation in *pol* show recombination with wild-type (*wt*) leukosis virus, yielding *wt* avian sarcoma virus with the *src* gene derived from the mutant sarcoma virus and *pol* and *env* contributed by the leukosis virus (Linial and Mason, 1973; Mason *et al.,* 1974). Two *ts* mutations located in different genes, and possibly even mutations in the same gene can also recombine to give *wt* virus (Wong and McCarter, 1973; Wyke *et al.,* 1975).

Recombination not only occurs between different RNA tumor viruses which infect a cell exogenously but also has been found to take place between markers of endogenous RNA tumor viruses and a superinfecting exogenous virus (Weiss *et al.,* 1973). Nondefective avian sarcoma viruses replicating in chicken cells which contain the genetic information of an endogenous RNA tumor virus acquire by genetic recombination the characteristic host range marker of this endogenous virus. However, a prerequisite for this type of recombination is that the endogenous marker be expressed (i.e., that RNA sequences of this marker be transcribed). Endogenous viral information that is not transcribed does not participate in recombination. Recombination between exogenous and endogenous RNA tumor viruses in a mammalian system is suggested by the work of Stephenson *et al.* (1974*a*), who found that passage of ecotropic MuLV in human cells selects for viral variants which carry the envelope glycoprotein of xenotropic MuLV. This glycoprotein facilitates entry into human cells and this makes it possible for the virus to grow in the heterologous host. However, these variants have retained the p12 protein of the ecotropic parent and thus may be recombinants between eco- and xenotropic murine leukemia viruses which were selected for in the human cells. A different possible recombinant between ecotropic and xenotropic MuLV was found by Fischinger *et al.* (1975). This agent shows the combined host range of the parental viruses and carries glycoprotein markers from both parents. The presumptive recombinant is genetically stable; whether it represents a crossover within *env* or a stable heterozygote is not known. Measurements of genetic complexity could decide this question. At least phenotypically, this virus is an amphotropic MuLV.

Recombination of endogenous viral markers has also been observed with avian leukosis viruses. In chicken cells which express the subgroup E host range marker of the endogenous leukosis virus (*chf*[+] cells), superinfection with an exogenous leukosis virus results in the release of progeny which carry the genetic information for the host range of the endogenous virus. The majority, if not all, of these new subgroup E viruses, termed collectively RAV-60, are recombinants between the exogenous leukosis virus (e.g., Rous-associated virus type 2, RAV-2) and endogenous viral information rather than being exclusively ˙endogenous viruses which were activated by the superinfecting exogenous leukosis virus (T. Hanafusa *et al.*, 1970*b*; Hayward and H. Hanafusa, 1975). Nucleic acid hybridization shows that RAV-60 has sequences in common with the exogenous virus (e.g., RAV-2) and with RAV-0, an endogenous avian leukosis virus produced spontaneously without the intervention of an exogenous agent in fibroblast cultures of certain chicken lines. Unlike RAV-0, however, RAV-60 is only partially represented in the genome of the cell, presumably because part of its genome is derived from RAV-2. Because RAV-60 originates by recombination, it must be expected that RAV-60 isolates derived from different recombinational events, even with the same exogenous virus, are nonidentical. RAV-60 isolates generated with different exogenous leukosis viruses will definitely be nonidentical.

4.2.2. Recombinants between RNA Tumor Viruses Arise by Crossing Over

Recombinants make up a sizable portion of mixed yields in avian RNA tumor virus infections. This high frequency of recombination suggested at first that genetic exchange was probably achieved by reassortment of genome segments (Vogt, 1971*b*; Kawai and Hanafusa, 1972*b*). High-frequency recombination with influenza viruses and with reoviruses is based on such a mechanism (Hirst, 1962; Fields and Joklik, 1969). Both of these viruses also have a segmented genome. However, the genome of RNA tumor viruses has now been shown to be nonsegmented. The 30–40 S pieces comprising the 60–70 S RNA are identical, and each contains a complete set of genes. Given this polyploid, nonsegmented structure, an exchange of 30–40 S unit genomes between genetically different parent viruses by reassortment would lead to heterozygotes but not to genetically stable recombinants. Heterozygotes of RNA tumor viruses have indeed been found, but have also been shown to be genetically unstable and to segregate into parental or recombinant genotypes (Weiss *et al.*, 1973; Wyke *et al.*, 1975). Because of the structural properties of the RNA tumor virus genome, recombination most likely involves crossing over (i.e., genetic exchange between homologous molecules of nucleic acid). Experimental evidence for crossing over between RNA tumor viruses is threefold (Vogt and Duesberg, 1973; Beemon *et al.*, 1974; Duesberg *et al.*, 1975*b*).

1. In crosses between nondefective avian sarcoma and leukosis viruses, the parental viruses differ in the size of their 30–40 S RNA. The RNA of the sarcoma virus is about 10–15% larger (class *a* RNA) than that of the leukosis virus (class *b* RNA). If recombinants arose by reassortment of 30–40 S RNA derived from the two parents, then all of these recombinants should contain class *a* and class *b* RNA together, since they unite the host range marker originally situated on the class *b* RNA of the leukosis virus with the transformation marker derived from class *a* RNA of the sarcoma virus. However, all sarcoma virus recombinants which have acquired the host range marker of the leukemia virus have class *a* RNA and little, if any, class *b*, suggesting that crossing over between sarcoma and leukosis virus genomes has taken place rather than reassortment.

An alternative explanation for this observation on the size of recombinant RNA has not been ruled out but is less likely: Class *b* RNA of parental leukosis virus could be augmented by cellular sequences to become size class *a*, and for geometric reasons only class *a* RNA could be incorporated into sarcoma viruses. In this event, however, recombinants should show a greater sequence complexity than the parental sarcoma viruses, and this is not the case.

2. The class *a* RNA of recombinants is often not exactly the same size as the class *a* RNA of the parental sarcoma virus. Recombinants selected for the same markers but derived from different recombinational events may have a 30–40 S RNA either slightly smaller or slightly larger than that of the parental sarcoma virus. The differences are detectable by gel electrophoresis. They represent RNA sequences of about 70,000 molecular weight; they are characteristic for individual recombinants, and are genetically stable. Again, reassort-

ment fails to explain this observation, but crossing over could account for it if the crossover were occasionally unequal, resulting in small deletions or duplications of genetic material to the genome of a recombinant. In this respect, it is of interest that one of the recombinants which showed a slightly smaller class *a* RNA than that of the parental virus was also relatively defective in replication, producing lowered quantities of virus (Duesberg *et al.*, 1975*b*).

 3. Recombinants derived from different recombination events but selected for the same markers have different oligonucleotide fingerprint patterns. Only a very limited sequence diversity between recombinants selected for the same markers would be expected if reassortment were the mechanism of genetic recombination. If there were maximally three 30–40 S pieces per 60–70 S RNA complex (Mangel *et al.*, 1974; Delius *et al.*, 1975), then the two pieces carrying the selected markers would have to be constant, allowing the third one to be derived from either parent. This situation could generate two oligonucleotide fingerprint patterns, but in the two crosses studied the fingerprints of the first five recombinants tested were all different. These differences could be explained by variable or multiple crossover points between the selected markers as well as crossover points outside the markers studied. In one of the recombinants an oligonucleotide not present in either parent was found. It is conceivable that this new oligonucleotide contains sequences of both parents and represents the point of crossover.

 The conclusion from all these data is that RNA tumor viruses undergo high-frequency crossingover. The molecular mechanism of this genetic exchange remains unknown, but two observations are relevant to it: (1) Double infections with RNA tumor viruses lead to the formation of heterozygotes which are genetically unstable and segregate into parental and recombinant progeny (Weiss *et al.*, 1973; Wyke *et al.*, 1975). The formation of such heterozygotes is to be expected because of the polyploidy of the RNA tumor virus genome. In crosses between sarcoma viruses (with size class *a* RNA) and leukosis viruses (with the smaller size class *b* RNA), heterozygotes should contain both class *a* and class *b* RNA, but so far no pure preparations of heterozygotes have been obtained, and this suggestion remains untested. (2) Recombinants do not arise in the first cycle of double infection but only after a second cycle (Wyke *et al.*, 1975). This observation is in accord with the hypothesis that heterozygotes are the obligatory precursors of recombinants and are generated in the first cycle of mixed infection. Recombinants would be derived from heterozygotes in the second cycle of infection (Vogt, 1973; Vogt and Duesberg, 1973; Weiss, 1973; Wyke *et al.,* 1975). The high frequency of crossover might then be explained by the fact that genetic exchange takes place between parental genomes which comprise the same 60–70 S RNA complex, presumably during reverse transcription of this complex.

4.2.3.   Deletion Mutants Show Specific Defects in Recombination

An interesting exception to the generality of recombination between RNA tumor virus markers is provided by the *rd* deletion mutants of avian sarcoma viruses RSV(−) and *NY*8. RSV(−) or *NY*8 grown together with an avian leukosis virus which can be thought of as *td* deletion cannot recombine to yield nondefective sarcoma virus (Hanafusa *et al.,* 1963; Kawai *et al.,* 1972; Weiss *et al.,* 1973; Kawai and Hanafusa, 1973). This fact may be explained by the position of the two deletions. As Wyke (1974) has suggested and as has been confirmed by recent mapping experiments, the *src* and the *env* functions are probably located adjacent to each other on the viral genome (Joho *et al.,* 1975; Wang *et al.,* 1975, 1976*a,b*). Therefore, if in one parent *env* is missing, and the other parent lacks *src,* the mating genomes will form opposing deletion loops. Assuming that recombinants arise by crossing-over, nondefective sarcoma virus could not be generated by such a mating pair. This hypothetical explanation has three corollaries: (1) RSV(−) and *NY*8 should be able to recombine in the *src* gene with nondefective avian sarcoma virus, (2) genetic exchange between RSV(−) or *NY*8 and *td* helper virus should occur outside the deletions, and (3) if deletions in two parental viruses are not contiguous or overlapping, nondefective recombinants may occur with certain mechanisms of recombination.

Evidence for (1) has recently been obtained by Hunter (1975, personal communication) and by Kawai and Hanafusa (1976) who have recombined B77 with RSV(−) and *NY*8 with the Schmidt-Ruppin strain of RSV (mutant *NY*68) and found replication-defective progeny with focus morphology characteristics of B77 or temperature sensitivity of the mutant *NY*68 of Schmidt-Ruppin RSV, respectively.

An example for corollary (2) may be provided by the isolation of RAV-61, an RNA tumor virus obtained from ringnecked pheasant cells. Ringnecked pheasant cells infected with RSV(−) frequently begin to release an infectious pseudotype of this defective sarcoma virus whose glycoprotein is controlled by viral genetic information indigenous to pheasant cells. From such pseudotypes an avian leukosis virus has been isolated. This helper virus replicates to high titers in several avian cell types, including pheasant cells. By this efficiency of replication, it can be sharply distinguished from the endogenous virus which is spontaneously released by ringnecked pheasant cells without the help of a superinfecting avian sarcoma virus and which replicates very poorly (Hanafusa and Hanafusa, 1973). It is therefore likely that RAV-61 is a recombinant between exogenous RSV(−) and endogenous viral sequences of ringnecked pheasant cells. It may be generated by a mechanism similar to that shown for RAV-60, a recombinant between exogenous avian leukosis virus and endogenous viral genes in chicken cells. Because of the recombinant nature of RAV-61, it is also probable that different isolates of this virus are genetically nonidentical, containing different proportions of exogenous and endogenous genomes (Fujita et al., 1974).

The genetic instability of RSVα(−) and of NY8α which are env⁻ and pol⁻ mutants but seem to recombine with helper leukosis virus for wt pol (Hanafusa and Hanafusa, 1968; Kawai and Hanafusa, 1973) can be explained either by corollary (2), if the pol⁻ mutation is not due to a deletion, or by corollary (3), if it is a deletion that is not contiguous with the env deletion in RSV(−) or NY8.

Defective MSV and other mammalian sarcoma viruses are also unable to acquire missing genetic functions by recombination with helper viruses. There is evidence from the size of the murine sarcoma virus genome that R and possibly C functions are deleted. These deletions may again be contiguous with the src deletion in the various helper viruses, thus barring recombination which would lead to nondefective sarcoma virus.

5. CONDITIONAL MUTANTS

In conditional mutants the manifestation of mutant character is dependent on experimentally controllable physiological parameters. It is expressed under nonpermissive conditions, but under permissive conditions the mutant virus behaves like wild type. All conditional mutants of RNA tumor viruses are temperature sensitive (ts). The conditionality of the mutant character offers two principal advantages: (1) Since the virus can be grown at the permissive temperature, mutants can be isolated in all viral genes, including those in which a nonconditional mutation would be lethal. (2) Shift experiments between permissive and nonpermissive conditions offer a flexibility in the physiological characterization of gene action not available with nonconditional mutants. The main disadvantage of conditional mutants is their leakiness. A variable fraction of the mutant virus may behave as *wt* under nonpermissive conditions, yet the leaky viruses are genetically unaltered and produce mutant progeny. Leakiness can be reduced but not eliminated by maximizing the differential between permissive and nonpermissive conditions to the extent which is practical with the cell culture system used. Selection of nonleaky mutants often also selects for multiple mutants which present their own difficulty, especially in genetic analysis.

Most conditional mutants of RNA tumor viruses studied in any detail have been isolated after mutagenization, but spontaneously occurring *ts* mutants have been observed (Temin, 1971; Friis *et al.*, 1971; Wong *et al.*, 1973; Somers and Kit, 1973).

5.1. *ts* Mutants of Avian Sarcoma Viruses

Several mutagens have been used in the isolation of avian sarcoma virus *ts* mutants, incorporative mutagens acting on replicating RNA (5-azacytidine, 5-fluorouracil) or DNA (bromodeoxyuridine), and nonincorporative mutagens acting on resting nucleic acids (*N*-methyl-*N'*-nitro-*N*-nitrosoguanidine, ultraviolet light, and ^{60}Co irradiation) (Toyoshima and Vogt, 1969; Martin, 1970; Biquard and Vigier, 1971; Kawai and Hanafusa, 1971; Bader, 1972; Wyke, 1973*a*; Linial and Mason, 1973; Friis and Hunter, 1973). Most mutants of avian sarcoma viruses have been isolated by picking single foci of transformed cells at random. The progeny of these virus clones are tested for transformation and replication at the permissive temperature (35–36°C) and nonpermissive temperature (41–41.5°C). This simple primary mutant characterization divides the mutants into three large classes: those which are temperature sensitive for transformation but show an unimpaired synthesis of virus progeny at 41°C (class T), those which produce greatly reduced amounts of viral progeny at 41°C but can still transform cells with the same efficiency as *wt* (class R), and those for which the nonpermissive temperature imposes a restriction on transformation and virus production alike (class C for coordinate).

For class T mutants, a selective isolation procedure has also been described. It is based on the preferential killing of *wt*-transformed cells by bromodeoxyuridine and light (Wyke, 1973*a*). Because of the polyploidy of the viral genome, it seems advisable to passage mutagenized stocks of virus at low multiplicities of infection and under permissive conditions in order to accumulate homozygote mutants. However, there are no data showing that this practice actually increases the frequency of mutant isolation.

Most avian sarcoma virus *ts* mutants obtained so far fall in the T class; very few have been found in the R class; and of the isolates in the C class, several have turned out to be multiple mutants with defects in R and T functions or in C and T functions. The reason for the preponderance of class T mutants is not clear. As judged from work with *td* deletion viruses, the T function occupies only a small fraction of the genome, probably not more that 15%, and if mutants were picked up at about equal frequency in all viral genes, class T mutants should be in the minority compared to mutations in the rest of the genome. The unbalanced distribution of mutants isolated in the three classes could derive from the fact that the nonpermissive temperature in this system is also the body temperature of the chicken, the environment in which these viruses normally replicate. Structural proteins of the virus may therefore have evolved a relatively high stability for 41°C, so that most amino acid exchanges do not lead to temperature sensitivity under these conditions. Another possibility is that recombination or complementation with endogenous viral genes repairs many defects in replication functions, although there is no experimental evidence that this happens in cells which do not transcribe endogenous viral genes.

The assignment of mutant isolates to the three classes T, R, and C is strictly operational and very simplistic. It is useful but should not be regarded rigidly, for it can lead to inconsistencies, especially in the R and C classes. For instance, mutant *LA*672 belongs formally to class R, yet it has a lesion in the reverse transcriptase, clearly a function required for both transformation and virus production.

A second parameter conventionally used to characterize mutants is the time point in the life cycle of the virus at which the mutant acts, early vs. late. In the avian sarcoma viruses, this distinction is made operationally and is not identical with the definition of early and late mutants in other viral systems. According to Wyke and Linial (1973), early avian sarcoma virus *ts* mutants do not become restricted in the mutated function if the shift to the nonpermissive temperature is delayed for a few hours after infection. Their action is therefore not only early but also transient. Many of these mutants also cannot be recovered if the infection is initiated at 41°C and then shifted to permissive temperatures a few hours later. This decay at the nonpermissive temperature is sometimes but not always linked to *ts* virion components. Late mutants are responsive to temperature shifts at any time after infection. Shift up will always bring about mutant character, and shift down to permissive conditions will restore the *wt* behavior of the virus. This definition of early vs. late has the advantage of being technically convenient, but remains unsatisfactory, because it is not tied to a specific event in the virus life cycle. Wyke (1975) has now proposed to use as a dividing line the integration of provirus, and to define this line along the studies of Humphries and Temin (1972, 1974), Boettiger and Temin (1970), and Balduzzi and Morgan (1970), who showed that in stationary cell cultures provirus is synthesized, but no viral RNA is transcribed. A *ts* mutant which could go through the early events of infection in stationary cultures at the nonpermissive temperature would be "late" and one lacking this ability would be called "early." Wyke reports that preliminary tests applying this definition of "early" vs. "late" to mutants which have been classified previously by shifts in replicating cell cultures revealed agreement between the two methods (Wyke and Linial, 1973; Wyke, 1975). The difficulty with the new definition of "early" and "late" is that the experimental tests used do not determine integration. In this chapter, the older definition of Wyke and Linial (1973) for early and late mutants based on shift experiments alone will therefore be retained.

A convention has been agreed to for the numbering of avian sarcoma virus *ts* mutants and has been published (Vogt *et al.,* 1974). This convention is adopted in this chapter. The minimal mutant designation consists of a two-letter laboratory code followed by a mutant number. Each laboratory follows its own numbering system. Additional information may be incorporated in the mutant designation; for instance, *ts LA*335 PR-C refers to an avian sarcoma virus *ts* mutant derived from subgroup C Prague strain of Rous sarcoma virus (PR-C). *LA* is one of the laboratory codes. The rules on mutant numbering apply also to nonconditional mutants.

5.1.1. Class T Mutants of Avian Sarcoma Viruses

Most *ts* avian sarcoma viruses of class T share basic physiological characteristics; they are unable to transform fibroblasts at 41°C but can synthesize progeny virus under these conditions. Aside from three somewhat enigmatic exceptions, all class T mutants are late and respond to temperature shift at any time after infection with the appropriate changes in their transformed or normal state. However, beyond

TABLE 6

Avian Sarcoma Virus *ts* Mutants of Class T

Mutant designation	Mutagen[a]	Parental wt virus[b]	Reference
*BK*1 to *BK*6	NG	SR RSV-A	Martin (1970, 1971)
*LA*22 to *LA*29	5AC	PR RSV-A	Wyke (1973*a*)
*LA*31 to *LA*35	5AC	PR RSV-A	
*PA*19	5FU	SR RSV-D	Biquard and Vigier (1972)
*NY*10 to *NY*19	NG	SR RSV-A	Kawai and Hanafusa (1971)
*NY*68	5FU	SR RSV-A	Kawai *et al.* (1972)
*OS*122	BUDR	SR RSV-D	Toyoshima *et al.* (1973)
*OS*260	UV	B77-C	
*OS*538	5AC	SR RSV-A	
*BE*1	BUDR	BH RSV	Bader (1972)
*LA*6 to *LA*8	5AC	B77-C	Friis (1972, unpublished)
*LA*12 to *LA*14	5AC	PR RSV-A	Vogt (1972, unpublished)
*LA*1 to *LA*5	5AC	PR RSV-A	Skoog (1974, unpublished)
*LA*30m	5AC	PR RSV-A	Wyke (1973*a*)
*MI*100	⁶⁰Co	SR RSV-B	Bookout and Sigel (1975)
*RO*1 and others	BUDR	BH RSV	Balduzzi (1976)

[a] Abbreviations: NG, *N*-methyl-*N'*-nitro-N-nitrosoguanidine; 5AC, 5-azacytidine; 5FU, 5-fluorouracil; BUDR, bromodeoxyuridine; UV, ultraviolet light; ⁶⁰Co, γ-irradiation.

[b] Abbreviations: SR RSV-A, -B, -D, Schmidt-Ruppin strain Rous sarcoma virus subgroup A, B, and D, respectively; PR RSV-A, Prague strain Rous sarcoma virus of subgroup A; BH RSV, Bryan high-titer Rous sarcoma virus; B77-C, avian sarcoma virus B77, subgroup C.

these basic common denominators there is considerable diversity among the class T mutants in the kinetics of temperature shift, in the transformed cell parameters which are affected, and in the metabolic requirements for retransformation upon downshift to permissive conditions. Table 6 gives a survey of avian sarcoma virus class T *ts* mutants.

5.1.2. In Cultures Infected with Class T *ts* Mutants of Avian Sarcoma Viruses Numerous Changes of Cellular Properties Are Temperature Dependent

Productive infection with an avian sarcoma virus affects many cellular properties. Those virus-induced cellular changes which are not due to the processes of virus replication alone and therefore are *not* found in cells infected with *td* deletion mutants are considered related to transformation. They can therefore be linked, directly or indirectly, to the action of *src*. These physiological parameters of transformation and their temperature dependence in class T mutants will now be discussed. They constitute a rather lengthy catalogue of often unrelated cellular changes.

Focus formation in fibroblast cultures is, of course, uniformly *ts* in class T mutants, because this parameter serves to define the T class. Temperature-shift experiments clearly show that the morphological transformation of fibroblasts is dependent on the continuous action of a viral gene (Toyoshima and Vogt, 1969; Martin, 1970, 1971; Kawai and Hanafusa, 1971; Friis *et al.*, 1971; Biquard and Vigier, 1971, 1972; Wyke and Linial, 1973; Bookout and Sigel, 1975).

Colony formation in agar is not uniformly *ts* in class T mutants. For instance, the T lesions in *LA*334 and *LA*25 do not affect this parameter, and a collection of class T mutants obtained from BH RSV contain some which promote the formation of agar colonies at 41°C (Friis *et al.*, 1971); Bauer *et al.*, 1975; Balduzzi, 1976). Nonconditional transformation mutants which lack focus-forming potential but can induce agar colony formation have also been described (Duesberg and Vogt, 1973a; Weiss *et al.*, 1973). However, most class T mutants show temperature sensitivity of colony formation, and this property extends to mammalian cells transformed by these mutants as well (Kawai and Hanafusa, 1971; Friis *et al.*, 1971; Wyke, 1973a; Graf and Friis, 1973; Bookout and Sigel, 1975; Chen *et al.*, in preparation).

The *in vivo* correlate of focus formation and colony formation in agar is induction of sarcomas in chickens, and since the body temperature of the chicken is the nonpermissive 41°C, this parameter can be studied. It has been found to be *ts* in the class T mutants tested (Friis *et al.*, 1971; Toyoshima *et al.*, 1973). Toyoshima and co-workers also carried out a shift experiment *in vivo* by exposing the chickens to lower temperature and found that this procedure greatly enhanced the formation of sarcomas by class T mutants. Temperature sensitivity of tumor formation has also been demonstrated by infection of the chorioallantoic membrane of the developing chick embryo (Biquard and Vigier, 1972).

High saturation density of growth in cell culture is another parameter of transformation which is usually *ts* in class T mutants. One exception is again *LA*25, which induces cell growth to high densities even at the nonpermissive temperature (Wyke and Linial, 1973; Kurth *et al.*, 1975). A collection of class T *ts* mutants isolated from BH RSV also contains such exceptional viruses which promote high cell density at the nonpermissive temperature (Balduzzi, 1976).

The properties of the cell surface and of the plasma membrane undergo extensive changes during transformation. Most of these changes have been shown to be *ts* in class T mutants. To these belong increased agglutinability by plant lectins such as concanavalin and wheat germ hemagglutinin (Burger and Martin, 1972; Biquard, 1973; Graf and Friis, 1973), appearance of cell membrane ruffles demonstrable by scanning electron microscopy (Ambros *et al.*, 1975), production of excess hyaluronic acid (Bader, 1972), and alteration of glycolipid patterns resulting in a marked reduction of hematoside in transformed cells (Hakomori *et al.*, 1973, 1977; see, however, Warren *et al.*, 1972).

Cell transformation by avian sarcoma viruses is also accompanied by the excretion of proteases (Unkeless *et al.*, 1973). Indirect evidence suggests that several such proteolytic enzymes exist which can be distinguished in different assay systems (Chen and Buchanan, 1975). The secretion of all proteolytic activity is *ts* in class T mutants *BK*5 and *NY*68, the only ones reported on so far.

Avian sarcoma virus-transformed cells contain a new antigen on their surface, referred to as TSSA (tumor-specific surface antigen) (Kurth and Bauer, 1972*a,b,* 1975). Class T mutants behave rather heterogeneously with respect to the elaboration of this antigen at 41°C (Bauer *et al.*, 1975; Kurth *et al.*, 1975). Apart from the fact that the acknowledged leaky mutant, *LA*25, which induces high population density and agar colony formation at 41°C, also stimulates the production of some TSSA, there are generally nonleaky class T mutants in which the ability to induce TSSA is undiminished at 41°C. At this time, too few mutants have been tested to allow a correlation with the genetically defined "cooperative transformation groups" of the T class (Wyke, 1973*b*; Wyke *et al.*, 1975), but induction of TSSA under nonpermissive conditions occurs in at least two of these groups. The presence of TSSA on phenotypically normal cells may suggest that TSSA, although necessary, is not sufficient for morphological transformation. It could also be argued that a mutated TSSA detected at 41°C is functionally deficient while retaining its antigenicity.

Further cell surface changes accompanying transformation include increases and decreases i. certain proteins associated with the plasma membrane and perhaps other cellular membranes. Although the molecular weights given by various authors for membrane and surface proteins affected by transformation differ, and different authors do not always emphasize all of the changes which may occur, there is a fairly good consensus that the major alterations in transformation are as follows: A "large external transformation specific" (LETS) protein of about 150,000–250,000 molecular weight disappears during transformation. Two membrane proteins of about 70,000–80,000 and 90,000–95,000 molecular weight, respectively, increase in amount. A decrease is reported in a membrane protein of about 40,000–50,000 molecular weight (Hynes, 1973; Gahmberg and Hakomori, 1973; Bussell and Robinson, 1973; Wickus and Robbins, 1973; Stone *et al.*, 1974; Vaheri and Ruoslahti, 1974; Robbins *et al.*, 1975; Isaka *et al.*, 1975; Yamada *et al.*, 1975). There seems to be no uniformity in mutant behavior with respect to the transformation-induced decrease in LETS protein: some mutants do not show this transformation-related decrease at the non-permissive temperature but others, e.g., *LA*334, *LA*31, and *OS*122, do, suggesting retention of some transformed properties at 41°C (Hynes and Wyke, 1975; Isaka *et al.*, 1975). The increase of the 70,000–80,000 and the 90,000–95,000 molecular weight protein species is found *ts* in all class T mutants studied. The decrease of the 40,000–50,000 molecular weight protein has been reported to be *ts* in class T mutants, but this is not a universal finding (Stone *et al.*, 1974; Robbins *et al.*, 1975; Isaka *et al.*, 1975). It is particularly noteworthy that the transformation-related changes in the LETS glycoprotein and in the 70,000–80,000 and 90,000–95,000 molecular weight proteins are also seen in cells of Japanese quail and of rat transformed by avian sarcoma virus class T mutants at the permissive temperature but not at the non-permissive temperature (Stone *et al.*, 1974; Chen *et al.*, 1977). Possibly related to the various changes of cellular membrane proteins seen during transformation is the observation that glycopeptides from transformed cell surfaces are larger. This increase in the size of trypsin-resistant glycopeptides is temperature dependent in the avian sarcoma virus class T mutant *BK*5 (Warren *et al.*, 1972).

Transformation by avian sarcoma viruses brings about an increase in the rate of hexose uptake over that in normal fibroblasts (Hatanaka and Hanafusa, 1970; Weber, 1973). This transformation-related alteration which seems to be due to an increase in the number of functional transport sites is not induced by class T mutants at the nonpermissive temperature (Kawai and Hanafusa, 1971; Martin *et al.*, 1971; Bader, 1972; Graf and Friis, 1973; Venuta and Rubin, 1973; Kletzien and Perdue, 1974, 1975; Bookout and Sigel, 1975; Hynes and Wyke, 1975.

Another physiological characteristic of transformed cells is a lower level of cyclic AMP. This change from the normal fibroblast is due to a reduction in adenylate cyclase activity in transformed cells. It is temperature dependent in chick embryo fibroblasts transformed by avian sarcoma virus class T mutants (Otten *et al.*, 1972; Anderson *et al.*, 1973*a,b*). However, several mechanisms seem to exist by which various strains of avian sarcoma virus and their *ts* mutants affect adenylate cyclase activity (Yoshida *et al.*, 1975).

A transformation-related change which at present cannot be linked directly to altered growth or surface properties of avian sarcoma cells is the increase in dimeric and oligomeric mitochondrial DNA (Nass, 1973). This change is also temperature dependent in chick embryo fibroblast cultures infected with class T *ts* mutants of avian sarcoma viruses.

Two interesting transformation-related effects of infection by avian sarcoma viruses have been observed in cultures of embryonic myoblasts (Holtzer *et al.*, 1975; Fiszman and Fuchs, 1975). As a result of infection either with class T mutant at the permissive temperature or with *wt* avian sarcoma virus over the entire physiological temperature range, mononucleate cells in these cultures become rounded, continue to divide, but do not fuse into myotubes. Multinucleate myotubes present at the time of infection become vacuolated and degenerate. At the nonpermissive temperature, both effects are suppressed in mutant-infected cultures. Myoblasts then show increasing fusion activity and form healthy myotubes. Upon shift to the permissive temperature, these myotubes degenerate. A shift of mutant-infected cultures to the nonpermissive temperature results in fusion of the transformed myoblast to form multinucleate myotubes. This observation indicates that transformation of chicken myogenic cells by avian sarcoma viruses does not erase the commitment of the cells to myogenesis but blocks the execution of the differentiated program.

Chick embryo fibroblasts infected by certain class T mutants of avian sarcoma viruses at the nonpermissive temperature also support induction of plaques by avian leukosis viruses of subgroups B and D (Kawai and Hanafusa, 1972*a*; Wyke and Linial, 1973). Although plaques can also be induced by these leukosis viruses in normal cells (Dougherty and Rasmussen, 1964; Graf, 1972), plaque formation in mutant infected cells seems to have less stringent requirements. After infection with a *ts* mutant, plaque formation can be observed when normal control cells are refractory to the cytopathic effect of leukosis viruses either because of physiological conditions or because of genetic constitution of the cell (Vogt, 1975, unpublished observation).

The large number of different transformation-related changes induced by avian sarcoma viruses is puzzling if considered in the context of evidence which suggests that transformation is caused by the reaction of a single viral gene (Wyke *et al.*, 1975). No doubt, many of these changes are indirect effects stemming from the viral gene action on cellular control mechanisms. It would be desirable to identify the primary effect of the *src* gene and differentiate it from the numerous secondary ones. Since most parameters of transformation are responsive to temperature shifts at any time in class T mutant-infected cultures, it is tempting to look for the transformed characteristic that appears first after a shift from the nonpermissive to the permissive temperature. However, since the techniques for measuring these changes have intrinsically different sensitivities and therefore are not comparable, the kinetics of shift are unlikely to establish the true time sequence and interdependence of transformation effects.

5.1.3. Temperature-Shift Experiments Suggest the Existence of a Virus-Coded Transforming Protein

Class T mutants have been further characterized physiologically by determining the metabolic requirements for retransformation following a downshift to the permissive temperature. The general experience has been that inhibitors of DNA and of DNA-dependent RNA synthesis do not interfere with retransformation, but inhibitors of protein synthesis do. This result is in accord with the hypothesis that the *src* gene codes for a transforming protein which in class T mutants is irreversibly inactivated at the nonpermissive temperature and needs to be resynthesized upon downshift to effect transformation (Kawai and Hanafusa, 1971; Biquard and Vigier, 1972; Bader, 1972; Hynes and Wyke, 1975). However, there are some notable exceptions to the rule that only protein synthesis is required to effect transformation upon shift to the permissive temperature. In certain mutants, some parameters of transformation do not require protein synthesis upon downshift, e.g., vacuolization and increased water uptake by a mutant of the Bryan high-titer strain of RSV, *BE*1, or increased agglutinability by concanavalin A in cells infected with *PA*19 and shifted from 41°C to 35°C (Bader, 1972; Biquard, 1973; Bader *et al.*, 1974). Such exceptions could be explained by postulating reversible temperature sensitivity of transforming protein at least in some of its apparently multiple functions. Exceptions in the other direction, namely, toward more complex metabolic requirements for retransformation, have also been recorded. DNA-dependent RNA synthesis is needed for alterations in the rates of hexose uptake, for increased hyaluronic acid synthesis, and for the transformation-related appearance of plasminogen activator in a downshift from 41°C to 35°C (Bader, 1972; Unkeless *et al.*, 1973; Friis, as quoted by Wyke, 1975). Sensitivity of morphological retransformation to actinomycin-D has been observed in mammalian cells with some class T mutants (Y. Chen, personal communication), but this observation needs further study. The requirement for RNA synthesis in the restoration of certain parameters of transformation may reflect an indirect effect of the viral transforming function: if these parameters of transformation depend on cellular mRNA synthesis, which in turn is activated by the transforming protein, a need for RNA synthesis in retransformation would be understandable.

5.1.4. The Genetic Lesion in Early Class T Mutants Is Not Understood

Three mutants in the T class are unusual, because the *ts* lesion is an early one. Transforming ability decays rapidly if infection is initiated at 41°C, and a shift to 35°C, even after only a few hours at 41°C, does not allow transformation to take place. Conversely, incubation at 35°C for the beginning hours of infection permits the mutants to pass through the transient *ts* phase. For early mutants, a later shift to 41°C is expected to prove nonrestrictive, but this is not the case with the three mutants in this category, because they are multiple mutants and carry a late-acting *ts* lesion in the *src* function in addition to the early one. This late mutation is responsive to nonpermissive conditions at any time after infection. These three mutants are *LA*30, *MI*1300, and *LA*338 (Wyke and Linial, 1973; Bookout and Sigel, 1975; Hunter and Vogt, 1976). They are apparently not affected in their replication at the nonpermissive temperature, and they can form *wt* recombinants with avian leukosis virus. *LA*30 and *MI*100 also have heat-sensitive virions. The genetic lesion in these viruses is somewhat of an enigma, because in the present understanding of avian sarcoma virus life cycle there is no place for an early function that is specific for transformation; all early events leading up to and including integration should be coordinately required for transformation and replication as well. There are two ways out of this puzzling situation: one is to propose an *ad hoc* explanation, the other is to reinterpret the data. Wyke (1975) has done the former and suggests that the *ts* function in *LA*30, *MI*100, and *LA*338 may determine the specific site of integration which the virus must use in order to transform. Integration in another site may still occur at the nonpermissive temperature but would result in virus replication only, in the absence of transformation. A reexamination and reinterpretation of the data would clearly have to confirm the claim that these mutants are not *ts* in replication. Usually replication tests are done at higher multiplicities than focus-forming tests, and may show greater leakiness. A coordinate replication and transformation defect in these mutants is suggested by the decay of focus formation if infection is initiated at 41°C. If virus were indeed released actively, then the cells infected after the downshift should become transformed and form a focus. The argument that this does not happen, because the cultures are confluent, have ceased DNA synthesis, and thus do not allow spread of the infection, would have to be tested experimentally in this system.*

5.1.5. Recombination Occurs between Different Class T *ts* Mutants at 41°C and Results in Cooperative Transformation

The ease with which class T *ts* mutants of avian sarcoma viruses can be obtained stimulated early attempts to demonstrate complementation between different mutants. Double infection with some mutant combinations was indeed found to result in an increase of phenotypically *wt*-transformed cells over the background of single infections. Kawai and co-workers concluded that the T function encompassed at least two complementation groups, and Wyke, after studying a larger number of mutants, presented data suggesting the existence of at least four such groups (Kawai *et al.*, 1972; Wyke, 1973*b*). The conclusion drawn from these data was that the transforming function was genetically complex and included up to four virus-coded polypeptides. However, class T *ts* mutants of avian sarcoma viruses replicate at 41°C, and thus the possibility existed that the enhanced transformation observed in the complementation experiments was not caused by cooperation of different functional viral polypeptides but by *wt* recombinants of the two *ts* parents. According to recent studies, this interpretation is probably the correct one, and the interaction between different class T mutants at 41°C resulting in *wt* properties has been renamed "cooperative transformation" (Wyke *et al.*, 1975). Double infection with mutants belonging to different cooperative transformation groups leads to a far higher incidence of genetically stable *wt* progeny at 41°C than does double infection with mutants of the same cooperative complementation group. The

---

* **Note added in Proof:** Tato, Beamand, and Wyke (personal communication, 1976) have now established that *LA*30 is an early coordinate mutant with a defect in *env*.

transformation seen at 41°C could thus be explained by the appearance of *wt* recombinants. These results remove the need for postulating the existence of several cistrons in the T function, because recombination may occur within one gene. The size of the *td* deletion (about 350,000 molecular weight of RNA), which includes all or most of the class T *ts* mutants of avian sarcoma viruses, also argues in favor of a single cistron rather than several ones (Bernstein *et al.*, 1976). Why class T *ts* mutants should fall into distinct cooperative transformation groups reflecting several discontinuities in the recombination frequencies is not clear. One would expect that recombination frequencies should vary continuously with the distance of markers and that the discontinuous groups seen with the mutant material so far will disappear once more mutants have been investigated. However, if crossover points or effective *ts* mutations are not randomly distributed over the genome, then the cooperative transformation groups may reveal some structural properties of the *src* gene or its product.

Cooperative transformation groups have been defined only with mutants of the Prague strain of Rous sarcoma virus. Attempts to obtain cooperative transformation with mutant combinations from different strains (e.g., Schmidt-Ruppin strain and Prague or Prague and Bryan high-titer strain) have given erratic results (Wyke, 1973*b*; Balduzzi, 1976). The suggested explanation for this inefficient recombination in the *src* genes of different avian sarcoma viruses is lack of homology in this region of the viral genome. However, this suggestion has recently become less attractive, because a DNA transcript of the *src* gene from Prague strain Rous sarcoma virus was found to be closely homologous by nucleic acid hybridization to the RNAs of three independent isolates of avian sarcoma viruses, B77, Fujinami sarcoma virus, and derivatives of the chicken tumor No. 1 isolate of Rous (Stehelin *et al.*, 1976*a*). Oligonucleotide fingerprints of the *src* region also show that it is highly conserved among different avian sarcoma viruses (Wang *et al.*, 1975). The absence of cooperative transformation between different avian sarcoma virus strains is therefore probably not due to a lack of genetic relationship in this region of the genome. Additional experimental data on cooperative transformation are needed and may suggest another explanation of its apparent strain specificity.

5.1.6. Class C and R Mutants of Avian Sarcoma Viruses

Mutants with temperature-sensitive lesions in a replication function or a coordinately required function will be considered together for

TABLE 7

Avian Sarcoma Virus *ts* Mutants of Classes R and C

Mutant designation	Mutagen[a]	Parental *wt* virus[b]	Reference
Class R			
*LA*3342	5AC	B77-C	Hunter *et al.* (1976)
*LA*672	5AC	PR RSV-A	Friis and Hunter (1973)
Class C			
*LA*335	5AC	PR RSV-C	Wyke (1973*a*)
*LA*337	5AC	PR RSV-C	Linial and Mason (1973)
*LA*336m	5AC	B77-C	Toyoshima and Vogt (1969), Verma *et al.* (1976)
*LA*338m	5AC	PR RSV-C	Wyke (1973*a*), Hunter and Vogt (1976)
*LA*339m	5AC	B77-C	Graf and Friis (1973)
*LA*343m	UV	PR RSV-C	Wyke and Linial (1973)

[a] Abbreviations: 5AC, 5-azacytidine; UV, ultraviolet light.
[b] Abbreviations: PR RSV-A, PR RSV-C, Prague strain Rous sarcoma virus subgroup A or C, respectively; B77-C, avian sarcoma virus B77, subgroup C.

practical reasons: some of the class C mutants are really multiple mutants with a lesion in replication and transformation (or coordinate) genes. Furthermore, mutants in the reverse transcriptase may fall into the R class, although synthesis of DNA provirus is clearly a function required for transformation and replication. It is therefore sometimes difficult to draw the line between the R and the C class. Avian sarcoma virus mutants classified as R or C are listed in Table 7.

5.1.7. *LA*335, *LA*336, and *LA*337 Have a Heat-Labile Virion DNA Polymerase

*LA*335 and *LA*337 are class C mutants; at 41°C, focus formation and virus production are greatly reduced (Wyke, 1973*a*; Linial and Mason, 1973). The mutants are early; transforming and replicating abilities decay within 8 h if infection is initiated at 41°C, and these viral functions cannot be recovered by a shift to 35°C after that time. Conversely, if infection is initiated at 35°C and allowed to proceed for 10–15 h, the *ts* phase is passed, and an upshift to 41°C after that period no longer affects transformation or replication. The virion DNA polymerase in *LA*335 and *LA*337 is heat labile, and at 41°C becomes irreversibly inactivated. The virions of the two mutants are also significantly more heat labile than *wt* PR RSV-C. This is probably a reflection of the temperature inactivation of the DNA polymerase. *LA*335 and *LA*337 cannot be complemented by *wt* leukosis virus infecting simultaneously the same cell at the nonpermissive temperature, presumably because under these conditions the polymerase cannot be shared by different viruses. However, recombination between leukosis virus and these mutants leading to *wt* sarcoma takes place at the permissive temperature. Therefore, the lesion in these *ts* mutants must be located in a gene which is also present in leukosis virus, and *pol* could fulfill this requirement.

Under nonpermissive conditions, *LA*335 and *LA*337 synthesize only about one-fifth of the DNA that is made at 35°C (Varmus *et al.*, 1975*a*). Compared to the reduction in the biological parameters, focus formation, and synthesis of progeny virus, this residual DNA synthesis may appear high. However, it is likely that the DNA polymerase starts transcription at 41°C but becomes inactivated before the synthesis of a complete provirus. The DNA made, although biochemically significant in quantity, would be biologically nonfunctional. The virion polymerase of *LA*335 and *LA*337 has been isolated and purified (Verma *et al.*, 1974). RNA- and DNA-dependent DNA synthesis is heat labile in the purified enzymes, and so is RNase H activity, but to a lesser degree, suggesting that DNA polymerase and RNase H activities reside in two different catalytic sites on these enzymes. The enzyme activities of *LA*335 and of *LA*337 are inactivated at different rates, indicating that the mutations in *LA*335 and *LA*337 are not identical. In neither mutant does the presence of a template-primer have a stabilizing effect on the enzyme, whereas such an effect is seen with *wt* polymerase (Verma *et al.*, 1974). The *LA*335 and *LA*337 enzymes may therefore be defective in template binding. The DNA polymerase of avian leukosis and sarcoma viruses contains two polypeptide subunits, 100,000 and 60,000 in molecular weight (Kacian *et al.*, 1971; Temin and Baltimore, 1972; Grandgenett *et al.*, 1973). The lower molecular weight subunit (α), which appears to be derived from the larger one (β), carried all enzymatic activities of the DNA polymerase (Verma and Gibson, 1975). It was isolated from *LA*335 and *LA*337 and found to be thermolabile. Therefore, at least this 60,000 molecular weight polypeptide is coded for by the viral genome (Verma, 1975).

The defect in the polymerase has been causally linked to the biological properties of the mutants—inability to transform and to replicate at 41°C—by the isolation of a series of genetic revertants (Mason *et al.,* 1974). These were selected for growth at 41°C, and restoration of this property was correlated in all cases, not only with *wt* focus formation but also with *wt* polymerase properties. This perfect correlation between enzymatic and biological characteristics indicates that the *ts* polymerase is the cause for the inability to form foci or to produce progeny at 41°C in *LA*335 or *LA*337. Similar conclusions can be drawn from studies on recombinants between *LA*335 or *LA*337 and Rous-associated virus type 6 (RAV-6). All of these recombinants have acquired the *env* marker of RAV-6, and most have also gained *wt pol.* However, a few have retained the *ts* marker in *pol*. Again, there is a perfect correlation between temperature sensitivity of the enzyme and temperature sensitivity of transformation and replication.

In summary, the studies on *LA*335 and *LA*337 show that at least the α subunit of the virion RNA-dependent DNA polymerase is coded for by the viral genome, and that a functioning polymerase is essential for virus-induced oncogenic transformation and for production of progeny particles.

Mutant *LA*336 isolated by Toyoshima and Vogt (1969) (and then called *ts*149) also appears to have a *ts* lesion in the virion DNA polymerase (Verma *et al.,* 1976; Mölling, as quoted by Wyke, 1975). As with *LA*335 and *LA*337, the *ts* phase of *LA*336 occurs early in infection and is transient, but the situation is complicated by the fact that *LA*336 is a multiple mutant which, besides an early coordinate lesion, also contains one of the common late *ts* mutations in the T function (Friis *et al.,* 1971). Unlike *LA*335 and *LA*337, the virions of *LA*336 are not significantly more temperature labile than parental *wt* avian sarcoma virus B77 (Friis *et al.,* 1971; Wyke and Linial, 1973). The purified virion DNA polymerase of *LA*336 is exceedingly heat labile in all three enzymatic activities, RNA- and DNA-dependent DNA synthesis and RNase H. However, in contrast to the polymerase of *LA*335 and *LA*337, the enzyme of *LA*336 can be stabilized by the presence of template-primer, which may explain why intact virions of *LA*336 are not detectably more heat labile than *wt* B77 at 41°C. During infection at 41°C, *LA*336 produces only about 4–10% the amount of viral DNA that is made at 35°C. Recombination studies have also been carried out with *LA*336 and avian leukosis virus RAV-6 (Blair *et al.,* 1976; Verma *et al.,* 1976). Among recombinants carrying the host range marker of RAV-6 (subgroup B), there were two which had lost the early coordinate *ts* phase and one which had retained it. The two former ones had also gained *wt* polymerase; the latter one had retained the *ts* enzyme.

5.1.8. *LA*672 Belongs to Class R But May Have A Defect in the Synthesis of DNA Polymerase

A mutant which may also have a temperature-sensitive lesion in the virion DNA polymerase, but with a physiology completely different from that of *LA*335, *LA*336, and *LA*337, is *LA*672 (Friis and Hunter, 1973; Friis *et al.,* 1975). This *ts* mutant of the Prague strain of RSV (subgroup A) belongs to the R class; it transforms at 41°C, but does not produce infectious progeny virus. The *ts* phase is late and continuous. Progeny synthesis can be manipulated at any time after infection by appropriate temperature shifts. *LA*672 synthesizes large quantities of noninfectious virions at 41°C; these lack DNA polymerase activity. However, the polymerase of *LA*672 synthesized at 35°C is not *ts,* nor are the virions produced under permissive conditions any more thermolabile than *wt* virus. The absence of polymerase activity from virus produced at 41°C must therefore be due to a defect in production or packaging of the enzyme. *LA*672 can be complemented by avian leukosis viruses at 41°C, but if cells infected with the polymerase mutants *LA*335 or *LA*337 are cocultivated with *LA*672 infected cells at 35°C for 48 h and then shifted to 41°C the progeny virus shows a greatly reduced infectivity at 41°C. This result suggests that the *ts* in *LA*672 lesion may affect the polymerase molecule directly rather than interfere with the packaging of an otherwise functional enzyme.

5.1.9. Many Class C Mutants Contain Several Mutations

Not all coordinate mutants of avian sarcoma viruses carry a single mutation in a gene whose function is necessary for transformation and for production of progeny virus alike. Coordinate temperature sensitivity can also be found in mutants which carry separate lesions in R and T functions. Coordinate mutants may further contain, besides the mutation in the C function, additional ones in T or R functions. Positive identification of such multiple mutants requires genetic analysis. Crosses with *wt* viruses can separate the various mutations by recombination. In some cases, simple physiological experiments can suggest multiple mutations as well. Temperature shifts reveal multiple mutations if the mutant properties in transformation and replication respond differently, for instance, if one indicates an early and transient lesion and the other one a late and continuous lesion. Wyke and Linial

(1973) have described such incongruity in shift patterns for avian sarcoma virus *ts* mutants *LA*338 and *LA*343, which therefore were suspected to carry several mutations. For *LA*338, this suggestion has been borne out by recent studies (Hunter and Vogt, 1976) which show that *LA*338 contains, besides early and late class T lesions (see above), also a replication lesion; this class R lesion is late, continuous, and can be complemented by avian leukosis virus. Probably related to the replication lesion in *LA*338 is the reduction in synthesis of nonglycosylated intracellular virion proteins seen at 41°C (Halpern *et al.*, 1974; Hunter and Vogt, 1976).

Although incongruous shift patterns in transformation and replication are indicative of multiple mutations, the reverse, namely that parallel behavior of these virus functions in shift experiments proves the presence of only one mutation, is of course not true. An example for a mutant whose shift pattern does not betray multiplicity of mutation is *LA*334. *LA*334 (formerly called *ts*75) was one of the first *ts* mutants of avian sarcoma viruses described in the literature (Toyoshima and Vogt, 1969). Its *ts* lesion is late and continuous for focus formation and production of viral progeny. Owada and Toyoshima (1973) have shown that *LA*334 can be recombined with avian leukosis virus to yield a pure class T mutant and can also be complemented for replication by avian leukosis virus at 41°C, but not for transformation. These data indicate that *LA*334 carries two separate late mutations, one in the T and one in the R function; the latter but not the former could be complemented or replaced by avian leukosis virus.

5.1.10. *LA*334 is *ts* in Virus Assembly

The R lesion in *LA*334 has been isolated by recombination and has been characterized in detail (Hunter and Vogt, 1976; Hunter *et al.*, 1976a). In a genetic cross with Prague strain RSV subgroup B (PR RSV-B), it was found that the host range marker and the *ts* replication marker of *LA*334 segregated, and that therefore the *ts* replication lesion does not reside in *env* as had been suggested previously (Katz and Vogt, 1971). From such a cross between *LA*334 and PR RSV-B, a recombinant was isolated which had retained the *ts* lesion in replication, but had become *wt* for transformation. This recombinant, referred to as *LA*3342, can complement the *env⁻* deletion mutant RSV(−) at 41°C and interferes with superinfecting viruses of the same subgroup at 41°C, two further indications that this *ts* mutant produces functional glycoproteins under nonpermissive conditions. Noninfectious virions synthesized by *LA*3342 at 41°C differ from 35°C virions in that they are slightly more dense in sucrose. They contain the same virion proteins as *wt* or *LA*3342 produced at 35°C, but in addition they incorporate four new virus-specific mutant polypeptides, mp-1 to mp-4. Three of these novel polypeptides, not detectable in *wt* virus or virions of *LA*3342 produced at 35°C, can be precipitated with antiviral serum and therefore are not cellular contaminants. They are probably the result of delayed or aberrant proteolytic cleavage, because the polyprotein precursor of the nonglycosylated internal virion proteins is processed only at a considerably reduced rate in *LA*3342-infected cells at 41°C. The polyprotein precursor itself is synthesized at 41°C, and after shift it can even be cleaved correctly and incorporated into virus particles of *LA*3342. These biochemical experiments point to a possible defect in assembly, a suggestion which is corroborated by electron microscopic studies. Thin sections of chick embryo fibroblasts infected with *LA*3342 at 41°C show grossly abnormal virus particles lacking electron-dense cores as well as multiple and enlarged budding structures. In many respects, this replication mutant of avian sarcoma viruses resembles the MuLV mutant *ts*3 described by Wong and McCarter (1974).

5.2. Conditional Mutants of Murine Leukemia and Sarcoma Viruses

Since most if not all murine sarcoma viruses (MSV) are defective for replication and, in turn, murine leukemia viruses (MuLV) replicate in but do not transform fibroblasts, the latter have been used to study R and C functions with *ts* mutants and the former have yielded *ts* mutants in the T function. The permissive temperature for the murine system is 31–33°C; the nonpermissive temperature is 39°C. Most mutants have been isolated after chemical mutagenization with bromodeoxyuridine, 5-azacytidine, or *N*-methyl-*N'*-nitro-*N*-nitrosoguanidine (Stephenson *et al.*, 1972; Scolnick *et al.*, 1972*b*), but some spontaneous *ts* mutants have also been found and proved useful (Wong *et al.*, 1973; Somers and Kit, 1973). All of the *ts* mutants of MuLV show a reduced ability to produce infectious progeny virus at 39°C, but it would be unjustified to regard them as class R mutants. Some of them may carry a mutation in a coordinate function; without an *in vitro* test for transformation such a coordinate mutation could not be identified. To some extent, such a test is supplied by pseudotype formation with MSV. Studies with such pseudotypes show indeed that there are MuLV mutants with an early *ts* phase required for transformation and replication.

5.2.1. *ts* Mutants of MuLV Have Lesions in R or in C Functions

Table 8 summarizes the physiological characteristics of the Ravscher MuLV mutants described by Stephenson and co-workers (Stephenson and Aaronson, 1973, 1974; Stephenson *et al.*, 1974*b*; Tronick *et al.*, 1975). Four physiological categories have been identified so far, two early ones (I and II in the table) and two late ones (III and IV). The terms "early" and "late" as used with the MuLV *ts* mutants are not comparable to those applied to the avian sarcoma viruses, because in MuLV infection they are based on synthetic capacities of the mutants at 39°C, not on temperature-shift experiments. Both of the late mutant categories of MuLV synthesize internal nonglycosylated virion proteins at the restrictive temperature. One of these categories (II) also produces noninfectious virions containing a *wt* DNA polymerase. Mutants in both early categories fail to synthesize virion proteins. Early and late categories can also be distinguished by their ability to form pseudotypes with MSV. Mutants in the late categories can produce MSV pseudotypes at 31°C which are infectious and can induce focus formation at 39°C. The conditions of focus formation in these tests do not require recruitment of neighboring cells and thus are independent of virus production and spread. Each focus is the result of

TABLE 8

Physiological Characteristics of Rauscher Murine Leukemia Virus *ts* Mutants[a]

Category	Representative mutant	Synthesis of infectious progeny at 39°C	Synthesis of group-specific antigens at 39°C	Synthesis of virions at 39°C	MSV pseudotype[b]	Heat-labile virion DNA polymerase	Complementation by murine sarcoma virus
I (early)	*ts*17	−	−	−	−	*wt*	−
II (early)	*ts*29	−	−	−	−	Labile	−
III (late)	*ts*25	−	+	−	+	*wt*	−
IV (late	*ts*28	−	+	+	+	*wt*	−

[a] From data of Stephenson and co-workers (Stephenson and Aaronson, 1973, 1974; Stephenson *et al.*, 1974*b*, 1975; Tronick *et al.*, 1975).
[b] Ability to perform early, postpenetration function needed for transformation in MSV pseudotypes at 39°C.

the initial infection with the sarcoma virus. Pseudotypes produced at 31°C with mutants of the early categories cannot induce foci at 39°C. It can be shown that the function which is defective in these pseudotypes is needed after penetration but before the virus–cell complex becomes stable and probably before integration (Stephenson and Aaronson, 1974). In one of the early mutant categories (II), the function required for transformation in the MSV pseudotype appears to be the DNA polymerase which is heat labile both in the MuLV mutant virion (ts29) and as partially purified enzyme (Tronick et al., 1975). The heat lability affects all three enzymatic activites of the enzyme RNA- and DNA-dependent polymerase and RNase H activity. The situation appears to be similar to that in the avian sarcoma virus ts mutant LA336, because the presence of template-primer combination exerts some protective effect on the enzyme at the elevated temperature.

In the other early mutant category of MuLV (category I in the table), the lesion interfering with transformation by the corresponding MSV pseudotype is also located after penetration and probably before integration of the virus. Since the DNA polymerase of this mutant category is not temperature labile in the virion or as partially purified enzyme preparation, there may be another nonstructural virion component with a specific early coordinate function. Alternatively, the lesion may be structural, interfering with efficient uncoating, and in this way set a block early in infection.

The situation in the early mutant categories of MuLV under nonpermissive conditions is reminiscent of the Fv-1-mediated block early in infection. Here too there is evidence for a virion component needed after penetration but probably before integration by both sarcoma and leukemia virus. Whether the function affected by Fv-1 is the polymerase or the component which is ts in category II is not known.

The late mutant category III (Table 8) represented by Rauscher MuLV mutants ts25 and ts26 is of interest, because it shows accumulation of the 70,000 molecular weight precursor of internal virion proteins p30, p15, and p12 at the nonpermissive temperature (Stephenson et al., 1975). After downshift to 31°C, virus synthesis is restored, and this recovery is not sensitive to cycloheximide. The polyprotein precursor collecting in infected cells at 39°C must therefore be cleaved correctly after the downshift and the products incorporated into infectious virions after the downshift. In these respects, the MuLV mutants of this late category resemble LA3342, a class R mutant of avian sarcoma virus B77. However, unlike LA3342, the MuLV mutants do not seem to release noninfectious particles under restrictive conditions, at least as measured by polymerase activity. It will be interesting to examine electron micrographs of cells infected with *ts*25 or *ts*26 at 39°C for aberrant or abortive viral muturation forms.

The early and late *ts* mutants of Rauscher MuLV show a greatly reduced ability to induce leukemia in mice, probably because of their impaired ability to replicate at the body temperature of the mouse, rather than because of an as yet undetected defect in an *onc* function responsible for leukemia (Greenberger *et al.*, 1974*b*).

The physiological properties of a collection of *ts* mutants from Moloney MuLV are summarized in Table 9 (Wong *et al.*, 1973; Wong and McCarter, 1973, 1974; Wong and MacLeod, 1975). A late and an early category have been distinguished by shift experiments. The early temperature sensitivity is transient, and shift to 39°C after a few hours at 31°C no longer constitutes a restrictive condition. Conversely, infection at 39°C does not permit virus to become stabilized in the cell, and upon downshift viral functions cannot be fully recovered. The titer increases which do occur under these conditions can be prevented by inhibitors of RNA and of protein synthesis, indicating that these viral macromolecules must be produced after the shift to permissive conditions. The virions and the DNA polymerase of the early mutants are, however, not more temperature labile than those of *wt* MuLV.

In the late mutants, temperature shifts can turn virus synthesis on or off any time after infection. Virus production after downshift is not sensitive to inhibitors of RNA or protein synthesis, suggesting that these viral macromolecules are synthesized at 39°C and can then be incorporated into infectious virus after shift. That the late mutants are defective in virus assembly can be best seen in electron micrographs, which at the nonpermissive temperature show the same aberrant forms

TABLE 9

Physiological Characteristics of Moloney MuLV *ts* Mutants[1]

Category	Representative mutant	Synthesis of noninfectious progeny at 39°C	Shift pattern	Ability to rescue MSV at 39°C	Heat-labile virion DNA polymerase
A	*ts*1	Reduced	Early, transient	Not tested	*wt*
B	*ts*3	Reduced	Late, continuous	Negative	*wt*

[a] Data compiled from Wong *et al.* (1973) and Wong and McCarter (1973, 1974).

of virus budding which were later found with the *ts* avian sarcoma virus *LA*3342. As expected, the late mutant is also unable to act as a helper virus for MSV at the nonpermissive temperature, and pseudotypes formed with the mutant at 31°C show a greatly reduced focus-forming ability at 39°C. This temperature sensitivity of focus formation is probably not due to a helper-dependent virion component which has an early coordinate function, but reflects inefficient recruitment of neighboring cells because of reduced synthesis of progeny virus.

Ts mutants of murine leukemia viruses show complementation and recombination. Complementation has been demonstrated between the early and the late Moloney MuLV mutants by Wong and McCarter (1973). Recombination to *wt* virus also occurs between these physiologically different mutants, but can also be demonstrated between similar mutants which may have a defect in the same gene (Stephenson *et al.*, 1974*b*). No significant and consistent differences in recombination frequencies have been observed in these experiments.

Ts mutants of leukemia viruses have been isolated and tested so far only in assay systems which register virus replication and coordinate functions, but not leukemogenic functions. Since there are now *in vitro* transformation tests available for Abelson and Friend MuLV viruses, it would be desirable to look for mutants in T functions (Sklar *et al.*, 1974; Rosenberg *et al.*, 1975; Clarke *et al.*, 1975). Such an investigation would not be a mere exercise in analogy to sarcoma viruses, because it is not known whether the *src* gene of sarcoma viruses has a counterpart in leukemia viruses where it would be responsible for the transformation of hematopoietic cells. It has been argued that leukemia viruses do not have a specific T function distinct from those required for replication (Dulbecco, 1973). If this hypothesis is correct, there should be no mutants of Abelson or Friend MuLV which are *ts* for maintenance of transformation but continue to replicate (with the aid of a helper) at the nonpermissive temperature. Conversely, the isolation of such mutants would provide evidence for specific transforming information in MuLV. Similar considerations make the search for avian leukosis virus class T *ts* mutants with the use of focal transformation assays a worthwhile proposition.

5.2.2. *ts* Mutants of MSV Also Suggest the Existence of a Specific Transformation Gene

Relatively few conditional mutants of MSV have been described; all show temperature dependence of transforming activity. Several such mutants have been isolated from the Kirsten strain of MSV after mutagenesis with 5-bromodeoxyuridine or 5-azacytidine (Scolnick *et al.*, 1972*b*, 1975*a*; Carchman *et al.*, 1974). These mutants cannot induce foci at 39°C, and fail to impart to infected cells the ability to grow into colonies in agar or on confluent layers of normal cells at this temperature. The transformation-related decrease of cyclic AMP is also temperature dependent. No complementation or cooperative transformation has been observed between ten *ts* mutants of Kirsten strain MSV. The available data from temperature-shift experiments suggest that these mutants have a defect in a function required for the maintenance of transformation. One would assume that this function is the *src* gene, but since MSV cannot replicate in solitary infection it is not possible to say that the R and C functions are unaffected at the nonpermissive temperature. Nonproducing cells infected by certain *ts* mutants of Kirsten MSV, e.g., *ts*6, become *wt* for transformation if they are superinfected with a MuLV helper: they remain transformed when shifted to 39°C, and they induce formation of cell colonies in agar or on confluent monolayers under nonpermissive conditions. If this effect represents true complementation, it would lead to the surprising conclusion that MuLV has a genetic function needed in the maintenance of MSV-induced transformation. One would then expect complementation and recombination between *ts*6 and those *ts* mutants of Kirsten MSV which are not complemented by MuLV. One would also anticipate recombination with the complementing MuLV, none of which takes place. Clearly, more work is needed on this type of complementation, which shows some resemblance to the transforming effect of MuLV seen in cultures of S$^+$L$^-$ cells and in T$^-$R$^-$ cultures (Bassin *et al.*, 1971*b*; Ball *et al.*, 1973*b*). Those *ts* mutants which are not complemented by MuLV for transformation can nevertheless be complemented for replication at 39°C. Thus virus synthesis occurs while transformation is blocked by the nonpermissive conditions. This fact suggests that the lesion of these mutants is in a true T function not required for the production of progeny viruses.

An interesting spontaneous mutant of MSV which is cold sensitive for the maintenance of transformation was isolated by Somers and Kit (1973). Cells transformed by this mutant assume normal morphology and behavior at 33°C but are transformed at 39°C. Colony formation on confluent monolayers and focus formation by the pseudotype MSV rescued from such cells with MuLV are also cold sensitive. This mutant was also used in the study of fucosyl glycolipids and their changes during transformation. In cells transformed by *wt* MSV, there is a characteristic change in the glycolipid pattern; the most complex glycolipid is much reduced in concentration as compared to the less complex ones which are presumably precursors. Cells infected with the cold-sensitive mutant show changes similar to *wt*-transformed cells at the permissive temperature, and at the nonpermissive temperature the glycolipid patterns of these cultures resemble those of normal cultures (Steiner *et al.*, 1974). The metabolic requirements for retransformation in cultures infected with the cold-sensitive mutant of MSV following shift from 33°C to 39°C do not extend to DNA or RNA synthesis but include protein and glycoprotein synthesis. Presence of the appropriate inhibitors (cycloheximide, 2-deoxy-D-glucose, or glucosamine) reversibly blocks retransformation as measured by increased hexose uptake and morphological changes occurring upon upshift (Somers *et al.*, 1973). The data are in agreement with the hypothesis that the transforming genetic information of MSV codes for a protein, and that either this primary transforming protein or one whose synthesis is dependent on it needs to be glycosylated.

6. BIOCHEMICAL APPROACHES TO RNA TUMOR VIRUS GENETICS

Biochemical techniques have become increasingly applicable to problems of RNA tumor virus genetics. Nucleic acid hybridization and radioimmunoassays have delineated relationships among RNA tumor viruses and have uncovered homologies between virus and cell. Results from oligonucleotide fingerprints have been decisive in determining the complexity and structure of the viral genome and the mechanism of recombination. The same techniques are now providing the first data on the genetic map of RNA tumor viruses. This section of the chapter will survey a selection of biochemical experiments with RNA tumor viruses as they relate to questions of genetics.

6.1. RNA Tumor Virus Species: Genetic Relationships and Distribution among Various Hosts

From a wide variety of nucleic acid hybridizations, one can deduce the general rule that there is extensive homology between RNA tumor virus genomes infecting the same species, and little if any homology between viruses infecting different host animals (Benveniste and

Todaro, 1973; Neiman *et al.*, 1974; Wright and Neiman, 1974; Haapala and Fischinger, 1973; Quintrell *et al.*, 1974). The high degree of nucleic acid homology found among RNA tumor viruses infecting the same species is correlated with close antigenic relationships, and viruses which are linked by these features are assigned the taxonomic status of a species (Vogt, 1976). This rule has some interesting exceptions in viruses which show homology even though they are indigenous to different host species and in host species which harbor more than two species of unrelated or minimally related viruses.

The endogenous type C viruses of baboons are antigenically related to a group of endogenous feline viruses represented by RD114, and show nucleic acid homology to these feline viruses (Sherr and Todaro, 1974; Sherr *et al.*, 1974; Todaro *et al.*, 1975; Lieber *et al.*, 1975c). Furthermore, DNA from normal cells of Old World monkeys contains nucleic acid sequences related to RD114, and DNA transcripts from endogenous baboon viruses hydridize to cat DNA. The favored interpretation of this unusual relationship between endogenous viruses of unrelated host species is that during the evolution of felines and of primates, possible in the Pleiocene, there was a horizontal transfer of endogenous type C virus from primates to felines, where the virus also became established in the germ line (Benveniste and Todaro, 1974a,b). Such a conclusion is, of course, speculative, and other readings of the data have not been excluded. An analogous situation was found by comparing the endogenous type C virus from pigs with murine type C viruses (Todaro *et al.*, 1974; Benveniste and Todaro, 1975; Sherr *et al.*, 1975; Lieber *et al.*, 1975a). Normal murine cells contain sequences related to endogenous porcine type C virus, but in this case the reverse is not true; there are no sequences related to murine viruses in normal pig cells. Porcine and murine type C viruses share, however, antigenic determinants on p30 and on virion DNA polymerase. After considering the distribution of the related viral sequences in several procine and murine species, Benveniste and Todaro (1975) have concluded that there was a horizontal transmission of endogenous viral sequences from rodents to pigs before the family Muridae had diverged, but after rats had split off from a common rodent ancestor.

In the preceding examples of related type C viruses in unrelated species, the virus was incorporated into the germ line of the presumed recipient in the horizontal transmission. There is another instance in which the data suggest horizontal transmission between an Asian mouse species (probably *Mus caroli*) and gibbons or possibly other apes and monkeys (Lieber *et al.*, 1975b). The type C viruses isolated from gibbons and from one woolly monkey have antigens and nucleic acid sequences in common with an endogenous xenotropic virus which can be induced in cultures of *Mus caroli* cells. In this case, however, sequences of the gibbon virus and its relatives are not present in normal gibbon cells. The infection in gibbons seems to be perpetuated without integration into the germ line, probably by a horizontal route (Scolnick *et al.*, 1974).

The general rule that the type C viruses that infect the same host species and are closely related in their p30 polypeptides and possibly in the DNA polymerase is broken in a number of cases. The situation in the mouse would still fit this rule, although there is some divergence among murine endogenous viruses: the ecotropic and the xenotropic murine type C viruses show clear differences in biological properties, and their genomes are only partially homologous (Aaronson and Stephenson, 1973; Levy 1973; Benveniste *et al.*, 1974; Callahan *et al.*, 1975). However, the p30 polypeptides of these viruses are very closely related and so are the DNA polymerases. In normal tissues of the domestic cat, sequences of two type C viruses are found, RD114 and feline leukemia virus (Quintrell *et al.*, 1974). Of these, RD114 or the very closely related CCC virus is readily inducible in normal feline cells (Fischinger *et al.*, 1973; Livingston and Todaro, 1973; Sarma *et al.*, 1973), but induction of feline leukemia virus in normal feline cells has not been observed, possibly because only part of the viral genome is present. These two viruses have no detectable genome homology and do not show extensive antigenic cross-reaction in p30 or in the DNA polymerase (McAllister *et al.*, 1972; Oroszlan *et al.*, 1972; Scolnick, 1972*a*). The fact that these viruses have remained distinct and separate despite their presence in the same host cell suggests that no recombination occurs between them. This genetic separation may result from the absence of homology between RD114 and feline leukemia virus. Another example of two unrelated type C viruses in the same host species is provided by the chicken, where normal cells harbor a complete and inducible genome of an avian leukosis virus but only part of the genome of reticuloendotheliosis virus (Weiss *et al.*, 1971; Varmus *et al.*, 1972; Neiman, 1973; Kang and Temin, 1974; Tereba *et al.*, 1975). The endogenous avian leukosis virus and reticuloendotheliosis virus belong to two unrelated groups (species) of type C viruses. They do not share virion antigens, they are apparently unable to undergo phenotypic mixing, and there is no sequence homology between their genomes (Theilen *et al.*, 1966; Maldonado and Bose, 1971; Halpern *et al.*, 1973; Kang and Temin, 1973; Moelling *et al.*, 1975). As more endogenous viruses are discovered, other host species harboring two or several unrelated species of type C viruses will no doubt be identified.

6.2. Occurrence and Origin of *src* Sequences

The work of *td* deletion mutants of avian sarcoma viruses shows that the sequences frequently lost by these mutants and presumably encompassing most of the *src* gene are not required for the synthesis of infectious viral progeny. The *src* gene is therefore dispensable and unneeded for the perpetuation of the virus. These two facts, namely that the *src* information is nonessential for the virus and that it is lost rather easily, suggest that the sequences are not genuinely viral but may be acquired from the cellular genome. This notion is supported by recent studies on murine and avian sarcoma viruses.

Scolnick and co-workers have analyzed the homologies of the MSV genome with MuLV and with endogenous type C viruses from rat cells (Scolnick *et al.,* 1973; Scolnick and Parks, 1974; Roy-Burman and Klement, 1975). Both the Harvey and the Kirsten MSV contain nucleic acid sequences of diverse origin. Part is homologous to MuLV and another part to endogenous, probably viral information from rat cells. However, the homology to endogenous rat sequences is not complete. It appears that these portions of the Harvey and Kirsten MSV genomes, although related to information present in normal rat cells, have diverged considerably from it. Whether this divergence is related to the transforming ability of MSV is not known. In the Harvey MSV, the rat-specific sequences are present only in the smaller of the two 30–40 S virion RNA species obtained from pseudotype preparations which contain MuLV and MSV (Maisel *et al.,* 1975). Harvey MSV was isolated after passage of Moloney MuLV in rats and Kirsten MSV after similar passage of Kirsten murine erythroblastosis virus (Harvey, 1964; Kirsten and Mayer, 1967). It is probable that during these passages in the heterologous host the rat-specific sequences, and with them the sarcoma-producing capacity, were acquired by the murine leukemia viruses. The Moloney MSV which emerged after passage of the Moloney MuLV in mice does not contain sequences homologous to a different host, as do the Harvey and Kirsten strains, but it does carry sarcoma-specific genetic material which is not present in the Moloney MuLV, again suggesting that the *src* gene of RNA sarcoma viruses represents additional genetic information not needed for virus reproduction. Significantly, the sarcoma-specific information of

Moloney MSV shows no homology to that of the Harvey strain of MSV, nor is there homology between sarcoma-specific sequences of the Moloney MSV and the gene responsible for fibroblast transformation in Abelson MuLV (Scolnick *et al.,* 1975*b*). It would be interesting to test whether there is recombination or complementation in the *src* functions of Harvey and Moloney sarcoma viruses and of Abelson MuLV.

The sarcoma-specific genetic information in avian sarcoma viruses has been studied with the aid of a specific complementary DNA probe referred to as cDNA$_{sarc}$ (Stehelin *et al.,* 1976*a,b*). This DNA probe contains the sequences deleted in *td* viruses and is prepared by hybridizing single-stranded DNA transcripts of nondefective avian sarcoma viruses to the virion RNA of a *td* deletion mutant derived from the same sarcoma virus. The nonhybridized DNA, separated from the hybridized material by hydroxylapatite chromatography, is sarcoma specific after several cycles of selective hybridization. cDNA$_{sarc}$ represents 15% of the avian sarcoma virus genome, about as much as would be expected from the size of the *td* deletion. Sequences homologous to cDNA$_{sarc}$ have been found in all strains of avian sarcoma viruses, but not in avian leukosis viruses, including various types of Rous-associated virus and myeloblastosis virus. MSV also lacks homology to the cDNA$_{sarc}$ of avian sarcoma viruses. cDNA$_{sarc}$ hybridizes completely with the RNA from all strains of avian sarcoma virus tested, including such independent isolates as avian sarcoma virus B77 and Fujinami sarcoma virus. Hybrids between cDNA$_{sarc}$ of Prague strain RSV and virion RNA of avian sarcoma virus B77, and between cDNA$_{sarc}$ of B77 and virion RNA of Prague strain RSV, show the same thermal stability as homologous hybrids, suggesting conservation of sarcoma sequences. As pointed out above, this observation on the homology of cDNA$_{sarc}$ from different avian sarcoma viruses is difficult to reconcile with genetic experiments which reveal reduced and unpredictable genetic recombination in the *src* gene of avian sarcoma viruses from different strains (Wyke *et al.,* 1975; Balduzzi, 1976).

cDNA$_{sarc}$ has been shown to hybridize to the DNA of normal cells obtained from various avian species, including Japanese quail, from which an endogenous type C virus has so far not been isolated and which does not contain sequences homologous to the rest of the avian sarcoma virus genome. The thermal stability of the hybrids between cDNA$_{sarc}$ and cellular DNA is reduced as compared to that of the cDNA annealed to homologous provirus. The reduction in the T_m is least with chicken DNA, and in other avian DNAs it is roughly correlated with the evolutionary distance from the chicken. The widespread occurrence of *src*-related sequences among avian DNAs again suggests that the host cell may be the ultimate source of the transforming genetic information in the sarcoma virus (Stehelin *et al.*, 1976*b*).

6.3. The Genetic Map of Avian Sarcoma Viruses Probably Reads *gag-pol-env-src-C*-poly(A)

Mapping of viral genes is traditionally accomplished with genetic crosses between appropriate markers and determination of recombination frequencies. This approach is theoretically feasible with RNA tumor viruses, because recombinants arise by crossing over. However, the technical problems in obtaining accurate recombination frequencies are formidable, and relatively little mapping information has been forthcoming since recombination was first demonstrated to occur between RNA tumor viruses (Friis *et al.*, 1975; Wyke *et al.*, 1975; Blair *et al.*, 1976). Biochemical methods for genetic mapping have been phenomenally successful in virus systems in which DNA restriction enzymes can be used to generate defined genome fragments (Lai and Nathans, 1975; Shenk *et al.*, 1975; Grodzicker *et al.*, 1975). For RNA genomes, such elegant techniques are not yet available, but even with less sophisticated methods it has now been possible to arrive at a provisional map of avian sarcoma viruses.

The 30–40 S RNA of RNA tumor viruses labeled with ^{32}P and then exhaustively digested with RNase T_1 yields, after two-dimensional separation of the products by chromatography and electrophoresis or by two-dimensional electrophoresis, a characteristic fingerprint pattern which can be visualized by autoradiography. In this technique, the small oligonucleotides which occur several times along the genome and which make up the bulk of the digestion products are not resolved. However, each RNA tumor virus genome yields about 20 larger oligonucleotides (from 12 to 30 nucleotides in size) which statistically occur only once in the 30–40 S RNA and constitute 3–5% of the total. These large oligonucleotides are well separated and make up the usable portion of the fingerprint pattern. These patterns of 20 or so large RNase T_1-resistant oligonucleotides are on the whole virus specific; although there are shared oligonucleotides, many are characteristic of a given virus, and no two biologically different viruses have the same RNA fingerprint. In order to construct a genetic map from such fingerprints, it is necessary to accomplish two things: (1) to determine the linear order of oligonucleotides along the viral genome (Wang *et al.*,

1975; Coffin and Billeter, 1976) and (2) to correlate specific oligonucleotides with biological functions of the virus (Lai *et al.*, 1973; Duesberg *et al.*, 1975*a*).

The oligonucleotides separated in the fingerprint patterns have
been arranged in a linear sequence along the 30–40 S RNA by exploiting the fact that the 3′ ends of most 30–40 S genomes consist of
poly(A), which binds to Millipore filters, oligo(dT)-cellulose, or
poly(U)-sepharose. The exclusive use of poly(A)-containing genomes in
mapping does not select for genetic variants in an RNA tumor virus
preparation, because genomes without poly(A) have the same fingerprints as those with poly(A). The ^{32}P-labeled viral RNA is fragmented
with dilute alkali to give RNA pieces which extend in size from about
5% up to the total length of the genome. The poly(A)-containing fragments are then separated from the rest of such a mixture by the selective binding properties of poly(A), so that a preparation of fragments is
obtained all of which have the 3′ end of the genome, but then extend to
varying degrees toward the 5′ end. This collection of fragments is then
fractionated according to size in sucrose density gradients. Individual
size classes of fragments are fingerprinted. It is found that a number of
oligonucleotides in the fingerprints increase with the size of the fragment, which indicates that the oligonucleotides are arranged in a linear
order and that a given oligonucleotide occupies a fixed position relative
to the poly(A)-containing 3′ end (Wang and Duesberg, 1974). Oligonucleotides close to the 3′ end are present in the fingerprint patterns of
small fragments. The farther an oligonucleotide is away from the
poly(A) of the 3′ end, the larger is the required size of the genome fragment which is to contain such an oligonucleotide. In this way, the large
RNase T_1 oligonucleotides of several avian leukemia and sarcoma
viruses have been ordered in a linear sequence from the 3′ to the 5′ end
of the genome (Wang *et al.*, 1975, 1976*a*,*b*; Coffin and Billeter, 1976).

Deletion mutants and recombinants have helped assigning specific
functions to some of the ordered oligonucleotides. If the fingerprint
pattern of *rd* or *td* deletions is compared with that of the parental nondefective sarcoma virus, certain oligonucleotides, specific for each type
of deletion, are found missing. *Td* deletions have been shown to lack
two to three oligonucleotides in comparison to sarcoma viruses. These
oligonucleotides can therefore be designated as transformation-specific
and are probably derived from the *src* gene (Lai *et al.*, 1973; Wang *et
al.*, 1975). An analogous comparison of the *env⁻ rd* deletion mutant
*NY*8 with its parent, the Schmidt-Ruppin strain of RSV, revealed that
all oligonucleotides of the mutant are present in the parental RNA fin-

gerprint but that the mutant lacks six oligonucleotides of the parent. These six can be tentatively assigned to the *env* function (Duesberg *et al.*, 1975*a*; Wang *et al.*, 1976*a*). Recombinants yield data on the correlation between chemical structure and biological function according to the following principle: if recombinants are selected for two markers, one from each parent, the oligonucleotides corresponding to these markers will be present in all recombinants from this genetic cross, but oligonucleotides of genes not selected for can be derived from either parent and will vary depending on the location of the crossover point. Given a sufficient number of recombinants selected for the same two markers from one genetic cross, it is possible to line up the linear oligonucleotide maps and determine those regions of the recombinant genomes which are invariably derived from one parent and those always contributed by the other parent. These invariant regions can be provisionally identified with the selected markers. Such an approach not only assigns biological functions to oligonucleotides but also determines the map location of these functions (Wang *et al.*, 1976*b*). Recombinant mapping is also possible using the linear sequence of oligonucleotides from one parent alone and finding homologous oligonucleotides in the fingerprints of several recombinants (Joho *et al.*, 1975). In this method, it is assumed that homologous oligonucleotides would occur in the same map position in parent and recombinant. This assumption was justified when it was found that neither parental nor recombinant genomes show permutation of gene sequences (Wang *et al.*, 1975, 1976*a,b*; Coffin and Billeter, 1976). From these studies with deletions and recombinants a genetic map of avian sarcoma viruses is emerging. Maps of *rd* and *td* deletion mutants show that following the poly(A) at the 3′ end there is a heteropolymeric sequence which appears to be conserved in all avian leukosis and sarcoma viruses and their mutants and recombinants. This sequence is referred to as the *C* (constant) region. Because of this immutability, it may have a function which requires the same sequence in all avian leukosis and sarcoma viruses; it could be involved in the circularization of the genome or in integration. In the nondefective and the *rd* sarcoma viruses, the *C* region is followed by the sarcoma-specific oligonucleotides representing the *src* gene. The next identifiable function toward the 5′ end of the genome is the series of *env*-specific oligonucleotides which occur in one uninterrupted block in the second fourth of the genome starting from the 3′ end. It is likely that *src* and *env* are located adjacent to each other, but the possibility that an as yet unidentified gene lies between them has not been definitely ruled out (Wang *et al.*, 1975, 1976*a*).

Maps of recombinants have been obtained with viruses which have been selected for the transforming ability of the sarcoma virus parent and the host range of the leukemia virus. All recombinants share with their sarcoma virus parents a series of three contiguous oligonucleotides which are preceded by the C region and which have previously been identified as transformation specific. These sarcoma virus-derived oligonucleotides are followed in the direction toward the 5′ end by at least five to six oligonucleotides which are in common with the leukemia virus parent and which from other studies are known to be *env* specific. Farther toward the 5′ end the patterns of the different recombinants diverge, reflecting the fact that these sequences are not selected for in the cross and can vary at random. In one series of recombinants, three out of four have 5′ halves of the genome homologous to the leukosis virus parent, and one shows a block of oligonucleotides on the 5′ end contributed by the sarcoma virus parent. This latter one must have arisen by double crossover; the former ones are ostensibly single crossovers, although a second crossover in the C region would not be detectable (Wang *et al.*, 1976b). In a second series of recombinants studied, three of five appear to be derived from double crossovers (Joho *et al.*, 1975).

Pol and *gag* have not yet been mapped, but by exclusion they are thought of as residing in the 5′ half of the genome. Because *in vitro* protein-synthesizing systems directed by viral RNA produce *gag* protein, it is likely that the information for this series of internal structural proteins is located at the 5′ end of the genome since internal initiation of protein synthesis presumably does not occur in animal cells (Jacobson *et al.*, 1970; Siegert *et al.*, 1972; Twardzig *et al.*, 1973; Naso *et al.*, 1973; Von der Helm and Duesberg, 1975). However, in some *in vitro* protein-synthesizing systems, precursors of viral glycoproteins and possibly other viral polypeptides are made besides *gag* proteins (Gielkens *et al.*, 1976). An independent mapping of *pol* is also in progress using recombinants of the *ts pol* mutants *LA*335 and *LA*337 with avian leukosis virus. Correlation of the *ts* or *wt* properties with host range and the presence of oligonucleotides from either parent should allow an approximate localization of *pol* (Duesberg *et al.*, 1976).

The genetic map which can be derived for an avian sarcoma virus from oligonucleotide fingerprints of deletions and recombinants reads therefore 5′-(*gag, pol*)-*env-src*-C-poly(A)-3′.

This biochemical map is in agreement with the limited genetic data available from recombination experiments. The three-factor cross described by Wyke (1975) suggests that *pol* is more closely linked to *env* than to *src* (Wyke *et al.*, 1975). Linkage between *env* and *pol* is suggested by the studies of Mason and co-workers, who found that in crosses between the polymerase *ts* mutants *LA*335 or *LA*337 and RAV-6 of subgroup B most recombinants with the subgroup B envelope marker had also acquired the *wt* polymerase marker of the avian leukosis virus (Mason *et al.*, 1974). Similar results were obtained with another cross between the *ts* polymerase mutant *LA*672 and *wt* leukosis virus (Friis *et al.*, 1975). Hunter and Vogt (1976) have further presented recombination data between *ts* replication mutant *LA*334, which probably has a lesion in *gag*, and *wt* PR RSV-B. The results show that the R lesion of *LA*334 is not linked to *env*, a conclusion which is in accord with the suggestion that *pol* is located between *env* and *gag*. However, the mutated *gag* lesion of *LA*334 appears linked to *src*; linkage between *src* and *gag* has also been seen in clones between PR RSV-B and RAV-1 and between B77 and RAV-1 (Hayman and Vogt, 1976). The recombination data from three-factor crosses thus support the following four statements: (1) *env* is linked to *pol*, (2) *src* is linked to *gag*, (3) *env* is not linked to *gag*, and (4) *pol* is not linked to *src*. Table 10 shows six different linear arrangements of the basic genetic elements; additional arrangements are possible, but they would be circular permutations of those shown in the table. Sequence (i) corresponds to the map deduced from oligonucleotide analysis. It is compatible with the four statements on linkage or nonlinkage, provided it is assumed that the genome becomes circularized: *env* is linked to *pol*, and *gag* would show linkage to *src*. The pairs *pol/src* and *env/gag* would not be expected to show close linkage in sequence (i), in accord with the genetic data. On the basis of similar considerations, sequences

TABLE 10

Genetic Elements of Avian Sarcoma Viruses
Arranged in Six Different Sequences

Sequence No.	Genetic elements				Incompatible with linkage statement No.
(i)	*gag*	*pol*	*env*	*src* 3′	—
(ii)	*gag*	*pol*	*src*	*env* 3′	1, 2, 3, 4
(iii)	*gag*	*env*	*pol*	*src* 3′	3, 4
(iv)	*gag*	*env*	*src*	*pol* 3′	1, 2, 3, 4
(v)	*gag*	*src*	*pol*	*env* 3′	3, 4
(vi)	*gag*	*src*	*env*	*pol* 3′	—

(ii) and (iv) are incompatible with all four genetic linkage statements. Sequences (iii) and (v) cannot be reconciled with the observed absence of linkage between the *pol/src* and *env/gag* marker pairs. Sequence (vi), however, is again compatible with the genetic data; it can be ruled out only on the basis of the biochemical evidence.

Further refinement of the map in the *gag* region comes from studies on processing of viral proteins. *Gag* includes the nonglycosylated internal proteins p27, p19, p15, and p12, which are derived from a 76,000 molecular weight precursor polyprotein (Vogt and Eisenman, 1973). The sequence of p27, p19, p15, and p12 within this precursor has now been determined by using pactamycin, an inhibitor of initiation of polypeptide synthesis (Vogt *et al.,* 1976). If an amino acid label is introduced a short time after the inhibitor, radioactivity is incorporated preferentially into the *C*-terminal portion of the polyprotein. Picornavirus proteins which are made from a polycistronic message have been ordered by this method (Taber *et al.,* 1971; Butterworth, 1973). The results of studies with avian myeloblastosis virus suggest the sequence *N*-p19-p27-p12-p15-*C*, in which the position of p12 is uncertain, and the order of p12 and p27 could be reversed. Applied to the genetic map, these data indicate that the gene for p19 is located at the 5′ end of the genome or very near to it, depending on the position of p10. P10, the smallest of the nonglycosylated internal proteins, is not derived from the 76,000 molecular weight precursor and has not been mapped as yet. The possibility that it maps at the 5′ end has not been ruled out. Applying this information to the map of an avian sarcoma virus, the sequence reads as follows: *gag*$_{p19-27-12-15}$-*pol*-(p10)-*env*-*src*-*C*-poly(A). The positions of p10 and of *pol* are guessed and need experimental confirmation.

7. CONCLUDING SPECULATIONS

In the present state of RNA tumor virus genetics, there are four areas which seem particularly inviting for predictions and speculations: (1) the mechanism of recombination, (2) the product of the *src* gene, (3) interaction of virus and cell genomes including integration and transduction, and (4) restriction enzyme mapping of the DNA provirus.

7.1. On Recombination

Building models for recombination has become a favorite pastime among RNA tumor virologists, and this activity has great heuristic value. In the context of this chapter, a presentation of detailed speculative models would be out of place, but some basic premises and their consequences shall be examined. Most models of recombination propose that reverse transcription generates recombinants. However, there is no evidence against the possibility that recombination could occur between completed DNA proviruses.

The two published models for recombination between RNA tumor viruses work with linear genomes (Vogt, 1973; Cooper and Wyke, 1975). If recombination occurs between linear genomes, then genes at opposite ends of the genome should not be linked. Considering the preliminary map of avian sarcoma viruses, *gag-pol-env-src-C*-poly(A), there should be a very high recombination frequency between *src* and *gag*. Studies by Hunter and Vogt (1976) and by Hayman and Vogt (1976), however, have suggested some linkage between these genes. This observation can be best explained by postulating that recombination occurs between circularized genomes. The two published models for recombination are also in contradiction with other experimental facts and would require major modifications. The best evidence suggests that the 30–40 S genomes are not linked in tandem, i.e., both oriented in the same 3′ to 5′ polarity, but are joined symmetrically at their 5′ ends with a reversion of polarity in the center of the dimer (Kung *et al.,* 1975*a*). Furthermore, the primer attachment site is at the 5′ and not at the 3′ end. This fact could be interpreted as generating a need for early circularization, since transcription proceeds in the 3′ → 5′ direction of the template (Taylor and Illmensee, 1975).

There are two main choices for circular intermediates in recombination. The 70 S RNA or its DNA transcript may circularize in its entirety to generate a dimeric circle. One could imagine that this happens as a consequence of reverse transcription: the transcripts started with the primer on the 5′ end of genome A would run into the 3′ end of genome A′ and continue in the 3′ → 5′ direction of the template. Transcripts started with primer positioned at the 5′ end of genome A′ would extent into the 3′ portion of genome A (Mason, 1974, personal communication). The result would be a figure-eight in which the 5′ end of genome A is physically linked to the 3′ end of genome A′ and, *vice versa,* the 5′ end of A′ is linked to the 3′ end of A. Monomers would be generated from this dimeric circle by single or odd-numbered recombinational events. One important and testable prediction of the dimeric circle model is that markers at the 5′ end of one parent will be genetically linked to markers at the 3′ end of the other parent. The second possibility for circular intermediates in recombination is that the 30–40 S genomes circularize individually (Hunter *et al.*, 1977). According to this hypothetical model, a given virus particle is thought to produce a single-stranded DNA transcript of minus polarity from each of the two unit genomes which are present in the virion. Plus-stranded DNA is synthesized on the minus-strand template in small pieces (Varmus *et al.*, 1975*b*; Gianni and Weinberg, 1975), and it is hypothesized that such pieces could be exchanged between the two circular unit genomes of the same virion, leading to heteroduplex recombinant molecules. Each recombinant would be produced by two (or a multiple of two) crossovers. In this monomeric circle model, the genes at the 5′ end and at the 3′ end of the *same* genome should be linked. The few data which are available from crosses between avian sarcoma and leukemia viruses suggest that *src* located at the 3′ end of the genome is linked to *gag* from the 5′ end of the *same* genome (Hunter and Vogt, 1976; Hayman and Vogt, 1976). Similar linkage between *gag* and *src* has been seen with simian sarcoma viruses, but data on the positions of these genes are not available, nor is it known whether simian sarcoma virus is capable of recombining with the various heterologous helper viruses which have been used for virus rescue (Scolnick and Parks, 1973). In both circular models, recombination frequencies should be highest between genes which are half genomes apart.

In the dimeric circle model, parental genomes with two different deletions could give rise to nondefective recombinant progeny if the deletions are not contiguous or overlapping. In the monomeric circle model, the generation of recombinant nondefective virus from two defective viruses carrying noncontiguous deletions may or may not be possible, depending on the molecular details which are being assumed (see Hunter *et al.*, 1977).

Whatever the correct model may be, it must be able to explain heterozygosity. If it is accepted that heterozygotes are real as opposed to trivial virus clumps, then this means that at least in the *env* marker, for which experimental evidence of heterozygosity exists, both genomes present in a virion can be expressed. Yet pseudotypes formed with avian leukosis helper virus and the *env⁻ rd* deletion mutant RSV(−) or *NY*8 do not produce infectious progeny in solitary infection. At least some of these pseudotypes must be heterozygotes containing a genome of RSV(−) and of the helper virus combined in the 60–70 S RNA complex. Evidence for such heterozygosity can be adduced from data which suggest that RSV(−) does recombine with other avian leukosis or sarcoma viruses. Hanafusa and Hanafusa (1968) observed probable recombination between RSV($-$) and leukosis virus in *pol,* and recombinants in *src* can be obtained after mixed infection with RSV($-$) and a nondefective avian sarcoma virus (Balduzzi, 1976; Hunter *et al.,* 1976*b*). Since recombinants most likely arise from heterozygotes, such heterozygotes must be formed between RSV($-$) and its helper virus. If both genomes in a heterozygote are expressed, many pseudotype particles of RSV($-$) should form infectious centers in solitary infection and not require independent secondary infection of the cell by a helper virus. A way out of this dilemma would be to postulate that although two parental genomes may be enclosed in the same virion, only one provirus which may combine genetic information from both parents becomes integrated. Sustained heterozygosity in a given marker may derive from the formation of a stable heteroduplex DNA molecule in the process of recombination. Such heteroduplices are envisaged in the monomeric circle model of Hunter *et al.* (1976*b*). The phenotypic manifestations of heterozygosity would then always be the result of a recombinational event which in turn generates the heteroduplex. The idea that the diploid virion produces only a single functional provirus is also in agreement with long-standing results on single-hit inactivation of avian RNA tumor viruses with agents affecting primarily nucleic acids (UV light, chemical mutagens, X-rays) (Rubin and Temin, 1959; Rubin, 1960; Friesen and Rubin, 1961; Hanafusa *et al.,* 1964*b*; Levinson and Rubin, 1966; Graf and Bauer, 1970; Toyoshima *et al.,* 1970; Friis *et al.,* 1971; Yoshikura, 1973*a,b*; Lovinger *et al.,* 1975*a*; Owada *et al.,* 1976; Bister *et al.,* 1977). However, since there appear to exist extensive areas of close physical contact between the two genomes of a virion (Delius *et al.,* 1975), a single lesion could conceivably affect these interactions in some way and cause inactivation of both genomes.

7.2. The Product of *src*

If one makes the simplifying assumption that *src* is not substantially larger than the *td* deletion, then the coding capacity of this transforming function would suffice for one or a few proteins with a combined molecular weight of 30,000–40,000. The still hypothetical gene product of *src* is referred to as the transforming protein. Evidence for the existence of a transforming protein is indirect: most class T *ts* mutants of avian sarcoma viruses and the cold-sensitive mutant of MSV require protein synthesis to effect retransformation upon shift to the permissive temperature. Presumably in these mutants the transforming protein is temperature labile and irreversibly inactivated under nonpermissive conditions, requiring resynthesis after shift. The function of the transforming protein would be to interfere with cellular control mechanisms. This action would lead to oncogenic transformation with its pleomorphic cellular changes. In this connection, the evidence suggesting that src may be derived from the cellular genome is of particular interest (Ball et al., 1973a; Scolnick et al., 1975a,b; Roy-Burman and Klement, 1975).

It is now an obvious task of cardinal importance to isolate the transforming protein and to show how it acts on the cell. The greatest technical obstacle to this goal is the lack of an assay for a transforming protein. A number of approaches are possible and will no doubt be tried. Use of intact cells as indicators of exogenously supplied transforming protein may run into problems of uptake, but this difficulty is probably not insurmountable. In vitro tests such as binding to DNA could perhaps be linked to the transforming properties of a candidate protein. At this time, there is no promising beginning in this area, but given the clear conceptual statement of the problem, the breakthrough is likely to be technical.

However, lest the idea of a transforming protein becomes codified, an alternative possibility should be considered. There is precedence for temperature-sensitive tRNAs (Smith et al., 1970). Could the src region perhaps code for one or several suppressor tRNAs which would induce changes in cellular proteins and could intervene with the correct function of some cellular regulatory mechanisms? For instance, one could imagine the existence of a cellular gene which is normally not expressed because it contains an amber triplet. If the virus introduces an appropriate suppressor tRNA, the protein is made. It may interfere with the regulation of cell growth and cause oncogenic transformation. In class T mutants, the suppressor tRNA would be ts in one of its functions; thus at the nonpermissive temperature the cellular protein in question would not be made, and the cell would assume normal properties. Upon shift to the permissive temperature, new protein synthesis may be required to effect retransformation. In this hypothetical situation, there would still be a "transforming protein," but it would be coded for by the cell; the virus would provide merely an accessory needed for the synthesis of this cellular protein. The size of src would be sufficient to code for several tRNAs, but some of it could be "spacer" sequences. Although this hypothesis suggesting that src does not code directly for a transforming protein is not considered likely, it cannot be definitely ruled out with the available experimental data.

7.3. Interaction between Virus and Cell Genomes

One of the products of reverse transcription is closed circular viral DNA. It is now widely assumed that this supercoiled DNA is the precursor of the integrated provirus (Smotkin *et al.,* 1975; Varmus *et al.,* 1975a; Guntaka *et al.,* 1975). However, the process of integration itself is not understood. Some of the basic questions should at least be stated here. Is integration site-specific or can provirus integrate anywhere in the host genome? If there is site specificity, how many sites are there per genome, and can these sites be saturated? Does the endogenous viral genome determine the site of integration? Is there an obligatory requirement for integration even in virus reproduction, or can some provirus function outside the cellular genome? Only fragmentary answers are available to these questions. There are indications for a limited number of integration sites which can be saturated. Preliminary data suggest that the number of integrated genomes cannot be increased *ad libitum* by increasing the multiplicity of infectivity or by exposing avian sarcoma virus-transformed cells to ever new kinds of exogenous sarcoma virus (Khoury and Hanafusa, 1975, unpublished observations; Varmus and Vogt, 1975, unpublished observations). Data have also been presented which suggest that the avian myeloblastosis virus genome is integrated in chicken cells adjacent to unique-sequence DNA, possibly the endogenous viral genome (Evans *et al.,* 1975). In Peking duck cells, cytoplasmic DNA of avian sarcoma virus is found long after infection (Varmus and Shank, 1976). This unintegrated provirus probably does not derive from reinfection of cells, and its occurrence in relatively large quantities raises the question of a possible function of free viral DNA.

The enzymatic machinery needed for integration is probably supplied by the cell. Cellular mutants should therefore exist which show various defects in integration, and such mutants could contribute substantially to our understanding of the integration process.

The possibility that sarcoma viruses and perhaps also leukemia viruses transduce cellular genes has already been mentioned. The transformation-specific genetic information of avian sarcoma viruses and of certain murine sarcoma viruses appears to be derived from the host cell (Scolnick *et al.,* 1975a; Stehelin *et al.,* 1976b). The acquisition of *src* sequences by transformation-defective virus from the cell is a rare event and has not been documented experimentally, except possibly in the isolation of sarcoma virus described by Ball *et al.* (1973a). It would be of great interest if *src* sequences could be acquired by a *td* virus reproducibly in a tissue culture system. Perhaps passage of *td* viruses in chemically transformed cells could give the desired result. Whether cellular sequences other than those related to sarcoma induction can be transduced by RNA tumor viruses is uncertain. Acquisition of cellular genetic material during passage in a heterologous host has been reported for avian sarcoma virus B77 (Shoyab *et al.,* 1975). However, alternative explanations of these data, especially the possibility that virus variants have been selected, need to be examined.

7.4. Analysis of the Viral Genome and of Integration Sites with DNA Restriction Enzymes

The highly developed technology of restriction enzyme mapping which has been so successfully applied to papova- and adenoviruses will probably gain importance for RNA tumor virus genetics in the next few years. The key prerequisites for genetic mapping with restriction enzymes are genome length, purified viral DNA in sufficient amounts, and a reliable and efficient infectivity test for viral DNA. Both conditions will probably soon be fulfilled (Smotkin *et al.,* 1975; Gianni *et al.,* 1976). Treatment of integrated provirus with restriction enzymes will generate fragments with cellular DNA attached to the termini of the provirus, and the properties of these fragments could provide an answer to the question of specific vs. nonspecific integration sites.

It is clear from these speculations that RNA tumor virus genetics is headed toward a complete molecular understanding of virus-induced oncogenesis and of the RNA tumor virus life cycle. Conventional genetic approaches generate suitable mutant and recombinant material, which then allows successful application of techniques in protein and nucleic acid chemistry to answer specific genetic questions.

ACKNOWLEDGMENTS

The author gratefully acknowledges many stimulating, instructive, and critical discussions with Stuart A. Aaronson, Martin C. Alevy, J. Michael Bishop, Klaus Bister, Peter H. Duesberg, Donald Fujita, Hidesaburo Hanafusa, Michael J. Hayman, Eric Hunter, Michael C. Lai, Jay A. Levy, William S. Mason, Carlo Moscovici, Roland R. Rueckert, Edward M. Scolnick, Harold E. Varmus, and Inder Verma.

Work of the author is supported by U.S. Public Health Service Research Grant No. CA 13213 and by Virus Cancer Program Contract No. NO1 CP 53518 awarded by the National Cancer Institute.

8. REFERENCES

Aaronson, S. A., 1973, Biologic characterization of mammalian cells transformed by a primate sarcoma virus, *Virology* **52**:562.

Aaronson, S. A., and Rowe, W. P., 1970, Nonproducer clones of murine sarcoma virus transformed BALB/3T3 cells, *Virology* **42**:9.

Aaronson, S. A., and Stephenson, J. R., 1973, Independent segregation of loci for activation of biologically distinguishable RNA C-type viruses in mouse cells, *Proc. Natl. Acad. Sci. USA* **70**:2055.

Aaronson, S. A., and Weaver, C. A., 1971, Characterization of murine sarcoma virus (Kirsten) transformation of mouse and human cells, *J. Gen. Virol.* **13**:245.

Aaronson, S. A., Jainchill, J. L., and Todaro, G. J., 1970, Murine sarcoma virus transformation of BALB/3T3 cells: Lack of dependence on murine leukemia virus, *Proc. Natl. Acad. Sci. USA* **66**:1236.

Aaronson, S. A., Bassin, R. H., and Weaver, C., 1972, Comparison of murine sarcoma viruses in nonproducer and S^+L^--transformed cells, *J. Virol.* **9**:701.

Aaronson, S. A., Stephenson, J. R., Hino, S., and Tronick, S. R., 1975, Differential expression of helper viral structural polypeptides in cells transformed by clonal isolates of wolly monkey sarcoma virus, *J. Virol.* **16**:1117.

Abelson, H. T., and Rabstein, L. S., 1970, Lymphosarcoma: Virus-induced thymic-independent disease in mice, *Cancer Res.* **30**:2213.

Ambros, V. R., Chen, L. B., and Buchanan, J. M., 1975, Surface ruffles as markers for studies of cell transformation by Rous sarcoma virus, *Proc. Natl. Acad. Sci. USA* **72**:3144.

Anderson, W. B., Johnson, G. S., and Pastan, I., 1973*a*, Transformation of chick-embryo fibroblasts by wild-type and temperature-sensitive Rous sarcoma virus alters adenylate cyclase activity, *Proc. Natl. Acad. Sci. USA* **70**:1055.

Anderson, W. B., Lovelace, E., and Pastan, I., 1973*b*, Adenylate cyclase activity is decreased in chick embryo fibroblasts transformed by wild-type and temperature sensitive Schmidt-Ruppin Rous sarcoma virus, *Biochem. Biophys. Res. Commun.* **52**:1293.

Bader, A. V., 1973, Role of mitochondria in the production of RNA-containing tumor viruses, *J. Virol.* **11**:314.

Bader, J. P., 1972, Temperature-dependent transformation of cells infected with a mutant of Bryan Rous sarcoma virus, *J. Virol.* **10**:267.

Bader, J. P., Ray, D. A., and Brown, N. R., 1974, Accumulation of water during transformation of cells by an avian sarcoma virus, *Cell* **3**:307.

Balduzzi, P. C., 1976, Cooperative transformation studies with temperature sensitive mutants of Rous sarcoma virus, *J. Virol.* **18**:332.

Balduzzi, P., and Morgan, H. R., 1970, Mechanism of oncogenic transformation by Rous sarcoma virus. I. Intracellular inactivation of cell-transforming ability of Rous sarcoma virus by 5-bromodeoxyuridine and light, *J. Virol.* **5**:470.

Balduzzi, P. C., and Murphy, H., 1975, Plaque assay of avian sarcoma viruses using casein, *J. Virol.* **16**:707.

Ball, J. K., Harvey, D., and McCarter, J. A., 1973*a*, Evidence for naturally occurring murine sarcoma virus, *Nature (London)* **241**:272.

Ball, J. K., McCarter, J. A., and Sunderland, S. M., 1973*b*, Evidence for helper independent murine sarcoma virus. I. Segregation of replication-defective and transformation-defective viruses, *Virology* **56**:268.

Baltimore, D., 1970, Viral RNA-dependent DNA polymerase, *Nature (London)* **226**:1209.

Baltimore, D., 1975, Tumor viruses: 1974, *Cold Spring Harbor Symp. Quant. Biol.* **39**:1187.

Baluda, M. A., and Goetz, I. E., 1961, Morphological conversion of cell cultures by avian myeloblastosis virus, *Virology* **15**:185.

Baluda, M. A., Shoyab, M., Markham, P. D., Evans, R. M., and Drohan, W. N., 1975, Base sequence complexity of 35 S avian myeloblastosis virus RNA determined by molecular hybridization kinetics, *Cold Spring Harbor Symp. Quant. Biol.* **39**:869.

Bassin, R. H., Tuttle, N., and Fischinger, P. J., 1970, Isolation of murine sarcoma virus-transformed mouse cells which are negative for leukemia virus from agar suspension cultures, *Int. J. Cancer* **6**:95.

Bassin, R. H., Phillips, L. A., Kramer, M. J., Haapala, D. K., Peebles, P. T., Nomura, S., and Fischinger, P. J., 1971a, Transformation of mouse 3T3 cells by murine sarcoma virus: Release of virus-like particles in the absence of replicating murine leukemia helper virus, *Proc. Natl. Acad. Sci. USA* **68**:1520.

Bassin, R. H., Tuttle, N., and Fischinger, P. J., 1971b, Rapid cell culture assay technique for murine leukaemia viruses, *Nature (London)* **229**:564.

Bassin, R. H., Duran-Troise, G., Gerwin, B. I., Gisselbrecht, S., and Rein, A., 1975, Murine sarcoma virus pseudotypes acquire a determinant specifying N or B tropism from leukaemia virus during rescue, *Nature (London)* **256**:223.

Bauer, H., Kurth, R., Rohrschneider, L., Pauli, G., Friis, R. R., and Gelderblom, H., 1975, The role of cell surface changes in RNA tumor virus-transformed cells, *Cold Spring Harbor Symp. Quant. Biol.* **39**:1181.

Beaudreau, G. S., Becker, C., Bonar, R. A., Wallbank, A. M., Beard, D., and Beard, J. W., 1960, Virus of avian myeloblastosis. XIV. Neoplastic response of normal chicken bone marrow treated with the virus in tissue culture, *J. Natl. Cancer Inst.* **24**:395.

Beemon, K., Duesberg, P., and Vogt, P., 1974, Evidence for crossing-over between avian tumor viruses based on analysis of viral RNAs, *Proc. Natl. Acad. Sci. USA* **71**:4254.

Beemon, K. L., Faras, A. J., Haase, A. T., Duesberg, P. H., and Maisel, J. E., 1976, Genomic complexities of murine leukemia and sarcoma, reticuloendotheliosis, and visna viruses, *J. Virol.* **17**:525.

Bellamy, A. R., Gillies, S. C., and Harvey, J. D., 1974, Molecular weight of two oncornavirus genomes: Derivation from particle molecular weights and RNA content, *J. Virol.* **14**:1388.

Bender, W., and Davidson, N., 1976, Mapping of poly(A) sequences in the electron microscope reveals unusual structure of type C oncornavirus RNA molecules, *Cell* **7**:595.

Benveniste, R. E., and Scolnick, E. M., 1973, RNA in mammalian sarcoma virus transformed nonproducer cells homologous to murine leukemia virus RNA, *Virology* **51**:370.

Benveniste, R. E., and Todaro, G. J., 1973, Homology between type-C viruses of various species as determined by molecular hybridization, *Proc. Natl. Acad. Sci. USA* **70**:3316.

Benveniste, R. E., and Todaro, G. J., 1974a, Evolution of type C viral genes. I. Nucleic acid from baboon type C virus as a measure of divergence among primate species, *Proc. Natl. Acad. Sci. USA* **71**:4513.

Benveniste, R. E., and Todaro, G. J., 1974*b*, Evolution of C-type viral genes: Inheritance of exogenously acquired viral genes, *Nature (London)* **252**:456.

Benveniste, R. E., and Todaro, G. J., 1975, Evolution of type C viral genes: Preservation of ancestral murine type C viral sequences in pig cellular DNA, *Proc. Natl. Acad. Sci. USA* **72**:4090.

Benveniste, R. E., Lieber, M. M., and Todaro, G. J., 1974, A distinct class of inducible murine type-C viruses that replicates in the rabbit SIRC cell-line, *Proc. Natl. Acad. Sci. USA* **71**:602.

Bernstein, A., MacCormick, R., and Martin, G. S., 1976, Transformation-defective mutants of avian sarcoma viruses: The genetic relationship between conditional and non-conditional mutants, *Virology* **70**:206.

Biggs, P. M., Milne, B. S., Graf, T., and Bauer, H., 1973, Oncogenicity of non-transforming mutants of avian sarcoma viruses, *J. Gen. Virol.* **18**:399.

Bilello, J. A., Strand, M., and August, J. T., 1974, Murine sarcoma virus gene expression: Transformants which express viral envelope glycoprotein in the absence of the major internal protein and infectious particles, *Proc. Natl. Acad. Sci. USA* **71**:3234.

Billeter, M. A., Parson, J. T., and Coffin, J. M., 1974, The nucleotide sequence complexity of avian tumor virus RNA, *Proc. Natl. Acad. Sci. USA* **71**:3560.

Biquard, J.-M., 1973, Agglutinability of Rous cells by concanavalin A: Study with a temperature-sensitive RSV mutant and inhibitors of macromolecular synthesis, *Intervirology* **1**:220.

Biquard, J.-M., and Vigier, P., 1971, Isolement ét etude d'un mutant conditionnel du virus de Rous à capacité transformante thermosensible, *C. R. Acad. Sci. Paris* **271(D)**:2430.

Biquard, J.-M., and Vigier, P., 1972, Characteristics of a conditional mutant of Rous sarcoma virus defective in ability to transform cells at high temperature, *Virology* **47**:444.

Bishop, J. M., and Varmus, H., 1975, Molecular biology of RNA tumor viruses, in: *Cancer,* Vol. 2 (F. F. Becker, ed.), pp. 3–48, Plenum Publishing Corporation, New York.

Bishop, J. M., Levinson, W. E., Quintrell, N., Sullivan, D., Fanshier, L., and Jackson, J., 1970*a*, The low molecular weight RNAs of Rous sarcoma virus. I. The 4S RNA, *Virology* **42**:182.

Bishop, J. M., Levinson, W. E., Sullivan, D., Fanshier, L., Quintrell, N., and Jackson, J., 1970*b*, The low molecular weight RNAs of Rous sarcoma virus. II. The 7 S RNA, *Virology* **42**:927.

Blair, D. G., Mason, W. S., Hunter, E., and Vogt, P. K., 1976, Temperature-sensitive mutants of avian sarcoma viruses: Genetic recombination between multiple or coordinate mutants and avian leukosis viruses, *Virology* **75**:48.

Boettiger, D., 1974, Virogenic nontransformed cells isolated following infection of normal rat kidney cells with B77 strain Rous sarcoma virus, *Cell* **3**:71.

Boettiger, D., 1975, Activation and repression of virus expression in mammalian cells infected by Rous sarcoma virus, *Cold Spring Harbor Symp. Quant. Biol.* **39**:1169.

Boettiger, D., and Temin, H. M., 1970, Light inactivation of focus formation by chicken embryo fibroblasts infected with avian sarcoma virus in the presence of 5-bromodeoxyuridine, *Nature (London)* **228**:622.

Boettiger, D., Love, D. N., and Weiss, R. A., 1975, Virus envelope markers in mammalian tropism of avian RNA tumor viruses, *J. Virol.* **15**:108.

Bolognesi, D. P., 1974, Structural components of RNA tumor virus, in: *Advances in Virus Research,* Vol. 19 (M. Lauffer, F. Bang, K. Maramorosch, and K. Smith, eds.), pp. 315–360, Academic Press, New York.

Bolognesi, D. P., Bauer, H., Gelderblom, H., and Gudrun, H., 1972, Polypeptides of avian RNA tumor virus. IV. Components of the viral envelope, *Virology* **47**:551.

Bonar, R. A., Sverak, L., Bolognesi, D. P., Langlois, A. J., Beard, D., and Beard, J. W., 1967, Ribonucleic acid components of BAI strain A (myeloblastosis) avian tumor virus, *Cancer Res.* **27**:1138.

Bookout, J. B., and Sigel, M. M., 1975, Characterization of a conditional mutant of Rous sarcoma virus with alterations in early and late functions of cell transformation, *Virology* **67**:474.

Bryant, M. L., and Klement, V., 1976, Clonal heterogeneity of wild mouse leukemia viruses: Host range and antigenicity, *Virology* **73**:532.

Burger, M. M., and Martin, G. S., 1972, Agglutination of cells transformed by Rous sarcoma virus by wheat germ agglutinin and concanavalin A, *Nature (London)* New Biol. **237**:9.

Bussell, R. H., and Robinson, W. S., 1973, Membrane proteins of uninfected and Rous sarcoma virus-transformed avian cells, *J. Virol.* **12**:320.

Butterworth, B. E., 1973, A comparison of virus-specific polypeptides of encephalomyocarditis virus, human rhinovirus-1A, and poliovirus, *Virology* **56**:439.

Butterworth, B. E., and Rueckert, R. R., 1972, Kinetics of synthesis and cleavage of encephalomyocarditis virus-specific proteins, *Virology* **50**:535.

Callahan, R., Lieber, M. M., and Todaro, G. J., 1975, Nucleic acid homology of murine xenotropic type C viruses, *J. Virol.* **15**:1378.

Canaani, E., and Duesberg, P., 1972, Role of subunits of 60 to 70 S avian tumor virus ribonucleic acid in its template activity for the viral deoxyribonucleic acid polymerase, *J. Virol.* **10**:23.

Canaani, E., Helm, K. V. D., and Duesberg, P., 1973, Evidence for 30–40 S RNA as precursor of the 60–70 S RNA of Rous sarcoma virus, *Proc. Natl. Acad. Sci. USA* **70**:401.

Carchman, R. A., Johnson, G. S., Pastan, I., and Scolnick, E. M., 1974, Studies on the levels of cyclic AMP in cells transformed by wild-type and temperature-sensitive Kirsten sarcoma virus, *Cell* **1**:59.

Chan, E. W., Schiop-Stansly, P. E., and O'Connor, T. E., 1974, Rescue of cell-transforming virus from a non-virus-producing bovine cell culture transformed by feline sarcoma virus, *J. Natl. Cancer Inst.* **52**:469.

Chen, L. B., and Buchanan, J. M., 1975, Plasminogen-independent fibrinolysis by proteases produced by transformed chick embryo fibroblasts, *Proc. Natl. Acad. Sci. USA* **72**:1132.

Chen, Y. C., and Vogt, P. K., 1977, Endogenous leukosis viruses in the avian family *Phasianidae. Virology* **76**:740.

Chen, Y. C., Hayman, M. J., and Vogt, P. K., 1977, Properties of mammalian cells transformed by temperature sensitive mutants of avian sarcoma virus, in preparation.

Cheung, K.-S., Smith, R. E., Stone, M. P., and Joklik, W. K., 1972, Comparison of immature (rapid harvest) and mature Rous sarcoma virus particles, *Virology* **50**:851.

Chi, Y. Y., and Bassel, A. R., 1975, Electron microscopy of viral RNA: Avian tumor virus RNA, *Virology* **64**:217.

Clarke, B. J., Axelrad, A. A., Shreeve, M. M., and McLeod, D. L., 1975, Erythroid colony induction without erythropoietin by Friend leukemia virus, *in vitro, Proc. Natl. Acad. Sci. USA* **72**:3556.

Coffin, J. M., and Billeter, M. A., 1976, A physical map of the Rous sarcoma virus genome, *J. Mol. Biol.* **100**:293.

Cooper, G. M., and Temin, H. M., 1974, Infectious Rous sarcoma virus and reticuloendotheliosis virus DNAs, *J. Virol.* **14**:1132.

Cooper, G. M., and Temin, H. M., 1975, Infectious DNA from cells infected with Rous sarcoma virus, reticuloendotheliosis virus or Rous-associated virus-O, *Cold Spring Harbor Symp. Quant. Biol.* **39**:1027.

Cooper, P. D., and Wyke, J. A., 1975, The genome of RNA tumor viruses: A functional requirement for a polyploid structure? *Cold Spring Harbor Symp. Quant. Biol.* **39**:997.

Courington, D., and Vogt, P. K., 1967, Electron microscopy of chick fibroblasts infected by defective Rous sarcoma virus and its helper, *J. Virol.* **1**:400.

Crittenden, L. B., 1968, Observations on the nature of a genetic cellular resistance to avian tumor viruses, *J. Natl. Cancer Inst.* **41**:145.

Crittenden, L. B., 1975, Two levels of genetic resistance to lymphoid leukosis, *Avian Dis.* **19**:281.

Crittenden, L. B., and Motta, J. V., 1975, The role of *tvb* locus in genetic resistance to RSV (RAV-O), *Virology* **67**:327.

Crittenden, L. B., Okazaki, W., and Reamer, R., 1963, Genetic resistance to Rous sarcoma virus in embryo cell cultures and embryos, *Virology* **20**:541.

Crittenden, L. B., Okazaki, W., and Reamer, R. H., 1964, Genetic control of responses to Rous sarcoma and strain RPL12 viruses in the cells, embryos, and chickens of two inbred lines, *Natl. Cancer Inst. Monogr.* **17**:161.

Crittenden, L. B., Stone, H. A., Reamer, R. H., and Okazaki, W., 1967, Two loci controlling genetic cellular resistance to avian leukosis-sarcoma viruses, *J. Virol.* **1**:898.

Crittenden, L. B., Wendel, E. J., and Motta, J. V., 1973, Interaction of genes controlling resistance to RSV (RAV-O), *Virology* **52**:373.

Dahlberg, J. E., Sawyer, R. C., Taylor, J. M., Faras, A. J., Levinson, W. E., Goodman, H. M., and Bishop, J. M., 1974, Transcription of DNA from the 70 S RNA of Rous sarcoma virus. I. Identification of a specific 4 S RNA which serves as primer, *J. Virol.* **13**:1126.

Dahlberg, J. E., Harada, F., and Sawyer, R. C., 1975, Structure and properties of an RNA primer for initiation of Rous sarcoma virus DNA synthesis *in vitro, Cold Spring Harbor Symp. Quant. Biol.* **39**:925.

Dales, S., and Hanafusa, H., with the assistance of Huima, T., 1972, Penetration and intracellular release of the genomes of avian RNA tumor viruses, *Virology* **50**:440.

Dalton, A. J., 1962, Micromorphology of murine tumor viruses and of affected cells, *Fed. Proc.* **21**:936.

Dawson, P. J., Tacke, R. B., and Fieldsteel, A. H., 1968, Relationship between Friend virus and an associated lymphatic leukaemia virus, *Br. J. Cancer* **22**:569.

Declève, A., Niwa, O., Gelmann, E., and Kaplan, H. S., 1975, Replication kinetics of N- and B-tropic murine leukemia viruses on permissive and nonpermissive cells *in vitro, Virology* **65**:320.

De Giuli, C., Kawai, S., Dales, S., and Hanafusa, H., 1975, Absence of surface projections on some noninfectious forms of RSV, *Virology* **66**:253.

Delius, H., Duesberg, P. H., and Mangel, W. F., 1975, Electron microscope measurements of Rous sarcoma virus RNA, *Cold Spring Harbor Symp. Quant. Biol.* **39**:835.

Dinowitz, M., 1975, Inhibition of Rous sarcoma virus by α-amanitin: Possible role of cell DNA-dependent RNA polymerase form II, *Virology* **66**:1.

Dougherty, R. M., and Di Stephano, H. S., 1965, Virus particles associated with "nonproducer" Rous sarcoma cells, *Virology* **27**:351.

Dougherty, R. M., and Rasmussen, R., 1964, Properties of a strain of Rous sarcoma virus that infects mammals, *Natl. Cancer Inst. Monogr.* **17**:337.

Duesberg, P. H., 1968, Physical properties of Rous sarcoma virus RNA, *Proc. Natl. Acad. Sci. USA* **60**:1511.

Duesberg, P. H., and Vogt, P. K., 1970, Differences between the ribonucleic acids of transforming and nontransforming avian tumor viruses, *Proc. Natl. Acad. Sci. USA* **67**:1673.

Duesberg, P. H., and Vogt, P. K., 1973*a*, RNA species obtained from clonal lines of avian sarcoma and avian leukosis virus, *Virology* **54**:207.

Duesberg, P. H., and Vogt, P. K., 1973*b*, Gel electrophoresis of avian leukosis and sarcoma viral RNA in formamide: Comparison with other viral and cellular RNA species, *J. Virol.* **12**:594.

Duesberg, P. H., Martin, G. S., and Vogt, P. K., 1970, Glycoprotein components of avian and murine RNA tumor viruses, *Virology* **41**:631.

Duesberg, P. H., Kawai, S., Wang, L.-H., Vogt, P. K., Murphy, H. M., and Hanafusa, H., 1975*a*, RNA of replication-defective strains of Rous sarcoma virus, *Proc. Natl. Acad. Sci. USA* **72**:1569.

Duesberg, P., Vogt, P. K., Beemon, K., and Lai, M., 1975*b*, Avian RNA tumor viruses: Mechanism of recombination and complexity of the genome, *Cold Spring Harbor Symp. Quant. Biol.* **39**:847.

Duesberg, P. H., Wang, L. H., Mellon, P., Mason, W. S., and Vogt, P. K., 1976, Towards a complete genetic map of Rous sarcoma virus, in: *Animal Virology* (D. Baltimore, A. S. Huang, and C. F. Fox, eds.), pp. 107–123, Academic Press, New York.

Duff, R. G., and Vogt, P. K., 1969, Characteristics of two new avian tumor virus subgroups, *Virology* **39**:18.

Dulbecco, R., 1973, Cell transformation by viruses and the role of viruses in cancer: The eleventh Marjory Stephenson memorial lecture, *J. Gen. Microbiol.* **79**:7.

Eckner, R. J., 1973, Helper-dependent properties of Friend spleen focus-forming virus: Effect of the *Fv-1* gene on the late stages in virus synthesis, *J. Virol.* **12**:523.

Eckner, R. J., and Steeves, R. A., 1971, Defective Friend spleen focus-forming virus: Pseudotype neutralization by helper-specific antisera, *Nature (London)* New Biol. **229**:241.

Eckner, R. J., and Steeves, R. A., 1972, A classification of the murine leukemia viruses: Neutralization of pseudotypes of Friend spleen focus-forming virus by type-specific murine antisera, *J. Exp. Med.* **136**:832.

Eiden, J. J., Quade, K., and Nichols, J. L., 1976, Interaction of tryptophan transfer RNA with Rous sarcoma virus 35 S RNA, *Nature (London)* **259**:245.

Eisenman, R., Vogt, V. M., and Diggelmann, H., 1975, Synthesis of avian RNA tumor virus structural proteins, *Cold Spring Harbor Symp. Quant. Biol.* **39**:1067.

Erikson, E., and Erikson, R. L., 1970, Isolation of amino acid acceptor RNA from purified avian myeloblastosis virus, *J. Mol. Biol.* **52**:387.

Erikson, E., and Erikson, R. L., 1971, Association of 4S ribonucleic acid with oncornavirus ribonucleic acids, *J. Virol.* **8**:254.

Erikson, E., Erikson, R. L., Henry, B., and Pace, N. R., 1973, Comparison of oligonucleotides produced by RNase T1 digestion of 7 S RNA from avian and murine oncornaviruses and from uninfected cells, *Virology* **53**:40.

Erikson, R. L., 1969, Studies on the RNA from avian myeloblastosis virus, *Virology* **37**:124.

Evans, R. M., Shoyab, M., and Baluda, M. A., 1975, Studies on characterization of the integration sites of avian RNA tumor virus-specific DNA, *Cold Spring Harbor Symp. Quant. Biol.* **39**:1005.

Fan, H., and Baltimore, D., 1973, RNA metabolism of murine leukemia virus: Detection of virus-specific RNA sequences in infected and uninfected cells and identification of virus-specific messenger RNA, *J. Mol. Biol.* **80**:93.

Fan, H., and Paskind, M., 1974, Measurement of the sequence complexity of cloned Moloney murine leukemia virus 60 to 70 S RNA: Evidence for a haploid genome, *J. Virol.* **14**:421.

Faras, A. J., 1975, The methionyl transfer RNAs of Rous sarcoma virus, *Virology* **63**:583.

Faras, A. J., Garapin, A. C., Levinson, W. E., Bishop, J. M., and Goodman, H. M., 1973, Characterization of the low-molecular-weight RNAs associated with the 70 S RNA of Rous sarcoma virus, *J. Virol.* **12**:334.

Faras, A. J., Dahlberg, J. E., Sawyer, R. C., Harada, F., Taylor, J. M., Levinson, W. E., Bishop, J. M., and Goodman, H. M., 1974, Transcription of DNA from the 70 S RNA of Rous sarcoma virus. II. Structure of a 4 S RNA primer, *J. Virol.* **13**:1134.

Fields, B. N., and Joklik, W. K., 1969, Isolation and preliminary genetic and biochemical characterization of temperature-sensitive mutants of reovirus, *Virology* **37**:335.

Fieldsteel, A. H., Kurahara, C., and Dawson, P. J., 1969, Moloney leukaemia virus as a helper in retrieving Friend virus from a non-infectious reticulum cell sarcoma, *Nature (London)* **223**:1274.

Fieldsteel, A. H., Dawson, P. J., and Kurahara, C., 1971, *In vivo* and *in vitro* recovery of defective Friend virus by various leukemia viruses, *Int. J. Cancer* **8**:304.

Fischinger, P. J., Peebles, P. T., Nomura, S., and Haapala, D. K., 1973, Isolation of an RD-114-like oncornavirus from a cat cell line, *J. Virol* **11**:978.

Fischinger, P. J., Nomura, S., and Bolognesi, D. P., 1975, A novel murine oncornavirus with dual eco- and xenotropic properties, *Proc. Natl. Acad. Sci. USA* **72**:5150.

Fiszman, M. Y., and Fuchs, P., 1975, Temperature-sensitive expression of differentiation in transformed myoblasts, *Nature (London)* **254**:429.

Friesen, B., and Rubin, H., 1961, Some physiochemical and immunological properties of an avian leucosis virus (RIF), *Virology* **15**:387.

Friis, R. R., 1971, Inactivation of avian sarcoma viruses with UV light: A difference between helper-dependent and helper-independent strains, *Virology* **43**:521.

Friis, R. R., and Hunter, E., 1973, A temperature-sensitive mutant of Rous sarcoma virus that is defective for replication, *Virology* **53**:479.

Friis, R. R., Toyoshima, K., and Vogt, P. K., 1971, Conditional lethal mutants of avian sarcoma viruses. I. Physiology of *ts*75 and *ts*149, *Virology* **43**:375.

Friis, R. R., Mason, W. S., Chen, Y. C., and Halpern, M. S., 1975, A replication defective mutant of Rous sarcoma virus which fails to make a functional reverse transcriptase, *Virology* **64**:49.

Fujita, D. J., Chen, Y. C., Friis, R. R., and Vogt, P. K., 1974, RNA tumor viruses of pheasants: Characterization of avian leukosis subgroups F and G, *Virology* **60**:558.

Furuichi, Y., Shatkin, A. J., Stavnezer, E., and Bishop, J. M., 1975, Blocked, methylated 5'-terminal sequence in avian sarcoma RNA, *Nature (London)* **257**:618.

Gahmberg, C. G., and Hakomori, S.-I., 1973, Altered growth behavior of malignant cells associated with changes in externally labeled glycoprotein and glycolipid, *Proc. Natl. Acad. Sci. USA* **70**:3329.

Gazdar, A. F., Russell, E., Sarma, P. S., Sarin, P. S., Hall, W., and Chopra, H. C., 1973, Properties of noninfectious and transforming viruses released by Murine sarcoma virus-induced hamster tumor cells, *J. Virol.* **12**:931.

Gazzolo, L., Moscovici, M. G., and Moscovici, C., 1974, Replication of avian sarcoma viruses in chicken macrophages, *Virology* **58**:514.

Gazzolo, L., Moscovici, M. G., Moscovici, C., and Vogt, P. K., 1975, Susceptibility and resistance of chicken macrophages to avian RNA tumor viruses, *Virology* **67**:553.

Gianni, A. M., and Weinberg, R. A., 1975, Partially single-stranded form of free Moloney viral DNA, *Nature (London)* **255**:646.

Gianni, A. M., Smotkin, D., and Weinberg, R. A., 1975, Murine leukemia virus: Detection of unintegrated double-stranded DNA forms of the provirus, *Proc. Natl. Acad. Sci. USA* **72**:447.

Gianni, A. M., Hutton, J. R., Smotkin, D., and Weinberg, R. A., 1976, Proviral DNA of Moloney leukemia virus: Purification and visualization, *Science* **191**:569.

Gielkens, A. L. J., Salden, M. H. L., and Bloemendal, H., 1974, Virus-specific messenger RNA on free and membrane-bound polyribosomes from cells infected with Rauscher leukemia virus, *Proc. Natl. Acad. Sci. USA* **71**:1093.

Gielkens, A. L. J., Van Zaane, D., Bloemers, H. P. J., and Bloemendal, H., 1976, Synthesis of Rauscher murine leukemia virus-specific polypeptides *in vitro, Proc. Natl. Acad. Sci. USA* **73**:356.

Goldé, A., 1970, Radio-induced mutants of the Schmidt-Ruppin strain of Rous sarcoma virus, *Virology* **40**:1022.

Goldé, A., and Latarjet, R., 1966, Dissociation, par irradiation, des fonctions oncogène et infectieuse du virus de Rous, souche de Schmidt-Ruppin, *C. R. Acad. Sci Paris* **262(D)**:420.

Graf, T., 1972, A plaque assay for avian RNA tumor viruses, *Virology* **50**:567.

Graf, T., and Bauer, H., 1970, Studies on the relative target size of various functions in the genome of avian tumor viruses, in: *"Defectivité, Démasquage et Stimulation des Virus Oncogènes,"* pp. 87–92, Editions du Centre National de la Recherche Scientifique, Paris.

Graf, T., and Friis, R. R., 1973, Differential expression of transformation in rat and chicken cells infected with an avian sarcoma virus *ts* mutant, *Virology* **56**:369.

Graf, T., Bauer, H., Gelderblom, H., and Bolognesi, D. P., 1971, Studies on the reproductive and cell-converting abilities of avian sarcoma viruses, *Virology* **43**:427.

Granboulan, N., Huppert, J., and Lacour, F., 1966, Examen au microscope electronique du RNA du virus de la myeloblastose aviaire, *J. Mol. Biol.* **16**:571.

Grandgenett, D. P., Gerard, G. F., and Green, M., 1973, A single subunit from avian myeloblastosis virus with both RNA-directed DNA polymerase and ribonuclease H activity, *Proc. Natl. Acad. Sci. USA* **70**:230.

Greenberger, J. S., Anderson, G. R., and Aaronson, S. A., 1974a, Transformation-defective virus mutants in a class of morphologic revertants of sarcoma virus transformed nonproducer cells, *Cell* **2**:279.

Greenberger, J. S., Stephenson, J. R., Aoki, T., and Aaronson, S. A., 1974b, Cell-surface antigens of murine sarcoma-virus-transformed nonproducer cells: Further evidence for lack of transplantation immunity, *Int. J. Cancer* **14**:145.

Grodzicker, T., Williams, J., Sharp, P., and Sambrook, J., 1975, Physical mapping of temperature-sensitive mutations of adenoviruses, *Cold Spring Harbor Symp. Quant. Biol.* **39**:439.

Guntaka, R. V., Mahy, B. W. J., Bishop, J. M., and Varmus, H. E., 1975, Ethidium bromide inhibits appearance of closed circular viral DNA and integration of virus-specific DNA in duck cells infected by avian sarcoma virus, *Nature (London)* **253**:507.

Haapala, D. K., and Fischinger, P. J., 1973, Molecular relatedness of mammalian RNA tumor viruses as determined by DNA-RNA hybridization, *Science* **180**:972.

Hakomori, S., Wyke, J. A., and Vogt, P. K., 1977, Glycolipids of chick embryo fibroblasts infected with temperature sensitive mutants of avian sarcoma viruses, *Virology* **76**:485.

Hall, W. T., Gazdar, A. F., Hobbs, B. A., and Chopra, H. C., 1974, Morphology of a "noninfectious" sarcoma virus, *J. Natl. Cancer Inst.* **52**:1337.

Halpern, M. S., Wade, E., Rucker, E., Baxter-Gabbard, K. L., Levine, A. S., and Friis, R. R., 1973, A study of the relationship of reticuloendotheliosis virus to the avian leukosis-sarcoma complex of viruses, *Virology* **53**:287.

Halpern, M. S., Hunter, E., Alevy, M. C., Friis, R. R., and Vogt, P. K., 1974, Immunological studies with avian RNA tumor viruses, in: *Advances in the Biosciences 12* (G. Raspé, ed.), pp. 567–576, Pergamon Press, New York.

Halpern, M. S., Bolognesi, D. P., Friis, R. R., and Mason, W. S., 1975, Expression of the major viral glycoprotein of avian tumor virus in cells of *chf(+)* chicken embryos, *J. Virol.* **15**:1131.

Halpern, M. S., Bolognesi, D. P., and Friis, R. R., 1976, Viral glycoprotein synthesis studied in an established line of Japanese quail embryo cells infected with the Bryan high-titer strain of Rous sarcoma virus, *J. Virol.* **18**:504.

Hanafusa, H., 1965, Analysis of the defectiveness of Rous sarcoma virus. III. Determining influence of a new helper virus on the host range and susceptibility to interference of RSV, *Virology* **25**:248.

Hanafusa, H., and Hanafusa, T., 1966, Determining factor in the capacity of Rous sarcoma virus to induce tumors in mammals, *Proc. Natl. Acad. Sci. USA* **55**:532.

Hanafusa, H., and Hanafusa, T., 1968, Further studies on RSV production from transformed cells, *Virology* **34**:630.

Hanafusa, H., and Hanafusa, T., 1971, Noninfectious RSV deficient in DNA polymerase, *Virology* **43**:313.

Hanafusa, H., Hanafusa, T., and Rubin, H., 1963, The defectiveness of Rous sarcoma virus, *Proc. Natl. Acad. Sci. USA* **49**:572.

Hanafusa, H., Hanafusa, T., and Rubin, H., 1964*a*, Analysis of the defectiveness of Rous sarcoma virus. II. Specification of RSV antigenicity by helper virus, *Proc. Natl. Acad. Sci. USA* **51**:41.

Hanafusa, H., Hanafusa, T., and Rubin, H., 1964*b*, Analysis of the defectiveness of Rous sarcoma virus. I. Characterization of the helper virus, *Virology* **22**:591.

Hanafusa, H., Miyamoto, T., and Hanafusa, T., 1970, A cell-associated factor essential for formation of an infectious form of Rous sarcoma virus, *Proc. Natl. Acad. Sci. USA* **66**:314.

Hanafusa, H., Baltimore, D., Smoler, D., Watson, K. F., Yaniv, A., and Spiegelman,

S., 1972, Absence of polymerase protein on virions of alpha-type Rous sarcoma virus, *Science* **177**:1188.

Hanafusa, H., Aoki, T., Kawai, S., Miyamoto, T., and Wilsnack, R. E., 1973, Presence of antigen common to avian tumor viral envelope antigen in normal chick embryo cells, *Virology* **56**:22.

Hanafusa, T., and Hanafusa, H., 1973, Isolation of leukosis-type virus from pheasant embryo cells: Possible presence of viral genes in cells, *Virology* **51**:247.

Hanafusa, T., Miyamoto, T., and Hanafusa, H., 1970a, A type of chick embryo cell that fails to support formation of infectious RSV, *Virology* **40**:55.

Hanafusa, T., Hanafusa, H., and Miyamoto, T., 1970b, Recovery of a new virus from apparently normal chick cells by infection with avian tumor viruses, *Proc. Natl. Acad. Sci. USA* **67**:1797.

Hanafusa, T., Hanafusa, H., Metroka, C. E., Hayward, W. S., Rettenmier, C. W., Sawyer, R. C., Dougherty, R. M., and Di Stefano, H. S., 1976, Pheasant virus: A new class of ribodeoxyvirus, *Proc. Natl. Acad. Sci. USA* **73**:1333.

Hartley, J. W., and Rowe, W. P., 1966, Production of altered cell foci in tissue culture by defective Moloney sarcoma virus particles, *Proc. Natl. Acad. Sci. USA* **55**:780.

Hartley, J. W., and Rowe, W. P., 1976, Naturally occurring murine leukemia viruses in wild mice: Characterization of a new "amphotropic" class, *J. Virol* **19**:19.

Hartley, J. W., Rowe, W. P., and Huebner, R. J., 1970, Host-range restrictions of murine leukemia viruses in mouse embryo cell cultures, *J. Virol.* **5**:221.

Harvey, J. J., 1964, An unidentified virus which causes the rapid production of tumours in mice, *Nature (London)* **204**:1104.

Harvey, J. J., and East, J., 1971, The murine sarcoma virus (MSV), *Int. Rev. Exp. Pathol.* **10**:265.

Hatanaka, M., and Hanafusa, H., 1970, Analysis of a functional change in membrane in the process of cell transformation by Rous sarcoma virus; alteration in the characteristics of sugar transport, *Virology* **41**:647.

Hatanaka, M., Kakefuda, T., Gilden, R. V., and Callan, E. A. O., 1971, Cytoplasmic DNA synthesis induced by RNA tumor viruses, *Proc. Natl. Acad. Sci. USA* **68**:1844.

Hayman, M. J., and Vogt, P. K., 1976, Subgroup specific antigenic determinants of avian RNA tumor virus structural proteins: Analysis of virus recombinants, *Virology* **73**:372.

Hayward, W. S., and Hanafusa, H., 1975, Recombination between endogenous and exogenous RNA tumor virus genes as analyzed by nucleic acid hybridization, *J. Virol.* **15**:1367.

Heine, U. I., Weber, G. H., Cottler-Fox, M., Layard, M. W., Stephenson, M. L., and Zamecnik, P. C., 1975, Analysis of oncornavirus RNA subunits by electron microscopy, *Proc. Natl. Acad. Sci. USA* **72**:3716.

Henderson, I. C., Lieber, M. M., and Todaro, G. J., 1974, Mink cell line Mv1Lu (CCL 64). Focus formation and the generation of "nonproducer" transformed cell lines with murine and feline sarcoma viruses, *Virology* **60**:282.

Hill, M., and Hillova, J., 1972, Virus recovery in chicken cells treated with Rous sarcoma cell DNA, *Nature (London) New Biol.* **237**:35.

Hill, M., and Hillova, J., 1974, RNA and DNA forms of the genetic material of C-type viruses and the integrated state of the DNA form in the cellular chromosome, *Biochim. Biophys. Acta* **355**:7.

Hill, M., Hillova, J., Dantchev, D., Mariage, R., and Goubin, G., 1975, Infectious viral DNA in Rous sarcoma virus-transformed nonproducer and producer animal cells, *Cold Spring Harbor Symp. Quant. Biol.* **39**:1015.

Hillova, J., Dantchev, D., Mariage, R., Plichon, M.-P., and Hill, M., 1974, Sarcoma and transformation-defective viruses produced with infectious DNA(s) from Rous sarcoma virus (RSV)-transformed chicken cells, *Virology* **62**:197.

Hirst, G. K., 1962, Genetic recombination with Newcastle disease virus, polioviruses, and influenza, *Cold Spring Harbor Symp. Quant. Biol.* **27**:303.

Holtzer, H., Biehl, J., Yeoh, G., Meganathan, R., and Kaji, A., 1975, Effect of oncogenic virus on muscle differentiation, *Proc. Natl. Acad. Sci. USA* **72**:4051.

Huang, A. S., Besmer, P., Chu, L., and Baltimore, D., 1973, Growth of pseudotypes of vesicular stomatitis virus with N-tropic murine leukemia virus coats in cells resistant to N-tropic viruses, *J. Virol.* **12**:659.

Huebner, R. J., Hartley, J. W., Rowe, W. P., Lane, W. T., and Capps, W. I., 1966, Rescue of the defective genome of Moloney sarcoma virus from a noninfectious hamster tumor and the production of pseudotype sarcoma viruses with various murine leukemia viruses, *Proc. Natl. Acad. Sci. USA* **56**:1164.

Humphries, E. H., and Temin, H. M., 1972, Cell cycle-dependent activation of Rous sarcoma virus-infected stationary chicken cells: Avian leukosis virus group-specific antigens and ribonucleic acid, *J. Virol.* **10**:82.

Humphries, E. H., and Temin, H. M., 1974, Requirement for cell division for initiation of transcription of Rous sarcoma virus RNA, *J. Virol.* **14**:531.

Hunter, E., and Vogt, P. K., 1976, Temperature-sensitive mutants of avian sarcoma viruses: Genetic recombination with wild type sarcoma virus and physiological analysis of multiple mutants, *Virology* **69**:23.

Hunter, E., Hayman, M. J., Rongey, R. W., and Vogt, P. K., 1976*a*, An avian sarcoma virus mutant which is temperature-sensitive for virion assembly, *Virology* **69**:35.

Hunter, E., Hayman, M. J., and Tereba, A., 1977, On the mechanism of genetic recombination among avian RNA tumor viruses, in preparation.

Hynes, R. O., 1973, Alteration of cell-surface proteins by viral transformation and by proteolysis, *Proc. Natl. Acad. Sci. USA* **70**:3170.

Hynes, R. O., and Wyke, J. A., 1975, Alterations in surface proteins in chicken cells transformed by temperature-sensitive mutants of Rous sarcoma virus, *Virology* **64**:492.

Ikeda, H., Hardy, W., Tress, E., and Fleissher, E., 1975, Chromatographic separation and antigenic analysis of proteins of oncornaviruses. V. Identification of a new murine viral protein p15(E), *J. Virol.* **16**:53.

Isaka, T., Yoshida, M., Owada, M., and Toyoshima, K., 1975, Alterations in membrane polypeptides of chick embryo fibroblasts induced by transformation with avian sarcoma viruses, *Virology* **65**:226.

Ishizaki, R., and Shimizu, T., 1970, Heterogeneity of strain R avian erythroblastosis virus, *Cancer Res.* **30**:2827.

Ishizaki, R., Langlois, A. J., Chabot, J., and Beard, J. W., 1971, Component of strain MC29 avian leukosis virus with the property of defectiveness, *J. Virol.* **8**:821.

Jacobson, A. B., and Bromley, P. A., 1975*a*, Molecular weight of RNA subunits of Rous sarcoma virus determined by electron microscopy, *J. Virol.* **15**:161.

Jacobson, A. B., and Bromley, P. A., 1975*b*, Determination of the molecular weight of the RNA subunits of Rous sarcoma virus by electron microscopy, *Cold Spring Harbor Symp. Quant. Biol.* **39**:845.

Jacobson, M. F., and Baltimore, D., 1968, Polypeptide cleavages in the formation of poliovirus proteins, *Proc. Natl. Acad. Sci. USA* **61**:77.

Jacobson, M. F., Asso, J., and Baltimore, D., 1970, Further evidence on the formation of poliovirus proteins, *J. Mol. Biol.* **49**:657.

Joho, R. H., Billeter, M. A., and Weissmann, C., 1975, Mapping of biological functions of RNA of avian tumor viruses: Location of regions required for transformation and determination of host range, *Proc. Natl. Acad. Sci. USA* **72**:4772.

Jolicoeur, P., and Baltimore, D., 1975, Effect of the *Fv-1* locus on the titration of murine leukemia viruses, *J. Virol.* **16**:1593.

Jolicoeur, P., and Baltimore, D., 1976, Effect of *Fv-1* gene product on synthesis of N-tropic and B-tropic murine leukemia viral RNA, *Cell* **7**:33.

Kacian, D. L., Watson, K. F., Burny, A., and Spiegelman, S., 1971, Purification of the DNA polymerase of avian myeloblastosis virus, *Biochim. Biophys. Acta* **246**:365.

Kakefuda, T., and Bader, J. P., 1969, Electron microscopic observations on the ribonucleic acid of murine leukemia virus, *J. Virol.* **4**:460.

Kang, C.-Y., and Temin, H. M., 1973, Lack of sequence homology among RNAs of avian leukosis-sarcoma viruses, reticuloendotheliosis viruses, and chicken endogenous RNA-directed DNA polymerase activity, *J. Virol.* **12**:1314.

Kang, C.-Y., and Temin, H. M., 1974, Reticuloendotheliosis virus nucleic acid sequences in cellular DNA, *J. Virol.* **14**:1179.

Karpas, A., and Milstein, C., 1973, Recovery of the genome of murine sarcoma virus (MSV) after infection of cells with nuclear DNA from MSV transformed non-virus producing cells, *Eur. J. Cancer* **9**:295.

Katz, E. and Vogt, P. K., 1971, Conditional lethal mutants of avian sarcoma viruses. II. Analysis of the lesion in *ts* 75, *Virology* **46**:745.

Kawai, S., and Hanafusa, H., 1971, The effects of reciprocal changes in temperature on the transformed state of cells infected with a Rous sarcoma virus mutant, *Virology* **46**:470.

Kawai, S., and Hanafusa, H., 1972a, Plaque assay for some strains of avian leukosis virus, *Virology* **48**:126.

Kawai, S., and Hanafusa, H., 1972b, Genetic recombination with avian tumor virus, *Virology* **49**:37.

Kawai, S., and Hanafusa, H., 1973, Isolation of defective mutant of avian sarcoma virus, *Proc. Natl. Acad. Sci. USA* **70**:3493.

Kawai, S., and Hanafusa, H., 1976, Recombination between temperature sensitive mutant and a deletion mutant of Rous sarcoma virus. *J. Virol* **19**:389.

Kawai, S., and Yamamoto, T., 1970, Isolation of different kinds of non-virus producing chick cells transformed by Schmidt-Ruppin strain (subgroup A) of Rous sarcoma virus, *Jap. J. Exp. Med.* **40**:243.

Kawai, S., Metroka, C. E., and Hanafusa, H., 1972, Complementation of functions required for cell transformation by double infection with RSV mutants, *Virology* **49**:302.

Keith, J., and Fraenkel-Conrat, H., 1975, Identification of the 5′ end of Rous sarcoma virus RNA, *Proc. Natl. Acad. Sci. USA* **72**:3347.

King, A. M. Q., 1976, High molecular weight RNAs from Rous sarcoma virus and Moloney murine leukemia virus contain two subunits, *J. Biol. Chem.* **251**:141.

King, A. M. Q., and Wells, R. D., 1976, All intact subunit RNAs from Rous sarcoma virus contain poly(A), *J. Biol. Chem.* **251**:150.

Kirsten, W. H., and Mayer, L. A., 1967, Morphologic responses to a murine erythro-blastosis virus, *J. Natl. Cancer Inst.* **39**:311.

Kleinschmidt, A. K., 1968, Monolayer techniques in electron microscopy of nucleic acid molecules, in: *Methods in Enzymology: Nucleic Acids,* Vol. 12 (L. Grossman and K. Moldave, eds.), Part B, pp. 361–377, Academic Press, New York.

Klement, V., Hartley, J. W., Rowe, W. P., and Huebner, R. J., 1969, Recovery of a hamster-specific, focus-forming, and sarcomagenic virus from a "noninfectious" hamster tumor induced by the Kirsten mouse sarcoma virus, *J. Natl. Cancer Inst.* **43**:925.

Klement, V., Nicolson, M. O., and Huebner, R. J., 1971, Rescue of the genome of focus forming virus from rat non-productive lines by 5′-bromodeoxyuridine, *Nature (London)* New Biol. **234**:12.

Kletzien, R. F., and Perdue, J. F., 1974, Sugar transport in chick embryo fibroblasts. II. Alterations in transport following transformation by a temperature-sensitive mutant of the Rous sarcoma virus, *J. Biol. Chem.* **249**:3375.

Kletzien, R. F., and Perdue, J. F., 1975, Regulation of sugar transport in chick embryo fibroblasts infected with a temperature-sensitive mutant of RSV, *Cell* **6**:513.

Krontiris, T. G., Soeiro, R., and Fields, B. N., 1973, Host restriction of Friend leukemia virus: Role of the viral outer coat, *Proc. Natl. Acad. Sci. USA* **70**:2549.

Kung, H.-J., Bailey, J. M., Davidson, N., Nicolson, M. O., and McAllister, R. M., 1974, Structure and molecular length of the large subunits of RD-114 viral RNA, *J. Virol.* **14**:170.

Kung, H.-J., Bailey, J. M., Davidson, N., Nicolson, M. O., and McAllister, R. M., 1975a, Structure, subunit composition, and molecular weight of RD-114 RNA, *J. Virol.* **16**:397.

Kung, H. J., Bailey, J. M., Davidson, N., Vogt, P. K., Nicolson, M. O., and McAllister, R. M., 1975b, Electron microscope studies of tumor virus RNA, *Cold Spring Harbor Symp. Quant. Biol.* **39**:827.

Kung, H.-J., Hu, S., Bender, W., Bailey, J. M., and Davidson, N., 1976, RD-114, Baboon and wooly monkey viral RNA's compared in size and structure, *Cell* **7**:609.

Kurth, R., and Bauer, H., 1972a, Cell-surface antigens induced by avian RNA tumor viruses: Detection by a cytotoxic microassay, *Virology* **47**:426.

Kurth, R., and Bauer, H., 1972b, Common tumor-specific surface antigens on cells of different species transformed by avian RNA tumor viruses, *Virology* **49**:145.

Kurth, R., and Bauer, H., 1975, Avian RNA tumor viruses. A model for studying tumor associated cell surface alterations, *Biochim. Biophys. Acta* **417**:1.

Kurth, R., Friis, R. R., Wyke, J. A., and Bauer, H., 1975, Expression of tumor-specific surface antigens on cells infected with temperature-sensitive mutants of avian sarcoma virus, *Virology* **64**:400.

Lai, C.-J., and Nathans, D., 1975, Mapping of the genes of simian virus 40, *Cold Spring Harbor Symp. Quant. Biol.* **39**:53.

Lai, M. M. C., and Duesberg, P. H., 1972, Adenylic acid-rich sequence in RNAs of Rous sarcoma virus and Rauscher mouse leukaemia virus, *Nature (London)* **235**:383.

Lai, M. M. C., Duesberg, P. H., Horst, J., and Vogt, P. K., 1973, Avian tumor virus RNA: A comparison of three sarcoma viruses and their transformation-defective derivatives by oligonucleotide fingerprinting and DNA-RNA hybridization, *Proc. Natl. Acad. Sci. USA* **70**:2266.

Langlois, A. J., and Beard, J. W., 1967, Converted-cell focus formation in culture by strain MC29 avian leukosis virus, *Proc. Soc. Exp. Biol. Med.* **126**:718.

Langlois, A. J., Veprek, L., Beard, D., Fritz, R. B., and Beard, J. W., 1971, Isolation of a nonfocus forming agent from strain MC29 avian leukosis virus, *Cancer Res.* **31**:1010.

Latarjet, R., and Chamaillard, L., 1962, Inactivation du virus de Friend par les rayons X et les ultraviolets, *Bull. Cancer* **49**:382.

Leis, J., Schincariol, A., Ishizaki, R., and Hurwitz, J., 1975, RNA-dependent DNA polymerase activity of RNA tumor viruses. V. Rous sarcoma virus single-stranded RNA-DNA covalent hybrids in infected chicken embryo fibroblast cells, *J. Virol.* **15**:484.

Leong, J.-A., Garapin, A.-C., Jackson, N., Fanshier, L., Levinson, W., and Bishop, J. M., 1972, Virus-specific ribonucleic acid in cells producing Rous sarcoma virus: Detection and characterization, *J. Virol.* **9**:891.

Levin, J. G., and Rosenak, M. J., 1976, Synthesis of murine leukemia virus proteins associated with virions assembled in actinomycin D-treated cells: Evidence for the persistence of viral messenger RNA, *Proc. Natl. Acad. Sci. USA* **73**:1154.

Levinson, W., and Rubin, H., 1966, Radiation studies of avian tumor viruses and of Newcastle disease virus, *Virology* **28**:533.

Levy, J. A., 1971, Demonstration of differences in murine sarcoma virus foci formed in mouse and rat cells under a soft agar overlay, *J. Natl. Cancer Inst.* **46**:1001.

Levy, J. A., 1973, Xenotropic viruses: Murine leukemia viruses associated with NIH Swiss, NZB, and other mouse strains, *Science* **182**:1151.

Levy, J. A., 1975, Host range of murine xenotropic virus: Replication in avian cells, *Nature (London)* **253**:140.

Levy, J. A., 1977, Murine xenotropic type C viruses. III. Phenotypic mixing with avian sarcoma viruses, *Virology* (in press).

Levy, J. A., Hartley, J. W., Rowe, W. P., and Huebner, R. J., 1973, Studies of FBJ osteosarcoma virus in tissue culture. I. Biologic characteristics of the "C"-type viruses, *J. Natl. Cancer Inst.* **51**:525.

Levy, J. A., Kazan, P. A., and Varmus, H. E., 1974, The importance of DNA size for successful transfection of chicken embryo fibroblasts, *Virology* **61**:297.

Lieber, M. M., Sherr, C. J., Benveniste, R. E., and Todaro, G. J., 1975a, Biologic and immunologic properties of porcine type C viruses, *Virology* **66**:616.

Lieber, M. M., Sherr, C. J., Todaro, G. J., Benveniste, R. E., Callahan, R., and Coon, H. G., 1975b, Isolation from the Asian mouse *Mus caroli* of an endogenous type C virus related to infectious primate type C viruses, *Proc. Natl. Acad. Sci. USA* **72**:2315.

Lieber, M. M., Benveniste, R. E., Sherr, C. J., and Todaro, G. J., 1975c, Isolation of a type C virus (FS-1) from the European wildcat (*Felis sylvestris*), *Virology* **66**:117.

Lilly, F., 1967, Susceptibility to two strains of Friend leukemia virus in mice, *Science* **155**:461.

Lilly, F., and Pincus, T., 1973, Genetic control of murine viral leukemogenesis, in: *Advances in Cancer Research,* Vol. 17 (G. Klein and S. Weinhouse, eds.), p. 231, Academic Press, New York.

Linial, M., and Mason, W. S., 1973, Characterization of two conditional early mutants of Rous sarcoma virus, *Virology* **53**:258.

Livingston, D. M., and Todaro, G. J., 1973, Endogenous type C virus from a cat cell clone with properties distinct from previously described feline type C virus, *Virology* **53**:142.

Lo, A. C. H., and Ball, J. K., 1974, Evidence for helper-independent murine sarcoma virus. II. Differences between the ribonucleic acids of clone-purified leukemia virus, helper-independent and helper-dependent sarcoma viruses, *Virology* **59**:545.

Love, D. N., and Weiss, R. A., 1974, Pseudotypes of vesicular stomatitis virus determined by exogenous and endogenous avian RNA tumor viruses, *Virology* **57**:271.

Lovinger, G. G., Ling, H. P., Klein, R. A., Gilden, R. V., and Hatanaka, M., 1974, Unintegrated murine leukemia viral DNA in newly infected cells, *Virology* **62**:280.

Lovinger, G. C., Ling, H. P., Gilden, R. V., and Hatanaka, M., 1975a, Effect of UV light on RNA-directed DNA polymerase activity of murine oncornaviruses, *J. Virol.* **15**:1273.

Lovinger, G. G., Klein, R., Ling, H. P., Gilden, R. V., and Hatanaka, M., 1975b, Kinetics of murine type C virus-specifiec DNA synthesis in newly infected cells, *J. Virol.* **16**:824.

Maisel, J., Klement, V., Lai, M. M.-C., Ostertag, W., and Duesberg, P., 1973, Ribonucleic acid components of murine sarcoma and leukemia viruses, *Proc. Natl. Acad. Sci. USA* **70**:3536.

Maisel, J., Scolnick, E. M., and Duesberg, P., 1975, Base sequence differences between the RNA components of Harvey sarcoma virus, *J. Virol.* **16**:749.

Maldonado, R. L., and Bose, H. R., 1971, Separation of reticuloendotheliosis virus from avian tumor viruses, *J. Virol.* **8**:813.

Maldonado, R. L., and Bose, H. R., 1973, Relationship of reticuloendotheliosis virus to the avian tumor viruses: Nucleic acid and polypeptide composition, *J. Virol.* **11**:741.

Mangel, W. F., Delius, H., and Duesberg, P. H., 1974, Structure and molecular weight of the 60-70 S RNA and the 30-40 S RNA of the Rous sarcoma virus, *Proc. Natl. Acad. Sci. USA* **71**:4541.

Martin, G. S., 1970, Rous sarcoma virus: A function required for the maintenance of the transformed state, *Nature (London)* **227**:1021.

Martin, G. S., 1971, Mutants of the Schmidt-Ruppin strain of Rous sarcoma virus, in: *The Biology of Oncogenic Viruses* (L. G. Silvestri, ed.), pp. 320–325, North-Holland, Amsterdam.

Martin, G. S., and Duesberg, P. H., 1972, The *a* subunit in the RNA of transforming avian tumor viruses. I. Occurrence in different virus strains. II. Spontaneous loss resulting in nontransforming variants, *Virology* **47**:494.

Martin, G. S., Venuta, S., Weber, M., and Rubin, H., 1971, Temperature-dependent alterations in sugar transport in cells infected by a temperature-sensitive mutant of Rous sarcoma virus, *Proc. Natl. Acad. Sci. USA* **68**:2739.

Mason, W. S., Friis, R. R., Linial, M., and Vogt, P. K., 1974, Determination of the defective function in two mutants of Rous sarcoma virus, *Virology* **61**:559.

McAllister, R. M., Nicolson, M., Gardner, M. B., Rongey, R. W., Rasheed, S., Sarma, P. S., Huebner, R. J., Hatanaka, M., Oroszlan, S., Gilden, R. J., Kabigting, A., and Vernon, L., 1972, C-type virus released from cultured human rhabdomyosarcoma cells, *Nature (London) New Biol.* **235**:3.

Meyers, P., Sigel, M. M., and Holden, H. T., 1972, Cross protection *in vivo* against avian sarcoma virus subgroups A, B, and C induced by Rous-associated viruses, *J. Natl. Cancer Inst.* **49**:173.

Miyamoto, K., and Gilden, R. V., 1971, Electron microscopic studies of tumor viruses. I. Entry of murine leukemia virus into mouse embryo fibroblasts, *J. Virol.* **7**:395.

Mizutani S., and Temin, H. M., 1973, Lack of serological relationship among DNA polymerases of avian leukosis-sarcoma viruses, reticuloendotheliosis viruses, and chicken cells, *J. Virol.* **12**:440.

Moelling, K., Gelderblom, H., Pauli, G., Friis, R., and Bauer, H., 1975, A comparative study of the avian reticuloendotheliosis virus: Relationship to murine leukemia virus and viruses of the avian sarcoma-leukosis complex, *Virology* **65**:546.

Montagnier, L., and Vigier, P., 1972, Un intermédiare ADN infectieux et transformant du virus du sarcome de Rous dans les cellules de Poule transformées par ce virus, *C. R. Acad. Sci. Paris* **274**(D):1977.

Montagnier, L., Goldé, A., and Vigier, P., 1969, A possible subunit structure of Rous sarcoma virus RNA, *J. Gen. Virol.* **4**:449.

Morgan, C., and Rose, H. M., 1968, Structure and development of viruses as observed in the electron microscope. VIII. Entry of influenza virus, *J. Virol.* **2**:925.

Moscovici, C., 1967, A quantitative assay for avian myeloblastosis virus, *Proc. Soc. Exp. Biol. Med.* **125**:1213.

Moscovici, C., 1975, Leukemic transformation with avian myeloblastosis virus: Present status, *Curr. Top. Microbiol. Immunol.* **71**:79.

Moscovici, C., and Vogt, P. K., 1968, Effects of genetic cellular resistance on cell transformation and virus replication in chicken hematopoietic cell cultures infected with avian myeloblastosis virus, *Virology* **35**:487.

Moscovici, C., and Zanetti, M., 1970, Studies on single foci of hematopoietic cells transformed by avian myeloblastosis virus (BAI-A), *Virology* **35**:487.

Moscovici, C., Gazzolo, L., and Moscovici, M. G., 1975, Focus assay and defectiveness of avian myeloblastosis virus, *Virology* **68**:173.

Naso, R. B., Wang, C. S., Tsai, S., and Arlinghaus, R. B., 1973, Ribosomes from Rauscher leukemia virus-infected cells and their response to Rauscher viral RNA and polyuridylic acid, *Biochim. Biophys. Acta* **324**:346.

Naso, R. B., Arcement, L. J., and Arlinghaus, R. B., 1975, Biosynthesis of Rauscher leukemia viral proteins, *Cell* **4**:31.

Nass, M. M. K., 1973, Temperature-dependent formation of dimers and oligomers of mitochondrial DNA in cells transformed by a thermosensitive mutant of Rous sarcoma virus, *Proc. Natl. Acad. Sci. USA* **70**:3739.

Neiman, P. E., 1973, Measurement of endogenous leukosis virus nucleotide sequences in the DNA of normal avian embryos by RNA-DNA hybridization, *Virology* **53**:196.

Neiman, P. E., Wright, S. E., McMillin, C., and MacDonnell, D., 1974, Nucleotide sequence relationships of avian RNA tumor viruses: Measurement of the deletion in a transformation-defective mutant of Rous sarcoma virus, *J. Virol.* **13**:837.

Nowinski, R. C., Watson, K. F., Yaniv, A., and Spiegelman, S., 1972, Serological analysis of the deoxyribonucleic acid polymerase of avian oncornaviruses. II. Comparison of avian deoxyribonucleic acid polymerases, *J. Virol.* **10**:959.

Ogura, H., and Friis, R., 1975, Further evidence for the existence of a viral envelope protein defect in Bryan high-titer strain of Rous sarcoma virus, *J. Virol.* **16**:443.

Oroszlan, S., Bova, D., Martin White, M. H., Toni, R., Foreman, C., and Gilden, R. V., 1972, Purification and immunological characterization of the major internal protein of the RD-114 virus, *Proc. Natl. Acad. Sci. USA* **69**:1211.

Ostertag, W., Cole, T., Crozier, T., Gaedicke, G., Kind, J., Kluge, N., Krieg, J. C., Roesler, G., Weimann, B. J., and Dube, S. K., 1975, Viral involvement in the differentiation of erythroleukemic mouse and human cells, in: *Differentiation and Control of Malignancy* (Waro Nakahara ed.), Univ. of Tokyo Press, Tokyo.

Otten, J., Bader, J., Johnson, G. S., and Pastan, I., 1972, A mutation in a Rous sarcoma virus gene that controls adenosine 3′,5′-monophosphate levels and transformation, *J. Biol. Chem.* **247**:1632.

Owada, M., and Toyoshima, K., 1973, Analysis on the reproducing and cell-transforming capacities of temperature sensitive mutant (*ts*334) of avian sarcoma virus B77, *Virology* **54**:170.

Owada, M., Ihara, S., Toyoshima, K., Kozai, Y., and Sugino, Y., 1976, Ultraviolet-inactivation of avian sarcoma viruses: Biological and biochemical analysis, *Virology* **69**:710.

Pal, B. K., and Roy-Burman, P., 1975, Phosphoproteins: Structural components of oncornaviruses, *J. Virol.* **15**:540.

Pal, B. K., McAllister, R. M., Gardner, M. B., and Roy-Burman, P., 1975, Compara-tive studies on the structural phosphoproteins of mammalian type C viruses, *J. Virol.* **16**:123.

Panet, A., Baltimore, D., and Hanafusa, T., 1975*a*, Quantitation of avian RNA tumor virus reverse transcriptase by radioimmunoassay, *J. Virol.* **16**:146.

Panet, A., Haseltine, W., Baltimore, D., Peters, G., Harada, F., and Dahlberg, J. E., 1975*b*, Specific binding of tryptophan transfer RNA to avian myeloblastosis virus RNA-dependent DNA polymerase (reverse transcriptase), *Proc. Natl. Acad. Sci. USA* **72**:2535.

Pani, P. K., 1975, Genetic control of resistance of chick embryo cultures to RSV(RAV 50), *J. Gen. Virol.* **27**:163.

Parkman, R., Levy, J. A., and Ting, R. C. 1970, Murine sarcoma virus: The question of defectiveness, *Science* **168**:387.

Payne, L. N., 1972, Interactions between host genome and avian RNA tumor viruses, in: *RNA Viruses and Host Genome in Oncogenesis* (P. Emmelot and P. Bentvelzen, eds.), pp. 93–115, North-Holland, Amsterdam.

Payne, L. N., and Biggs, P. M., 1964, Differences between highly inbred lines of chickens in the response to Rous sarcoma virus of the chorioallantoic membrane and of embryonic cells in tissue culture, *Virology* **24**:610.

Payne, L. N., and Biggs, P. M., 1970, Genetic resistance of fowl to MH2 reticuloendo-thelioma virus, *J. Gen. Virol.* **7**:177.

Payne, L. N., and Pani, P. K., 1971, Evidence for linkage between genetic loci control-ling response of fowl to subgroup A and subgroup C sarcoma viruses, *J. Gen. Virol.* **13**:253.

Payne, L. N., Pani, P. K., and Weiss, R. A., 1971, A dominant epistatic gene which inhibits cellular susceptibility to RSV(RAV-O), *J. Gen. Virol.* **13**:455.

Payne, L. N., Crittenden, L. B., and Weiss, R. A., 1973, A brief definition of host genes which influence infection by avian RNA tumor viruses, in: *Possible Episomes in Eukaryotes, Proceedings of the Fourth Lepetit Colloquium, 1972* (L. Silvestri, ed.), pp. 94–97, North-Holland, Amsterdam.

Peebles, P. T., Bassin, R. H., Haapala, D. K., Phillips, L. A., Nomura, S., and Fisch-inger, P. J., 1971, Rescue of murine sarcoma virus from a sarcoma-positive leukemia-negative cell line: Requirement for replicating leukemia virus, *J. Virol.* **8**:690.

Peebles, P. T., Haapala, D. K., and Gazdar, A. F., 1972, Deficiency of viral ribonucleic acid-dependent deoxyribonucleic acid polymerase in noninfectious virus-like particles released from murine sarcoma virus-transformed hamster cells, *J. Virol.* **9**:488.

Peebles, P. T., Fischinger, P. J., Bassin, R. H., and Papageorge, A. G., 1973, Isolation of human amnion cells transformed by rescuable murine sarcoma virus, *Nature (London) New Biol.* **242**:98.

Phillips, L. A., Hollis, V. W., Jr., Bassin, R. H., and Fischinger, P. J., 1973,

Characterization of RNA from noninfectious virions produced by sarcoma positive leukemia-negative transformed 3T3 cells, *Proc. Natl. Acad. Sci. USA* **70**:3002.

Pincus, T., Hartley, J. W., and Rowe, W. P., 1971*a*, A major genetic locus affecting resistance to infection with murine leukemia viruses. I. Tissue culture studies of naturally occurring viruses, *J. Exp. Med.* **133**:1219.

Pincus, T., Rowe, W. P., and Lilly, F., 1971*b*, A Major genetic locus affecting resistance to infection with murine leukemia viruses. II. Apparent identity to a major locus described for resistance to Friend murine leukemia virus, *J. Exp. Med.* **133**:1234.

Pincus, T., Hartley, J. W., and Rowe, W. P., 1975, A major genetic locus affecting resistance to infection with murine leukemia viruses. IV. Dose–response relationships in *Fv-1* sensitive and resistant cell cultures, *Virology* **65**:333.

Piraino, F., 1967, The mechanism of genetic resistance of chick embryo cells to infection by Rous sarcoma virus-Bryan strain (BS-RSV), *Virology* **32**:700.

Purchase, H. G., and Okazaki, W., 1964, Morphology of foci produced by standard preparation of Rous sarcoma virus, *J. Natl. Cancer Inst.* **32**:579.

Quade, K., Smith, R. E., and Nichols, J. L., 1974*a*, Evidence for common nucleotide sequences in the RNA subunits comprising Rous sarcoma virus 70 S RNA, *Virology* **61**:287.

Quade, K., Smith, R. E., and Nichols, J. L., 1974*b*, Poly(riboadenylic acid) and adjacent nucleotides in Rous sarcoma virus RNA, *Virology* **62**:60.

Quigley, J. P., Rifkin, D. B., and Reich, E., 1972, Lipid studies of Rous sarcoma virus and host cell membranes, *Virology* **50**:550.

Quintrell, N., Varmus, H. E., Bishop, J. M., Nicholson, M. O., and McAllister, R. M., 1974, Homologies among the nucleotide sequences of the genomes of C-type viruses, *Virology* **58**:568.

Rao, P. R., Bonar, R. A., and Beard, J. W., 1966, Lipids of the BAI strain A avian tumor virus and of the myeloblast host cell, *Exp. Mol. Pathol.* **5**:374.

Rasheed, S., Gardner, M. B., and Chan, E., 1976, Amphotropic host range of naturally occurring wild mouse leukemia viruses, *J. Virol.* **19**:13.

Rho, H. M., and Green, M., 1974, The homopolyadenylate and adjacent nucleotides at the 3′-terminus of 30-40 S RNA subunits in the genome of murine sarcoma-leukemia virus, *Proc. Natl. Acad. Sci. USA* **71**:2386.

Richert, N. J., and Hare, J. D., 1972, Distinctive effects of inhibitors of mitochondrial function on Rous sarcoma virus replication and malignant transformation, *Biochem. Biophys. Res. Commun.* **46**:5.

Riggin, C. H., Bondurant, M., and Mitchell, W. M., 1975, Physical properties of Moloney murine leukemia virus high-molecular-weight RNA: A two subunit structure, *J. Virol.* **16**:1528.

Roa, R. C., and Bose, S. K., 1974, Inhibition by ethidium bromide of the establishment of infection by murine sarcoma virus. *J. Gen. Virol.* **25**:197.

Robbins, P. W., Wickus, G. G., Branton, P. E., Gaffney, B. J., Hirschberg, C. B., Fuchs, P., and Blumberg, P. M., 1975, The chick fibroblast cell surface after transformation by Rous sarcoma virus, *Cold Spring Harbor Symp. Quant. Biol.* **39**:1173.

Robinson, H. L., 1967, Isolation of noninfectious particles containing Rous sarcoma virus RNA from the medium of Rous sarcoma virus-transformed nonproducer cells, *Proc. Natl. Acad. Sci. USA* **57**:1655.

Robinson, W. S., and Robinson, H. L., 1971, DNA polymerase in defective Rous sarcoma virus, *Virology* **44**:457.

Robinson, W. S., Pitkanen, A., and Rubin, H., 1965, The nucleic acid of the Bryan strain of Rous sarcoma virus: Purification of the virus and isolation of the nucleic acid, *Proc. Natl. Acad. Sci. USA* **54**:137.

Robinson, W. S., Robinson, H. L., and Duesberg, P. H., 1967, Tumor virus RNA's, *Proc. Natl. Acad. Sci. USA* **58**:825.

Rohrschneider, L. R., Kurth, R., and Bauer, H., 1975, Biochemical characterization of tumor-specific cell surface antigens on avian oncornavirus transformed cells, *Virology* **66**:481.

Rosenberg, N., Baltimore, D., and Scher, C. D., 1975, *In vitro* transformation of lymphoid cells by Abelson murine leukemia virus, *Proc. Natl. Acad. Sci. USA* **72**:1932.

Rowe, W. P., 1971, The kinetics of rescue of the murine sarcoma virus genome from a nonproducer line of transformed mouse cells, *Virology* **46**:369.

Rowson, K. E. K., and Parr, I. B., 1970, A new virus of minimal pathogenicity associated with Friend virus. I. Isolation by end-point dilution, *Int. J. Cancer* **5**:96.

Roy-Burman, P., and Klement, V., 1975, Derivation of mouse sarcoma virus (Kirsten) by acquisition of genes from heterologous host, *J. Gen. Virol.* **28**:193.

Rubin, H., 1960, Growth of rous sarcoma virus in chick embryo cells following irradiation of host cells or free virus, *Virology* **11**:28.

Rubin, H., 1965, Genetic control of cellular susceptibility of pseudotypes of Rous sarcoma virus, *Virology* **26**:270.

Rubin, H., and Temin, H. M., 1959, A radiological study of cell–virus interaction in the Rous sarcoma, *Virology* **7**:75.

Rymo, L., Parsons, J. T., Coffin, J. M., and Weissmann, C., 1974, *In vitro* synthesis of Rous sarcoma virus-specific RNA is catalyzed by a DNA-dependent RNA polymerase, *Proc. Natl. Acad. Sci. USA* **71**:2782.

Sarma, P. S., Log, T., and Huebner, R. J., 1970, Trans-species rescue of defective genomes of murine sarcoma virus from hamster tumor cells with helper feline leukemia virus, *Proc. Natl. Acad. Sci. USA* **65**:81.

Sarma, P. S., Baskar, J. F., Gilden, R. V., Gardner, M. B., and Huebner, R. J., 1971, *In vitro* isolation and characterization of the GA strain of feline sarcoma virus, *Proc. Soc. Exp. Biol. Med.* **137**:1333.

Sarma, P. S., Tseng, J., Lee, Y. K., and Gilden, R. V., 1973, Virus similar to RD114 virus in cat cells, *Nature (London) New Biol.* **244**:56.

Scheele, C. M., and Hanafusa, H., 1971, Proteins of helper-dependent RSV, *Virology* **45**:401.

Scher, C. D., and Siegler, R., 1975, Direct transformation of 3T3 cells by Abelson murine leukaemia virus, *Nature (London)* **253**:729.

Schincariol, A. L., and Joklik, W. K., 1973, Early synthesis of virus-specific RNA and DNA in cells rapidly transformed with Rous sarcoma virus, *Virology* **56**:532.

Scolnick, E. M., and Parks, W. P., 1973, Isolation and characterization of a primate sarcoma virus: Mechanism of rescue, *Int. J. Cancer* **12**:138.

Scolnick, E. M., and Parks, W. P., 1974, Harvey sarcoma virus: A second murine type C sarcoma virus with rat genetic information, *J. Virol.* **13**:1211.

Scolnick, E. M., Parks, W. P., Todaro, G. J., and Aaronson, S. A., 1972a, Immunological characterization of primate C-type virus reverse transcriptases, *Nature New Biol.* **235**:35.

Scolnick, E. M., Stephenson, J. R., and Aaronson, S. A., 1972b, Isolation of temperature-sensitive mutants of murine sarcoma virus, *J. Virol.* **10**:653.

Scolnick, E. M., Rands, E., Williams, D., and Parks, W. P., 1973, Studies on the nucleic acid sequences of Kirsten sarcoma virus: A model for formation of a mammalian RNA-containing sarcoma virus, *J. Virol.* **12**:458.

Scolnick, E. M., Parks, W., Kawakami, T., Kohne, D., Okabe, H., Gilden, R., and Hatanaka, M., 1974, Primate and murine type-C viral nucleic acid association kinetics: analysis of model systems and natural tissues, *J. Virol.* **13**:363.

Scolnick, E. M., Goldberg, R. J., and Parks, W. P., 1975a, A biochemical and genetic analysis of mammalian RNA-containing sarcoma viruses, *Cold Spring Harbor Symp. Quant. Biol.* **39**:885.

Scolnick, E. M., Howk, R. S., Anisowicz, A., Peebles, P. T., Scher, C. D., Parks, W. P., 1975b, Separation of sarcoma virus-specific and leukemia virus-specific genetic sequences of Moloney sarcoma virus, *Proc. Natl. Acad. Sci. USA* **72**:4650.

Shanmugam, G., Bhaduri, S., and Green, M., 1974, The virus-specific RNA species in free and membrane-bound polyribosomes of transformed cells replicating murine sarcoma-leukemia viruses, *Biochem. Biophys. Res. Commun.* **56**:697.

Shenk, T. E., Rhodes, C., Rigby, P. W. J., and Berg, P., 1975, Mapping of mutational alterations in DNA with S_1 nuclease: The location of deletions, insertions and temperature-sensitive mutations in SV40, *Cold Spring Harbor Symp. Quant. Biol.* **39**:61.

Sherr, C. J., and Todaro, G. J., 1974, Radioimmunoassay of the major group specific protein of endogenous baboon type C viruses: Relation to RD-114/CCC group and detection of antigen in normal baboon tissue, *Virology* **61**:168.

Sherr, C. J., Lieber, M. M., Benveniste, R. E., and Todaro, G. J., 1974, Endogenous baboon type C virus (M7): Biochemical and immunologic characterization, *Virology* **58**:492.

Sherr, C. J., Fedele, L. A., Benveniste, R. E., and Todaro, G. J., 1975, Interspecies antigenic determinants of the reverse transcriptases and p30 proteins of mammalian type C viruses, *J. Virol.* **15**:1440.

Shoyab, M., Markham, P. D., and Baluda, M. A., 1975, Host induced alteration of avian sarcoma virus B-77 genome, *Proc. Natl. Acad. Sci. USA* **72**:1031.

Siegert, W., Konings, R. N. H., Bauer, H., and Hofschneider, P. H., 1972, Translation of avian myeloblastosis virus RNA in a cell-free lysate of *Escherichia coli*, *Proc. Natl. Acad. Sci. USA* **69**:888.

Sklar, M. D., White, B. J., and Rowe, W. P., 1974, Initiation of oncogenic transformation of mouse lymphocytes *in vitro* by Abelson leukemia virus, *Proc. Natl. Acad. Sci. USA* **71**:4077.

Smith, J. D., Barnett, L., Brenner, S., and Russell, R. L., 1970, More mutant tyrosine transfer ribonucleic acids, *J. Mol. Biol.* **54**:1.

Smotkin, D., Gianni, A. M., Rozenblatt, S., and Weinberg, R. A., 1975, Infectious viral DNA of murine leukemia virus, *Proc. Natl. Acad. Sci. USA* **72**:4910.

Somers, K., and Kit, S., 1973, Temperature-dependent expression of transformation by a cold-sensitive mutant of murine sarcoma virus, *Proc. Natl. Acad. Sci. USA* **70**:2206.

Somers, K. D., May, J. T., and Kit, S., 1973, Control of gene expression in rat cells transformed by a cold-sensitive murine sarcoma virus (MSV) mutant, *Intervirology* **1**:176.

Steeves, R. A., Eckner, R. J., Bennett, M., Mirand, E. A., and Trudel, P. J., 1971,

Isolation and characterization of a lymphatic leukemia virus in the Friend virus complex, *J. Natl. Cancer Inst.* **46**:1209.

Stehelin, D., Guntaka, R. V., Varmus, H. E., and Bishop, J. M., 1976*a*, Purification of DNA complementary to nucleotide sequences required for neoplastic transformation of fibroblasts by avian sarcoma viruses, *J. Mol. Biol.* **101**:349.

Stehelin, D., Varmus, H. E., Bishop, J. M., and Vogt, P. K., 1976*b*, DNA related to the transforming genes of avian sarcoma viruses is present in normal avian NDA, *Nature (London)* **260**:170.

Steiner, S. M., Melnick, J. L., Kit, S., and Somers, K. D., 1974, Fucosyl-glycolipids in cells transformed by a temperature-sensitive mutant of murine sarcoma virus, *Nature (London)* **248**:682.

Stephenson, J. R., and Aaronson, S. A., 1971, Murine sarcoma and leukemia viruses: Genetic differences determined by RNA-DNA hybridization, *Virology* **46**:480.

Stephenson, J. R., and Aaronson, S. A., 1973, Characterization of temperature-sensitive mutants of murine leukemia virus, *Virology* **54**:53.

Stephenson, J. R., and Aaronson, S. A., 1974, Temperature-sensitive mutants of murine leukemia virus. III. Mutants defective in helper functions for sarcoma virus fixation, *Virology* **58**:294.

Stephenson, J. R., Reynolds, R. K., and Aaronson, S. A., 1972, Isolation of temperature-sensitive mutants of murine leukemia virus, *Virology* **48**:749.

Stephenson, J. R., Anderson, G. R., Tronick, S. R., and Aaronson, S. A., 1974*a*, Evidence for genetic recombination between endogenous and exogenous mouse RNA type C viruses, *Cell* **2**:87.

Stephenson, J. R., Tronick, S. R., and Aaronson, S. A., 1974*b*, Temperature-sensitive mutants of murine leukemia virus. IV. Further physiological characterization and evidence for genetic recombination, *J. Virol.* **14**:918.

Stephenson, J. R., Tronick, S. R., and Aaronson, S. A., 1975, Murine leukemia virus mutants with temperature-sensitive defects in precursor polypeptide cleavage, *Cell* **6**:543.

Stoltzfus, C. M., and Snyder, P. N., 1975, Structure of B77 sarcoma virus RNA: Stabilization of RNA after packaging, *J. Virol.* **16**:1161.

Stone, K. R., Smith, R. E., and Joklik, W. K., 1974, Changes in membrane polypeptides that occur when chick embryo fibroblasts and NRK cells are transformed with avian sarcoma viruses, *Virology* **58**:86.

Stone, M. P., Smith, R. E., and Joklik, W. K., 1975, 35S *a* and *b* RNA subunits of avian RNA tumor virus strains cloned and passaged in chick and duck cells, *Cold Spring Harbor Symp. Quant. Biol.* **39**:859.

Sveda, M. M., Fields, B. N., and Soeiro, R., 1974, Host restriction of Friend leukemia virus; fate of input virion RNA, *Cell* **2**:271.

Taber, R., Rekosh, D., and Baltimore, D., 1971, Effect of pactamycin on synthesis of poliovirus proteins: A method for genetic mapping, *J. Virol.* **8**:395.

Takano, T., and Hatanaka, M., 1975, Fate of viral RNA of murine leukemia virus after infection, *Proc. Natl. Acad. Sci. USA* **72**:343.

Taylor, J. M., and Illmensee, R., 1975, Site on the RNA of an avian sarcoma virus at which primer is bound, *J. Virol.* **16**:553.

Taylor, J. M., Varmus, H. E., Faras, A. J., Levinson, W. E., and Bishop, J. M., 1974, Evidence for non-repetitive subunits in the genome of Rous sarcoma virus, *J. Mol. Biol.* **84**:217.

Taylor, J. M., Cordell-Stewart, B., Rohde, W., Goodman, H. M., and Bishop, J. M.,

1975, Reassociation of 4 S and 5 S RNA's with the genome of avian sarcoma virus, *Virology* **65**:248.

Temin, H., 1960, The control of cellular morphology in embryonic cells infected with Rous sarcoma virus *in vitro, Virology* **10**:182.

Temin, H. M., 1961, Mixed infection with two types of Rous sarcoma virus, *Virology* **13**:158.

Temin, H. M., 1962, Separation of morphological conversion and virus production in Rous sarcoma virus infection, *Cold Spring Harbor Symp. Quant. Biol.* **27**:407.

Temin, H. M., 1963, Further evidence for a converted, non-virus-producing state of Rous sarcoma virus-infected cells, *Virology* **20**:235.

Temin, H. M., 1971, The role of the DNA provirus in carcinogenesis by RNA tumor viruses, in: *The Biology of Oncogenic Viruses* (L. Silvestri, ed.), pp. 176–187, North-Holland, Amsterdam.

Temin, H., and Baltimore, D., 1972, RNA-directed DNA synthesis and RNA tumor viruses, in: *Advances in Virus Research,* Vol. 17 (K. Smith, M. Lauffer, and F. Bang, eds.), pp. 129–185, Academic Press, New York.

Temin, H. M., and Mizutani, S., 1970, RNA-dependent DNA polymerase in virions of Rous sarcoma virus, *Nature (London)* **226**:1211.

Tennant, R. W., Myer, F. E., and McGrath, L., 1974a, Effect of the *Fv-1* gene on leukemia virus in mouse cell heterokaryons, *Int. J. Cancer* **14**:504.

Tennant, R. W., Schulter, B., Yang, W.-K., and Brown, A., 1974b, Reciprocal inhibition of mouse leukemia virus infection by *Fv-1* allele cell extracts, *Proc. Natl. Acad. Sci. USA* **71**:4241.

Tereba, A., Skoog, L., and Vogt, P. K., 1975, RNA tumor virus specific sequences in nuclear DNA of several avian species, *Virology* **65**:524.

Theilen, G. H., Zeigel, R. F., and Twiehaus, M. J., 1966, Biological studies with RE virus (strain T) that induces reticuloendotheliosis in turkeys, chickens, and Japanese quail, *J. Natl. Cancer Inst.* **37**:731.

Todaro, G. J., Benveniste, R. E., Lieber, M. M., and Sherr, C. J., 1974, Characterization of a C type virus released from the porcine cell line PK(15), *Virology* **58**:65.

Todaro, G. J., Benveniste, R. E., Callahan, R., Lieber, M. M., and Sherr, C. J., 1975, Endogenous primate and feline type C viruses, *Cold Spring Harbor Symp. Quant. Biol.* **39**:1159.

Tooze, J., 1973, RNA tumour viruses: Morphology, composition and classification, in: *The Molecular Biology of Tumour Viruses* (J. Tooze, ed.), pp. 502–584, Cold Spring Harbor Laboratory, Cold Spring Harbor, N.Y.

Toyoshima, K., and Vogt, P. K., 1969, Temperature-sensitive mutants of an avian sarcoma virus, *Virology* **39**:930.

Toyoshima, K., Friis, R. R., and Vogt, P. K., 1970, The reproductive and cell-transforming capacities of avian sarcoma virus B77: Inactivation with UV light, *Virology* **42**:163.

Toyoshima, K., Owada, M., and Kozai, Y., 1973, Tumor producing capacity of temperature sensitive mutants of avian sarcoma viruses in chicks, *Biken J.* **16**:103.

Toyoshima, K., Nomaguchi, H., Owada, M., Ihara, S., and Yoshida, M., 1975, Hereditary modification of avian sarcoma viruses by quail cell passage, in: *VIIth International Symposium on Comparative Leukemia Research Program and Abstracts,* p. 139.

Trávníček, M., 1968, RNA with amino acid-acceptor activity isolated from an oncogenic virus, *Biochim. Biophys. Acta* **166**:757.

Tronick, S. R., Stephenson, J. R., Verma, I. M., and Aaronson, S. A., 1975, Thermolabile reverse transcriptase of a mammalian leukemia virus mutant temperature sensitive in its replication and sarcoma virus helper functions, *J. Virol.* **16**:1476.

Tsuchida, N., Robin, M. S., and Green, M., 1972, Viral RNA subunits in cells transformed by RNA tumor viruses, *Science* **176**:1418.

Tsuchida, N., Long, C., and Hatanaka, M., 1974, Viral RNA of murine sarcoma virus produced by a hamster–mouse somatic cell hybrid, *Virology* **60**,200.

Twardzik, D., Simonds, J., Oskarsson, M., and Portugal, F., 1973, Translation of AKR-murine leukemia viral RNA in an *E. coli* cell-free system, *Biochem. Biophys. Res. Commun.* **52**:1108.

Unkeless, J. C., Tobia, A., Ossowski, L., Quigley, J. P., Rifkin, D. B., and Reich, E., 1973, An enzymatic function associated with transformation of fibroblasts by oncogenic viruses. I. Chick embryo fibroblast cultures transformed by avian RNA tumor viruses, *J. Exp. Med.* **137**:85.

Vaheri, A., and Ruoslahti, E., 1974, Disappearance of a major cell-type specific surface glycoprotein antigen (SF) after transformation of fibroblasts by Rous sarcoma virus, *Int. J. Cancer* **13**:579.

van Zaane, D., Gielkens, A. L. J., Dekker-Michielsen, M. J. A., and Bloemers, H. P. J., 1975, Virus-specific precursor polypeptides in cells infected with Rauscher leukemia virus, *Virology* **67**:544.

Varmus, H. E., and Shank, P. R., 1976, Unintegrated viral DNA is synthesized in the cytoplasm of avian sarcoma virus-transformed duck cells by viral DNA polymerase, *J. Virol.* **18**:567.

Varmus, H. E., Weiss, R. A., Friis, R. R., Levinson, W., and Bishop, J. M., 1972, Detection of avian tumor virus-specific nucleotide sequences in avian cell DNAs, *Proc. Natl. Acad. Sci. USA* **69**:20.

Varmus, H. E., Bishop, J. M., and Vogt, P. K., 1973*a*, Synthesis and integration of Rous sarcoma virus-specific DNA in permissive and non-permissive hosts, in: *Virus Research, Proceedings of the Second ICN-UCLA Symposium on Molecular Biology* (C. Fox and W. Robinson, eds.), pp. 373–383, Academic Press, New York.

Varmus, H. E., Vogt, P. K., and Bishop, J. M., 1973*b*, Integration of deoxyribonucleic acid specific for Rous sarcoma virus after infection of permissive and nonpermissive hosts, *Proc. Natl. Acad. Sci. USA* **70**:3067.

Varmus, H. E., Guntaka, R. V., Fan, W. J. W., Heasley, S., and Bishop, J. M., 1974, Synthesis of viral DNA in the cytoplasm of duck embryo fibroblasts and in enucleated cells after infection by avian sarcoma virus, *Proc. Natl. Acad. Sci. USA* **71**:3874.

Varmus, H. E., Guntaka, R. V., Deng, C.-T., and Bishop, J. M., 1975*a*, Synthesis, structure and function of avian sarcoma virus-specific DNA in permissive and non-permissive host cells, *Cold Spring Harbor Symp. Quant. Biol.* **39**:987.

Varmus, H. E., Guntaka, R. V., Deng, C.-T., Domenik, C., and Bishop, J. M., 1975*b*, Synthesis and function of avian sarcoma virus-specific DNA in permissive and non-permissive host cells, in: *Proceedings XI International Cancer Congress, Florence, Italy, 1974* (P. Bucalossi, U. Veronesi, and N. Casinelli, eds.), pp. 272–276, American Elsevier, New York.

Venuta, S., and Rubin, H., 1973, Sugar transport in normal and Rous sarcoma virus-transformed chick-embryo fibroblasts, *Proc. Natl. Acad. Sci. USA* **70**:653.

Verma, I. M., 1975, Studies on reverse transcriptase of RNA tumor viruses. I. Localization of thermolabile DNA polymerase and RNase H activities on one polypeptide, *J. Virol.* **15**:121.

Verma, I. M., and Gibson, W., 1975, Role of reverse transcriptase in the life cycle of RNA tumor viruses, in: *DNA Synthesis and its Regulation, Proceedings of the Fifth ICN-UCLA Symposium on Molecular and Cell Biology* (M. Gullian, P. Hanowalt, and C. Fox, eds.), pp. 730–752, W. A. Benjamin, Menlo Park, Calif.

Verma, I. M., Mason, W. S., Drost, S. D., and Baltimore, D., 1974, DNA polymerase activity from two temperature-sensitive mutants of Rous sarcoma virus is thermolabile, *Nature (London)* **251**:27.

Verma, I. M., Varmus, H., and Hunter, E., 1976, Characterization of early temperature-sensitive mutants of avian sarcoma viruses—Biological properties and thermal lability of the reverse transcriptase *in vitro* and synthesis of viral DNA in infected cells, *Virology,* **74**:16.

Vogt, P. K., 1965, A heterogeneity of Rous sarcoma virus revealed by selectively resistant chick embryo cells, *Virology* **25**:237.

Vogt, P. K., 1967*a*, A virus released by "nonproducing" Rous sarcoma cells, *Proc. Natl. Acad. Sci. USA* **58**:801.

Vogt, P. K., 1967*b*, Phenotypic mixing in the avian tumor virus group, *Virology* **32**:708.

Vogt, P. K., 1967*c*, Virus-directed host response in the avian leukosis and sarcoma complex, in: *Perspectives in Virology,* Vol. 5 (M. Pollard, ed.), pp. 199–228, Academic Press, New York.

Vogt, P. K., 1970, Envelope classification of avian RNA tumor viruses, in: *Comparative Leukemia Research 1969 (Bibl. Haematol.,* No. 36) (R. M. Dutcher, ed.), pp. 153–167, Karger, New York.

Vogt, P. K., 1971*a*, Spontaneous segregation of nontransforming viruses from cloned sarcoma viruses, *Virology* **46**:939.

Vogt, P. K., 1971*b*, Genetically stable reassortment of markers during mixed infection with avian tumor viruses, *Virology* **46**:947.

Vogt, P. K., 1973, The genome of avian RNA tumor viruses: A discussion of four models, in: *Possible Episomes in Eukaryotes, Proceedings of the Fourth Lepetit Colloquium, 1972* (L. Silvestri, ed.), pp. 35–41, North-Holland, Amsterdam.

Vogt, P. K., 1976, The oncovirinae—A definition of the group, in: *WHO Centre for Collection and Evaluation of Data on Comparative Virology* (P. Thein, ed.), pp. 327–339, Munich, 1976.

Vogt, P. K., and Duesberg, P. H., 1973, On the mechanism of recombination between avian RNA tumor viruses, in: *Virus Research, Proceedings of the Second ICN-UCLA Symposium on Molecular Biology* (C. Fox and W. Robinson, eds.), pp. 505–511, Academic Press, New York.

Vogt, P. K., and Ishizaki, R., 1965, Reciprocal patterns of genetic resistance to avian tumor viruses in two lines of chickens, *Virology* **26**:664.

Vogt, P. K., Weiss, R. A., and Hanafusa, H., 1974, Proposal for numbering mutants of avian leukosis and sarcoma viruses, *J. Virol.* **13**:551.

Vogt, P. K., Hunter, E., Hayman, M., and Duesberg, P. H., 1977, A new nonconditional replication defective mutant of Rous sarcoma virus, in preparation.

Vogt, V. M., and Eisenman, R., 1973, Identification of a large polypeptide precursor to avian oncornavirus proteins, *Proc. Natl. Acad. Sci. USA* **70**:1734.

Vogt, V. M., Eisenman, R., and Diggelmann, H., 1975, Generation of avian myeloblastosis virus structural proteins by proteolytic cleavage of a precursor polypeptide, *J. Mol. Biol.* **96**:471.

Von der Helm, K., and Duesberg, P. H., 1975, Translation of Rous sarcoma virus

RNA in a cell-free system from ascites Krebs II cells, *Proc. Natl. Acad. Sci. USA* **72**:614.

Walker, T. A., Pace, N. R., Erikson, R. L., Erikson, E., and Behr, F., 1974, The 7 S RNA common to oncornaviruses and normal cells is associated with polyribosomes, *Proc. Natl. Acad. Sci. USA* **71**:3390.

Wang, L.-H., and Duesberg, P., 1974, Properties and location of poly(A) in Rous sarcoma virus RNA, *J. Virol.* **14**:1515.

Wang, L.-H., Duesberg, P., Beemon, K., and Vogt, P. K., 1975, Mapping RNase T$_1$-resistant oligonucleotides of avian tumor virus RNAs: Sarcoma-specific oligonucleotides are near the poly(A) end and oligonucleotides common to sarcoma and transformation-defective viruses are at the poly(A) end, *J. Virol.* **16**:1051.

Wang, L.-H., Duesberg, P. H., Kawai, S., and Hanafusa, H., 1976a, The location of envelope-specific and sarcoma-specific oligonucleotides on the RNA of Schmidt-Ruppin Rous sarcoma virus, *Proc. Natl. Acad. Sci. USA* **73**:447.

Wang, L.-H., Duesberg, P. H., Mellon, P., and Vogt, P. K., 1976b, Distribution of envelope specific and sarcoma specific nucleotide sequences from different parents in the RNAs of avian tumor virus recombinants, *Proc. Natl. Acad. Sci. USA* **73**:1073.

Warren, L., Critchley, D., and MacPherson, I., 1972, Surface glycoproteins and glycolipids of chicken embryo cells transformed by a temperature-sensitive mutant of Rous sarcoma virus, *Nature (London)* **235**:275.

Waters, L. C., Mullin, B. C., Bailiff, E. G., and Popp, R. A., 1975, tRNA's associated with the 70 S RNA of avian myeloblastosis virus, *J. Virol.* **16**:1608.

Weber, G. H., Heine, U., Cottler-Fox, M., Garon, C. F., and Beaudreau, G. S., 1975, Nucleic acids of RNA tumor viruses: Identification and ultrastructure, *Virology* **64**:205.

Weber, M. J., 1973, Hexose transport in normal and in Rous sarcoma virus-transformed cells, *J. Biol. Chem.* **248**:2978.

Weiss, R., 1967, Spontaneous virus production from "non-virus producing" Rous sarcoma cells, *Virology* **32**:719.

Weiss, R. A., 1969a, The host range of Bryan strain Rous sarcoma virus synthesized in the absence of helper virus, *J. Gen. Virol.* **5**:511.

Weiss, R. A., 1969b, Interference and neutralization studies with Bryan strain Rous sarcoma virus synthesized in the absence of helper virus, *J. Gen. Virol.* **5**:529.

Weiss, R. A., 1972, Helper viruses and helper cells, in: *RNA Viruses and Host Genome in Oncogenesis* (P. Emmelot and P. Bentvelzen, eds.), pp. 117–135, North-Holland, Amsterdam.

Weiss, R. A., 1973, Transmission of cellular genetic elements by RNA tumor viruses, in: *Possible Episomes in Eukaryotes* (L. Silvestri, ed.), pp. 130–141, North-Holland, Amsterdam.

Weiss, R. A., Friis, R. R., Katz, E., and Vogt, P. K., 1971, Induction of avian tumor viruses in normal cells by physical and chemical carcinogens, *Virology* **46**:920.

Weiss, R. A., Mason, W. S., and Vogt, P. K., 1973, Genetic recombinants and heterozygotes derived from endogenous and exogenous avian RNA tumor viruses, *Virology* **52**:535.

Weiss, R. A., Boettiger, D., and Love, D. N., 1975, Phenotypic mixing between vesicular stomatitis virus and avian RNA tumor viruses, *Cold Spring Harbor Symp. Quant. Biol.* **39**:913.

Weiss, R. A., and Wong, A. L., 1977, Phenotypic mixing between avian and mammalian RNA tumor viruses: Envelope pseudotypes of Rous sarcoma virus, *Virology* (in press).

Weissmann, C., Parsons, J. T., Coffin, J. W., Rymo, L., Billeter, M. A., and Hofstetter, H., 1975, Studies on the structure and synthesis of Rous sarcoma virus RNA, *Cold Spring Harbor Symp. Quant. Biol.* **39**:1043.

Wickus, G. G., and Robbins, P. W., 1973, Plasma membrane proteins of normal and Rous sarcoma virus-transformed chick-embryo fibroblasts, *Nature (London) New Biol.* **245**:65.

Wong, P. K. Y., and McCarter, J. A., 1973, Genetic studies of temperature-sensitive mutants of Moloney-murine leukemia virus, *Virology* **53**:319.

Wong, P. K. Y., and McCarter, J. A., 1974, Studies of two temperature-sensitive mutants of Moloney murine leukemia virus, *Virology* **58**:396.

Wong, P. K. Y., and MacLeod, R., 1975, Studies on the budding process of a temperature sensitive mutant of murine leukemia virus with a scanning-electron microscope *J. Virol.* **16**:434.

Wong, P. K. Y., Russ, L. J., McCarter, J. A., 1973, Rapid, selective procedure for isolation of spontaneous temperature-sensitive mutants of Moloney leukemia virus, *Virology* **51**:424.

Wright, S. E., and Neiman, P. E., 1974, Base-sequence relationships between avian ribonucleic acid endogenous and sarcoma viruses assayed by competitive ribonucleic acid–deoxyribonucleic acid hybridization, *Biochemistry* **13**:1549.

Wyke, J. A., 1973*a*, The selective isolation of temperature-sensitive mutants of Rous sarcoma virus, *Virology* **52**:587.

Wyke, J. A., 1973*b*, Complementation of transforming functions by temperature-sensitive mutants of avian sarcoma virus, *Virology* **54**:28.

Wyke, J. A., 1974, The genetics of C-type RNA tumor viruses, *Int. Rev. of Cytology* **38**:67.

Wyke, J. A., 1975, Temperature sensitive mutants of avian sarcoma viruses, *Biochim. Biophys. Acta* **417**:91.

Wyke, J. A., and Linial, M., 1973, Temperature-sensitive avian sarcoma viruses: A physiological comparison of twenty mutants, *Virology* **53**:152.

Wyke, J. A., Bell, J. G., and Beamand, J. A., 1975, Genetic recombination among temperature-sensitive mutants of Rous sarcoma virus, *Cold Spring Harbor Symp. Quant. Biol.* **39**:897.

Yamada, K. M., Yamada, S. S., and Pastan, I., 1975, The major cell surface glycoprotein of chick embryo fibroblasts is an agglutinin, *Proc. Natl. Acad. Sci. USA* **72**:3158.

Yoshida, M., Owada, M., and Toyoshima, K., 1975, Strain specificity of changes in adenylate cyclase activity in cells transformed by avian sarcoma viruses, *Virology* **63**:68.

Yoshii, S., and Vogt, P. K., 1970, A mutant of Rous sarcoma virus (type O) causing fusiform cell transformation, *Proc. Soc. Exp. Biol. Med.* **135**:297.

Yoshikura, H., 1973*a*, Ultraviolet inactivation of murine leukemia virus and its assay in permissive and non-permissive cells, *Int. J. Cancer* **11**:739.

Yoskikura, H., 1973*b*, Host range conversion of murine sarcoma-leukaemia complex, *J. Gen. Virol.* **19**:321.

Závada, J., 1972, Pseudotypes of vesicular stomatitis virus with the coat of murine leukaemia and of avian myeloblastosis viruses, *J. Gen. Virol.* **15**:183.

CHAPTER 9

Genetics and Paragenetic Phenomena of Paramyxoviruses

Michael A. Bratt

Department of Microbiology
University of Massachusetts Medical School
Worcester, Massachusetts 01605

and

Lawrence E. Hightower

Microbiology Section, Biological Science Group
University of Connecticut
Storrs, Connecticut 06268

1. INTRODUCTION

This is the companion chapter to Chapter 10, "Genetics of Orthomyxoviruses." These two groups of viruses, paramyxoviruses and orthomyxoviruses, known since the turn of the century, possess many similarities of structure and biological properties but molecular biologies which differ greatly (see Choppin and Compans, 1975; Compans and Choppin, 1975). The orthomyxoviruses undergo extensive recombination or chromosomal reassortment, and numerous reviews of their genetics have been written. For paramyxoviruses, there is no evidence for recombination, and their genetic properties have never been reviewed. Finally, although we have worked on paramyxoviruses for 15 years, we have never worked on any aspect of orthomyxoviruses.

We have therefore approached these two groups of viruses in very different ways. The chapter on orthomyxovirus genetics takes cognizance of the many reviews, and concentrates on an aspect which has only briefly been covered in these earlier reviews—temperature-sensitive mutants and their use in understanding the molecular biology and biology of these viruses. It is to be hoped that our naivete will bring some light to this complex but important area of investigation.

This chapter on paramyxoviruses covers most aspects of the genetic and paragenetic phenomena of these viruses. As a result, it has been necessary to place a heavy emphasis on virus populations, the important distinction between mutants and variants, and the use of proper criteria for the conduct of these studies.

The paramyxoviruses include Newcastle disease virus (NDV), five different types of parainfluenza virus, and mumps virus. In addition, the viruses of measles, canine distemper, and rinderpest are considered as paramyxoviruses, although they differ from the former in that current evidence suggests that they neither possess a virion-associated neuraminidase nor require neuraminidase-sensitive receptors on susceptible cell surfaces. Our knowledge of the structure, molecular biology, and biology of these viruses is derived mainly from studies on NDV, parainfluenza virus type 1 [Sendai, or hemagglutinating virus of Japan (HVJ)], and parainfluenza virus type 5 (SV5), but in recent years we have seen increasing numbers of studies on measles virus. In this chapter, it is assumed that these viruses serve as reasonable models of paramyxovirus infection. Only where obvious differences are known will specific references be made.

The goal of virological studies is the understanding and control of disease processes. The complex variables involved in the infection of the whole animal—viral variation and selection, tissue tropisms, and the protective mechanisms of the host, including both interferon and immune responses—have forced the isolated study of the biological and molecular biological aspects of virus–cell interactions in tissue culture systems. Of considerable importance in such studies is the use of genetics to establish correlations and causal relationships between genome changes and biological properties, and interactions among the biological properties themselves. However, a serious limitation in the study of paramyxoviruses is the lack of evidence for genetic recombination for any member of this group. Thus standard genetic procedures for mapping and ordering viral genomes cannot be used. Complementation analyses with temperature-sensitive mutants are beginning to be used to localize functional defects within specific genes, but other new methods for studying genetic fine structure will have to be sought. These limitations are to some extent compensated for by an abundance of biochemical and biological properties in proportion to the amount of genetic information. This high biology/protein/gene ratio renders these viruses ideal candidates for phenotypic analyses of mutants, variants, and strains.

In this chapter, we emphasize the need to reduce the variables to as few as possible and to distinguish between system-specific and general principles. Many workers including ourselves have in the past adopted comparative approaches employing different strains of a given virus in a single cell type, or a single strain of virus in a number of cell types. Such studies usually lead to no correlations at all, or to correlations which last only until the next variable is changed. In this chapter, we have almost completely ignored such studies because of their inherent complexity. We have also emphasized the difficulties in establishing causal relationships using variants of unknown genetic composition. Only through the use of models employing mutants is there a high likelihood of success in establishing such relationships. This is not to say that we disagree with the conclusion of Estupinan and Hanson (1971b) that disease processes in the animal may involve interaction among populations of genetically differing viruses. However, to understand the workings of these multivariable systems, we must first understand what happens in more readily defined systems.

2. PROPERTIES RELEVANT TO GENETIC ANALYSES

Since genetic studies of paramyxoviruses are restricted to analyses of phenotypic behavior, it is necessary to consider the viral properties which provide the framework for the genetic and paragenetic phenomena to be described. Also necessary is a brief description of our current knowledge of (1) the amounts and arrangement of genetic material within the paramyxovirus genome; (2) the numbers and sizes of viral genes, messenger RNAs, and polypeptides; (3) the mechanisms of synthesis and control of these virus-specific macromolecules; and (4) the interactions between these virus-specific macromolecules and their effects on host cells. Our current knowledge of the structure, molecular biology, and biology of these viruses has been excellently reviewed by Choppin and Compans (1975) and previously by Kingsbury (1973a). Therefore, in the interest of brevity we have left out most of the specific details and the background references contained in those reviews. More recent findings and references are given in somewhat greater detail. Perhaps relevant, also, are the chapters on the reproduction (Wagner,

1975) and genetics (Pringle, this volume) of rhabdoviruses which appear in this series. While the rhabdoviruses lack the extensive biological phenomena of the paramyxoviruses, these two groups share many common features of their molecular biology.

2.1. Summary of Virus Structure and the Infectious Process

2.1.1. Virions

Paramyxoviruses are pleomorphic, roughly spherical particles with diameters of 150–300 nm. Virions consist of helically arranged nucleocapsids containing the genome RNA, surrounded by an envelope or limiting membrane. This envelope consists of a lipid bilayer, an underlying protein layer, and glycoprotein spikes which protrude from the surface of the particles. The vast majority of the proteins of the virion are virus specified, the lipids are selected almost quantitatively from those of the host cell, and the specificity of carbohydrates of both glycolipids and glycoproteins is determined by host cell transferases.

2.1.2. Infection and Virus Production

Infection begins with attachment to receptors. This is followed by penetration of the cellular membrane, which in most instances probably involves fusion of viral envelope and cellular membrane, but in some instances may involve phagocytosis. Access of the nucleocapsid to the cytoplasm would be a natural consequence of entry by fusion, but would need to occur as a separate step if phagocytosis were a mechanism of entry. The initial synthetic event in infection is primary transcription of mRNA, using the virion-associated transcriptase and the RNA of the genome as template. This mRNA is then translated into viral proteins. Some of the newly synthesized proteins are required for viral RNA replication. Replication creates more templates for mRNA transcription (secondary transcription) and amplified protein synthesis, as well as genomes for progeny virus. While viral genomes are accumulating in nucleocapsids, other viral proteins are being processed into the cellular membrane. Nucleocapsids then associate with regions of altered cellular membrane, and bud out, surrounded by this altered cellular membrane.

As will be discussed below, there appears to be little if any temporal control over the synthesis of individual viral proteins and RNAs after the initial translation of primary transcripts. Therefore, designation of the synthetic events in infection as either "early" or "late" has little meaning in this system unless one chooses to define the macromolecular synthesis which occurs after the initial translation of primary transcripts as "late" and that which occurs prior to this time as "early." Obviously, however, some properties of infected cells, such as virus production, hemadsorption (Section 2.5.1), and fusion from within (Section 2.5.3), which depend on the accumulation of sufficient amounts of virus-specific products, can be defined as "late" functions.

2.1.3. Effects on Host Cells

Depending on the virus–cell system, the host cell may either be killed or continue to live and produce virus in considerably varying amounts. The molecular events involved in cell killing or sparing remain to be elucidated. Other biological effects of infection will be discussed below.

2.2. Identification and Synthesis of Viral Proteins

2.2.1. Virion Proteins

The most probable numbers of viral polypeptides lie in the range of six to nine for each of the paramyxoviruses (Choppin and Compans, 1975). However, final determination of the uniqueness of polypeptides within individual peaks on gels requires tryptic peptide analysis. Indeed, where this has been done in the case of NDV (Hightower *et al.*, 1975), evidence was obtained for only six distinct polypeptides.

2.2.2. Virus-Specific Proteins in the Infected Cell

The identification of virus-specific proteins in infected cells has been hampered by the continued synthesis of host-specified proteins. Where host cell backgrounds have been low enough, or eliminated by difference analyses (Hightower and Bratt, 1974; Lamb *et al.*, 1976), the virus-specific proteins detected correspond mainly to those found in virions or to precursors of the glycoproteins (Hightower and Bratt, 1974; Hightower *et al.*, 1975; Lamb *et al.*, 1976; Nagai *et al.*, 1976; Portner and Kingsbury, 1976). Other potentially virus-specific polypeptides identified in infected cells but not in virions (nonstructural proteins) have been reported for both NDV (Hightower and Bratt, 1974; Bratt *et al.,* 1975) and Sendai virus (Zaides *et al.,* 1975; Lamb and Mahy, 1975; Lamb *et al.,* 1976). No evidence for uniqueness of these has been established, however. In fact, when analyzed in the NDV-infected cell, all potential virus-specific polypeptides other than the six found in virions and the F_0 glycopolypeptide were shown to share tryptic peptides with the major nucleocapsid polypeptide, NP, suggesting that they were not unique (Hightower *et al.,* 1975).

2.2.3. Virus-Specific Protein Synthesis

No abrupt inhibition of host cell protein synthesis (Hightower and Bratt, 1974, 1975; Bratt *et al.,* 1975) or abrupt dissociation of host cell polyribosomes (C. W. Clinkscales and M. A. Bratt, unpublished) occurs in NDV-infected chick embryo cells. Instead, the synthesis of NDV proteins gradually replaces that of host proteins. Nothing is known about the mechanism of this replacement. The process seems to be similar for Sendai virus, although total protein synthesis actually appears to increase in this case (Zaides, *et al.,* 1975; Lamb *et al.,* 1976). Furthermore, there is no evidence for temporal control of individual viral polypeptides. Throughout infection, all polypeptides seem to be synthesized in approximately the same relative proportions (Hightower and Bratt, 1974; Bratt *et al.,* 1975; Lamb *et al.,* 1976). Control of synthesis of individual polypeptides must exist, however, since they are synthesized in greatly varying proportions.

2.3. Identification and Synthesis of Viral RNA

2.3.1. Virion RNA

The RNA from virions is single stranded and sediments under standard conditions at 50 S. The best molecular weight estimates for these molecules are those of Kolakofsky *et al.* (1974*a,* 1975), who obtained values of 5–5.4 $\times$ 10^6 using a variety of techniques. The majority of the RNA molecules in virions possess antimessage polarity, but reports from several laboratories have indicated highly variable amounts of intermolecular self-annealing (see Kingsbury, 1973*a;* Choppin and Compans, 1975). While the biological significance of these findings remains obscure, Kolakofsky and Bruschi (1975) have provided a hint of their origin. They found even larger amounts of self-annealing for the 50 S RNA of nucleocapsids isolated from infected cells as compared to that from released virions. In spite of these unexplained findings, the most appealing model continues to be one in which infectious particles are those which contain RNA of antimessage sense, since (1) no one has ever obtained infectious RNA from these viruses and (2) virions contain a transcriptase activity (presumably essential for RNA viruses whose genomes possess antimessage polarity). Nevertheless, it must be pointed out that while no one has reported messenger activity for any 50 S RNA preparations—Kingsbury (1973*b*) was unable to obtain cell free translation of 50 S RNA from Sendai virions—the possibility that some messenger-sense 50 S molecules might possess mRNA activity or even infectious potential has not been definitively ruled out.

2.3.2. Intracellular Single-Stranded RNA Species

Virus-specific RNA from the infected cell sediments in three size classes—50 S, 35 S, and 18–22 S. As mentioned above, single-stranded RNA which sediments at 50 S has both message and antimessage polarity (Kolakofsky and Bruschi, 1975). A single-stranded 33 S RNA of message polarity has been shown in annealing experiments by Roux and Kolakofsky (1975) to correspond to 40% of the Sendai virus genome. A comparable single-stranded 35 S RNA (B. B. Spanier and M. A. Bratt, submitted for publication) has been shown to function as the mRNA for the largest NDV protein, L (Morrison *et al.,* 1975; B. B. Spanier, C. W. Clinkscales, M. A. Bratt, and T. G. Morrison, unpublished).

Most of the 22 S RNA of both Sendai virus and NDV has recently been shown to consist of apparently single-stranded aggregates of the 18 S RNAs (Roux and Kolakofsky, 1975; Weiss and Bratt, 1976). Annealing studies show that the 18 S RNAs of Sendai virus (Roux and Kolakofsky, 1975) and NDV (B. B. Spanier and M. A. Bratt, unpublished) correspond to 60% of their respective genomes. For NDV, these 18 S RNAs can be separated into five discrete peaks on formamide gels (Weiss and Bratt, 1976). The estimated molecular weights of these RNAs are sufficient to code for the five smallest unique polypeptides, and their combined estimated molecular weights also correspond to 60% of the genome (Weiss and Bratt, 1976).

Cell-free translation of the 18 S RNA from paramyxovirus-infected cells was first accomplished by Kingsbury (1973*b*). One of the products was identified by tryptic peptide analysis as authentic Sendai virus NP polypeptide. Subsequently, Morrison *et al.* (1975) and Davies *et al.* (1976) reported cell free synthesis of authentic HN and NP polypeptides of NDV, and NP and M polypeptides of Sendai virus, respectively. More recently, all of the known NDV polypeptides expected to be encoded by the 18 S mRNAs—HN, F, NP, 47K, and M—have been authentically synthesized in a cell free system (C. W. Clinkscales, M. A. Bratt, and T. G. Morrison, submitted for publication).

Like most mammalian mRNAs, the 18 S RNAs of NDV and Sendai virus possess poly(A) sequences. In the case of Sendai virus, the poly(A) sequences have been shown to have a 3′-end location (Marx *et al.,* 1975), similar to most eukaryotic mRNAs. Poly(A) sequences also seem to be present on the 35 S mRNA of NDV (B. B. Spanier, C. W. Clinkscales, M. A. Bratt, and T. G. Morrison, unpublished). Boersma and Stone (1976) have also reported that the 5′ ends of NDV mRNA, like most other mammalian mRNAs, are both capped and methylated.

2.3.3. Intracellular RNA Synthesis

Nothing is known about the factors controlling 50 S RNA replication and messenger transcription, although the two processes can be uncoupled. Replication appears to be blocked by inhibitors of protein synthesis and in cells coinfected with defective interfering particles, and, as described below, only transcription is detected *in vitro*.

Partially base-paired RNA structures sedimenting from 22 S to 50 S have been isolated from infected cells. The conformation of these partially base-paired structures is probably significantly different from that in the infected cell. Nevertheless, it has been possible to ascribe a transcriptive function to the most rapidly sedimenting species and a replicative function to slower-sedimenting species on the basis of their behavior under the various conditions where replication does not occur (Portner and Kingsbury, 1972; B. B. Spanier and M. A. Bratt, submitted for publication).

2.3.4. *In Vitro* Transcription

Virions contain a transcriptase activity which, when activated by nonionic detergents, can catalyze transcription from the virion RNA template. The products of such reactions have been identified mainly as the 18 S RNAs and their 22 S aggregates. These RNAs possess many of the properties of intracellular 18–22 S RNA, including the presence of poly(A), which appears to be added without transcription. In addition, Colonno and Stone (1975*b*) provided evidence for methylation of the *in vitro* transcripts of NDV. It is unclear whether all five of NDV's 18 S RNAs are transcribed *in vitro*. Recent studies in our laboratory have revealed that the poly(A)-containing molecules are probably limited to only two or three of the five 18 S species (S. R. Weiss and M. A. Bratt, unpublished). In addition, while *in vitro* transcripts have been translated in a cell-free system, the only unique product identified thus far is the nucleocapsid protein, NP (T. G. Morrison, S. R. Weiss, B. B. Spanier, and M. A. Bratt, unpublished).

2.3.5. Primary Transcription

In vitro transcription is presumably a facsimile of the first synthetic event in infection—transcription from the genome template by the virion transcriptase. The latter has been designated *primary transcription* to distinguish it from *secondary transcription,* the amplified transcription which occurs as replication increases the number of templates and new transcriptase molecules are synthesized. Primary transcription can be detected if replication is blocked by inhibitors of protein synthesis from the time of infection (Robinson, 1971). Measured in this manner, primary transcripts include the 35 S mRNA which is not detected among the *in vitro* transcripts (B. B. Spanier and M. A. Bratt, submitted for publication).

2.4. Relationships among Viral Genomes, mRNAs, and Proteins

The combined estimated molecular weights of the 35 S mRNAs of both Sendai virus (Roux and Kolakofsky, 1975) and NDV (B. B. Spanier and M. A. Bratt, submitted for publication). B. B. Spanier, C. W. Clinkscales, M. A. Bratt, and T. G. Morrison, unpublished) and the five 18 S NDV mRNAs discernable on formamide gels (Weiss and Bratt, 1976) are strikingly similar to the estimated molecular weight of $5.0–5.4 \times 10^6$ for the paramyxovirus genome (Kolakofsky *et al.,* 1974*a*, 1975). Estimated in this way, the 35 S RNA corresponds to 40% of the genome, and the five 18 S RNA species to 60%. Annealing studies provide additional evidence in that the 18 S RNAs of Sendai virus (Roux and Kolakofsky, 1975) and NDV (B. B. Spanier, and M. A. Bratt, unpublished) each correspond to 60% of their respective genomes, while the combined 18 S and

35 S RNAs of Sendai virus correspond to 100% of the genome (Roux and Kolakofsky, 1975).

The combined estimated molecular weight of the six unique NDV polypeptides is 4.9×10^5 (Hightower *et al.*, 1975), or 85–90% of the genome's estimated maximum coding capacity of 5.5–6×10^5. Therefore, most of the viral proteins have been identified, although the possibility of additional polypeptides, present in insufficient amounts for detection, still exists. Alternatively, however, there is considerable appeal in the correlation of six mRNA peaks, corresponding to the entire genome and each having a more-than-sufficient estimated size to serve as a monocistronic message for one of the six unique polypeptides. The uncertainty in all of these calculations lies in (1) the molecular weight estimates, (2) whether the separated mRNAs contain even one or possibly two unique species, and (3) whether all the virus-specific polypeptides have indeed been identified. The larger coding capacity of the mRNAs in relation to the viral proteins suggests at least two other potential complications. First, even if the individual peaks contain unique species, one or more of them might code for more than a single protein. Second, there is still the possibility that proteins other than F are processed from larger precursor molecules.

Studies on the mRNAs and proteins of paramyxoviruses other than NDV should be of considerable value in sorting out these relationships. An important first step will be the use of tryptic peptide analyses to establish the uniqueness of Sendai virus proteins in virions and infected cells. These studies would allow evaluation of (1) the existence of at least one Sendai polypeptide, P (Marx *et al.*, 1974; Zaides *et al.*, 1975; Lamb *et al.*, 1976), without correspondence in NDV; (2) the possibility that one of the polypeptides in Sendai virions is indeed actin, derived from the host (Lamb *et al.*, 1976)—a possibility already excluded for NDV (Hightower *et al.*, 1975); and (3) the possible existence of additional nonstructural polypeptides in the infected cell (Zaides *et al.*, 1975; Lamb and Mahy, 1975; Lamb *et al.*, 1976).

2.5. Properties of Virions and Infected Cells

Because of their replicative pattern and the fact that the multiplication of paramyxoviruses involves extensive modification of the host cell, many of the properties characteristic of these viruses are shared by virions and infected cells. In some cases, however, it is difficult to determine whether a particular property is associated with the cell itself, or with newly synthesized virus particles on the cell surface. Many properties can be studied within the complexity of the infectious process, or, alternatively, under conditions of isolation which allow the investigator to focus on a given property. Despite this advantage, there are a number of properties for which evidence of viral or host specificity is either poor or not available. Genetic studies should be particularly useful in establishing the viral or host origin in these cases.

2.5.1. Hemagglutination and Hemadsorption

Paramyxoviruses attach to cells by means of a glycoprotein, HN, which constitutes some of the spikes on the surface of the virion. These spikes also react with neutralizing antibody. Distribution of these spikes over the virion surface allows simultaneous attachment to two cells. At appropriate virus/red blood cell concentrations, lattice formation can occur. This process, known as hemagglutination, has been used as a model in the study of viral attachment.

Late in the infectious process, the infected cell develops the ability to adsorb red blood cells (hemadsorption), presumably as a result of alteration of the cell surface by the hemagglutinin.

2.5.2. Neuraminidase

Another property recently ascribed to this HN glycoprotein is the enzymatic activity neuraminidase. This enzyme presumably releases virus particles from soluble mucoproteins, red blood cells, and infected cells, as a result of splitting N-acetylneuraminic (sialic) acid, thought to constitute a part of the receptor on these substrates. This property is also associated with both virions and infected cells.

2.5.3. Fusion

The ability to cause cell fusion is associated with both virions and infected cells. Fusion from without (FFWO) (or early fusion) is a direct response of cells to input virus particles, since it occurs rapidly after infection by high multiplicities of virus which need be neither infectious nor capable of synthesizing virus-specific RNA or protein (Bratt and Gallaher, 1969, 1970). Studies on Sendai virus (Homma and Ohuchi, 1973; Homma, 1975; Scheid and Choppin, 1974, 1975, 1976) have provided convincing evidence correlating this fusion activity with the F glycoprotein. This glycoprotein probably constitutes a second type of spike on the surface of virions.

Late in infection, the infected cell may become capable of fusing with other cells. This fusion, designated "fusion from within" (FFWI), does not require high multiplicities of virus, but does require viral RNA and protein synthesis as well as viral infectivity, and presumably occurs as a result of alterations of the cell membrane (Bratt and Gallaher, 1969, 1970). As discussed in previous publications (Bratt and Gallaher, 1972; Poste and Waterson, 1975), the designations of FFWO and FFWI have direct parallels in the bacteriophage phenomena of lysis from without and lysis from within (Doermann, 1948). It should be pointed out that neither in the case of bacterial lysis nor in that of animal cell fusion has it been definitively proven that the components and mechanisms of early and late lysis or fusion are identical, but this is not an unreasonable possibility.

2.5.4. Hemolysis and Cytolysis

Interaction between paramyxoviruses and red blood cells can result in cell lysis (hemolysis). Along with other types of evidence, the parallel inactivation of cell-fusing and hemolytic activities of NDV by red blood cells (Clavell and Bratt, 1972b) and parallel activation of these activities by proteases in the case of Sendai virus (Homma and Ohuchi, 1973; Homma, 1975; Scheid and Choppin, 1974, 1975) strongly suggest that these activities are related. The latter evidence with Sendai virus relates both of these activities to the F glycoprotein.

Cell lysis rather than FFWO occurs when tissue culture cells are exposed to Sendai virus or NDV in the absence of calcium ions (Okada and Murayama, 1966; W. R. Gallaher and M. A. Bratt, unpublished)—conditions similar to those required for hemolysis of red blood cells (Clavell and Bratt, 1972a). It is not known whether a comparable lytic function paralleling FFWI can occur late in infection.

2.5.5. RNA Synthesis and Modification

Relatively little is known about the RNA-synthesizing and -modifying activities. *In vitro,* these activities include the transcriptase, the poly(A) adding activity, the methylating activity, and a capping activity if the latter exists. Marx *et al.* (1974) suggested that at least the nucleocapsid protein, NP, and the P (polymerase) protein are necessary for *in vitro* transcription by Sendai virus. Whether Sendai virus's newly recognized (L) protein (Zaides *et al.*, 1975; Lamb and Mahy, 1975; Lamb *et al.*, 1976) is also involved, as has been suggested for NDV (Colonno and Stone, 1975a) and/or possibly other proteins, remains to be determined. Similarly, the enzyme activities involved in primary transcription (including the factors which allow 35 S RNA synthesis here, but not *in vitro*) and those involved in secondary transcription must be determined. Preliminary evidence with transcriptive complexes isolated from Sendai virus-infected cells also has implicated both the P and NP polypeptides (Stone *et al.*, 1972).

Also remaining to be answered is the question of whether there are individual initiation sites for each of the mRNAs. Alternatively, the genome RNA might contain a single initiation site with individual mRNAs being formed by cleavage (which would require still another enzymatic activity) or some other mechanism. Evidence for a single initiation site has been obtained by Ball and White (1976) and Abraham and Banerjee (1976) for the RNAs of the rhabdovirus VSV. Comparable evidence has recently been obtained for both Sendai virus (K. Glazier, R. Raghow, and D. W. Kingsbury, personal communication) and NDV (L. A. Ball, L. E. Hightower, and P. Collins, unpublished).

Finally, the question whether the same enzymes are involved in replication and transcription must be answered. The apparent absolute need for protein synthesis for replication to occur must also be explained. This requirement is apparently also manifest when cell-free extracts are prepared from NDV and Sendai virus-infected cells, for there, too, only evidence for transcriptive activity is found (Scholtissek and Rott, 1969; Mahy *et al.*, 1970; Stone *et al.*, 1971, 1972). In addition, the factors which allow the synthesis of both complete genome-sized messenger-sense molecules, to be used as templates for genome RNA synthesis, and 18–35 S mRNAs remain to be elucidated.

2.5.6. Other Enzymes

Other enzymatic activities reported to be associated with virions include esterases and leucine aminopeptidases (Neurath, 1964); ATPases (Neurath, 1965; Kohn and Klibansky, 1967); protein kinases (Roux and Kolakofsky, 1974; Lamb, 1975), which may function in the phosphorylation of paramyxovirus proteins (Lamb, 1975; Lamb and Mahy, 1975); a transfer RNA nucleotidyltransferase (Kolakofsky,

1972); and an RNA-dependent DNA polymerase activity, associated with NDV isolated from persistently infected L cells (Furman and Hallum, 1973). Functions and origins of all of these are obscure at this time.

2.5.7. Interference and Defectiveness

Paramyxoviruses are susceptible to, and induce, a number of different types of viral interference, including (1) surface interference, a phenomenon involving reduced attachment and penetration of homologous virus; (2) interferon; and (3) intrinsic interference (induced by heterologous virus), which involves neither a block at the surface nor interferon, and may be mediated at the level of replication (see Choppin and Compans, 1975). In addition, as will be described in Sections 3.5.5 and 6.5, paramyxoviruses, like most other viruses, have the ability to shed defective virus particles which (1) possess reduced amounts of viral RNA, (2) interfere with the synthesis of normal virus, and (3) apparently block replication but not transcription of standard virus (Portner and Kingsbury, 1971).

2.5.8. Persistent Infection

Recent studies have suggested that persistent infection by paramyxoviruses may have an important role *in vivo* since variants of measles virus have been isolated from patients with subacute sclerosing panencephalitis (SSPE) (ter Meulen *et al.,* 1972*b*), and a variant of Sendai virus may have been isolated from a patient with multiple sclerosis (ter Meulen *et al.,* 1972*a*). Whether the latter virus or the recently isolated multiple sclerosis-associated agent (which is far smaller than a paramyxovirus, as indicated by its ability to pass through 50-nm filters; Koldovsky *et al.,* 1975) is causally involved in this disease remains to be determined. While the exact causal relationship in such instances (is the virus responsible for the disease, is the virus merely activated by the disease, or is the isolated virus only a fortuitous contaminant?) has not been established, these findings have revitalized interest in persistent infections. It has long been recognized that paramyxoviruses are particularly well suited to the establishment of persistent infections in culture. Tissue-culture models of persistence include steady-state infections in which all or most of the cells are infected and producing either little or no virus (Rustigian, 1966*a,b*), models in which relatively large amounts of virus continue to be produced (Choppin, 1964; Walker, 1968), and "carrier state" infections in which only a fraction of the cells appear to be infected and producing virus at any one time (Walker, 1968; Thacore and Youngner, 1969). Extensive consideration of the virus populations involved in persistent infection is given in Section 8.

2.5.9. Virulence

Virulence in the whole animal is obviously a complex function of variables such as virus population, routes of infection, tissue tropisms, and host responses. In tissue culture, its correlate is simply the extent of cytopathic effect or cell killing. While by no means absolute, there is a reasonable correlation between plaquing ability in tissue culture—no plaques vs. plaques, or small plaques vs. large plaques—and avirulence or virulence in the whole animal (e.g., Granoff, 1964a; Rapp, 1964; Schloer and Hanson, 1968, 1971; Daniel and Hanson, 1968).

As will be discussed in Section 3.1, passage in tissue culture, without the imposition of specific selective pressures for virulence, quite naturally leads to selection of variants with lowered virulence. This type of blind passage in tissue culture, in fact, is the backbone of procedures designed to attenuate virus for vaccine use. Selection for lowered virulence must also take place in natural populations, as exhibited, for instance, in the case of decreasing virulence for NDV isolates at later and later stages in a recent epizootic in California (Utterback and Schwartz, 1973; G. M. Schloer, personal communication). Since such correlations exist between tissue culture and *in vivo* infection, studies in culture can be used to focus on viral and cellular factors without the complications imposed by host responses. Obviously, however, studies will ultimately have to focus on the whole animal.

Studies in many laboratories have been directed at elucidating viral or cellular contributions to virulence in culture through the use of different strains of virus and/or different host cells. Choppin's laboratory has focused on the importance of cell membrane composition (*cf.* Choppin and Compans, 1975). Studies by Alexander *et al.* (1973a,b) and Reeve *et al.* (1971) have emphasized the importance of the balance between utilization and synthesis of virus-specific products. Bratt (1969) found that avirulent strains of NDV tend to synthesize lower amounts of mRNA (18–22 S) relative to 50 S RNA than do virulent strains, although the opposite was not always true. Reeve and Waterson (1970), Reeve *et al.* (1970), Reeve and Poste (1971), Poste and Waterson (1975), and Bratt and Gallaher (1972) have shown that avirulent strains of NDV do not cause FFWI, while virulent strains may or may not do so. These studies and that of Kohn and Fuchs (1969) failed to show any correlation between virulence and ability to induce FFWO. The recent studies of Nagai *et al.* (1976) on NDV strains of differing virulence suggest the importance of glycoprotein cleavage, in particular the role of endogenous cellular proteolytic enzymes, and the susceptibility of viral glycoproteins to them as possible determinants of virulence. All of these factors may indeed be important. However, even in these simplified systems the variables for the virus and the cell are considerable and the likelihood of identifying the key determinants of virulence is not encouraging. Indeed, it seems unlikely that any one factor, let alone one viral protein, will be found to be responsible. As discussed below, however, the use of specific mutants may prove useful in sorting out these factors. In this regard, Portner *et al.* (1975), on the basis of studies with a *ts* mutant of Sendai virus, have suggested that the synthesis of the HN glycopeptide may be an important factor in cell killing.

3. VIRUS POPULATIONS

Perhaps more than for any other group of viruses, an understanding of paramyxovirus genetics and paragenetic phenomena requires a knowledge of the variety of, and variability within, the virus populations. First, some viruses within this group exhibit a high degree of genetic instability which is reflected not only in relatively high spontaneous rates of production of mutants and variants but also in the existence of numerous naturally occurring strains as exemplified by the hundreds of biologically different NDV strains maintained at the NDV repository at the University of Wisconsin under the direction of Dr. Robert P. Hanson. In contrast, the number of known mumps virus and measles virus strains is very small. Second, a given virus population will contain not only infectious particles but also noninfectious particles, which can be either genetically inactive or simply non-plaque-forming but capable of entering cells and contributing genetic information, as has been described for NDV (see Section 3.3.2). In addition, virus stocks can contain small noninfectious particles which possess no RNA. Each of these types of noninfectious particles, whose origin may lie either in the inherent inaccuracy of the viral maturation process or in the relatively high lability of virions, is capable of affecting the outcome of infection by infectious particles.

3.1. Adaptation and Selection in Culture

Virus populations employed in the laboratory inevitably must differ extensively from those occurring in nature. The differences can be due either to the conscious effort of the investigator to obtain a specific type of virus population or to adaptation and selection resulting from passage in culture.

The virus populations isolated during epidemics or epizootics can be extremely heterogeneous. This has clearly been shown by Granoff (1964a), Estupinan and Hanson (1971a,b), Schloer (1974, and personal communication), and Schloer et al. (1975), who found that virus populations isolated during NDV epizootics consist of mixtures of virus differing in genotype and phenotype. As Estupinan and Hanson (1971a,b) and Schloer (personal communication) have suggested, such mixed populations may be extremely important to the biologist interested in studying disease processes in the whole animal.

However, newly isolated virus populations may be unsatisfactory for experimentation. The investigator imposes his will on them when, upon finding that the virus "grows poorly" in culture (either because of inherently poor growth in the animal or because of the choice of tissue culture cells), he adapts (or directly selects) them to produce higher titers or more severe cytopathic effects. Such forced adaptation is probably counter to the natural progression toward lowered virulence which is observed when virus is passed in tissue culture. Furthermore, the careful investigator, in his desire to obtain reproducible results, clones his virus. This is particularly important for the geneticist hoping to isolate and analyze the behavior of mutant viruses which are isogenic with "wild-type" virus except for single genomic changes.

With paramyxoviruses, however, the use of cloned virus may provide no guarantee of homogeneity. Durand and Eisenstark (1962) found that spontaneously occurring plaque-size variants or mutants of NDV remained relatively stable through multiple passage in tissue culture, but during a single passage in embryonated eggs gave rise to considerable plaque heterogeneity. Other markers were relatively more stable, suggesting that the embryonated egg exerts a specific selective pressure for heterogeneity of plaque size. In contrast, Granoff (1964a) and Thiry (1964) found that cloned NDV rapidly gave rise to mutants or variants of several different types, including small plaque mutants which were relatively stable when passaged in either tissue culture or embryonating eggs. Whether these differences are due to the use of different strains is unclear. Nevertheless, it is clear that spontaneous changes occur in these viruses at relatively high frequencies.

This capacity for mutation and change makes the probability of selection of variants extremely likely during continuous passage, and guarantees significant divergence even for cloned populations. The tendency to become less virulent on continuous passage has been used extensively in the attenuation of viruses for the development of vaccines. Similarly, virus isolated from persistent infections is almost invariably different from that in the initiating population (although cloned virus has only rarely been used to initiate these infections). The changes observed include such diverse properties as temperature sensitivity, reduced virulence, and alterations in neuraminidase. However, as will be described in Sections 8 and 9, in most instances it is unclear to what extent these changes are directly associated with, or attributable to, the establishment and/or maintenance of persistence rather than simply to continuous passage.

3.2. Growth of Stocks

Potential variation introduced as described above, or through host-induced modification as discussed in Section 3.4, makes the choice of conditions for the growth of virus stocks an important decision. Additional important factors related to particle/infectivity ratios and purification will be considered in Section 3.3.

Long before the universality of defective viruses had been established, we made a conscious decision to grow all our NDV stocks in the following way: Virus obtained from other laboratories and mutants or variants which we have isolated are cloned two to three times by choosing widely separated plaques. After the final cloning, a seed stock is prepared and used to start all new stocks. Thus continuous passage is avoided. Stocks are grown by infecting eggs at relatively low multiplicities of infection (10^3–10^4 infectious units compared to the 10^8 cells in the chorioallantoic membrane of embryonated hen's eggs). This procedure represents a compromise between increasing the chances of obtaining defective particles by high-multiplicity passage (see Section 6.5) and allowing for the amplification of existing or newly mutated variants, by requring several rounds of multiplication. The latter problem can be monitored by carefully testing each new stock. Using these procedures, we have obtained uniform stocks involving as many as 35 preparations for a given virus, for almost 10 years.

Careful consideration of such factors and a conscious decision to grow virus stocks suited to the types of experiments for which they will be used would go a long way toward eliminating differences between findings in different laboratories and even within the same laboratory.

3.3. Particle Size Variation

3.3.1. Large and Small Hemagglutinins

Unpurified stocks of paramyxoviruses such as NDV contain variable amounts of particles which possess some but not all virus properties, such as neuraminidase and/or hemagglutinating activity, and which on sedimentation analysis behave as if they were smaller than infectious particles (hereafter referred to as the small and large hemagglutinating particles, respectively). Infectivity, hemolytic activity, and capacity to induce FFWO are associated with the large hemagglutinating particles, which therefore include, but are not limited to, normal and complete virions. By contrast, the small hemagglutinating particles (1) lack infectivity, but can interfere with infection by infectious virus (M. A. Bratt, unpublished); (2) are nonhemolytic, but are capable of interfering with hemolysis (Granoff and Henle, 1954; Hosaka, 1970; Clavell and Bratt, 1972a); and (3) are nonfusing, but are capable of interfering with FFWO (Hosaka, 1970; W. R. Gallaher and M. A. Bratt, unpublished).

Recently, LaMontagne et al. (1975) have observed these two populations of NDV particles in the electron microscope and found that the small hemagglutinating particles are indeed about half the size of the large particles. They also found that the specific activity of neuraminidase associated with the small particles was similar to that of the large particles, while the hemagglutinating activity per milligram of protein was two to three times greater. Such a result would be expected for smaller particles still able to make a bridge between red blood cells. The small hemagglutinating particles had a fatty acid composition similar to that of the large particles but differed from the latter in lacking RNA, nucleoprotein antigen, and the nucleocapsid protein, NP.

Roman and Simon (1976a) have recently shown that the relative proportions of these particles, and, in general, their size and density distribution, vary considerably for NDV grown in embryonated eggs, isolated chorioallantoic membranes, and tissue culture cells of various types. The significance of these differences is not clear, and their

interpretation is impeded by the fact that the virus grown in tissue culture was not virus spontaneously released into the extracellular fluids,
but cell-associated virus obtained by freezing and thawing cells.
Recognition of this problem brings us to the question of the origin of
the small hemagglutinating particles, which has also been considered
earlier by Simon (1972). LaMontagne *et al.* (1975) have suggested that
these particles may directly bud in this form from infected cells. An
alternative explanation is that they are formed by degradation of larger
particles. This could explain the larger proportion of small particles in
egg-grown virus than in tissue culture-grown virus observed by Roman
and Simon (1976a), since the egg-grown virus was harvested after much
longer incubation times, perhaps allowing more degradation to occur.
In this regard, it should be pointed out that Hosaka (1970) was able to
artificially prepare small hemagglutinating particles by sonicating
Sendai virus. Whatever the origin of the small hemagglutinating particles may be, it is clear that for most experiments they should be
eliminated by differential centrifugation.

3.3.2. Infectivity, Plaque-Forming Ability, and Noninfectious Particles

The larger hemagglutinating particles of paramyxoviruses always
possess relatively high particle-to-infectivity ratios. The origins of these
noninfectious particles, as in the case of the small hemagglutinating
particles, may be traced to such factors as conditions of production,
purification, and storage. Recognizing that truly noninfectious particles
exist, it is important to point out a subtler distinction between these and
particles which, although potentially infectious, for some reason at a
given time show no discernable sign of infection such as the production
of virus or a plaque. In his early studies on the genetic behavior of
NDV, Granoff (1959b) made the important observation of phenotypically mixed particles (see Section 6.2) in the single-cycle yields of cultures mixedly infected at very low multiplicities. Subsequently, Granoff
(1961b) showed that after mixed infection of cultures at multiplicities of
only 0.03 and 0.18 PFU/cell for each of two NDV strains, 9.7% of the
single-cycle yields were phenotypically mixed, and 8.6% of the infected
cells yielded both genotypes, in contrast to an expected value of 1.2%
mixedly infected cells. Obviously, particles which did not register as
plaque-forming units were able to contribute toward the production of
progeny virus. In addition, Marcus (1959) found that the titer of cell-
killing particles of NDV was also considerably higher than the titer

measured as plaque-forming particles. Recognition of the existence of potentially infectious but non-plaque-forming virus must be considered in such diverse areas as cloning of virus and in the discussion of heterozygotes (Section 6.3) and multiplicity reactivation (Section 6.4).

3.3.3. Cell-Associated Virus

In contrast with most nonenveloped viruses which mature and accumulate within cells, many enveloped viruses mature by budding through an altered plasma membrane and accumulate within cells to only limited extents. A prime example of this is to be found in the early study of Rubin *et al.* (1957) on the multiplication of NDV in chick embryo lung epithelium. They compared virus spontaneously released into the medium and cell-associated virus (CAV) released by alternate cycles of freezing and thawing. They found little evidence for accumulation of virus in cells. If neutralizing antibody was added to the cultures and then removed prior to freezing and thawing, 85–95% of the CAV was inactivated, indicating that most of this virus was located at the cell surface. To this day it has remained unclear whether CAV measured by freezing and thawing or sonication represents virus which (1) has accumulated within the cell, (2) is on the surface but not yet released, or (3) has readsorbed after release.

Thacore and Youngner (1969, 1970) showed that the apparent abortive infection of mouse L cells by the Herts strain of NDV was really a "covert" infection. Measuring CAV, they found that these cells indeed produce considerable amounts of virus but don't release it. A variant of this virus was able to release itself. Interestingly, these viruses exhibited the opposite behavior after adsorption to chicken red blood cells—80% of the infectivity of the Herts strain which had adsorbed to red blood cells would elute, compared to only 20% for the variant. Differences in thermal stability of the neuraminidase activity of the two viruses were subsequently demonstrated (Thacore and Youngner, 1971). While other differences between the two viruses were also detected, this result suggests the possibility that the different behavior of these viruses is due to changes in the HN glycoprotein, although how this might be related to different elution behavior from L cells and red blood cells remains obscure. An alternative explanation (which might still be related to the behavior of the HN glycoprotein) is that the two viruses differ in the extent to which interaction with red blood cells inactivates virus (Clavell and Bratt, 1972b). Alternatively, the differential release from infected L cells exhibited by the Herts stain and its variant could involve differences in requirements for protease activation of infectivity in a manner similar to the protease activation mutants of Sendai virus (Section 5.1) (Scheid and Choppin, 1976) or the different strains of NDV (Nagai *et al.,* 1976). A necessary protease might be available only after the Herts strain-infected cells are disrupted. The variant might not require access to this protease or might sufficiently disrupt the cell to release it.

Whatever the reason for these findings, it is clear that the measurement of CAV can be a valuable tool in evaluating infection. However, while it may give increased viral yields in certain cases, it presents serious potential dangers if the physical properties of virus are to be measured. Clearly, freezing and thawing or sonicating cells could have the effect of increasing particle/infectivity ratios either by inactivating already infectious virus or by breaking it down into smaller particles (Hosaka, 1970). It could potentially also create membrane vesicles both larger and smaller than normal virions which might or might not contain viral nucleocapsids and possess infectivity. Examples of potential problems with this will be discussed below in the sections on defective particles (Section 6.5) and multiploid particles (Section 6.4).

3.4. Host-Induced Modification

"Host-induced modification" refers to transient phenotypic changes in viral populations occurring during a single passage in cells of a different type, which are fully reversible on passage in the original cell type. It should not be confused with genotypic selection, which can also depend on cell type and conditions of culture, but which usually occurs more slowly and is not as readily reversible.

Differences in heat sensitivity were reported by Marcus (1960) for NDV grown in embryonated eggs and HeLa cells. Drake and Lay (1962) also found that NDV grown in cultured chick embryo cells differed in heat sensitivity from virus grown either in embryonated eggs or in isolated chorioallantoic membranes, and also in sensitivity to acid and ultraviolet irradiation. Differences in heat and pH sensitivity might be explained by differences in host cell components—lipids or carbohydrates—in the virus. Differences in the slopes of the ultraviolet light inactivation curves are less easily explained. Subsequently, Stenback and Durand (1963) found significant differences in the density of NDV grown in avian and mammalian cells and suggested that this might be due to differences in the lipid composition of these viruses. Simpson and Hauser (1966) reported that the infectivity of NDV grown in chick embryo cells in culture was inactivated by phospholipase C, while virus grown in the allantoic cavity was not. Klenk and Choppin (1969, 1970a,b) subsequently demonstrated that SV5 grown in different cell types differs both quantitatively and qualitatively in lipid composition, and that the lipid composition of the virus closely reflects that of the host cell plasma membrane.

Differences in biological behavior are also found when paramyxoviruses are grown in different cell types. In the early 1960s, Ishida and Homma (1960, 1961) and Matsumoto and Maeno (1962) found that infectivity for various cell types and hemolytic activity was changed when HVJ was grown in different hosts. Additional reports of differences in hemolytic activity, cell-fusing activity (FFWO), infectivity, and adsorption characteristics for HVJ (Sendai) and NDV grown in different cells have subsequently appeared (Kohn and Fuchs, 1969; Young and Ash, 1970, 1974; Homma, 1971, 1972, 1975; Homma and Ohuchi, 1973; Homma and Tamagawa, 1973; Scheid and Choppin, 1974, 1975, 1976). Such changes might have been attributed to changes in the lipid or carbohydrate composition of the virus, accompanying passage in different cells. Indeed, both hemolytic activity and ability to induce FFWO require association with lipids (Kohn, 1965; Kohn and Klibansky, 1967; Hosaka and Shimizu, 1972; Hosaka, 1975). However, for Sendai virus both of these activities have been shown to be associated with the F glycoprotein. Homma and Ohuchi (1973), Homma (1975), and Scheid and Choppin (1974, 1975, 1976) have shown that virus grown in certain cells contains F_0 (the precursor of the F protein), while virus grown in other cells possesses the product of cleavage, F. Treatment of virus grown in the former cells with proteases results in simultaneous cleavage of the F_0 glycoprotein and aquisition of infectivity, hemolytic activity, and cell-fusing activity. Host-dependent differences in glycoprotein cleavage have also been associated with differences in biological activities for a number of avirulent strains of NDV (Nagai et al., 1976). Whether such differences in cleavage can account for all differences in behavior of NDV grown in different cell types (Young and Ash, 1970, 1974; Kohn and Fuchs, 1969) remains to be determined. Furthermore, whether strain-specific differences in cell-fusing and hemolytic activity can also be explained on the basis of differences in sensitivity to cleavage of the precursor, as Choppin and Compans (1975) have suggested, remains to be determined. Similarly, differences in ability of virulent strains of NDV to induce fusion from within—induction in BHK-21 cells and chick embryo cells on the one hand, and no induction in MDBK cells on the other (Bratt and Gallaher, 1972)—might be determined by differences in proteolytic cleavage.

Another example of host cell-dependent variation is the ability to produce transient changes in the genomes of paramyxoviruses, as, for example, in the cell-specific differences in production of defective virus particles reported for Sendai virus (Kingsbury and Portner, 1970), SV5 (Choppin and Compans, 1975), and possibly also NDV (Roman and Simon, 1976*b*).

3.5. Distinctions between Genetically Different Populations

With the propensity for genetic diversity and rapid change, the definition of the types of genetically differing populations is particularly important. Genetically differing entities range from different serotypes such as NDV and measles virus, through different strains of a given serotype, to variants, single-step mutants, and defective particles. Additional variety is provided by the use of different host cells which show greatly varying responses to viral infection and have the potential for altering virus populations through host-induced modification (Section 3.4).

3.5.1. Relationships among Paramyxoviruses—Different Serotypes

The majority of the paramyxoviruses tested thus far contain genome RNAs which vary little from the standard 50 S size and estimated molecular weight of $5.0\text{--}5.4 \times 10^6$ (Kolakofsky *et al.*, 1974*a*, 1975). Base compositions for NDV (Duesberg and Robinson, 1965; Kingsbury, 1966*a*), Sendai virus (Iwai *et al.*, 1966; Blair and Robinson, 1968), SV5 (Compans and Choppin, 1968; Bussell *et al.*, 1974), measles virus and canine distemper virus (Bussell *et al.*, 1974), and an SSPE variant of measles virus (Yeh, 1973) are strikingly similar to each other and suggest possible genetic similarity. However, cross-annealing studies using potentially complementary RNAs of NDV, mumps virus, and Sendai virus reveal little if any homology (Blair and Robinson, 1968; East and Kingsbury, 1971).

Historically, Newcastle disease virus and mumps virus have been reported to show antigenic cross-reactions (see Chanock and Coates, 1964), but, as already mentioned, annealing studies provide no evidence of genetic similarity. Antigenetic cross-reactions have also been reported for measles, canine distemper, and rinderpest viruses (see Chanock and Coates, 1964; Warren, 1960; Örvell and Norrby, 1974). In fact, Örvell and Norrby (1974) could not detect antigenic differences between the nucleocapsids of these three viruses. Nevertheless, definitive proof that these are true reflections of genetic homology must await cross-annealing studies. In this regard, the search for genetic similarity would be most effective if annealing studies employed genome RNAs and individual mRNAs. One would expect external components such as the glycoproteins to vary the most, while internal structural components such as nucleocapsid proteins would vary the least, as in the case of influenza viruses (see Compans and Choppin, 1975). This appears to be the case for antigens of measles, canine distemper, and rinderpest viruses (Örvell and Norrby, 1974). Annealing studies employing the messages for the genetically more stable elements should provide a more precise measure of genetic similarity. Another possible explanation for reported antigenic cross-reactions, which would not require genetic similarity, would be similarities in glycoprotein antigens due mainly to the carbohydrate portion of the molecules. Such an explanation might account for the finding of Brostrom et al. (1971) which suggests a serological relationship for the isolated neuraminidases of NDV and Sendai virus, since, as mentioned above, the RNAs of these viruses show no cross-annealing.

3.5.2. Strains

The term "strains" denotes independently isolated viruses which show extensive cross-reaction and constitute a serotype (Schloer, 1974; Schloer et al., 1975; Lief et al., 1975; Payne and Baublis, 1973). Genetic homology among such strains is extensive, as in the case of NDV, where cross-annealing studies have indicated 95% homology (Kingsbury, 1966b; Blair and Robinson, 1968; Bratt, unpublished), and also for the 6/94 strain and another strain of Sendai virus (Kolakofsky, et al., 1974b). Again, annealing studies employing individual mRNAs of the glycoproteins, for instance, might reveal lesser degrees of homology.

Although extensive cross-reaction defines a serotype, systematic studies on antigenic relationships within a serotype employing neutralization kinetics, neutralization end points, or hemagglutination inhibition can yield anomalous results, as found with NDV (Upton et al., 1953; Schloer, 1974; Schloer et al., 1975; Bratt and Gallaher, 1972; Bratt, unpublished), Sendai virus (Lief et al., 1975), and measles virus

(Payne and Baublis; 1973). The anomaly is that certain specific antisera may show greater apparent cross-reaction with heterologous strains than with the homologous strain. This anomaly has variously been interpreted as being due to differences in quantity of surface antigens, differences in avidity, and differences in reactivity. For NDV, Bratt and Gallaher (1972) and Bratt (unpublished) have related this phenomenon to other surface interactions of virus and cells. Nevertheless, it is possible to prepare strain-specific sera by cross-adsorption (Granoff, 1959a), and sometimes using unadsorbed sera as well. Using such sera, antigenic differences between strains of a single serotype have been found (Upton *et al.,* 1953; Chanock and Coates, 1964; Payne and Baublis, 1973; Gomez-Lillo *et al.,* 1974; Schloer, 1974; Schloer *et al.,* 1975; Lief *et al.,* 1975).

3.5.3. Variants

For the purpose of this discussion, any virus which differs from a cloned or uncloned parental virus by an unknown number of genetic changes will be considered as a "variant." Included among these must be all genetically differing viruses (1) isolated from stocks which have never, or not recently, been cloned, (e. g., the plaque-type variants found in uncloned populations of various strains (Section 5.2)) (2) obtained after extensive passage of even cloned virus, and (3) isolated from persistent infections. These undefined variants carry with them inherent dangers for studies designed to identify causal relationships and to ascribe phenotypic changes to specific genetic defects. They have potential for these uses only when repeated completely independent isolates show identical correlations of properties, and even then the correlation must be viewed with extreme caution.

3.5.4. Mutants

In the paramyxovirus literature, the term "mutant" is more often than not used loosely to describe the general class of viral variants described above. At best the effect is confusing, and at worst it leads to misinterpretation. The term "mutant" should be reserved for a virus which is likely to be isogenic with a cloned parental virus (by convention, usually referred to as "wild type") with the exception of a single base change. Obviously, the great potential for change among these viruses (Sections 3.1 and 3.2) makes it clear that successful isolation of mutants likely to fit these criteria requires as few passages as possible between cloning and mutant selection.

An additional criterion for point mutations is usually an ability to revert to wild type at a frequency not grossly different from the original mutation frequency. Techniques with paramyxovirus are not yet sophisticated enough to allow a distinction to be made between same-site and other-site reversions to wild type. Obviously, reversion rates for mutants like *ts* mutants will be considerably lower than their original rates of isolation since the initial *ts* mutations can potentially be in any part of the genome coding for a protein, while the back mutation must usually be within the same gene as the original mutation, if not at the same site.

3.5.5. Defective Virus

As for other animal viruses, passage of paramyxoviruses at high multiplicities of infection can result in the production of noninfectious particles designated as defective interfering particles or incomplete virus (see Choppin and Compans, 1975; Huang, 1973; see also Huang and Baltimore in Volume 10 of this series). These particles tend to be smaller than normal particles and contain genomes with characteristic sizes significantly smaller than the normal 50 S RNA. As such, they may represent specific deletions. Defective particles are considered in Section 6.5.

4. ORIGINS OF MUTANTS AND VARIANTS

4.1. Spontaneous vs. Mutagenized Isolates

The studies of Granoff (1961a) and Thiry (1963, 1964) showed that plaque-type mutants can be isolated from cloned NDV populations at frequencies ranging from 0.001% to 1.0%. In some instances, these high values reflect a selective effect for plaque size heterogeneity during a single passage in embryonated eggs observed by Durand and Eisenstark (1962), as described in Section 3.1. We isolated spontaneous *ts* mutants of NDV at a frequency of 2% (Tsipis and Bratt, 1976). This relatively high frequency is probably a reflection of the ability of *ts* mutations to occur in most if not all of the viral genes. It should be pointed out, however, that high frequencies are not restricted to paramyxoviruses or animal viruses, but rather seem to be characteristic of RNA genomes, since RNA phages also have very high mutation frequencies (see Weissmann *et al.*, 1973).

Treatment of virus with mutagens can increase the isolation frequency for mutants of particular markers by as much as ten- to a hundredfold over spontaneous levels (Granoff, 1961*a*; Thiry, 1963, 1964). These increases were shown to be due to induced mutation frequencies rather than to selection of preexisting mutants. Our frequency of *ts* mutant isolation was increased only twofold when mutagens were used (Tsipis and Bratt, 1976). In such cases, it would be difficult to determine whether the mutants isolated are the result of the mutagen or simply spontaneous mutations. Therefore, the use of mutagens may dramatically increase the probability of isolating virus with multiple mutations, as has been the problem with influenza virus (see Hightower and Bratt, this volume). For example, both Granoff (1961*a*) and Thiry (1964) reported that small plaque mutants obtained from stocks treated with the mutagen nitrous acid or hydroxylamine were considerably more stable than spontaneous mutants. The greater stability of these mutants could be the result of multiple-site mutations. For this reason, if mutagenesis must be used, the conditions should be chosen so as to increase mutation rates only slightly so that the possibility that a virus will carry more than one mutation can be kept to a minimum.

4.2. Mutagens

Potential mutagens fall into two classes: (1) those which when used to treat virions cause changes in the nucleotide bases of the viral genome and (2) base analogues or reagents which when added to infected cells are presumably incorporated into the viral nucleic acids. The mutagenic effect of the latter is thought to be due to a direct mispairing of bases, but may also result from increased susceptibility of the produced virus to external stimuli such as visible or ultraviolet light, nitrous acid, or other reagents as discussed by Thiry (1966).

The use of base analogues carries with it the serious danger of obtaining many isolates of the same mutant. If virus is grown in 5-fluorouracil, for instance, a mispairing of bases may occur in an early round of replication, with the result that many of the virus particles released from the cell will contain the same mutation. Isolation of a number of mutants from the same mutagenesis experiment can then result in numerous isolations of the same identical mutant. If these viruses contain the same multiple mutations, their use could lead to false impressions of covariation (Section 5) or could suggest causal relationships between completely unrelated properties. Similarly, if many identical isolates of the same *ts* mutant were obtained in this way, they would lead to false creation of a complementation group whose members all show identical functional defects. To avoid this problem when using this type of mutagen, only one mutant of any given type should be chosen from each mutagenesis experiment. Obviously, mutants isolated under these conditions but which are within different complementation groups and/or show different functional defects can be safely used.

Reagents which are probably mutagenic for paramyxoviruses include nitrous acid (Granoff, 1961*a*; Thiry, 1963; 1964; Preble and Youngner, 1973*b*; Tsipis and Bratt, 1976; Scheid and Choppin, 1976), hydroxylamine, ethylethane sulfonate, and dimethylsulfate (Thiry, 1963), and nitrosoguanidine (Portner *et al.,* 1974; Tsipis and Bratt, 1976; A. Hamburger, C. S. Raine, R. B. Johnson, and B. N. Fields, personal communication). The most commonly used base analogue is 5-fluorouracil (Yamazi and Black, 1972; Bergholz *et al.,* 1975; Haspel *et al.,* 1975*a*; Tsipis and Bratt, 1976). 5-Azacytidine was used by Haspel *et al.* (1975*a*). Proflavin was used by Yamazi and Black (1972) and Haspel *et al.* (1975*a*). An extensive discussion of the effects of these and other base analogues is given by Thiry (1966).

Of considerable interest is the tendency of some mutagens to induce particular types of mutations. Granoff (1961*a*) obtained small plaque mutants after nitrous acid treatment of NDV, but while back mutations were found to occur spontaneously, nitrous acid did not increase the frequency of these back mutations. Thiry (1963) also found that "red" plaque mutants (Section 5) and small plaque mutants were regularly obtained after either nitrous acid or hydroxylamine treatment. Again, back mutations could not be obtained with these reagents. In contrast, she found that two alkylating agents, ethylethane sulfonate and dimethylsulfate, induced no plaque size mutations, and no "red" plaque mutations, but induced back mutations from "red" plaque to the standard plaque genotype. In analyzing the phenotypes of the plaque size mutations, she also found evidence for covariation. Plaque size mutants obtained after hydroxylamine and nitrous acid treatment tended to be affected also in a property involving the quantity of hemagglutinin produced by the infected cell. The plaque size mutants obtained after treatment with hydroxylamine also tended to be altered in properties related to interferon production and sensitivity to an inhibitor in agar (Thiry, 1964). While the mechanisms of action of these mutagens are thought to involve specific alterations of specific nucleotide bases (see Granoff, 1961a; Thiry, 1963, 1964), it is difficult to understand why mutations in both directions would not be induced by the same mutagen. Also difficult to understand is the apparent specificity in inducing particular mutations but not others. Possible causes of this apparent specificity have been discussed by both Granoff (1961a) and Thiry (1963, 1964) but no definitive explanation is available. However, the possibility has been considered that secondary structure of phage RNA might impose some specificity on mutagenesis by nitrous acid and hydroxylamine (cf. Weissmann et al., 1973), and provides a potential explanation for these findings.

5. TYPES OF MUTANTS AND VARIANTS

Mutants or variants obtained by selection or screening for alterations in a particular property often on further analysis reveal changes in any number of other properties. A single-site point mutation can simultaneously change a number of properties (covariation) if it occurs in a gene whose product has more than one function or can be measured in more than one way. For instance, an NDV mutant showing altered thermostability in its neuraminidase may also show altered thermostability in its hemagglutinin (see Pierce and Haywood, 1973). This presumably would be attributable to the fact that both properties are associated with the HN protein (see Sections 2.5.1 and 2.5.2). Similarly, an NDV mutant selected for altered thermostability of infectivity can also be altered antigenically and in plaque-forming ability (Granoff, 1964b). Again, each of these phenotypic changes could be a reflection of one and the same change in the HN protein since (1) inactivation of this protein will prevent infection, (2) neutralization involves combination of antibody with this protein, and (3) plaque formation requires synthesis of the HN protein and its interaction with adjacent cells. However, every mutation within such a gene need not necessarily affect all of the functions or measurable properties in the same way.

Another way in which a single point mutation can result in multiple phenotypic changes is if it occurs in a gene on which other genes are dependent. For example, as will be seen in Section 7, temperature-sensitive mutants which are defective in RNA synthesis will usually be deficient in antigen formation, hemadsorption, and fusion from within—pleiotropic effects of inability to synthesize the mRNAs for the proteins involved in each of these properties. Mutants defective in the gene for any one of these other proteins would not necessarily show alterations in the other properties. Finally, variants with multiple mutations may also show multiple, but not necessarily related, phenotypic defects. These distinctions are of considerable importance for viruses in general, and for paramyxoviruses in particular, not only because the terms "variant" and "mutant" have been so loosely used in the paramyxovirus literature but also because the high ratio of properties to genes (Section 2.5) allows considerable opportunity for pleiotropy and covariation. These considerations emphasize the importance of distinguishing among (1) the marker origi- nally selected or screened for, (2) any other properties which might be affected, and (3) the gene in which the mutation has occurred.

These considerations are also of importance in reference to a phenomenon such as "leakiness." This term is properly used only to describe the originally selected property. For example, a *ts* mutant which appears adequately inhibited in multiplication in a single cycle, but produces virus (still *ts*) under multiple-cycle conditions, can be described as leaky under the multiple-cycle conditions. However, if a mutant selected for temperature-sensitivity of growth shows reduced, but not completely inhibited, RNA synthesis at the nonpermissive tempera- ture ($RNA^{+/-}$ rather than RNA^-), it would be incorrect to describe it as "leaky" for RNA synthesis; it merely has a reduced RNA phenotype. Similarly, a hypothetical mutant selected for reduced neuraminidase activity but found also to be partially defective in hemagglutinating activity should not be described as leaky for the latter activity; it merely shows reduced hemagglutinating activity.

Selection of, or screening for, mutants can be either direct (for a specific property as in Section 5.1) or indirect as in the case of screen- ing for plaque-type mutants or variants (Sections 5.1 and 5.2) or temperature-sensitive mutants (Section 7).

5.1. Selection for Specifically Altered Properties

In spite of the variety of biological properties for which specific mutants might be directly selected, only limited steps have been taken in that direction. As previously mentioned, selection of mutants with altered thermostability of neuraminidase activity (and, simultaneously, hemagglutinating activity) probably involved direct selection for muta- tions in NDV's HN glycoprotein (see Pierce and Haywood, 1973). Similarly, the selection of thermostable mutants or variants of NDV

(Goldman and Hanson, 1955; Granoff, 1959*a*, 1964*a,b*; Picken, 1964), which in one case (Granoff, 1964*b*) were also found to be altered in sensitivity to neutralization by antibody, probably also represents direct selection for an altered HN protein. Selection of measles virus with reduced sensitivity to neutralizing antibody (Payne and Baublis, 1973) probably also resulted in the isolation of mutants or variants with an altered hemagglutinating protein.

To date, however, the best examples of direct selection are the protease activation mutants of Sendai virus isolated by Scheid and Choppin (1976). As mentioned in Sections 2.5 and 3.4, for Sendai virus, infectivity, cell fusing, and hemolytic activities require cleavage of the F_0 glycoprotein to F. For wild-type virus, cleavage and acquisition of these properties occur in embryonated eggs but not in MDBK cells. As a consequence of this, MDBK-grown virus is unable to go through the multiple cycles of multiplication required to produce a plaque. Cleavage of F_0 and concomitant activation of MDBK cell-grown virus can be obtained by treatment with trypsin but not with elastase or chymotrypsin. Furthermore, if incorporated into the overlay medium, trypsin will allow plaque formation in MDBK cells. Scheid and Choppin (1976) selected mutants able to grow in multiple cycles and form plaques in MDBK cells in the presence of either elastase or chymotrypsin. The two chymotrypsin-activated mutants could also plaque in the presence of elastase, but had lost the ability to do so in the presence of trypsin. They had also lost the ability to grow in the embryonated egg unless elastase or chymotrypsin was added with the virus. One of the eight elastase-activated mutants showed properties similar to the chymotrypsin-activated mutants except that it multiplied poorly in MDBK cells in the presence of chymotrypsin. In contrast, the remaining seven elastase-activated mutants were still able to multiply in MDBK cells in the presence of trypsin but not chymotrysin. These had also maintained the ability to multiply in the embryonated egg without added protease. The one chymotrypsin-activated mutant which was tested had the same protease specificity for activation of hemolytic activity as described above for infectivity and multiplication. For the mutants tested, the polypeptide patterns of egg- and MDBK-grown virus were consistent with a requirement of cleavage of F_0 for activation of these properties.

These protease activation mutants have thus (1) provided a means of specifically selecting mutations in the F gene, (2) indirectly allowed for the selection of host range mutants, and (3) provided strong supporting evidence for the role of F in infectivity and hemolysis.

5.2. Plaque-Type Mutants and Variants

With the development of the plaque assay, plaque-type mutants became an obvious tool for studying genetic variation. For the paramyxoviruses, there were mainly two types: size (large, small, minute plaques, etc.) and morphology ("red" vs. "white" or turbid vs. clear plaques).

5.2.1. Plaque Size

Large and small plaque-forming variants have been consistently found in uncloned stocks of various strains of NDV (Granoff, 1961a, 1964a; Durand and Eisenstark, 1962; Thiry, 1963; Schloer and Hanson, 1968; Schloer, 1974; Estupinan and Hanson, 1971a) and measles virus (Rapp, 1964; Gould, 1974). On cloning, these plaque size variants tend to breed true, although Durand and Eisenstark (1962) had difficulties in obtaining homogeneous stocks during egg passage of NDV. Gould (1974) was unable to obtain a stable clone of a small plaque variant of measles virus.

As described previously, both Granoff (1961a) and Thiry (1963) were able to significantly increase the isolation frequency of small plaque mutants from large plaque clones by treatment with nitrous acid or hydroxylamine. However, mutagenization would not increase the frequency of revertants from small to large plaque-formers above the relatively low spontaneous level. In fact, mutagenesis of small plaque mutants allowed the isolation of minute plaque mutants (Thiry, 1963).

This brings us to the question of the factors responsible for these plaque size differences. While it seems clear that small plaque mutants can result from single-step mutations, it is unlikely that a specific viral gene is responsible for plaque size. It is more reasonable to assume that changes in almost any viral gene can slow down the rate of multiplication or spread to other cells—factors as diverse as slowed rates of transcription or production of an inefficiently adsorbing hemagglutinin, for instance. The tendency to mutate only in the direction of smaller plaques, and the finding that on a second round of mutagenesis minute mutants—representing a further decrease in plaque size—can be isolated, suggests that the smaller plaque type is merely an indication of lowered efficiency of multiplication or spread. Unfortunately, no information is available on the relative rates of multiplication of otherwise isogenic plaque size mutants. The differing behavior of NDV variants observed by Schloer and Hanson (1971) cannot be evaluated because there is no way to determine the extent of genetic differences between these variants. Thiry (1964), however, did find that a fairly large proportion of her small plaque mutants produced significantly lower amounts of hemagglutinin.

Relative plaque size is of interest beyond its usefulness as a genetic marker because of its correlation with virulence *in vivo*. In analyzing 14 strains of NDV, Schloer and Hanson (1968) found a correlation between the tendency to make large plaques and *in vivo* virulence measured in several ways. This correlation applies also to small plaque variants of measles virus (Rapp, 1964), NDV (Schloer and Hanson, 1971), and NDV mutants (Granoff, 1961*a*, 1964*a,b*; Thiry, 1964). As might be expected, the studies on NDV mutants show that the correlation is not absolute, but there is a tendency for small plaque mutants of NDV to be less virulent in chick embryos or mice.

The tendency to change mainly in the direction of smaller plaques was also observed by Schloer and Hanson (1971), and the usually accompanying decrease in virulence suggested to these authors that such changes may be associated with strain attenuation in nature. Evidence for such changes in plaque type was found during the progression of the 1971–1973 NDV epizootic in California (Schloer, personal communication), and attenuation was simultaneously observed (Utterback and Schwartz, 1973; Schloer, personal communication).

5.2.2. Red Plaques

Animal virus plaques are commonly identified after the addition of the vital dye neutral red to the agar overlay. They appear as unstained or white areas (where dead cells have not accumulated the dye) against the background of stained living cells. As others have noted for both NDV (Thiry, 1963) and measles virus (Rapp, 1964; Atherton *et al.*, 1965), plaques usually show a transient hyperaccumulation of dye before the standard white plaque forms. Although attempts were made by each group, only Thiry (1963) was able to obtain mutants which maintained a red plaque phenotype. One mutant caused hyperaccumulation of dye under agar between 4 and 6 days after infection (if the dye was added at 4 days). The red plaques would subsequently disappear, leaving no alterations in the monolayer. In liquid medium, the cytopathic effects occurred 2–3 days later than in wild-type infection, and large amounts of virus were produced until that time (the possibility that wild-type revertants were responsible for this lysis was considered but not explored). This mutant also showed lowered pathogenicity in mice.

Red plaque variants of two other NDV strains have been studied by Schloer and Hanson (1971) and Estupinan and Hanson (1971a,b). Unlike Thiry's (1963) mutant, Schloer and Hanson's (1971) red plaque variant showed a prolonged period of hyperaccumulation of the dye, but this was then followed by lysis and whitening of the plaque (whether this was due to white plaque revertants is unclear). This variant seemed to be as virulent in embryonated eggs as the white plaque variant with which it was compared. The white and red plaque variants of Estupinan and Hanson (1971b) differed from each other in that the former was genetically stable while the latter continuously shed white plaque revertants. The significance of these results is unclear since the extent of the genetic differences between the original two variants is unknown.

The factors responsible for the red plaque phenotype are not known, nor is it clear whether mutations within only one gene, or more, can give this phenotype. Allison and Mallucci (1965) showed that both the transient red plaque stage of wild-type virus and the red plaque characteristic of Thiry's (1963) spontaneous red plaque mutant are due to increased accumulation of the dye in the lysosomes of the infected cell. Vamos (1966), also using Thiry's (1963) wild-type virus and spontaneous red plaque mutant, was unable to correlate red plaque formation with any viral property other than a lack of early inhibition of amino acid incorporation seen in wild-type infection. No causal relationship was established, however. Further attempts to correlate the red plaque phenotype with other viral properties using NDV variants were unsuccessful (Schloer and Hanson, 1971).

5.2.3. Turbid Plaques

Granoff (1959a, 1961a) described the isolation of a turbid variant (mutant?) which appears at a frequency of 10^{-2} in stocks of the RO (California, 1944) strain of NDV. In contrast to the majority of viruses in those stocks which produced standard white plaques, the variant produced a plaque with ill-defined borders, and lysed only a fraction of the cells, leaving some stainable cells intact. Nitrous acid treatment would neither increase the frequency of turbid plaques in the original stock cultures nor change the frequency of intermediate forms, which appeared at a rate of 0.02% in cloned turbid plaque stocks. This mutant, which was used by Granoff in his mixed infection experiments (Granoff, 1959a,b, 1962; Kingsbury and Granoff, 1970), was found to have a lowered plating efficiency in acid agar and lower virulence than the wild-type strain, but has not been further characterized.

6. GENETIC AND PARAGENETIC PHENOMENA

6.1. Recombination

Our knowledge of paramyxovirus genetic structure and replicative patterns provides little encouragement for the possibility of either the existence or detection of true genetic recombination for these viruses. First, most if not all of their intracellular life is spent in the cytoplasm, away from the enzymes involved in cellular DNA recombination. It is not even known whether such enzymes would be able to work on RNA genomes, were they available to them. However, the possibility of a mechanism for recombination of cytoplasmic RNA is held open by the limited evidence for recombination for poliovirus (Cooper, this volume). Second, a genome of covalently linked single-stranded RNA would seem to eliminate the possibility of genetic reassortment available to myxoviruses (Hightower and Bratt, this volume) and reoviruses (Cross and Fields, this volume). Furthermore, a genome size of 5–5.4×10^6 daltons, although over twice that of poliovirus, might permit only low levels of recombination even if mechanisms were available for it to occur. Finally, any true recombination would probably be obscured either by the relatively high reversion frequencies for many markers or by the high frequency of heterozygote formation, to be discussed below.

In his pioneering study on mixed infection with two strains of NDV, Granoff (1959a) was unable to show genetic recombination. His subsequent use of plaque-type mutants of one of these strains (Granoff, 1961a) may have eliminated some of the potential problems embodied in the use of different strains. However, in both of these studies, failure to obtain recombination could be due to localization of all markers within a small part of the genome; e.g., the markers in the first study (Granoff, 1959a)—plaque type, heat stability of hemagglutinin and infectivity, and serotype—could all be measures of the hemagglutinin. With the introduction of temperature-sensitive mutants and their potential for saturating most of the genome, Kirvaitis and Simon (1965) thought they detected recombination for NDV. However, Dahlberg and Simon (1969a) subsequently demonstrated that the supposed recombinant progeny were, in fact, complementing heterozygotes which segregated parental *ts* genotypes on subsequent passage—similar to Granoff's earlier demonstration of heterozygotes among progeny of mixed infection (Granoff, 1959*b*, 1962). The high frequency of heterozygotes (values as high as 15% of progeny of mixed infection) could potentially obscure low levels of recombination in all such studies. Therefore, it must be concluded that genetic recombination has not been detected for NDV. Similarly, no evidence for recombination has been detected where it has been looked for with measles virus (F. L. Black and Y. Yamazi, personal communication; A. Hamburger, C. S. Raine, R. B. Johnson, and B. N. Fields, personal communication).

6.2. Phenotypic Mixing

Cells mixedly infected with two compatible viruses often produce progeny virus containing the nucleic acid of one or the other of the parental types, but enclosed in capsids or envelopes containing proteins of either both parents or only the heterologous parent (the latter often being referred to as "pseudotypes"). This results in an acquisition of properties of the heterologous virus, referred to as "phenotypic mixing," which is transient since subsequent passage reveals that each particle possessed the genotype of only one parent. A possible exception is the little-understood case where apparent heterozygotes of NDV (see Section 6.4) continue to yield phenotypically mixed progeny of each parental genotype for several generations (Granoff, 1959*b*, 1962).

Granoff (1959*b*, 1962) demonstrated phenotypic mixing for paramyxoviruses using two different strains of NDV. The phenotypically mixed particles possessed a thermal stability intermediate between those of the parental viruses. In addition, a fraction of the progeny were neutralizable by antisera prepared against each of the parental types. Subsequently, Norrby (1965) reported phenotypic mixing between two unrelated paramyxoviruses. When cells chronically infected with measles virus but producing no virus were superinfected with Sendai virus, virions containing Sendai virus genomes but the adsorption and elution characteristics of both paramyxoviruses were produced.

Actually, the first demonstration of phenotypic mixing with a paramyxovirus involved NDV and the orthomyxovirus influenza A (Granoff and Hirst, 1954). Subsequently, Choppin and Compans (1970) and McSharry *et al.* (1971) provided another example of phenotypic mixing involving a paramyxovirus (SV5) and a virus of another type (the rhabdovirus, VSV). They found VSV genomes in envelopes neutralizable by VSV antiserum alone, by SV5 antiserum alone, or by either antiserum. The VSV genomes were shown to be encapsidated in typical bullet-shaped particles. However, they contained SV5 antigens and could adsorb to and elute from chicken erythrocytes, indicating the presence of SV5 hemagglutinin and neuraminidase activities. McSharry *et al.* (1971) demonstrated that VSV genomes and nucleocapsids could have the spike glycoproteins of either VSV or SV5, but that the membrane protein, M, must be that of VSV. This suggested that recognition between nucleocapsid and altered cell membrane requires a specific interaction between the nucleocapsid protein and the membrane protein. Whether such restrictions are exhibited in other cases of phenotypic mixing involving paramyxoviruses remains to be determined.

The finding that virus budding can occur with glycoproteins of antigenically unrelated viruses is of considerable interest since host proteins are not normally incorporated into virions. This suggests a basic difference between viral and host glycoproteins. In this regard, it is interesting to note that cells infected by a *ts* mutant of Sendai virus (Portner *et al.,* 1975) release virus particles at the nonpermissive temperature which lack both hemagglutinating and neuraminidase activity and which contain no HN glycoprotein, but which appear structurally similar to normal virus particles when observed in the electron microscope. It would be interesting to know whether these particles which lack the HN glycopeptide contain host cell glycopeptides instead—a possibility suggested by a heterogeneous distribution of polypeptides seen in these particles but not seen in normal virus. As the authors suggest, however, these extra polypeptides might simply represent host glycoproteins nonspecifically adsorbed to the particles because of the absence of neuraminidase (Portner, *et al.,* 1975). Alternatively, the presence of the F glycopeptide might be sufficient to allow budding and also give the virus a normal appearance.

6.3. Heterozygotes and Multiploid Particles

Granoff (1959*b*, 1962), and Kingsbury and Granoff (1970) reported that 10% or more of the progeny of dual infection by two different cloned strains of NDV yielded progeny of both parental types on subsequent passage. These mixed yielders were designated as heterozygotes and thought to consist of particles containing the complete genomes of both parental types. A similar finding was obtained by Dahlberg and Simon (1969a) using large and small plaque mutants of another NDV strain. Dahlberg and Simon (1969a) also found that the apparent recombinants which Kirvaitis and Simon (1965) had obtained from dual infection with complementing temperature-sensitive mutants were, instead, complementing heterozygotes.

Hypothetical explanations for these findings include the possibilities that the heterozygotes are (1) clumps consisting of virions of each of the two parental types; (2) virions which contain more than one complete genome of each type and each of which functions independently; (3) virions which contain more than one complete genome of each type, only one of which can function alone, while all others are dependent on it; or (4) virions which contain the complete genome of one parental type and only a portion of the other type of genome. Each of these possibilities has been considered by one or more of the following authors: Granoff (1959b, 1962), Kingsbury and Granoff (1970), Dahlberg and Simon (1969a,b) Simon (1972), and Roman and Simon (1976a). In our opinion, none of the experiments which have been done makes it possible to clearly distinguish among these possibilities. Therefore, rather than describing them in detail, we will present the evidence from various sources which tends to eliminate all but the third possibility—which is not very different from the original conclusion of Granoff (1959b) and is similar to that suggested by Roman and Simon (1976a).

Many of the studies (Granoff, 1959b; Dahlberg and Simon, 1969b; Kingsbury and Granoff, 1970; Roman and Simon, 1976a) have used UV inactivation data in an attempt to obtain a solution to this problem. NDV is inactivated by ultraviolet light with kinetics that appear to be single hit (see, among others, Levinson and Rubin (1966), Bratt and Rubin (1968), Clavell and Bratt (1971), and Roman and Simon (1976a)). Dahlberg and Simon's report (1969b) of multi-hit inactivation (particularly of the most rapidly sedimenting particles) could not be repeated by Roman and Simon (1976a), and can therefore be discounted. A result similar to that of Dahlberg and Simon (1969b) was obtained in a study of Sendai virus by Hosaka et al. (1966), but clumped virus was not excluded. Therefore, to the extent that the single-hit inactivation data can be considered valid for NDV, the infectivity of each virus particle is embodied in a single functional genome. This should be true of the progeny of dual as well as single infections. Thus possibilities (1) and (2) which employ at least two independently functioning genomes can be eliminated.

Possibility (4) would seem to be eliminated by Granoff's original finding that the progeny of the heterozygotes possess all the measured properties of either one or the other parental type (Granoff, 1959*b*), although as mentioned in Section 6.1 all of the properties he studied could have been a function of the HN protein alone.

This would leave only the third possibility, in which heterozygotes and possibly many of the virus particles in any population of NDV contain more than one genome of which only a specific one is required for infectivity. In support of this hypothesis is the finding that NDV stocks grown in embryonated eggs, and particularly in tissue culture, show considerable particle size heterogeneity in velocity sedimentation analyses (Kingsbury and Granoff, 1970; Roman and Simon, 1976*a*). [The extreme heterogeneity seen by Roman and Simon (1976*a*) may be the result of analyzing virus obtained by freezing and thawing cells rather than that spontaneously released from cells; see Sections 3.3.1 and 3.3.3.] In fact, the majority of infectious virus from tissue culture-grown virus (the source of the heterozygotes) sediments much faster than the major peak of infectivity.

Assuming that more rapid sedimentation is a consequence of the possession of more genomes—a reasonable assumption as described below—one would predict that the most rapidly sedimenting particles would have the highest fraction of heterozygotes. However, Kingsbury and Granoff (1970) found similar proportions of heterozygotes throughout their gradients. The problem in interpreting these data lies in the inherent inability of these gradients to provide distinctly separated populations, and in there being no data for the number of genomes or nucleocapsids in the various-sized particles. In fact, the finding that when the progeny of mixed infection are UV inactivated to a level of 1% survival (< 5 hits) the proportion of heterozygotes is similar to that found in unirradiated virus (Granoff, 1959*b*) suggests that all particles may contain large numbers of genomes, of which only one is capable of performing all the functions required for successful infection.

Assuming that there are multiple genome equivalents in most of these particles, it might be asked why the particles appear to contain only one fully functional genome. Given Granoff's finding (1959*b*, 1961*b*) that these virus populations contain large numbers of fully activatable but non-plaque-forming particles (Section 3.3.2), one would expect that the probability of having two independently functional genomes in any one particle would be very low. One might also question the basis for the difference between functional and nonfunctional genomes. We feel that a reasonable hypothesis is that the amount of transcriptase might be the limiting factor. It would also be necessary to impose the requirement that the functioning transcriptase carried in at the time of infection can operate only in a *cis* fashion; activation of the nonfunctioning genomes—a *trans* function—would require the synthesis of replicase or more transcriptase.

Is there any evidence that two or more 50 S RNAs can be contained in one particle? As mentioned by Simon (1972) and Choppin and Compans (1975), there have been reports from several laboratories, including principally that of Hosaka *et al.* (1966), suggesting that virions of paramyxoviruses can contain multiples of the 1 μm unit lengths of nucleocapsids; contour lengths as great as 20 μm were reported. However, upon release from virions, nucleocapsids are usually only 1 μm in length. This suggests that they exist as separate unit lengths within the virus, or that the longer nucleocapsids consist of tandemly arranged subunits. Such high numbers should be viewed with caution since Hosaka *et al.* (1966) did not completely rule out the possibility that they were looking at clumped virus. They showed that the large particles were not artifacts of the purification procedure, but did not rule out the possibility that clumps were formed prior to purification. In addition, sonication was reported to convert the larger particles to smaller particles with smaller nucleocapsids. Nevertheless, the possibility that virus particles contain linked or unlinked multimers of nucleocapsid could provide a physical basis for the finding of heterozygotes.

6.4. Multiplicity Reactivation

Multiplicity reactivation is the phenomenon whereby high-multiplicity infection by irradiated virus results in virus production greater than predicted from the remaining infectious virus. Barry (1962) studied the effects of high-multiplicity infection with UV-irradiated NDV by measuring single-cycle yields of hemagglutinin and infectious virus. He concluded that virus production under these conditions could only be attributed to virus which had not received a lethal hit, thus indicating a lack of reactivation. In that same year, however, Drake (1962) looked for reactivation at high multiplicities by measuring the fraction of cells registering as infectious centers rather than single-cycle yields. He obtained evidence for low but consistent levels of reactivation which would not have been detectable using the procedures of Barry (1962).

Kirvaitis and Simon (1965) were able to provide conclusive evidence that reactivation exists, by a clever experiment using artificially clumped UV-irradiated virus. They found that if UV-irradiated virus was artificially clumped by incubation in $MgCl_2$ (to a level where each clump contained about 50 particles), it produced 3–16 times more plaques than similarly treated virus which was sonicated prior to the plaque assay. This procedure allowed a sufficient number of particles to infect a single cell.

Classically, multiplicity reactivation involves recombination among viruses lethally irradiated in different parts of their genomes, allowing for the production of normal infectious virus. In the absence of demonstrated recombination for paramyxoviruses (Section 6.1), it seems unlikely that these viruses would exhibit this phenomenon, although the possibility cannot be definitely excluded. Other types of reactivation which do not involve interchange of genetic material can be considered, however. First, at the high multiplicities of infection used in these experiments, a normally infectious virus which has received a lethal hit might still have the potential to provide the necessary function to activate the potentially infectious but non-plaque-forming virus detected by Granoff (1959b, 1961b), as described in Section 3.3.2. Alternatively, two viruses lethally irradiated in different parts of their genomes might possess the ability to complement each other, with the result that progeny virus could be produced. Such progeny would then be able to go through the necessary rounds of complementation-assisted multiplication necessary to form a plaque. For this model, no individually infectious virus need be produced, although infectious virus of a form similar to the complementing heterozygotes (discussed in Sections 6.1 and 6.3) might be produced. In order to distinguish between activation of non-plaque-forming virus and complementation-mediated plaque formation involving either no virus production or some form of heterozygote, the plaques produced in these experiments would have to be analyzed for the presence and type of virus.

Iinuma (1974) has reported that UV-irradiated NDV has higher infectivity titers when assayed in Sendai virus carrier cultures of HeLa cells than when assayed on normal HeLa cells. A possible explanation for this phenomenon—perhaps a form of cross reactivation—might also be that Sendai virus provides a function necessary to activate the potentially infectious, non-plaque-forming virus in a manner similar to that suggested for multiplicity reactivation.

Important to all these considerations is a knowledge of how UV irradiation affects the virus. First of all, Clavell and Bratt (1971) and Meager and Burke (1972) have shown that the infectivity of NDV decreases far more rapidly than can be accounted for by breaks in 50 S genome RNA. Second, UV irradiation causes the synthesis of foreshortened mRNA molecules (Clavell and Bratt, 1971). Finally, and perhaps most important, as in the case of VSV (Ball and White, 1976; Abraham and Banerjee, 1976; Ball, personal communication) for both Sendai virus (K. Glazier, R. Raghow, and D. W. Kingsbury, personal communication) and NDV (L. A. Ball, L. E. Hightower, and P. Collins, unpublished) UV irradiation sequentially affects transcription of the viral mRNAs (the evidence for single initiation sites referred to in Section 2.5.5). The latter evidence in fact suggests that complementation cannot occur between two viruses that have each received a lethal hit, since complete messages from the distal end of neither genome could be made.

6.5.   Defective or Incomplete Virus

There is considerable evidence in the literature (see Choppin and Compans, 1975) for the production of Sendai virus, SV5, and measles and mumps viruses of varying particle/infectivity ratios. In some of these cases, increased ratios have been associated with high-multiplicity infection. The best example of this is provided by the studies (Kingsbury et al., 1970; Kingsbury and Portner, 1970; and Portner and Kingsbury, 1971, 1972) on the production of incomplete particles during Sendai virus infection. These incomplete particles have properties similar to the defective interfering particles of VSV and other viruses (Huang, 1973; see also Huang and Baltimore in Vol. 10 of this series), and are probably comparable to those of VSV in particular. They (1) are not infectious, (2) are slower sedimenting and smaller than standard virus, (3) possess antimessage-sense RNAs considerably smaller than the normal 50 S RNA of paramyxoviruses and (4) interfere with replication of normal virus by a process which does not involve interferon (Kingsbury et al., 1970). Interference appears to be associated with the inhibition of 50 S RNA synthesis (Portner and Kingsbury, 1971, 1972).

Kingsbury and Portner (1970) showed that the relative abundance of incomplete progeny is a reflection of their proportion in the inoculum. Cells infected with many incomplete particles produce high incomplete/standard virus ratios. Cells infected mainly by standard virus at high or low multiplicity infection promote the multiplication of existing incomplete virus, but do not play a role in the *de novo* genesis of these particles. Instead, genesis appears to involve random errors in replication. This concept was supported by the finding that for six plaque isolates obtained after six successive passages in chick embryo lung cells at multiplicities of 0.01 PFU/cell, only two produced incomplete virus after six subsequent undiluted passages in chick embryo lung cells. Cell specificity of genesis was suggested by the finding that the same six isolates all produced incomplete virus after comparable passages in embryonated eggs. Since the plaque isolates were not really cloned, it is unclear whether the incomplete particles were the result of genesis or amplification of existing incomplete particles. However, failure to produce incomplete virus on passage of 4/6 clones in chick embryo lung cells but production by these same clones in embryonated eggs suggests that genesis of new populations of incomplete particles may have taken place.

Of interest is the apparent specificity of the RNAs of the incomplete virus. If they are specific fragments of the viral genome, they represent specific deletion mutants which can potentially be used in mapping viral mRNAs and genomes, as has been possible for the defective interfering particles of VSV (see Wagner, 1975). Perhaps they might also be used in complementation studies with *ts* mutants (although this has not proven possible with VSV; see Wagner, 1975; Pringle, this volume).

Evidence that the RNAs of the incomplete particles are specific genome fragments is thus far limited to their discrete sizes, and the strain specificity in their production. The original strain of Sendai observed by Kingsbury *et al.* (1970) produced incomplete particles containing 25 S and 19 S RNAs. Another Sendai strain generated particles with 19 S RNA, while a third failed to produce incomplete particles (Kingsbury and Portner, 1970). Famulari and Fleissner (1976) obtained incomplete virus particles possessing 22 S RNA when egg-passaged Sendai was used to infect MDBK cells; here, too, there was evidence for cell specificity, for on passage in MDBK cells the incomplete particles disappeared. It is thus clear that while genesis of these RNAs may occur at random, it results in specific size classes. Of course, the presence of discrete size classes does not necessarily imply that all molecules within a specific size class correspond to a unique portion of the genome, although the experience with VSV (already mentioned) suggests that these incomplete RNAs will represent specific genome fragments. Exploitation of such deletions may be of considerable importance in the future.

Roman and Simon (1976*b*) have recently shown that variable amounts of noninfectious NDV are produced during serial passage in chick embryo cells but not in embryonated eggs. These noninfectious particles (referred to as "defective interfering particles") are similar to those of VSV (see Huang, 1973; Wagner 1975) and the incomplete particles of Sendai virus (Kingsbury *et al.,* 1970); they interfere with infection by standard virus, and this interfering potential is destroyed by ultraviolet irradiation. They differ, however, in cosedimenting with infectious virus rather than as smaller particles. Although no determinations of RNA size or polarity were made for these particles, the possibility that they contain either normal antimessage RNA with a small deletion or RNA of message sense was considered. These findings raise interesting questions about differences in egg-grown and chick embryo cell-grown NDV (if high multiplicities of infection and serial passage are used). However, their significance cannot be evaluated since these chick embryo cell-grown particles were apparently prepared by freezing and thawing infected cells as described in the accompanying report (Roman and Simon, 1976*a*). Potential problems with this procedure have already been mentioned (Sections 3.3.3 and 6.3).

7. TEMPERATURE-SENSITIVE MUTANTS

Analyses of *ts* mutants of paramyxoviruses are in a relatively early stage and the available data permit few generalizations. Those which can be made are contained in Section 7.4 (see Table 1 for a listing of the phenotypes of characterized mutants). Progress has been hampered by a variety of difficulties and technical problems, including (1) low multiplicities of infection, (2) available temperature ranges, (3) difficulties in preparing high-titered virus stocks, and (4) criteria for establishing complementation groups.

1. Multiplicity of infection: Reproducible and meaningful single-cycle growth curves, estimates of RNA synthesis, and complementation indices require infection of 100% of the cells with each virus. The low yields of virus and the resultant low titers of viral stocks make it difficult (and for measles virus often impossible) to obtain uniform infection. The solution often adopted—measuring various properties in multiple cycles after low-multiplicity infection—is not really satisfactory.

2. Temperature: The choice of permissive and nonpermissive temperatures involves a compromise between obtaining as great a range as possible and not going so far from the temperature optimum of the virus–cell system to severely inhibit virus multiplication. In most of the studies to be described, the chosen temperature range allows for nearly equal plating efficiencies—a qualitative measure of ability to undergo multiple-cycle multiplication—for the wild-type virus at the permissive and nonpermissive temperatures. More important, however, are the relative viral yields in a single cycle, for it is under these conditions that functional studies must be done in tissue culture. Even for the wild-type virus, the relative yields will usually depend on the time of assay. At the nonpermissive temperature (invariably supraoptimal), the virus usually multiplies more rapidly but for a shorter period of time, and reaches slightly lower levels than at the (usually suboptimal) permissive temperature. Perhaps because they are usually measured quite late, the yield ratio for nonpermissive to permissive temperatures even for the wild-type virus ranges from 0.1 to 0.5. For other properties, the opposite may be true, as in the case where we found that [^{3}H]uridine incorporation into wild-type virus-specific RNA at the nonpermissive temperature is 2.6 times that at the permissive temperature (Tsipis and Bratt, 1976). For this reason, meaningful results will be obtained only if, in every determination, the relative behavior of a mutant at nonpermissive and permissive temperatures is in turn considered relative to the similar ratio for wild-type virus. It should go without saying that mere comparisons of mutant and wild-type behavior at the nonpermissive temperature alone cannot yield unambiguous results.

3. Input virus: For paramyxoviruses, the inability to adequately remove input virus which remains reversibly attached to the infected cell surface is a serious complicating factor. It presents difficulties in single-cycle growth experiments and complementation experiments for two related reasons. First, yields for paramyxoviruses even at the permissive temperature are often not much higher than the 5–10 PFU/cell necessary to ensure infection of most of the cells. Second, residual input virus remaining reversibly associated with cells at the nonpermissive temperature may be confused with virus produced during infection. This can lead to artifactually high

nonpermissive/permissive yield ratios and the impression that a given mutant is less temperature sensitive than it really is. In complementation experiments, high levels of contaminating input virus could completely obscure low levels of complementation. Furthermore, for NDV, strain-specific and multiplicity-dependent differences in elution of input virus have been shown to exist (Bratt and Gallaher, 1972; Poste and Waterson, 1975), suggesting the possibility of mutant-specific differences which could further complicate the problem.

4. Criteria for establishing complementation groups: Finally, there is the problem of choosing the complementation level which will be used as a measure of true complementation. A. Hamburger, C. S. Raine, R. B. Johnson and B. N. Fields (personal communication) used a complementation index of 5. We (Tsipis and Bratt, 1976) have used a value of 3. All of the other studies have considered indices greater than 1.0 as indicative of complementation. In theory, indices greater than 1.0 could represent complementation. However, because of the difficulties with input virus described immediately above, it is difficult to know what value to accept when high levels of complementation are not obtained. This ambiguity could result in significantly different interpretations and might either obscure or exaggerate possible differences due to intracistronic complementation.

7.1. Temperature-Sensitive Mutants of NDV

Temperature-sensitive mutants of three different strains of NDV have been isolated in three different laboratories (Dahlberg and Simon, 1968; Preble and Youngner, 1973b; Tsipis and Bratt, 1975, 1976). Poor growth of NDV in chicken embryo cells at temperatures below 35°C and the ability of virus and cells to withstand temperatures as high as 43°C have allowed the use of 35–36°C and 42.5–43°C as permissive and nonpermissive temperatures, respectively.

Studies in our laboratory (Tsipis and Bratt, 1975, 1976) have been directed toward isolating temperature-sensitive mutants of NDV for functional studies. The latter study describes the current status of 15 of these mutants, although nine additional mutants have been characterized in almost as great detail (Tsipis and Bratt, unpublished). All 24 mutants have been included in Table 1 (see Section 7.4). A permissive temperature of 36°C was chosen, and mutants producing very few plaques (plating efficiencies of 10^{-3}–10^{-4}) or very small plaques at 41.8°C were selected. Virus treated with mutagens yielded only slightly higher frequencies of mutants (3–5%) than untreated stocks (2%). Of the 49 mutants we have isolated, five were spontaneous, 15 were obtained after treatment with nitrous acid, 26 after treatment with nitrosoguanidine, and three after growth in 5-fluorouracil. The majority of plaques produced by the small plaque mutants at 41.8°C yielded either no virus or virus which was still temperature sensitive. This suggests that the small plaques might be due to leakiness in multiple-cycle growth. This leakiness was deemed to be unimportant for functional studies which would be carried out under single-cycle conditions. Indeed, the majority of even these "leaky" mutants showed relative 41.8°C/36°C yields of progeny virus in single-cycle experiments of 0.1–1.0% (the same range exhibited by the standard mutants).

The mutants have been divided into five nonoverlapping complementation groups (A–E). Members of an additional complementation group (BC) containing noncomplementing mutants failed to complement both groups B and C. The possibilities that the latter group might represent either double mutants within the B and C cistrons or single mutants which are defective in a protein which must interact with both the B and C proteins were considered. An alternative and more appealing possibility is suggested by the low levels of complementation between groups B and C, which could be a reflection of intracistronic complementation. Groups B, C, and BC could thus represent mutations in different portions of the gene for a single protein. Such behavior might not be difficult to imagine for a bifunctional protein such as the HN protein, which has both hemagglutinating and neuraminidase activities. In fact, one of the B mutants was shown to be temperature sensitive for hemadsorption.

When RNA-synthesizing capacity (actinomycin D-resistant incorporation of [³H]uridine between 4 and 9 h postinfection) was measured, the mutants in groups A and the one mutant in group E were found to be temperature sensitive for RNA synthesis. The use of this relatively long labeling period should have allowed the detection of RNA synthesized at any time during the viral growth cycle. All of the mutants in groups B, C, BC, and D were RNA positive by this criterion, in some cases showing enhanced incorporation of [³H]uridine at 41.8°C (relative to 36°C) that was even greater than exhibited by wild-type virus.

As might have been anticipated, all of the RNA⁻ mutants and some of the RNA⁺ mutants exhibited thermal stabilities similar to the wild type. Other RNA$^+$ mutants in groups B, BC, and C were considerably more labile. Also, as expected, all of the RNA$^-$ mutants were temperature sensitive for both fusion from within and hemadsorption—both late functions dependent on synthesis of virus-specific proteins. None of the RNA$^+$ mutants was temperature sensitive for both hemadsorption and fusion from within. As mentioned above, one of the B group mutants was temperature sensitive for hemadsorption, while other members of the group either were temperature sensitive for fusion from within or showed no temperature sensitivity for either function. The group C mutants exhibited no fusion from within at either the permissive or nonpermissive temperature. The group D mutants were all temperature sensitive for fusion.

Recent studies (Bratt, unpublished) employing these mutants and CHO cells growing in suspension have confirmed the RNA phenotypes (of the 18 mutants tested thus far) in both pulse and accumulation studies throughout infection. In addition, at least two mutants in the D group appear to be temperature sensitive for fusion itself rather than for the synthesis of the fusion protein. Thus there is the possibility that the D-group mutants may possess a defect in the fusion protein (F). Furthermore, the facts that a B-group mutant is temperature sensitive for hemadsorption, that groups B and C show only low levels of complementation with each other and no complementation with the BC mutants, and that mutants within these three groups show reduced thermostability, suggest the possibility that these groups may represent mutations in the bifunctional HN protein. Groups A and E are clearly involved in RNA synthesis.

This distribution of NDV mutants among two RNA$^-$ complementation groups and four RNA$^+$ complementation groups (but possibly representing only two distinct polypeptides, if intracistronic complementation is indeed occurring) is strikingly similar to the distribution of two RNA$^-$ and three RNA$^+$ groups for VSV as described in the chapter by Pringle (this volume). Such a result might be expected since NDV contains only one more polypeptide than possessed by VSV, and the paramyxovirus and rhabdovirus groups show extensive similarity in their patterns of transcription, translation, and replication (see Section 2) (Wagner, 1975; Choppin and Compans, 1975).

Dahlberg and Simon (1968) reported the isolation of 48 mutants of NDV after treating wild-type stocks with nitrous acid. Twelve of the mutants having 42.5°C/37°C plating efficiencies between 10^{-4} and 10^{-6} were reported to fall into five nonoverlapping complementation groups. No further characterizations of these mutants have been published, although further characterization of nine complementation groups was reported by Dahlberg (1968). As described in Sections 6.1 and 6.4, some of these mutants were subsequently used in studies on complementing heterozygotes and mutliploid particles (Dahlberg and Simon, 1969a,b).

Preble and Youngner (1973b) isolated four spontaneous mutants and four mutants after treatment with nitrous acid which had low 43°C/37°C plating efficiencies and relative yields. All of these mutants were described as unable to synthesize virus-specific RNA at the nonpermissive temperature, although no data were given. As in the case of the RNA⁻ NDV mutants of Tsipis and Bratt (1976), these mutants were similar to wild-type virus in thermal stability of infectivity (as well as hemagglutinin and neuraminidase). Upon injection into chick embryos, only one mutant showed a reduced rate of killing at 36°C. No further characterization of these mutants has been described.

As described in Section 8, a series of variants isolated from persistently infected L cells also appear to be temperature sensitive for growth and for RNA synthesis (Preble and Youngner, 1972, 1973a). Three variants were unable to synthesize virus-specific RNA after a shift from 37°C to 42°C; two others continued to synthesize RNA for several hours after the shift (Preble and Youngner, 1973a). Thus two different types of defects might be involved. Stanwick and Hallum (1976) have subsequently shown that the *in vitro* assayed transcriptase activity of three additional variants from these persistently infected L cells is less stable at 42°C then that of the virus originally used to establish the persistent infection. Evaluation of these results must be done with caution, since the viruses are indeed variants, not mutants. It might be useful, however, to compare the *in vitro* and *in vivo* RNA-synthesizing capacity of the mutants of some of these variants which have partially reverted in their temperature sensitivity of growth (Preble and Youngner, 1973b).

7.2. Temperature-Sensitive Mutants of Sendai Virus

Portner *et al.* (1974) isolated ten mutants of Sendai virus which all showed low plating efficiencies and yield ratios after infection of chick embryo lung cells at 38°C and 30°C, the nonpermissive and permissive temperatures, respectively. Mutants were isolated at frequencies of 1.5% and 1.0%, respectively, after treatment of virus with nitrosoguanidine or growth in 5-fluorouracil. Seven complementation groups were found, including five groups each with a single mutant, one group with two mutants, and another with three mutants.

RNA synthesis by these mutants was measured as actinomycin D-resistant [³H]uridine incorporation during a 1-h pulse only at the non-permissive temperature after 48 h incubation—the time of maximal virus-specific RNA synthesis in this system. Comparisons of incorporation at both permissive and nonpermissive temperatures throughout infection, and direct comparisons with wild-type virus under similar conditions, were not included in this report, but unpublished experiments of this type (A. Portner and D. W. Kingsbury, personal communication) support the published conclusions. The sole member of one group (G) was designated RNA⁺. Members of the remaining groups were tested and designated as RNA⁻. Temperature-shift experiments were also done. Cultures were incubated at the permissive temperature for 48 h and then shifted to the nonpermissive temperatures for various periods of time before a 1-h labeling period at that temperature. While mutants in groups A, B, and C would synthesize virus-specific RNA under these conditions, the group D mutant would not. The group E and F mutants synthesized amounts which decreased significantly with increasing periods of incubation after the shift to the nonpermissive temperature. These findings suggested to the authors that groups D, E, and F are mutants within genes directly involved in RNA synthesis, while the mutants in groups A, B, and C may not be. The RNA⁻ categorization of the latter groups might reflect defects in functions required prior to initiating RNA synthesis—perhaps defects in structural components of the virions. The only such property tested for in these mutants was hemagglutination at permissive and nonpermissive temperatures. None of the nine members of groups A–F was defective in this property.

In contrast with the mutants in groups A–F, the one RNA⁺ mutant (*ts*271) constituting group G was clearly temperature sensitive for hemagglutination. It showed reversible agglutination and disruption at permissive and nonpermissive temperatures, respectively. Both hemagglutinating and neuraminidase activities were found to be more labile than the activities of wild-type virus at 54°C. Furthermore, while the neuraminidase of the mutant did not seem to be temperature sensitive, it exhibited lower than wild-type activities at both permissive and nonpermissive temperatures.

Subsequently, Portner *et al.* (1975) showed that during infection by this mutant at the nonpermissive temperature, noninfectious particles were produced. These particles lacked both hemagglutinating and neuraminidase activity, were less dense and more fragile than wild-type virus, were unable to attach to cells, and lacked both cell-fusing and hemolytic activity—activities which depend on viral attachment to cells. They also lacked the HN glycoprotein. Infected cells also lacked the hemagglutinating and neuraminidase activity, suggesting that the HN protein was not present in a functional form. Attempts to determine whether the absence of the HN protein was the result of failure to be synthesized or failure of this glycoprotein to go through the normal maturation process were inconclusive. However, all of these results are consistent with, and provide convincing support for, the dual function of the HN protein.

An interesting and unexpected conclusion from these results is that virus particle morphogenesis and budding from cells can occur in the absence of HN glycoprotein structure or function. Furthermore, since infectious virus particles are produced at the nonpermissive temperature but not at the permissive temperature, the authors concluded that the various stages of processing of the HN protein are dependent on correct conformation, but that once the virus particle has been allowed to form correctly at the permissive temperature it is stable and exhibits only the temperature-sensitive hemagglutinating activity and lower neuraminidase activity as described above.

Another interesting finding was that cells infected by this mutant and incubated at the nonpermissive temperature did not show the characteristic cytopathic effects and cell death which usually occur after 4 days. Instead, the cells could be maintained for a long time and could be carried through several passages. However, when cells maintained at the nonpermissive temperature were shifted down to the permissive temperature, inhibition of cellular protein synthesis and cellular destruction rapidly ensued. No explanation is available for this result, which suggests that the HN protein may play a role in the cell-killing phenomenon.

7.3. Temperature-Sensitive Mutants of Measles Virus

Temperature-sensitive mutants of measles virus have been isolated by four groups: Black and Yamazi (1971), Yamazi and Black (1972), Bergholz et al. (1975), Haspel et al. (1975a), and A. Hamburger, C. S. Raine, R. B. Johnson, and B. N. Fields (personal communication). Additional experiments with some of these mutants have also been described (Yamazi et al., 1975; Rapp et al., 1974; Haspel and Rapp, 1975; Haspel et al., 1975b).

One nitrosoguanidine mutant and nine mutants from a single preparation of virus grown in the presence of 5-fluorouracil were isolated from the Edmonston strain of measles virus by A. Hamburger,

C. S. Raine, R. B. Johnson, and B. N. Fields (personal communication). Efficiencies of plating and relative yields of virus at $39°C/33°C$ (nonpermissive/permissive) were in the range of $10^{-2}-10^{-4}$. Titers of wild-type and mutant virus were high enough to adequately infect all cells at multiplicities of 2–10 PFU/cell. Varying multiplicities of infection had little effect on virus yield. No evidence for recombination amoung the mutants could be found. The mutants were placed in four unambiguous nonoverlapping complementation groups (using a complementation index of > 5 to define complementation). Because most of the mutants were obtained from a single 5-fluorouracil mutagenesis experiment, and because all of the mutants within a complementation group showed identical defects, there is the possibility that some of the members of a given complementation group represent double or even triple isolates from the same mutational event.

Unlike other studies with measles virus, in this study virus-specific RNA synthesis could be detected in the presence of actinomycin D during a labeling period between 4 and 6 h after infection and incubation at the nonpermissive temperature. Mutants could also be tested in this system, but no comparisons were made with RNA synthesis at the permissive temperature. By these limited criteria, the four mutants in group A could be shown to incorporate only 10% as much [³H]uridine into virus-specific RNA as detected in wild-type infection. In contrast, the two mutants in group B and the one D mutant behaved similarly to wild type; the three group C mutants appeared to be intermediate. Tentative classification of the group A mutants as RNA⁻ and the other groups as RNA⁺ might be made on the basis of these limited criteria.

The defect in group B mutants could tentatively be ascribed to their hemagglutinin because cells infected by these mutants and incubated at nonpermissive temperatures showed considerably slowed and diminished synthesis of hemadsorbing cell surfaces. The infectivity of these B group mutants was also considerably less thermostable than that of wild-type virus. All other mutants tested in the A, C, and D groups had thermostabilities similar to that of wild-type virus. A surprising result was the ability of the RNA⁻ group A mutants, along with all other mutants, to synthesize virus-specific antigens and produce similar ultrastructural changes in the infected cells at nonpermissive as well as permissive temperatures. It is unclear how mutants with a greatly limited ability to synthesize RNA can still produce viral antigens, hemadsorbing cell surfaces, and ultrastructural changes. The possibility must be considered that this discrepancy is due to the assay of virus-specific RNA at 6 h postinfection, while the other properties are being assayed after 2 days. After 6 h, RNA synthesis might increase to levels sufficient to provide the mRNAs necessary for the synthesis of the proteins involved in these properties.

The studies on the temperature-sensitive mutants isolated by Bergholz *et al.* (1975) and Haspel *et al.* (1975a) share problems related to low-multiplicity infection. Although the solutions sought to alleviate these problems were somewhat different, they will be considered together. The mutants of Bergholz *et al.* (1975) were isolated from the Edmonston strain of measles virus, either spontaneously (one mutant) or after multiplication in the presence of 5-fluorouracil (eight mutants). All had plating efficiencies and nonpermissive/permissive yield ratios of between 10^{-3} and 10^{-4}. Haspel *et al.* (1975a) isolated 24 mutants from a variant of the Schwartz vaccine strain after growth in 5-fluorouracil (18 mutants), proflavin (four mutants), or 5-azacytidine (two mutants). These had a somewhat broader range of plating efficiencies but yield ratios not unlike those of the previously described mutants.

The problems inherent in doing complementation studies at low multiplicities of infection were handled in a similar manner by both groups. None of the mutants of Haspel *et al.* (1975a) produced syncytia at the nonpermissive temperature. This allowed a form of complementation to be measured by looking for fusion from within. Pairs of mutants were clumped in the presence of polyornithine (increasing the probability of dual infection) and cultures infected at multiplicities of 0.01. After incubation at the nonpermissive temperature, the cultures were qualitatively scored for fusion. On the basis of these tests the mutants were placed in three complementation groups: Group I contained 21 mutants; group II contained one mutant isolated after growth in 5-fluorouracil and one grown in proflavin; group III consisted of a single mutant from proflavin-treated cells. Subsequently, complementation was confirmed by several crosses in which yields were measured.

Bergholz *et al.* (1975) placed their nine mutants into three complementation groups—A (the spontaneous mutant), B (seven 5-fluorouracil mutants), and C (one 5-fluorouracil mutant). They used a combination of complementation analyses involving screening for viral antigens (seven out of nine of the mutants synthesized no detectable antigens at the nonpermissive temperature, so a form of complementation analysis could be obtained by screening for antigen formation in mixed infection with these mutants), and in some cases they used viral yields from mixed infection. Although the limits of the antigen assay were not described, and measuring antigen formation is not equivalent to measuring virus production, these procedures produced complementation groups which is most cases appeared to be functionally homogeneous.

Different solutions were sought by each group to determine the RNA-synthesizing capacity of these mutants. Inability to detect significant amounts of virus-specific RNA with the mutants prompted Bergholz et al. (1975) to look for actinomycin D-resistant [³H]uridine incorporation in the presence of cycloheximide (which enhances [³H]uridine incorporation in some extent). The RNA labeled between 60 and 68 h postinfection at the nonpermissive temperature was then analyzed on sucrose gradients. Virus-specific RNA could be detected only with the two antigen-producing mutants (the sole member of group C and one out of the seven members of group B). Because these results were obtained after infection at low multiplicities and well after a single cycle, and because under these conditions the two mutants designated as RNA⁺ synthesized only 2–3% as much virus-specific RNA as found in wild-type infected cells, these results must be viewed with caution.

The solution to this problem by Haspel et al. (1975a) was to use a very indirect assay which may or may not be a measure of RNA synthesis. They reported that cells infected at low multiplicity with any of the mutants and incubated at the nonpermissive temperature would, if shifted down to the permissive temperature at 24 h, produce infectious progeny by 48 h. They then reasoned that addition of an inhibitor of RNA synthesis at the time of shift-down would prevent subsequent virus production, if RNA had not been previously made at the nonpermissive temperature. 5-Azacytidine was added at the time of shiftdown. Whether the proposed mechanisms are operative is open to question. Furthermore, the limits of the assay cannot be assesed. Nevertheless, the procedures allowed the tentative classification of the two mutants in group II as RNA⁺ and the mutants in groups I and III as RNA⁻ (the number of mutants tested from group I was not stated). That this distinction might really reflect RNA-synthesizing capacity is suggested by the fact that only the two group II mutants produced either viral antigen or hemadsorbing cell surfaces at the nonpermissive temperature.

Although the results of the relatively unorthodox procedures adopted by both Bergholz et al. (1975) and Haspel et al. (1975a) are relatively consistent with the other paramyxovirus studies already described, several additional aspects should be mentioned. First, all of the mutants described by Bergholz et al. (1975) were more thermolabile than wild-type virus. This problem has been encountered in none of the other studies, and when increased thermolability has been found it has usually been limited to one complementation group or groups thought to represent the viral hemagglutinin. Second, the majority of the 5-fluorouracil mutants described by both Haspel *et al.* (1975*a*) and Bergholz *et al.* (1975) were found to be clustered in a single complementation group (87% and 75%, respectively), unlike the more equal distribution encountered by Hamburger *et al.* (1976). Again, since only single mutagenesis experiments were used in each case, it seems extremely likely that many of these mutants represent repeated isolations of identical mutants arising from the same mutational event.

Haspel and Rapp (1975), Haspel *et al.* (1975*b*), and Bergholz *et al.* (1975) were also interested in possible attenuation of the neurovirulence of their *ts* mutants in newborn hamsters. Bergholz *et al.* (1975) found that whereas intracerebral inoculation of their wild-type virus killed all experimental animals, injection of 3–40 times as much mutant virus resulted in survival rates of 30–100%. Haspel *et al.* (1975*b*) and Haspel and Rapp (1975) found that whereas wild-type infection produces a rapid and fatal encephalitis in newborn Syrian golden hamsters, group I showed varying degrees of attenuation, group II appeared to have maintained its virulence, and the mutant in group III, while apparently somewhat attenuated, produced a hydrocephalus not observed with wild-type virus. The last phenomenon was also occasionally observed with group I mutants.

Black and Yamazi (1971) and Yamazi and Black (1972) isolated seven proflavin mutants and one 5-fluorouracil mutant from the "Rapp" strain derived originally from the Edmonston strain. Relative yields were 1% or less, but plating efficiencies were not described. Only scanty information is available on the characterization of these mutants (Yamazi and Black, 1972; Yamazi *et al.*, 1975; F. L. Black, personal communication). Here, too, complementation studies were hampered by the low titers of stocks which resulted in low multiplicities of infection. Evidence could be obtained for nonoverlapping complementation with only three of the mutants. The data for the other mutants were interpreted as indicating their possession of multiple defects. Three out of six of the mutants were reported as RNA$^-$, although no details of the experimental procedures were available. All of the mutants appeared to have maintained the same thermostability as the wild-type virus except one of the RNA$^+$ mutants which was less stable at 39.5°C. Yamazi *et al.* (1975) interpreted their results of temperature-shift experiments as indicating that the mutants were blocked at different stages in the replicative cycle. However, these results are difficult to interpret because of the relative instability of all the mutants, and the abovementioned likelihood that many contained multiple lesions.

7.4. Summary

From the preceding sections it should be obvious that studies on *ts* mutants are in very early stages, fraught with numerous technical difficulties, and often open to differing interpretations. In spite of this, a few general principles emerge from the summary of properties for mutants from the most complete studies on NDV, Sendai virus, and measles virus, contained in Table 1. (Discussion of some of the unusual procedures has been left to the previous sections and the footnotes in the table.)

First, it is obvious that both RNA^+ and RNA^- groups exist. The distribution of mutants described here is 50/27 for RNA^-/RNA^+, but these numbers may be misleading. The majority of our mutants beyond those included in the table are RNA^+ (Tsipis and Bratt, unpublished). Furthermore, possible multiple isolations of mutants arising from the same mutational event may have produced artifactually large complementation groups and may have skewed this ratio in the direction of RNA^- mutants. It should be pointed out, however, that the majority of *ts* mutants of VSV are also RNA^- and also fall mainly in one complementation group (Pringle, this volume).

Second, with the exception of the measles virus mutants described by A. Hamburger, C. S. Raine, R. B. Johnson, and B. N. Fields (personal communication), all of the mutants categorized as RNA^- show no properties which require virus-specific protein synthesis. In contrast, RNA^+ mutants show a variety of phenotypes.

Third, with the exception of the Sendai virus mutants of Portner *et al.* (1974), no more than two RNA^- groups have been found by any group. An interesting possibility suggested by this finding is that the extra Sendai virus group is a reflection of the presence of the P (polymerase) polypeptide found in Sendai virions but not in those of NDV (see Sections 2.4 and 2.5.5). Alternatively, considering the similar behavior of groups D, E, and F, the complementations observed between them might be either intracistronic or perhaps artifactually high for the reasons discussed in Section 7. The likelihood of this is diminished by the moderately high levels of complementation observed between the mutants in groups D and F.

Fourth, the association of increased virion thermolability with

TABLE 1

Properties of *ts* Mutants Tentatively Separated into RNA⁻ and RNA⁺ Groups

Columns 2–7 pertain to the RNA⁻ grouping; columns 8–13 to the RNA⁺ grouping. "Fusion," "Hemadsorption," and "Antigen synthesis" are properties at nonpermissive temperature.

Virus	Group (RNA⁻)	Number of mutants	Thermal stability same as wild type	Fusion	Hemadsorption	Antigen synthesis	Group (RNA⁺)	Number of mutants	Thermal stability same as wild type	Fusion	Hemadsorption	Antigen synthesis
NDV[a]	A	5(7)	+	−	−		B	4(7)	+,−	+,−	+,−	
	E	1	+	−	−		BC[f]	2(3)	+,−	+,−	+	
							C	1(2)	+,−	−[g]	+	
							D	2(4)		−	+	
Sendai virus[b]	A[h]	1					G	1	−	−	−[i]	−[i]
	B[h]	2										
	C[h]	3										
	D	1										
	E	1										
	F	1										
Measles virus[c]	A	4	+		+	+	B	2	−		−	+
							C	3	+		+	+
							D	1	+		+	+
Measles virus[d]	A	1	−	−	−	−	B	1	−	±	−	+
	B	6	−	−	−	−	C	1	−	±	−	+
Measles virus[e]	I	21	+	−	−	−	II	2	+	−	+	+
	III	1	+	+	−	−						

[a] Tsipis and Bratt (1976). The numbers in parentheses include unpublished data on nine additional mutants.
[b] Portner et al. (1974, 1975).
[c] Hamburger et al. (1976). RNA synthesis measured 6 h. postinfection; other properties measured after 2–3 days.
[d] Bergholz et al. (1975). Unusual complementation, low multiplicities of infection, and detection of only low levels of RNA synthesis in the presence of cycloheximide.
[e] Haspel et al. (1975a). Unusual complementation, low multiplicities of infection, and indirect assay for RNA synthesis.
[f] Group BC fails to complement with groups B and C, which themselves show only low levels of complementation.
[g] No fusion at permissive temperature, either.
[h] May not be defective in RNA synthesis *per se*.
[i] No HN protein detected in virions or cells.

mutants in RNA$^+$ complementation groups in general, and groups thought to represent the viral hemagglutinin in particular, [the exception being all of the mutants—including the RNA$^-$ mutants—isolated by Bergholz *et al.* (1975)], strongly suggests that thermostability is mainly a property of the attachment protein.

Along with the discrepancies just described and the problems associated with the unorthodox procedures often employed in these studies, there are two additional problems which must ultimately be resolved. First, the finding of overlapping complementation groups of NDV (Tsipis and Bratt, 1976), while possibly explainable by intracistronic complementation, must be studied further. Second, the possibility that some of the Sendai virus RNA$^-$ mutants (Portner *et al.*, 1974) are not really altered in a protein involved in RNA synthesis, as suggested by these workers, must be investigated.

Temperature-sensitive mutants are obviously a useful approach to studying infection in tissue culture. For this approach to be of greater value for paramyxovirologists, it will be necessary for more cooperative efforts and information exchange between the groups working on them. Many of the other chapters in this volume attest to the value of such cooperation. Of value also would be the development of other conditional systems.

8. PERSISTENT INFECTION

The goals of studies on persistent infection in tissue culture are to determine the mechanisms of establishment, maintenance, and cure when it occurs. Factors considered potentially important in one or more of these processes include (1) cell type, (2) culture conditions, (3) the presence or absence of antibody, (4) interferon, (5) defective interfering virus, (6) temperature-sensitive or other types of variants, and (7) possibly DNA intermediates. For the most part, the studies are basically phenomenological analyses which compare either the persistently infected cell with uninfected or acutely infected cells or the virus populations which induce persistent infection with virus released from such cultures. The variety of results obtained, in part because of the use of different cell types and virus strains in the same or different laboratories, and perhaps in part because different factors may be involved in different systems, has served to emphasize the need to sort out the virus-specific or cell-specific phenomena from any general principles. Consider, for example, the virus-specific and cell-specific factors uncovered in studies on the role of interferon in persistent infection by NDV. The study of Henle *et al.* (1959) suggested the importance of interferon in the establishment and maintenance of persistent infection of L cells by paramyxoviruses, including NDV. Subsequently, Rodriguez *et al.* (1967), working with the same system, showed that the egg-passaged virus induced large amounts of interferon during the abortive infection of L cells which could lead to persistent infection. In contrast, virus isolated from the persistently infected cultures (but passed twice in embryonated eggs) induced no interferon and resulted in virulent infection when plated on L cells. This result would seem to emphasize the importance of interferon in the establishment of persistent infection. In contrast, Thacore and Youngner (1969), working with another strain of NDV, found that their wild-type virus (which produced the abortive infection and could lead to the establishment of persistent infection in the L cells) induced less interferon in L cells than did the variant of this virus released from the persistently infected cells. This led them to conclude that interferon plays no role in the abortive infection, although they saw a significant role for it in the maintenance of persistent infection. Whether or not these differences were due to differences in amounts of noninfectious interferon-inducing particles as suggested by Rodriguez *et al.* (1967) (perhaps due to differences in virus stock preparations) is unclear. Recently, however, Youngner and Quagliana (1975), using the same NDV strain employed previously by Thacore and Youngner (1969), established persistent infection in BHK-21 cells and, finding no evidence of interferon production, concluded that interferon is not essential to either the establishment or maintenance of persistent infection. Of course, it is still possible that interferon is important in persistent infection of the L cell and not in the BHK-21 cell.

These examples serve to illustrate the difficulties in distinguishing between system-specific findings and general principles. They have also introduced the concept of viral variants produced during persistent infection. Since persistent infection is the topic of a future chapter in this series, the only factors which will be considered here are the genetic properties of the viruses involved.

8.1. Variants from Persistent Infection

The major fact to emerge from studies on persistent infection is that the virus produced in persistent infection in all cases differs significantly from the virus population which was used to initiate it. In addition to the need for distinguishing between system-specific and general principles, there is the equally important need to identify those changes in the virus population which are directly related to the establishment or maintenance of persistent infection, and to distinguish them from virus population changes which may simply represent adaptation as a result of passage in culture.

8.1.1. Reduced Virulence

The NDV obtained from the persistent infections of L cells mentioned above was, in both cases, more virulent for L cells (Rodriguez *et al.,* 1967; Thacore and Youngner, 1969). In the former case the virus gave smaller, less distinct plaques in chick embryo cell cultures than did the virus used to initiate the persistent infection (Henle *et al.,* 1958; Rodriguez *et al.,* 1965), and, similarly, in the latter case the isolated virus made smaller plaques in chick embryo cells and was less virulent in embryonated eggs (Thacore and Youngner, 1969). In fact, reduced virulence as indicated by the formation of smaller plaques in tissue culture or disease manifestations in embryonated eggs or animals has been found for all of the following paramyxoviruses obtained from persistent infection: NDV (Henle *et al.,* 1958; Thacore and Youngner, 1969; Preble and Youngner, 1973*b*; Youngner and Quagliana, 1975), measles virus (Rustigian 1966*a,b*; Minagawa, 1971*a,b*; Norrby, 1967; Rapp *et al.,* 1974), mumps virus (Walker and Hinze, 1962), and Sendai virus (Kimura *et al.,* 1975).

Undoubtedly relevant to reduced virulence are two factors which have received considerable attention—the production of defective interfering particles and temperature—sensitive variants. Defective interfering particles have been most thoroughly studied with the rhabdovirus, VSV (Huang, 1973). However, evidence has accumulated for the presence of large amounts of noninfectious particles in persistent infections by measles virus (Norrby, 1967; Rustigian, 1966*a,b,* the 6/94 variants of Sendai virus (Lewandowski *et al.,* 1974), and also NDV (Rodriguez and Henle, 1965; Rodriguez *et al.,* 1967). Data relating to the role of *ts* variants in persistent infections will be described in Section 8.1.3.

8.1.2. Other Changes

The most extensively studied system of persistent infection in terms of the virus populations involved is that of NDV and L cells begun by Thacore and Youngner (1969) and continued to the present time (Thacore and Youngner, 1970, 1971, 1972; Preble and Youngner, 1972; 1973a,b, 1975; Youngner and Quagliana, 1975; Furman and Hallum, 1973; Stanwick and Hallum, 1976). Using the Herts strain of NDV, it was shown that clones of virus released from persistently infected L cells differed from the parent virus in (1) elution from red blood cells, (2) thermal stability, (3) virulence, (4) interferon induction in L cells, (5) release of infectious virus from L cells (Thacore and Youngner, 1969), (6) rate and extent of virus production in chick embryo cells, (7) time of detection of virus-specific RNA and effects on total cell RNA and protein synthesis in chick embryo cells (Thacore and Youngner, 1970), and (8) thermostability of the neuraminidase associated with virions (Thacore and Youngner, 1972). Preble and Youngner (1972) found that many isolates from the same persistent infection taken 2 years after those described in the initial study (Thacore and Youngner, 1969) had the same properties, although sometimes in a more exaggerated form. Clearly these changes are too numerous to be due to a single mutation as pointed out by the authors, and thus the isolated virus must be a variant of the virus population initiating the persistent infection. However, many of these coselected changes are strain specific, for as shown by Preble and Youngner (1973b) they do not occur in L cells persistently infected with two other strains of NDV. It would be interesting to know whether some of the same properties are coselected in the BHK-21 cells persistently infected by the Herts strain (Youngner and Quagliana, 1975). This would give an indication of whether cell specificity is involved, too. It would also be important to determine whether these coselected changes are a feature of persistent infection by the Herts strain or merely of continuous passage (see Section 3.1).

8.1.3. Temperature Sensitivity

The most actively pursued aspect of persistent infection is the finding that the variant viruses released from the persistently infected cells always seem to be temperature sensitive. This has been shown to be the case in the system described above (Preble and Youngner, 1972, 1973a,b) where L cells were persistently infected with the Herts and two other NDV strains, or with temperature-resistant revertant clones derived from the temperature-sensitive clones. It was also shown for Herts strain infection of BHK-21 cells and MDCK cells (Youngner and

Quagliana, 1975). These authors have concluded, therefore, that the temperature-sensitive property is independent of the other changes in the variants already described.

Temperature sensitivity is also characteristic of virus released from persistent infections of measles virus (Minagawa, 1971a,b; Haspel *et al.*, 1973; Gould, 1974) and Sendai virus (Nagata *et al.*, 1972; Kimura *et al.*, 1975). The temperature-sensitive defect in the case of Sendai virus seems to be in a late event, possibly protein processing or viral maturation.

All the NDV variants appear defective in RNA synthesis (Preble and Youngner, 1972, 1973a,b; Youngner and Quagliana, 1975). The demonstration that the temperature sensitivity of two clones could revert to wild type (Preble and Youngner, 1973b) suggests that in these two instances the temperature sensitivity is determined by a single mutation. However, the different behavior of different clones following temperature shifts shows that at least two types of temperature-sensitive defects may exist (Preble and Youngner, 1973a). The authors have also considered that some of the *ts* variants are at least double mutants—a possibility which can only be ruled out if revertants can be obtained. Thus there is the possibility that functions other than RNA synthesis may also become temperature sensitive under these conditions. For instance, double *ts* mutants could carry a mutation in the gene for a protein not involved in RNA synthesis, which would be obscured if the other *ts* lesion made the virus RNA$^-$.

Preble and Youngner (1973a) were unable to determine whether the temperature sensitivity in RNA synthesis represented a defect in transcriptase activity. A recent study by Stanwick and Hallum (1976) has demonstrated that—for three clones of virus from these same persistent infections—the activity of the virion-associated transcriptase is lower than in the wild-type virus. Furthermore, this activity is more sensitive to thermal inactivation than that of wild-type virus. Whether this type of lesion is responsible for all the *ts* properties of all of the NDV clones remains to be determined.

Preble and Youngner (1973b, 1975) have suggested that the selection of temperature-sensitive variants during persistent infection is not a random event, and that such variants may well play an important role in the persistent infection. Whether the lesion must be in RNA synthesis is open to question, since this does not appear to be true in the case of the Sendai virus persistent infections (Nagata *et al.*, 1972; Kimura *et al.*, 1975). Furthermore, it must be noted that not only were Preble and Youngner's (1973b) variants from persistent infection all

RNA⁻ but all of the spontaneous and nitrous acid-induced mutants which they isolated were also RNA⁻, whereas RNA⁺ temperature-sensitive mutants have clearly been obtained in a number of different laboratories and with several paramyxoviruses including NDV (Section 7.4).

8.2. Possible Involvement of DNA

Furman and Hallum (1973) provided preliminary evidence for an RNA-dependent DNA polymerase activity in stocks of NDV grown in embryonated eggs after isolation from persistently infected L cells (the original isolates of Thacore and Youngner, 1969). No such activity was found in the parental egg-passaged virus. These authors posed the interesting question of whether such an activity (and possibly DNA intermediates) might play a role in the maintenance of persistence. Since the original data demonstrated only that a small portion of the synthesized DNA was NDV specific, and the possibility of contamination by oncorna viruses in these preparations was never completely eliminated, this remains an unconfirmed but interesting and attractive hypothesis.

Whether the activity was indeed NDV specific or due to a contaminant may be of little importance. In either case there is the suggestion that a heterologous viral RNA might have the opportunity to be transcribed into DNA, and possibly in that form be incorporated into the host cell genome. Whether this mechanism is indeed available remains an unanswered question. However, there is preliminary but as yet uncorroborated evidence suggesting that for measles virus (Zhdanov and Parfanovich, 1974; Zhdanov, 1975) and respiratory syncytial virus (which, although possibly related to the paramyxoviruses, has otherwise been excluded from this chapter) (Simpson and Iinuma, 1975), DNA sequences specific for these RNA viruses could be isolated from persistently infected cells. When used in transfection experiments, the treated cells apparently produced viral products and/or virus with properties similar to those of the original virus. Our enthusiasm for these interesting results and their possible implications must be guarded until they can be confirmed and extended. If DNA intermediates are indeed a reality for these viruses, the possibility for obtaining recombination at that level might then exist.

8.3. Summary and Conclusions

The repeated isolation of temperature-sensitive variants from persistent paramyxovirus infections suggests that such variants are indeed characteristic of these infections. This does not, however, establish a causal relationship. In particular, it is unclear whether or not the selection of *ts* variants is simply the result of continuous passage in culture. The fact that these variants, like the specifically isolated *ts* mutants (see Section 7), show attenuation in tissue culture or animals is also not surprising, since passage in tissue culture is a classical method of obtaining attenuated virus for vaccine use. In fact, passage of paramyxoviruses at temperatures below the normal temperature optimum for virus or cells is known to select for variants ("cold variants") which multiply better at low temperatures and poorer at higher temperatures than wild-type virus (Ghendon and Markhushin, 1966; Hozinski *et al.,* 1966 Potash *et al.* 1970). It must be remembered, too, that in the NDV-L cell systems described above, the temperature of incubation is considerably lower than that of the virus in its natural host. The study of Haspel *et al.* (1973) is also of interest in this regard. These authors found that hamster cells latently infected with measles virus released only low levels of virus when maintained at 37°C but could be induced to release more virus either on cocultivation with other cells or after being incubated at 33.5°C. The virus released at 33.5°C was considerably less cytopathic in cell culture and more temperature sensitive than that released from the cocultivated cells incubated at the higher temperature. This system is somewhat different from those previously described, because after subsequent passage the cultures ultimately released more virus spontaneously at 37°C, and the differences between virus released in cocultivation and at 33.5°C diminished. Nevertheless, it should serve as a sentinel for the possible role of low-temperature selection of *ts* variants during persistent infection.

The major problem of identifying causal relationships between the types of changes exhibited by the isolated variants and the establishment (and/or maintenance) of persistent infection is the time element. By the time it is clear that persistent infection has been established, sufficient time has passed for extensive selection which may be unrelated to persistence. Only with the development of procedures which will allow elucidation of the early events will there be hope for understanding these processes. Certainly the same problems must also be faced in attempts to establish etiology (and/or mechanisms) in the case of chronic or slow virus infections in animals and man. There, too, the changes occurring between time of establishment and virus isolation may be extensive. Furthermore, the changes may be of a type which prevents the virus from reestablishing the same type of infection—as is the case for the variants from persistent infection of L cells with the Herts strain of NDV (Preble and Youngner, 1973b). Thus the possibility of establishing a direct etiological relationship by the application of Koch's postulates—often difficult in the case of acute infection—may be even more remote in the case of chronic and persistent infections.

9. OTHER DIRECTIONS

There has been considerable interest in attenuated variants for vaccine use. These have usually turned out to be temperature sensitive whether or not they were specifically selected for this. The value of these studies is obvious. Of more limited value are studies in which *ts* mutants, whose defects are either known or not known, are tested for disease-producing potential in animals. Clearly such mutants can be expected to show varying degrees of attenuation, but the significance and causes of this may be difficult if not impossible to determine. Such "shot in the dark" procedures may on occasion reveal interesting phenomena, such as the hydrocephalus induction by the measles virus mutant described by Haspel and Rapp (1975) and Haspel *et al.* (1975b) and the unusual phenomena exhibited by some of the reovirus mutants (Cross and Fields, this volume).

A more valuable approach might be the use of mutants with specific defects which do not depend on temperature. An example would be the protease activation mutants of Sendai virus described by Scheid and Choppin (1976). As recognized by these authors, such mutants may be of value in the analysis of tissue tropisms and may even provide mechanisms for these tropisms. Similar approaches could involve mutants with altered cell-fusing properties or other specific defects. These mutants need not necessarily be conditional lethal or even conditional. An approach of this type is being used by C. H. Madansky and M. A. Bratt (unpublished). They have isolated nonconditional mutants which, although able to grow as well as wild-type virus, show reduced cytopathology in tissue culture. The specific defects in these viruses are as yet unknown, but some may be less virulent in embryonated eggs.

Finally, the finding that paramyxovirus mRNAs are sequentially transcribed beginning at a single initiation point (see Sections 2.5.5 and 6.4) might provide a method for mapping *ts* mutant complementation groups on the viral genome. Virus treated with ultraviolet light for various periods of time could be used to complement *ts* mutants. UV irradiation should initially reduce the ability of virus to complement with complementation groups representing genes mainly at the 5′ end of the genome. Longer periods of irradiation would gradually reduce the ability to complement groups representing genes closer and closer to the 3′ end of the molecule. Other mapping procedures for specific mRNAs could involve hybridization with defective or incomplete viral RNAs, or possibly even heteroduplex mapping to locate specific mutations. The latter will of course depend on the existence of enzymes capable of recognizing mispairing at the single-base level. Through a combination of these and other new techniques, it should be possible to (1) distinguish between viral and host contributions to various properties of virions and infected cells, (2) ascribe individual biological properties to the appropriate viral proteins (3) correlate these proteins with the messenger RNAs which code for them, and (4) locate the genes for each on the viral genome. This unique opportunity to bridge the gap between genetic structure and biological function also carries with it a promise for future success in unraveling specific disease processes.

ACKNOWLEDGMENTS

We wholeheartedly thank Charles H. Madansky, C. Worth Clinkscales, and Trudy G. Morrison for numerous helpful discussions and criticisms. We also thank Bernard N. Fields, David W. Kingsbury, Philip I. Marcus, and Judith E. Tsipis for critically reading a version of the manuscript, and the numerous workers in the field who provided preprints which have since been published. Work in the authors' laboratories is supported by research grants from the National Science Foundation (BMS75-05024) (M. A. B.), the National Institute of Allergy and Infectious Diseases (AI-12467) (M. A. B.), and the National Institute of Heart and Lung (HL-19490) (L. E. H.).

10. REFERENCES

Abraham, G., and Banerjee, A. K., 1976, Sequential transcription of the genes of vesicular stomatitis virus, *Proc. Natl. Acad. Sci. USA* **73**:1504.

Alexander, D. J., Reeve, P., and Poste, G., 1973*a*, Studies on the cytopathic effects of Newcastle disease virus: RNA synthesis in infected cells, *J. Gen. Virol.* **18**:369.

Alexander, D. J., Hewlett, G., Reeve, P., and Poste, G., 1973*b*, Studies on the cytopathogenicity of strain Herts 33 in five cell types, *J. Gen. Virol.* **21**:323.

Allison, A. C., and Mallucci, M. D., 1965, Histochemical studies on lysosomes and lysosome enzymes in virus-infected cell cultures, *J. Exp. Med.* **121**:463.

Atherton, J. G., Chaparas, S. D., Cremer, M., and Gordan, I., 1965, Mechanism of polykaryocytosis associated with noncytopathic infection by measles virus. *J. Bacteriol.* **90**:213.

Ball, L. A., and White, C. N., 1976, Order of transcription of genes of vesicular stomatitis virus, *Proc. Natl. Acad. Sci. USA* **73**:442.

Barry, R. D., 1962, Failure of Newcastle disease virus to undergo multiplicity reactivation, *Nature (London)* **193**:96.

Bergholz, C. M., Kiley, M. P., and Payne, F. E., 1975, Isolation and characterization of temperature-sensitive mutants of measles virus, *J. Virol.* **16**:192.

Black, F. L., and Yamazi, Y., 1971, Temperature sensitive mutants of measles virus, *Bacteriol. Proc.* 218.

Blair, C. D., and Robinson, W. S., 1968, Replication of Sendai virus. I. Comparison of the viral RNA and virus-specific RNA synthesis with Newcastle disease virus, *Virology* **35**:537.

Boersma, D. P., and Stone, H. O., 1976, Methylation of Newcastle disease virus messenger RNAs *in vivo, Abst. Am. Soc. Microbiol.* p. 223.

Bratt, M. A., 1969, RNA synthesis in chick embryo cells infected with different strains of NDV, *Virology* **38**:485.

Bratt, M. A., and Gallaher, W. R., 1969, Preliminary analysis of the requirements for fusion from within and fusion from without by Newcastle disease virus, *Proc. Natl. Acad. Sci. USA* **64**:536.

Bratt, M. A., and Gallaher, W. R., 1970, Comparison of fusion from within and fusion from without by Newcastle disease virus, *In Vitro* **6**:3.

Bratt, M. A., and Gallaher, W. R., 1972, Biological parameters of fusion from within and fusion from without, in: *Membrane Research* (C. F. Fox, ed.), p. 383, Academic Press, New York.

Bratt, M. A., and Rubin, H., 1968, Specific interference among strains of Newcastle disease virus. II. Comparison of interference by active and inactive virus, *Virology* **35**:381.

Bratt, M. A., Collins, B. S., Hightower, L. E., Kaplan, J., Tsipis, J. E., and Weiss, S. R., 1975, Transcription and translation of Newcastle disease virus RNA, in: *Negative Strand Viruses,* Vol. 1 (B. W. J. Mahy and R. D. Barry, eds.), pp. 387–408, Academic Press, London.

Brostrom, M. A., Bruening, G., and Bankowski, R. A., 1971, Comparison of neuraminidases of paramyxoviruses with immunologically dissimilar hemagglutinins, *Virology* **46**:856.

Bussell, R. H., Waters, D. J., Seals, M. K., and Robinson, W. S., 1974, Measles, canine distemper and repiratory syncytial virions and nucleocapsids. A comparative study of their structure, polypeptide and nucleic acid composition, *Med. Microbiol. Immunol.* **160**:105.

Chanock, R. M., and Coates, H. V., 1964, Myxoviruses—A comparative description, in: *Newcastle Disease Virus: An Evolving Pathogen* (R. P. Hanson, ed.), pp. 270–298, University of Wisconsin Press, Madison.

Choppin, P. W., 1964, Multiplication of a myxovirus (SV5) with minimal cytopathic effects and without interference, *Virology* **23**:224.

Choppin, P. W., and Compans, R. W., 1970, Phenotypic mixing of envelope proteins of the parainfluenza virus SV5 and vesicular stomatitis virus, *J. Virol.* **5**:609.

Choppin, P. W., and Compans, R. W., 1975, Reproduction of paramyxoviruses, in: *Comprehensive Virology,* Vol. IV (H. Fraenkel-Conrat and R. R. Wagner, eds.), pp. 95–178, Plenum press, New York and London.

Clavell, L. A., and Bratt, M. A., 1971, Relationship between ribonucleic acid-synthesizing capacity of ultraviolet-irradiated Newcastle disease virus and its ability to induce interferon, *J. Virol.* **8**:500.

Clavell, L. A., and Bratt, M. A., 1972a, Hemolytic interaction of Newcastle disease virus and chicken erythrocytes. II. Determining factors, *Appl. Microbiol.* **23**: 461.

Clavell, L. A., and Bratt, M. A., 1972b, Hemolytic interaction of Newcastle disease virus and chicken erythrocytes. III. Cessation of the reaction as a result of inactivation of hemolytic activity by erythrocytes, *Virology* **44**:195.

Colonno, R. J., and Stone, H. O., 1975a, Isolation of a transcriptive complex from Newcastle disease virus, *Abst. Am. Soc. Microbiol.,* p. 250.

Colonno, R. J., and Stone, H. O., 1975b, Methylation of messenger RNA of Newcastle disease virus *in vitro* by a virion-associated enzyme, *Proc. Natl. Acad. Sci. USA* **72**:2611.

Compans, R. W., and Choppin, P. W., 1968, The nucleic acid of parainfluenza virus SV5, *Virology* **35**:289.

Compans, R. W., and Choppin, P. W., 1975, Reproduction of myxoviruses, in: *Comprehensive Virology,* Vol. IV (H. Fraenkel-Conrat and R. R. Wagner, eds.), pp. 179–252, Plenum Press, New York.

Dahlberg, J. E., 1968, Ph.D. thesis, Purdue University.

Dahlberg, J. E., and Simon, E. H., 1968, Complementation in Newcastle disease virus, *Bacteriol. Proc.,* p. 162.

Dahlberg, J. E., and Simon, E. H., 1969a, Recombination in Newcastle disease virus (NDV): The problem of complementing heterozygotes, *Virology* **38**:490.

Dahlberg, J. E., and Simon, E. H., 1969b, Physical and genetic studies of Newcastle disease virus: Evidence for multiploid particles, *Virology* **38**:666.

Daniel, M. D., and Hanson, R. P., 1968, Differentiation of representative Newcastle disease virus strains by their plaque-forming ability on monolayers of chick embryo fibroblasts, *Avian Dis.* **12**:423.

Davies, J. W., Portner, A., and Kingsbury, D. W., 1976, Synthesis of Sendai virus polypeptides by a cell-free extract from wheat germ, *J. Gen. Virol.* **33**:117.

Doermann, A. H., 1948, Lysis and lysis inhibition with *Escherichia coli* bacteriophage, *J. Bacteriol.* **55**:257.

Drake, J. W., 1962, Multiplicity reactivation of Newcastle disease virus, *J. Bacteriol.* **84**:352.

Drake, J. W., and Lay, P. A., 1962, Host-controlled variation in NDV, *Virology* **17**:56.

Duesberg, P. H., and Robinson, W. S., 1965, Isolation of the nucleic acid of Newcastle disease virus (NDV), *Proc. Natl. Acad. Sci.* USA **54**:794.

Durand, D. P., and Eisenstark, A., 1962, Influence of host cell type on certain properties of NDV in tissue culture, *Am. J. Vet. Res.* **23**:338.

East, J. L., and Kingsbury, D. W., 1971, Mumps virus replication in chick embryo lung cells: Properties of RNA species in virions and infected cells, *J. Virol.* **8**:161.

Estupinan, J., and Hanson, R. P., 1971a, Methods of isolating six mutant classes from the Hickman strain of Newcastle disease virus, *Avian Dis.* **15**:798.

Estupinan, J., and Hanson, R. P., 1971b, Mutation frequency of red and clear plaque types of the Hickman strain of Newcastle disease virus, *Avian Dis.* **15**:805.

Famulari, N. G., and Fleissner, E., 1976, High-titer replication of nondefective Sendai virus in MDBK cells, *J. Virol.* **17**:597.

Furman, P. A., and Hallum, J. V., 1973, RNA-dependent DNA polymerase activity in preparations of a mutant of Newcastle disease virus arising from persistently infected L cells, *J. Virol.* **12**:548.

Ghendon, Y., and Markhushin, S., 1966, Virus production in tissue culture at low temperatures, *Archiv Ges. Virusforsch.* **19**:334.

Goldman, E. L., and Hanson, R. P., 1955, The isolation and characterization of heat-resistant mutants of the Najarian strain of NDV. *J. Immunol.* **74**:101.

Gomez-Lillo, M., Bankowski, R. A., and Wiggins, A. D., 1974, Antigenic relationships among viscerotropic velogenic and domestic strains of Newcastle disease virus, *Am. J. Vet. Res.* **35**:471.

Gould, E., 1974, Variants of measles virus, *Med. Microbiol. Immunol.* **160**:211.

Granoff, A., 1959a, Studies on mixed infection with Newcastle disease virus. I. Isolation of Newcastle disease virus mutants and tests for genetic recombination between them, *Virology* **9**:636.

Granoff, A., 1959b, Studies on mixed infection with Newcastle disease virus. II. The occurrence of Newcastle disease virus heterozygotes and study of phenotypic mixing involving serotypes and thermal stability, *Virology* **9**:649.

Granoff, A., 1961a, Induction of Newcastle disease virus mutants with nitrous acid, *Virology* **13**:402.

Granoff, A., 1961b, Studies on mixed infection with Newcastle disease virus. III. Activation of non plaque-forming virus by plaque forming virus, *Virology* **14**:143.

Granoff, A., 1962, Heterozygosis and phenotypic mixing with Newcastle disease virus, *Cold Spring Harbor Symp. Quant. Biol.* **27**:319.

Granoff, A., 1964a, Nature of the Newcastle disease virus population, in: *Newcastle Disease Virus: An Evolving Pathogen* (R. P. Hanson, ed.), pp. 107–118, University of Wisconsin Press, Madison.

Granoff, A., 1964b, pp. 223–225 in discussion of "Thermostability of Newcastle disease virus," by J. C. Picken Jr., in: *Newcastle Disease Virus: An Evolving Pathogen* (R. P. Hanson, ed.), pp. 167–188, University of Wisconsin Press, Madison.

Granoff, A., and Henle, W., 1954, Studies on the interaction of the large and small hemagglutinating components of Newcastle disease virus with red cells, *J. Immunol.* **72**:329.

Granoff, A., and Hirst, G. K., 1954, Experimental production of combination forms of virus. IV. Mixed influenza A–Newcastle disease virus infections, *Proc. Soc. Exp. Biol. Med.* **86**:84.

Haspel, M. V., and Rapp, F., 1975, Measles virus: An unwanted variant causing hydrocephalus, *Science* **187**:450.

Haspel, M. V., Knight, P. R., Duff, R. G., and Rapp, F., 1973, Activation of a latent measles virus infection in hamster cells, *J. Virol.* **12**:690.

Haspel, M. V., Duff, R., and Rapp, F., 1975a, The isolation and preliminary characterization of temperature-sensitive mutants of measles virus, *J. Virol.* **16**:1000.

Haspel, M. V., Duff, R., and Rapp, F., 1975b, Experimental measles encephalitis: A genetic analysis, *Infect. Immun.* **12**:785.

Henle, G., Dienhardt, F., Bergs, V. V., and Henle, W., 1958, Studies on persistent infections of tissue cultures. I. General aspects of the system. *J. Exp. Med.* **108:** 537.

Henle, W., Henle, G., Dienhardt, F., and Bergs, V. V., 1959, Studies on persistent infections of tissue cultures. IV. Evidence of the production of an interferon in MCN cells by myxoviruses, *J. Exp. Med.* **110:**525.

Hightower, L. E., and Bratt, M. A., 1974, Protein synthesis in Newcastle disease virus-infected chicken embryo cells, *J. Virol.* **13:**788.

Hightower, L. E., and Bratt, M. A., 1975, Protein metabolism during the steady state of Newcastle disease virus infection. I. Kinetics of amino acid and protein accumulation, *J. Virol.* **15:**696.

Hightower, L. E., Morrison, T. G., and Bratt, M. A., 1975, Relationships among the polypeptides of Newcastle disease virus, *J. Virol.* **16:**1599.

Homma, M., 1971, Trypsin action on the growth of Sendai virus in tissue culture cells. I. Restoration of the infectivity for L cells by direct action of trypsin on L cell-borne Sendai virus, *J. Virol.* **8:**614.

Homma, M., 1972, Trypsin action on the growth of Sendai virus in tissue culture cells. II. Restoration of the hemolytic activity of L cell-borne Sendai virus by trypsin, *J. Virol.* **9:**829.

Homma, M., 1975, Host-induced modification of Sendai virus, in: *Negative Strand Viruses,* Vol. 2 (B. W. J. Mahy and R. D. Barry, eds.), pp. 685–697, Academic Press, London.

Homma, M., and Ohuchi, M., 1973, Trypsin action on the growth of Sendai virus in tissue culture cells. III. Structural differences of Sendai viruses grown in eggs and tissue culture cells, *J. Virol.* **12:**1457.

Homma, M., and Tamagawa, S., 1973, Restoration of the fusion activity of L cell borne Sendai virus by trypsin, *J. Gen. Virol.* **19:**423.

Hosaka, Y., 1970, Biological activities of sonically treated Sendai virus, *J. Gen. Virol.* **8:**43.

Hosaka, Y., 1975, Artifical assembly of active envelope particle of HVJ (Sendai virus), in: *Negative Strand Viruses,* Vol. 2 (B. W. J. Mahy and R. D. Barry, eds.) pp. 885–903, Academic Press, London.

Hosaka, Y., and Shimizu, K., 1972, Artifical assembly of envelope particles of HVJ (Sendai virus). I. Assembly of hemolytic and fusion factors from envelopes solubilized by Nonidet P_{40}, *Virology* **49:**627.

Hosaka, Y., Kitano, H., and Ikeguchi, S., 1966, Studies on the pleomorphism of HVJ virions, *Virology* **29:**205.

Hozinski, V. I., Seibil, V. B., Pantelyeva, N. S., Mazurova, S. M., and Novikova, E. A., 1966, The rct_{40} and T_{50} markers and the characteristics of some variants of measles virus, *Acta Virol.* **10:**20.

Huang, A. S., 1973, Defective interfering viruses, *Annu. Rev. Microbiol.* **27:**101.

Iinuma, M. 1974, Superinfection of HVJ carrier HeLa cells with ultraviolet-irradiated Newcastle disease virus, *Jpn. J. Microbiol.* **16:**53.

Isaacs, A., and Donald, H. B., 1955, Particle counts of hemagglutinating viruses, *J. Gen. Microbiol.* **12:**241.

Ishida, N., and Homma, M., 1960, A variant of Sendai virus, infectious to egg embryos but not to L cells, Tohoku, *J. Exp. Med.* **73:**56.

Ishida, N., and Homma, M., 1961, Host-controlled variation observed with Sendai virus grown in mouse (L) cells, *Virology* **14:**486.

Iwai, Y., Iwai, M., Okumoto, M., Hosokawa, Y., and Asai, T., 1966, Properties of the nucleic acid isolated from HVJ, *Bikens J.* **9**:241.

Kimura, Y., Ito, Y., Shimokata, K., Nishiyama, Y., Nagata, I., and Kitoh, J., 1975, Temperature-sensitive virus derived from BHK cells persistently infected with HVJ (Sendai virus), *J. Virol.* **15**:55.

Kingsbury, D. W., 1966a, Newcastle disease virus RNA. I. Isolation and preliminary characterization of RNA from virus particles, *J. Mol. Biol.* **18**:195.

Kingsbury, D. W., 1966b, Newcastle disease virus RNA. II. Preferential synthesis of RNA complementary to parental RNA by chick embryo cells, *J. Mol. Biol.* **18**:204.

Kingsbury, D. W., 1973a, Paramyovirus replication, *Curr. Top. Microbiol.* **59**:1.

Kingsbury, D. W., 1973b, Cell-free translation of paramyxovirus messenger RNA, *J. Virol.* **12**:1021.

Kingsbury, D. W., and Granoff, A., 1970, Studies on mixed infection with Newcastle disease virus. IV. On the structure of heterozygotes, *Virology* **42**:262.

Kingsbury, D. W., and Portner, A., 1970, On the genesis of incomplete Sendai virions, *Virology* **42**:872.

Kingsbury, D. W., Portner, A., and Darlington, R. W., 1970, Properties of incomplete Sendai virus and subgenomic viral RNAs, *Virology* **42**:857.

Kirvaitis, J., and Simon, E. H., 1965, A radiobiological study of the development of Newcastle disease virus, *Virology* **26**:545.

Klenk, H. D., and Choppin, P. W., 1969, Lipids of plasma membranes of monkey and hamster kidney cells and of parainfluenza virions grown in these cells, *Virology* **38**:255.

Klenk, H.-D., and Choppin, P. W., 1970a, Plasma membrane lipids and parainfluenza virus assembly, *Virology* **40**:939.

Klenk, H.-D., and Choppin, P. W., 1970b, Glycosphingolipids of plasma membranes of cultured cells and an enveloped virus (SV5) grown in these cells. *Proc. Natl. Acad. Sci. USA* **66**:57.

Kohn, A., 1965, Polykaryocytosis induced by Newcastle disease virus in monolayers of animal cells, *Virology* **26**:228.

Kohn, A., and Fuchs, P., 1969, Cell fusion by various strains of Newcastle disease virus and their virulence, *J. Virol.* **3**:539.

Kohn, A., and Klibansky, D., 1967, Studies on the inactivation of the cell-fusing property of NDV by phospholipase A, *Virology* **31**:385.

Kolakofsky, D., 1972, tRNA nucleotidyl transferase and tRNA in Sendai virions, *J. Virol.* **14**:33.

Kolakofsky, D., and Bruschi, A., 1975, Antigenomes in Sendai virions and Sendai virus infected cells, *Virology* **66**:185.

Kolakofsky, D., Boy de la Tour, E., and Deluis, H., 1974a, Molecular weight determination of Sendai and Newcastle disease virus RNA, *J. Virol.* **13**:261.

Kolakofsky, D., Spahr, P. F., and Koprowski, H., 1974b, Comparison of 6/94 virus and Sendai virus RNA by RNA-RNA hybridization, *J. Virol.* **13**:935.

Kolakofsky, D., Boy de la Tour, E., and Deluis, H., 1975, Molecular weight determination of parainfluenza virus RNA in: *Negative Strand Viruses,* Vol. 1 (B. W. J. Mahy and R. D. Barry, eds.), pp. 243–257, Academic Press, London.

Koldovsky, V., Koldovsky, P., Henle, G., Henle, W., Ackermann, R., and Haase, G., 1975, Multiple sclerosis-associated agent: Transmission to animals and some properties of the agent, *Infect. Immun.* **12**:1355.

Lamb, R. A., 1975, The phosphorylation of Sendai virus proteins by a virus particle-associated protein kinase, *J. Gen. Virol.* **26**:249.

Lamb, R. A., and Mahy, B. W. J., 1975, Characterization of the polypeptides and RNA of Sendai virus, in: *Negative Strand Viruses,* Vol. 1 (R. D. Barry and B. W. J. Mahy, eds.), pp. 65–87, Academic Press, London.

Lamb, R. A., Mahy, B. W. J., and Choppin, P. W., 1976, The synthesis of Sendai virus polypeptides in infected cells, *Virology* **69**:116.

LaMontagne, J. R., Schiller, J. G., Thacore, H. R., Feingold, D. S., and Youngner, J. S., 1975, Infective and noninfective hemagglutinating particles of Newcastle disease virus: Biological and chemical characterization, *J. Virol.* **16**:1191.

Levinson, W., and Rubin, H., 1966, Radiation studies of avian tumor viruses and Newcastle diseases virus, *Virology* **28**:533.

Lewandowski, L. J., Lief, F. S., Verini, M. A., Pienkowski, M. M., ter Meulen, V., and Koprowski, H., 1974, Analysis of a viral agent isolated from multiple sclerosis brain tissue: Characterization as a parainfluenza type 1, *J. Virol.* **13**:1037.

Lief, F. S., Loh, W., ter Meulen, V., and Koprowski, H., 1975, Antigenic variation among parainfluenza type 1 (Sendai) viruses: Analysis of 6/94 virus, *Intervirology* **5**:1.

McSharry, J. J., Compans, P. W., and Choppin, P. W., 1971, Proteins of vesicular stomatitis virus (VSV) and of phenotypically-mixed VSV-SV5, *J. Virol.* **8**:722.

Mahy, B. W. J., Hutchinson, J. E., and Barry, R. D., 1970, Ribonucleic acid polymerase induced in cells infected with Sendai viruses, *J. Virol.* **5**:663.

Marcus, P. I., 1959, Host-cell interaction of animal viruses. II. Cell-killing particle enumeration: Survival curves at low multiplicities, *Virology* **9**:546.

Marcus, P. I., 1960, Characterization of Hela cell-derived Newcastle disease virus (NDV), *Bacteriol. Proc.* 91–92.

Marx, P. A., Portner, A., and Kingsbury, D. W., 1974, Sendai virion transcriptase complex: Polypeptide composition and inhibition by virion envelope proteins, *J. Virol.* **13**:298.

Marx, P. A., Jr., Pridgen, C., and Kingsbury, D. W., 1975, Location and abundance of poly(A) sequences in Sendai virus messenger RNA molecules, *J. Gen. Virol.* **27**:247.

Matsumoto, T., and Maeno, K., 1962, A host-induced modification of hemagglutinating virus of Japan (HVJ, Sendai virus) in its hemolytic and cytopathic activity, *Virology* **17**:563.

Meager, A., and Burke, D. C., 1972, Production of interferon by ultraviolet irradiated Newcastle disease virus, *Nature (London)* **235**:280.

Minagawa, T., 1971a, Studies on the persistent infection with measles virus in the Hela cells. I. Clonal analysis of cells of carrier cultures, *Jap. J. Microbiol.* **15**:325.

Minagawa, T., 1971b, Studies on the persistent infection with measles virus in the Hela cells. II. The properties of carried virus, *Jap. J. Microbiol.* **15**:333.

Morrison, T. G., Weiss, S. R., Hightower, L. E., Spanier-Collins, B., and Bratt, M. A., 1975, Newcastle disease virus protein synthesis, in: *In Vitro Transcription and Translation of Viral Genomes* (A. L. Haenni and G. Beaud, eds.), pp. 281–289, INSERM 47 Institute National de la Sante ed de la Recherche Medicale, Paris.

Nagai, Y., Klenk, H. D., and Rott, R., 1976, Proteolytic cleavage of the viral glycoproteins and its significance for the virulence of Newcastle disease virus, *Virology* **72**:494.

Nagata, I., Kimura, Y., Ito, Y., and Tanaka, T., 1972, Temperature-sensitive phenomenon of viral maturation observed in BHK cells persistently infected with HVJ, *Virology* **49**:453.

Neurath, A. R., 1964, Association of Sendai virus with esterase and leucine amino peptidase activity; its probable relationship to "hemolysin," *Z. Naturforsch. Ser. B* **19**:810.

Neurath, A. R., 1965, Study on the adenosine diphosphatase (adenosine triphosphatase) associated with Sendai virus, *Acta Virol.* **9**:313.

Norrby, E. C. J., 1965, Characteristics of the progeny derived from multiplication of Sendai virus in a measles virus carrier cell line, *Arch. Ges. Virusforsch.* **17**:436.

Norrby, E., 1967, A carrier cell line of measles virus in LU 106 cells, *Arch. Ges. Virusforsch.* **20**:215.

Okada, Y., and Murayama, F., 1966, Requirement of calcium for the cell fusion reaction of animal cells by HVJ, *Exp. Cell Res.* **44**:527.

Örvell, C., and Norrby, E., 1974, Further studies on the immunologic relationships among measles, distemper, and rinderpest viruses, *J. Immunol.* **113**:1850.

Payne, E., and Baublis, 1973, Decreased reactivity of SSPE strains of measles virus with antibody, *J. Infect. Dis.* **127**:505.

Picken, J. C., Jr., 1964, Thermostability of Newcastle disease virus, in: *Newcastle Disease Virus: An Evolving pathogen* (R. P. Hanson, ed.), pp. 167–188, University of Wisconsin Press, Madison.

Pierce, J. S., and Haywood, A. M., 1973, Thermal inactivation of Newcastle disease virus. I. Coupled inactivation rates of hemagglutinating and neuraminidase activities, *J. Virol.* **11**:168.

Portner, A., and Kingsbury, D. W., 1971, Homologous interference by incomplete Sendai virus particles: Changes in virus-specific ribonucleic acid synthesis, *J. Virol.* **8**:388.

Portner, A., and Kingsbury, D. W., 1972, Identification of transcriptive and replicative intermediates in Sendai virus-infected cells, *Virology* **47**:711.

Portner, A., and Kingsbury, D. W., 1976, Regulatory events in the synthesis of Sendai virus polypeptides and their assembly into virions, *Virology* **73**:79.

Portner, A., Marx, P. A., and Kingsbury, D. W., 1974, Isolation and characterization of Sendai virus temperature-sensitive mutants, *J. Virol.* **13**:298.

Portner, A., Scroggs, R. A., Marx, P. A., and Kingsbury, D. W., 1975, A temperature-sensitive mutant of Sendai virus with an altered hemagglutinin-neuraminidase polypeptide: Consequences for virus assembly and cytopathology, *Virology* **67**:179.

Poste, G., and Waterson, A. P., 1975, Cell fusion by Newcastle disease virus, in: *Negative Strand Viruses,* Vol. 2 (B. W. J. Mahy and R. D. Barry, eds.), pp. 905–922, Academic Press, London.

Potash, L., Lees, R. S., Greenberger, J. L., Hoyrup, A., Denney, L. D., and Chanock, R. M., 1970, A mutant of parainfluenza type 1 virus with decreased capacity for growth at 38°C and 39°C, *J. Infect. Dis.* **121**:640.

Preble, O. T., and Youngner, J. S., 1972, Temperature-sensitive mutants isolated from cells persistently infected with Newcastle disease virus, *J. Virol.* **9**:200.

Preble, O. T., and Youngner, J. S., 1973a, Temperature-sensitive defect of mutants isolated from L cells persistently infected with Newcastle disease virus, *J. Virol.* **12**:472.

Preble, O. T., and Youngner, J. S., 1973b, Selection of temperature-sensitive mutants during persistent infection: Role in maintenance of persistent Newcastle disease virus infections of L cells, *J. Virol.* **12**:481.

Preble, O. T., and Youngner, J. S., 1975, Temperature-sensitive viruses and the etiology of chronic and inapparent infections, *J. Infect. Dis.* **131**:467.

Rapp, F., 1964, Plaque differentiation and replication of virulent and attenuated strains of measles virus, *J. Bacteriol.* **88**:1448.

Rapp, F., Haspel, M. V., Duff, R., and Knight, P., 1974, Measles virus latency and neurovirulence, in: *Mechanisms of Virus Disease* (W. S. Robinson and C. F. Fox, ed., pp. 199–212, W. A. Benjamin, Menlo Park, Calif.

Reeve, P., and Poste, G., 1971, Studies on the cytopathogenicity of Newcastle disease virus: Relationship between virulence, polykaryorytosis and plaque size, *J. Gen. Virol.* **11**:17.

Reeve, P., and Waterson, A. P., 1970, The growth cycle of avirulent strains of Newcastle disease virus, *Microbiology* **2**:5.

Reeve, P., Rosenblum, M., and Alexander, D., 1970, Growth in chick chorioallantoic membranes of strains of Newcastle disease virus of differing virulence, *J. Hyg.* **68**:61.

Reeve, P., Alexander, D. J., Pope, G., and Poste, G., 1971, Studies on the cytopathic effects of Newcastle disease virus: Metabolic requirements, *J. Gen. Virol.* **11**:25.

Robinson, W. S., 1971, Sendai virus RNA synthesis and nucleocapsid formation in the presence of cycloheximide, *Virology* **44**:494.

Rodriguez, J. E., and Henle, W., 1965, Studies on persistent infection of tissue cultures. V. The initial stages of infection of L (MCN) cells by Newcastle disease virus, *J. Exp. Med.* **119**:895.

Rodriguez, J. E., ter Meulen, V., and Henle, W., 1967, Studies on persistent infections of tissue culture. VI. Reversible changes in Newcastle disease virus populations as a result of passage in L cells or chick embryos, *J. Virol.* **1**:1.

Roman, J. A., and Simon, E. H., 1976a, Morphologic heterogeneity in egg- and monolayer-propagated Newcastle disease virus, *Virology* **69**:287.

Roman, J. A., and Simon, E. H., 1976b, Defective interfering particles in monolayer-propagated Newcastle disease virus, *Virology* **69**:298.

Roux, L., and Kolakofsky, D., 1974, Protein kinase associated with sendai virions, *J. Virol.* **13**:545.

Roux, L., and Kolakofsky, D., 1975, Isolation of RNA transcripts from the entire Sendai viral genome, *J. Virol.* **16**:1426.

Rubin, H., Franklin, R. M., and Baluda, M., 1957, Infection and growth of Newcastle disease virus (NDV) in cultured chick embryo lung epithelium, *Virology* **3**:587.

Rustigian, R., 1966a, Persistent infection of cells in culture by measles virus. I. Development and characteristics of HeLa sublines persistently infected with complete virus, *J. Bacteriol.* **92**:1792.

Rustigian, R., 1966b, Persistent infection of cells in culture by measles virus. II. Effect of measles virus antibody on persistently infected HeLa sublines and recovery of HeLa clonal line persistently infected with incomplete virus, *J. Bacteriol.* **92**:1805.

Scheid, A., and Choppin, P. W., 1974, Identification of biological activities of paramyxovirus glycoproteins: Activation of cell fusion, hemolysis and infectivity by proteolytic cleavage of an inactive precursor protein of Sendai virus, *Virology* **57**:475.

Scheid, A., and Choppin, P. W., 1975, Isolation of paramyxovirus glycoproteins and identification of their biological properties, in: *Negative Strand Viruses,* Vol. 1 (B. W. J. Mahy and R. D. Barry, eds.), pp. 177–192, Academic Press, London.

Scheid, A., and Choppin, P. W., 1976, Protease activation mutants of Sendai virus: Activation of biological properties by specific proteases, *Virology* **69**:265.

Schloer, G., 1974, Antigenic relationships among Newcastle disease virus mutants obtained from laboratory strains and from recent California isolates, *Infect. Immun.* **10**:724.

Schloer, G. M., and Hanson, R. P., 1968, Relationships of plaque size and virulence for chickens of 14 representitive Newcastle virus strain, *J. Virol.* **2**:40.

Schloer, G. M., and Hanson, R. P., 1971, Virulence and *in vitro* characteristics of four mutants of Newcastle disease virus, *J. Infect. Dis.* **124**:289.

Schloer, G., Spalatin, J., and Hanson, R. P., 1975, Newcastle disease virus antigens and strain variations, *Am. J. Vet. Res.* **36**:505.

Scholtissek, C., and Rott, R., 1969, Ribonucleic acid nucleotidyl transferase induced in chick fibroblasts after infection with Newcastle disease virus, *J. Gen. Virol.* **4**:565.

Simon, E. H., 1972, The distribution and significance of multiploid virus particles, *Prog. Med. Virol.* **14**:36.

Simpson, R. W., and Hauser, R. E., 1966, Influence of lipids on the viral phenotype. I. Interaction of myxoviruses and their lipid constituents with phospholipases, *Virology* **30**:684.

Simpson, R. W., and Iinuma, M., 1975, Recovery of infectious proviral DNA from mammalian cells infected with respiratory syncytial viruses, *Proc. Natl. Acad. Sci. USA* **72**:3230.

Stanwick, T. L., and Hallum, J. V., 1976, Comparison of RNA polymerase associated with Newcastle disease virus and a temperature sensitive mutant of Newcastle disease virus isolated from persistently infected L cells, *J. Virol.* **17**:68.

Stenback, W. A., and Durand, D. P., 1963, Host influence on the density of Newcastle disease virus (NDV), *Virology* **20**:545.

Stone, H. O., Portner, A., and Kingsbury, D. W., 1971, Ribonucleic acid transcriptases in Sendai virions and infected cells, *J. Virol.* **8**:174.

Stone, H. O., Kingsbury, D. W., and Darlington, R. W., 1972, Sendai virus-induced transcriptase from infected cells: Polypeptides in the transcriptive complex, *J. Virol.* **10**:1037.

ter Meulen, V., Koprowski, H., Iwasaki, Y., Käckell, Y. M., and Müller, D., 1972*a*, Fusion of cultured multiple sclerosis brain cells with indicator cells: Presence of nucleocapsids and virions and isolation of parainfluenza type virus, *Lancet* **2**:1.

ter Meulen, V., Katz, M., and Müller, D., 1972*b*, Subacute sclerosing panencephalitis. A review, *Curr. Top. Microbiol. Immunol.* **57**:1.

Thacore, H., and Youngner, J. S., 1969, Cells persistently infected with Newcastle disease virus. I. Properties of mutants isolated from persistently infected L cells, *J. Virol.* **4**:244.

Thacore, H., and Youngner, J. S., 1970, Cells persistently infected with Newcastle disease virus. II. Ribonucleic acid and protein synthesis in cells infected with mutants isolated from persistently infected L cells, *J. Virol.* **6**:42.

Thacore, H., and Youngner, J. S., 1971, Cells persistently infected with Newcastle disease virus. III. Thermal stability of hemagglutinin and neuraminidase of a mutant isolated from persistently infected L cells, *J. Virol.* **7**:53.

Thacore, H., and Youngner, J. S., 1972, Viral ribonucleic acid synthesis by Newcastle disease virus mutants isolated from persistently infected L cells: Effect of Interferon, *J. Virol.* **9**:503.

Thiry, L., 1963, Chemical mutagenesis of Newcastle disease virus, *Virology* **19**:225.

Thiry, L., 1964, Some properties of chemically induced small-plaque mutants of Newcastle disease virus, *Virology* **24**:146.

Thiry, L., 1966, Viruses grown in the presence of base analogs: Specific alteration of susceptibility to inactivation by radiations, mutagens, and photodyes, *Virology* **28**:543.

Tsipis, J. E., and Bratt, M. A., 1975, Temperature-sensitive mutants of Newcastle disease virus, in: *Negative Strand Viruses,* Vol. 2 (B. W. J. Mahy and R. D. Barry, eds.), pp. 777–784, Academic Press, London.

Tsipis, J. E., and Bratt, M. A., 1976, Isolation and preliminary characterization of temperature sensitive mutants of Newcastle disease virus, *J. Virol.* **18:**848.

Upton, E., Hanson, R. P., and Brandly, C. A., 1953, Antigenic differences among strains of Newcastle disease virus, *Proc. Soc. Exp. Biol. Med.* **84:**691.

Utterback, W. W., and Schwartz, J. H., 1973, Epizootiology of velogenic viscerotropic Newcastle disease in southern California, *J. Am. Vet. Med. Assoc.* **163:**1080.

Vamos, E., 1966, On the "red" character of a mutant of Newcastle disease virus (NDV), *Archiv. Ges. Virusforsch.* **18:**96.

Wagner, R. R., 1975, Reproduction of rhabdoviruses, in: *Comprehensive Virology,* Vol. 4 (H. Fraenkel-Conrat and R. R. Wagner, eds.), pp. 1–93, Plenum Press, New York.

Walker, D. L., 1968, Persistent viral infection in cell cultures, in: *Medical and Applied Virology* (M. Sanders and E. H. Lennette, eds.), pp. 99–110, Warren H. Green, St. Louis.

Walker, D. L., and Hinze, H. C., 1962, A carrier state of mumps virus in human conjunctiva cells. I. General Characteristics, *J. Exp. Med.* **116:**739.

Warren, J., 1960, The relationships of the viruses of measles, canine distemper, and rinderpest, *Adv. Virus. Res.* **7:**27.

Weiss, S. R., and Bratt, M. A., 1976, The 18–22 S RNAs of Newcastle disease virus, *J. Virol.* **18:**316.

Weissmann, C., Billeter, M. A., Goodman, H. M., Hindley, N., and Weber, H., 1973, Structure and function of phage RNA, *Annu. Rev. Biochem.* **42:**303.

Yamazi, Y., and Black, F. L., 1972, Isolation of temperature-sensitive mutants of measles virus, *Med. Biol. (Tokyo)* **84:**47 (in Japanese).

Yamazi, Y., Black, F. L., Honda, H., Todome, Y., Suganuma, M., Watari, E., Iwaguchi, H., and Nagashima, M., 1975, Characterization of temperature-sensitive mutants of measles virus: Temperature-shift experiments, *Jap. J. Med. Sci. Biol.* **28:**223.

Yeh, J., 1973, Characterization of virus-specific RNAs from subacute schlerosing panencephalitis virus-infected CV-1 cells, *J. Virol.* **12:**962.

Young, N. P., and Ash, R., 1970, Polykaryocytes induction by Newcastle disease virus propagation on different hosts, *J. Gen. Virol.* **7:**81.

Young, N. P., and Ash, R. J., 1974, Influence of viral envelope on Newcastle disease virus infection, *Appl. Microbiol.* **28:**26.

Youngner, J. S., and Quagliana, D. O., 1975, Temperature-sensitive mutants isolated from hamster and canine cell lines persistently infected with Newcastle disease virus, *J. Virol.* **16:**1332.

Zaides, V. M., Selimova, L. M., Zhirnov, O. P., and Bukrinskaya, A. G., 1975, Protein synthesis in Sendai virus-infected cells, *J. Gen. Virol.* **27:**319.

Zhdanov, V. M., 1975, Integration of viral genomes, *Nature (London)* **256:**471.

Zhdanov, V. M., and Parfanovich, M. I., 1974, Integration of measles virus nucleic acid into the cell genome. *Arch. Ges. Virusforsch.* **45:**225.

CHAPTER 10

Genetics of Orthomyxoviruses

Lawrence E. Hightower

Microbiology Section, Biological Sciences Group
University of Connecticut
Storrs, Connecticut 06268

and

Michael A. Bratt

Microbiology Department
University of Massachusetts Medical School
Worcester, Massachusetts 01605

1. INTRODUCTION

1.1. Scope of This Chapter

The influenza viruses of man and animals comprise the orthomyxovirus group (Melnick, 1973). Originally, these viruses were grouped with the viruses which now constitute the paramyxovirus group under the designation "myxoviruses" (Andrewes *et al.,* 1955). Members of both groups possess RNA genomes and lipid-containing envelopes (ether lability), and exhibit strong affinities for various mucoid substances. Despite these common properties, the elucidation of the genome strategy of these viruses has revealed dramatic differences between paramyxoviruses and influenza viruses. Most of these differences stem from the physical nature of the genome: continuous single-stranded RNA in paramyxoviruses and a segmented single-stranded RNA genome in orthomyxoviruses. Orthomyxoviruses also have a nuclear phase in their reproduction which is absent in paramyxoviruses. Long before molecular studies revealed the disparate nature of these groups, clear differences in their genetic interactions were apparent. Over a quarter century ago, Burnet and Lind (1951) observed that recombinant viruses were produced with unexpectedly high frequency after mixed infection with two different strains of influenza virus. "High-frequency recombination," as it was usually described, can now be more aptly termed "genetic reassortment," in light of our current knowledge of the segmented genome. Both terms are used in the contemporary literature and we will use them interchangeably here. Genetic recombination (or reassortment) has yet to be convincingly demonstrated in the paramyxovirus group. Both the early genetic studies which used naturally occurring strains and variants and recent studies using temperature-sensitive mutants of influenza viruses have been dominated by phenomena related to genetic reassortment. Complementation has played only a minor role in influenza virus genetics, and, in fact, complementation analyses are complicated by the occurrence of reassortment during mixed infections. On the other hand, complementation analyses are virtually the only method available for grouping mutants of paramyxoviruses. From a genetic viewpoint, it is apparent that paramyxoviruses have more in common with rhabdoviruses than with orthomyxoviruses, while the latter more closely resemble reoviruses in their genetic behavior. The similarities between influenza viruses and reoviruses have been emphasized in a review of the molecular biology and genome strategy of segmented viruses (Shatkin, 1971) and in the chapter on reovirus genetics in this volume by Cross and Fields.

We are now well into the third decade of research in influenza virus genetics, and the combination of a voluminous literature and the numerous diverse paths that current studies are following makes it almost impossible to review this field in anything less than a separate book. The early genetic studies have been extensively reviewed (Kilbourne, 1963; Hoyle, 1968) and the reader is referred to these excellent summaries.

Reviews of contemporary genetic studies are also available. These studies have progressed in a variety of areas including the origin and evolution of pandemic strains of influenza viruses (Webster, 1972; Webster and Granoff, 1974), antigenic variation (Webster and Laver, 1971), the isolation of temperature-sensitive variants and genetic recombinants for use in the production of live vaccine strains (see Maassab, 1975, and Richman et al., 1975 for recent references), the use of antigenic hybrids for the elucidation of virion structure and biological activities of the viral proteins (Kilbourne *et al.,* 1967), and the isolation and characterization of temperature-sensitive mutants (Fenner, 1969, 1970; Ghendon, 1972). These last reviews include influenza viruses in a general overview of conditional lethal mutants of animal viruses.

In the present chapter, we have limited ourselves to areas which have not been extensively reviewed during the last 5 years, primarily the isolation and characterization of temperature-sensitive mutants of influenza viruses. We have attempted to provide a critical summary of research in this rapidly developing area and to explore the implications of these studies for understanding the biological activities and genome strategy of influenza viruses.

1.2. Historical Perspective

A proper perspective of the present state of experimentation in influenza virus genetics cannot be attained without a brief accounting of at least some of the milestones which mark previous frontiers of research in this field. The first evidence for genetic interactions came from studies by Burnet and Lind (1949) on interference phenomena. These workers observed genetic recombination among influenza viruses (1951), and performed the first quantitative studies of this phenomenon (1952). Their finding that mixed infections between the MEL and WSE strains of influenza virus yielded recombinants with frequencies as high as 37% marked the beginning of the long campaign to understand "high-frequency recombination." Two related genetic phenomena, multiplicity reactivation (genetic recombination among inactivated viruses, Henle and Liu, 1951) and cross-reactivation (recombination between an inactivated and an active virus, Burnet and Lind, 1954; Baron and Jensen, 1955), were also discovered in the early 1950s. In fact, virtually all of the major genetic phenomena of influenza viruses were observed prior to the development of adequate cell culture systems, a tribute to the tenacity of these early workers.

Technological advances in the cultivation of influenza viruses were crucial for further progress in genetic analyses. Simpson and Hirst (1961) used chicken embryo cell cultures to develop plaque assay systems for the WSN strain of influenza A and fowl plague virus. Both viruses figure prominently in current studies of temperature-sensitive mutants. Additional plaque assay systems were developed for the human isolate A_2 (influenza A [H2N2]) which multiplied in monkey kidney cells (Choppin, 1963) and NWS (a neurotropic variant of the WSN strain) which Sugiura and Kilbourne (1965) were able to grow in an aneuploid line of human conjunctival cells (clone 1-5C-4). The latter assay system was particularly valuable because all of the recombinant types produced during mixed infection with strains NWS and CAM formed plaques on the 1-5C-4 line. When the progeny from a single growth cycle of NWS and CAM in mixedly infected cells were scored on 1-5C-4 cells, recombination frequencies as high as 34% were obtained (Sugiura and Kilbourne, 1966). Thus the early observations of high-frequency recombination by Burnet and Lind could be confirmed in cell culture.

In addition to advances in the cultivation of the viruses, progress has also been made in our understanding of populations of influenza viruses. Virus populations sometimes contain a mixture of both spherical and filamentous particles. After Kilbourne and Murphy's demonstration (1960) that the filamentous morphology was an exchangeable genetic trait, particle morphology became a useful marker in recombination studies.

In 1955, Burnet and colleagues suggested that the defective particles which comprise about 90% of the particles in so-called standard virus populations (Isaacs and Donald, 1955) may interact with each other or with complete virus during mixed infections. Hirst (1973) has provided evidence that non-plaque-forming particles, the major population in most influenza virus stocks, participate in genetic interactions. The quantitative interpretation of genetic experiments would be simplified by minimizing the contributions of non-plaque-forming particles. Toward this end, virus populations which contain relatively few incomplete particles, and which are capable of producing relatively high titers of infectious virus even in cells that usually support only abortive infections, have been produced in MDBK cells (Choppin, 1969).

The production of antigenically hybrid viruses (Kilbourne *et al.*, 1967; Tumova and Pereira, 1965) such as the recombinants of equine and human influenza viruses is an important technological as well as conceptual contribution. These recombinant viruses demonstrate the genetic compatibility of human and animal influenza viruses and they have provided valuable tools for studying the structure and biological activity of virions. The practical value of genetic experiments is perhaps best illustrated by Kilbourne's (1969) use of recombination to quickly generate high-yield vaccine strains which combined the desirable growth properties of a laboratory-adapted strain such as $A_0/PR/8$ with the antigenic characteristics of an epidemic strain. Finally, the isolation of temperature-sensitive mutants, initiated by Simpson and Hirst (1968) for the WSN strain, opened a new era of research in influenza virus genetics.

1.3. Organization of this Chapter

A summary of the molecular biology of influenza viruses is presented in Section 2. We have emphasized the physical and biochemical studies of the genome, identification of gene products, and the replicative strategy of the genome, all of which provide important background information for understanding the genetic interactions of influenza viruses. Since the molecular studies of these viruses must eventually be compatible with theories on the mechanisms of the genetic interactions of influenza virus, we have not attempted to achieve a rigid separation between genetic hypotheses and molecular concepts. Accordingly, the results of a number of genetic studies have been presented in Section 2 in the context of current knowledge about the structure of the genome and how it replicates.

For a more detailed current review of the reproduction of myxoviruses, the reader is referred to Compans and Choppin's excellent summary in Vol. 4 of this series and to the recent book *The Influenza Viruses and Influenza* (Kilbourne, 1975). Extensive reviews of the biological and chemical characterization of the proteins of influenza viruses are also available (Laver, 1973; White, 1974). In this chapter, we will follow the convention of referring to the genomic RNA as virion (vRNA) or negative-strand RNA and the RNA with message sense as complementary (cRNA) or positive-strand RNA. Specific strains of influenza virus will be identified only where their molecular or genetic aspects differ significantly from the common properties of most strains of influenza viruses.

Critical summaries of the studies of temperature-sensitive mutants of influenza viruses have been organized according to the groups which originally isolated each set of mutants. This format is dictated by the current state of knowledge of the mutants. Since few mutants have been extensively characterized, most influenza virus mutants cannot be readily grouped according to phenotype. Comparative studies of the various sets of mutants have not been undertaken either, partly because the variety of parental strains and cell culture systems used do not lend themselves easily to these kinds of analyses. Therefore, attempts to compare recombination groups exhibiting similar phenotypic properties are tenuous at best. Despite these ambiguities, significant progress has been made in the characterization of the temperature-sensitive mutants over the past several years, and it may be useful now to summarize the current state of affairs.

2. MOLECULAR BIOLOGY OF THE GENOME

2.1. The Genome

2.1.1. Chemical Nature and Size

Purified virus particles contain RNA (approximately 0.78% of the dry weight) but not detectable amounts of DNA (Ada and Perry, 1954). Analyses of the base composition, RNase sensitivity, and variations in the sedimentation coefficient of viral RNA as a function of salt concentration indicate that it is predominantly single stranded (Duesberg and Robinson, 1967).

Direct measurements of the size of the complete genome have not been possible since the nucleic acid extracted from virus particles is not infectious. Like other negative-strand viruses, the influenza genome requires a virion-associated polymerase for successful infection. Less direct size estimates are currently based on the separation of the RNA extracted from purified virions on polyacrylamide gels. An important reservation in all size estimates of the genome is that the majority of particles in most influenza virus preparations are non-plaque-formers, and the RNA derived from these particles, which must be the bulk of the RNA observed on gels, may not be representative of the genome complement of complete particles. Virus populations produced in cells such as MDBK, which give high yields of infectious particles and apparently little incomplete virus, should provide more reliable sources of genome RNA.

The most recent size estimates (Table 1) are based on the separation of single-stranded RNA on acrylamide–agarose–urea gels by the methods of Floyd et al. (1974). The consensus is that the RNA extracted from purified virions of influenza type A can be separated into eight size classes (three large segments, three intermediate segments, and two small segments) using improved methods of slab gel electrophoresis (Bean and Simpson, 1976; Content, 1976; Pons, 1976; Ritchey et al., 1976). Palese and Schulman (1976) obtained slightly different patterns for influenza A. The exact number of RNA segments

Table 1

Relationship between Viral Proteins and Genome RNAs

	Virion RNAs (10^{-5})							
	(1)	(2)	(3)	(4)	(5)	(6)	(7)	(8)
A/FPV (Inglis *et al.,* 1976)	11.9	10.2	10.0	8.3	6.8	5.8	3.2	2.8
A/WSN (Pons, 1976)	11.6	10.6^a	10.6^a	8.5	6.7	5.6	3.4	2.3
Polypeptides $(10^{-3})^{b,c}$	P_3	P_1	P_2	HA	NP	NA	M	NS
A/FPV (Inglis *et al.,* 1976)	85	96	87	75	53	45	25	23
A/WSN (Lamb and Choppin, 1976; Palese and Schulman, 1976; Pons, 1976)	85	96	87	80	60–65	58–72	26	25

a Two species were partially resolved.
b Molecular weight estimates of glycopolypeptides based on electrophoretic mobility are often anomalous.
c Our tentative assignments of individual polypeptides to specific RNA segments are based upon the correlations determined for strain A/PR/8/34 [HON1] by Ritchey *et al.,* 1976*b*.

resolved by gel electrophoresis varied from seven to nine depending on the multiplicity of infection used to produce the virus population for RNA extractions.

Size estimates for the complete genome of influenza A viruses based on these gel analyses range from 5.29×10^6 (Ritchey *et al.,* 1976) to 5.9×10^6 (Pons, 1976), assuming that each segment has a unique nucleotide sequence, each is essential for infectivity, and only one copy of each segment is present in a complete genome. The assumption that all eight of the segments detected on gels are unique has recently been confirmed by oligonucleotide mapping (McGeoch *et al.,* 1976).

Virtually all of the recent analyses of the genome RNA have employed type A influenza viruses; however, Ritchey *et al.* (1976*a*) have compared the gel patterns of RNAs extracted from types B and C as well as influenza A. Like type A, influenza B contains eight RNA segments with a total molecular weight of 6.43×10^6. At least four segments having a total molecular weight of 4.67×10^6, were obtained from influenza type C virions. This may well be a minimum estimate for the type C genome, and an analysis of the complexity of the RNA in discrete gel bands would be useful in identifying potentially heterogeneous regions.

2.1.2. Biochemical Evidence of a Segmented Genome

The general similarity in the polyacrylamide gel electropherograms of RNA extracted by a variety of procedures (including the studies described in Section 2.1.1 and previous gel studies by Duesberg, 1968; Pons and Hirst, 1968; Choppin and Pons, 1970; Skehel, 1971*b*; Bishop *et al.*, 1971; Lewandowski *et al.*, 1971; Bromley and Barry, 1973) supports the hypothesis that the genome RNA is not randomly fragmented during extraction but rather exists in a segmented form within the virion. End-group analysis of the virion RNA provides additional support for this hypothesis. The 5′ termini of the RNA molecules in each of three size classes obtained by velocity sedimentation are adenosine tetraphosphate (pppAp) (Young and Content, 1971). Uridine is present at the nonphosphorylated 3′ termini in all three classes Lewandowski (1971). It is unlikely that these termini would result from the endonucleolytic cleavage of a single polyribonucleotide.

Additional biochemical evidence for the segmented nature of the genome and for the uniqueness of the large, intermediate, and small size classes of genome RNA has been provided by hybridization and thermal denaturation studies. As a result of cross-hybridization experiments among the three size classes of single-stranded RNA extracted from virions and the corresponding size classes of base-paired RNA from infected cells, Content and Duesberg (1971) concluded that base sequences present in the smallest class are absent in larger molecules. This result would not be expected if the small molecules arose by degradation of larger ones. Distinct oligonucleotide sequences have also been identified in all eight of the genome RNA segments of influenza A (McGeoch *et al.*, 1976). Finally, the several species of double-stranded RNA isolated from fowl plague virus-infected cells possess distinct thermal transition profiles, suggesting they correspond to unique segments (Bromley and Barry, 1973).

2.1.3. Biological Evidence of a Segmented Genome

Attempts to understand the mechanism of high-frequency recombination resulted in proposals by Burnet (1956) and Hirst (1962) that recombination in influenza virus must occur via a mechanism of random reassortment of subgenomic segments, each capable of independent replication. If recombination occurred by conventional mechanisms of breakage and reunion as in the DNA bacteriophages, frequencies of 1–2% would be predicted for a single polynucleotide the size of the influenza virus genome. The facility with which both influenza type A (Barry, 1961) and type B (Kilbourne, 1955) undergo multiplicity reactivation also supports the theory of a segmented genome.

Additional biological evidence is derived from studies of the sequential inactivation of viral functions. Chemical inactivation of influenza virus by exposure to ethylene iminoquinone is accompanied by a sequential loss in the capacity of the altered genome to produce active hemagglutinin, neuraminidase, and finally ribonucleoprotein antigen in infected cells (Scholtissek and Rott, 1964). In contrast, these functions are inactivated at approximately the same rate for Newcastle disease virus, which has a continuous single-stranded RNA genome. The finding that ultraviolet irradiation of influenza virus results in a preferential reduction in the accumulation of the largest species of viral RNA and proteins in infected cells (Joss *et al.*, 1969) is also consistent with the hypothesis that the segments are capable of independent expression.

McCahon *et al.* (1975) have used influenza virus's propensity for genetic reassortment to advantage in marker rescue experiments between γ-irradiated fowl plague virus and human virus A/BEL/42 which does not plaque on chick embryo cells. Recombinant viruses were analyzed for six genetic markers (hemagglutinin and neuraminidase antigens, chick embryo lethality, plaque accessory factor, specific infectivity, and temperature sensitivity of reproduction), all of which were found to assort independently of one another and in a random manner. The target size for the hemagglutinin and neuraminidase antigens determined experimentally correlated well with their predicted gene size, based on the known molecular weights of the proteins. Again, these observations are compatible with the existence of a segmented genome, or at least with the existence of genes which act as independent units at some point during replication.

2.2. Gene Products

2.2.1. Viral Proteins

With minor exceptions, similar species of viral proteins are found in cells infected by a variety of different influenza viruses. The polypeptide products of influenza A/WSN and fowl plague virus, parental types for most of the mutants to be discussed, are summarized in Table 1 along with current molecular weight estimates. The designations of the polypeptides are based on probable biological functions (Kilbourne *et al.*, 1972). Current estimates of the number of primary gene products range from seven (P1, P2, HA, NA, NP, M, NS) with a total molecular weight of 4.1×10^5 to nine (P1, P2, P3, HA, NA, NP,

M, NS1, NS2) with a total molecular weight of approximately 5.1 $\times$ 10^5, still within the estimated coding capacity of the genome.

In Table 1, we have correlated each of the eight viral proteins which we consider the most likely to be primary gene products with the virion RNA segment possessing the appropriate coding capacity. The validity of constructing such a table rests upon the hypothesis that each virion RNA segment codes for a monocistronic messenger RNA, which in turn directs the synthesis of a single viral protein. Firm support for this hypothesis has recently been provided by Ritchey and co-workers (1976*b*). Using improved systems of polyacrylamide gel electrophoresis for both proteins and single-stranded RNAs, these investigators were able to distinguish all of the proteins (except NA which is distinguished serologically) and genome RNA segments of influenza A/PR/8 from those of strain A/Hong Kong. By taking advantage of the ability of these two strains to readily undergo genetic reassortment during mixed infections, Ritchey *et al.* were able to isolate recombinant progeny viruses containing only one or two genes from one parent and the balance of the genome from the other parent. Analysis of the RNA and proteins of these recombinants allowed the gene products of specific RNA segments to be identified. The correlations shown in Table 1 were derived for the A/PR/8 strain. The correlation between proteins and genome RNAs for the A/HK/8/68 [H3N2] strain was similar except that RNA segment (6) coded for NP, and segment (5) coded for NA. Therefore, some variability among strains exists, and the suggested correlations for A/WSN and A/FPV are only speculative. An additional high molecular weight polypeptide, designated P3 in Table 1 has been identified by high resolution polyacrylamide gel analysis of the proteins of strains A/PR/8, A/ HK (Ritchey *et al.*, 1976*b*), A/WSN (Lamb and Choppin, 1976), and A/ FPV (Inglis *et al.*, 1976). In addition, Inglis and co-workers (1976) have established the uniqueness of the three P proteins of FPV by two-dimensional tryptic peptide analysis. Following, the one segment-one gene hypothesis, we have omitted the NS2 protein (10,000–15,000 molecular weight) from Table 1 because a genome segment of corresponding coding capacity has not been routinely observed.

The largest glycoprotein HA (hemagglutinating activity) is synthesized as a primary gene product; however, HA is sometimes cleaved to form two polypeptides, HA1 and HA2. Cleavage of this glycoprotein depends on several factors including the particular host cell, the virus strain, and serum plasminogen levels. Neither hemagglutinating activity nor the specific infectivity of influenza virions is affected by the cleavage of HA. This glycoprotein forms one of the two morphologically distinct types of spike structure on the surface of the influenza virion. Each spike is composed of a trimer of HA held together by noncovalent bonds (Griffith, 1975). Each HA molecule is composed of HA1 and HA2, either separate or uncleaved, which are joined by disulfide bonds. The active site (or sites) for binding to erythrocytes or susceptible cells, for hemagglutinin-inhibiting antibodies, and for neutralizing antibodies is situated on this spike.

The NA glycoprotein is responsible for the neuraminidase activity of virions and infected cells. It too forms a spike structure on the surface of virions. This spike has a molecular weight of 180,000–270,000 and probably consists of four monomers of the NA glycoprotein. The monomers are linked in pairs by disulfide bonds, and pairs of dimers are noncovalently associated. Only one size class of NA glycoprotein has been detected in different strains of influenza virus except for the recombinant strain A/X-7 (H0N2) in which two species, NA1 and NA2, have been detected. The possibilities that these two species represent conformational alternatives or alterations in the carbohydrate moiety of the same gene product have not been eliminated.

The nonglycosylated membrane protein M is the most abundant polypeptide in virions, comprising approximately one-third of the total mass of virion protein. The electron-dense internal layer observed in electron photomicrographs of virions and modified regions of plasma membrane of infected cells is probably formed by aggregates of M (Apostolov and Flewett, 1969; Compans and Dimmock, 1969; Bachi *et al.*, 1969). The M protein may have the structural functions of adding rigidity to the virion envelope and providing recognition sites between viral-modified regions of the plasma membrane and the viral ribonucleoprotein complex. Gregoriades (1973) has taken advantage of the hydrophobic nature of M in order to selectively extract this protein from both virions and infected cells with acidified chloroform–methanol solutions.

The major polypeptide component of viral ribonucleoprotein complexes isolated from either virions or infected cells is NP, the nucleocapsid protein. NP binds avidly *in vitro* to viral RNAs of both positive and negative polarity. Two of the largest viral proteins P_1 and P_2, were previously shown to be associated with ribonucleoprotein complexes which possess transcriptase activity (Bishop *et al.*, 1972; Caliguiri and Compans, 1974), and recently, all three of the P proteins of fowl plague virus have been detected in active ribonucleoprotein complexes (Inglis *et al.*, 1976). The P proteins are considered likely candidates for the polymerase activity. However, a direct dependence of polymerase activity on the presence of P has not been demonstrated by *in vitro* reconstitution experiments like those involving the L protein of vesicular stomatitis virus (Emerson and Wagner, 1973).

Two additional polypeptides, NS1 and NS2 (nonstructural), accumulate in infected cells but are not detected in virions. Neither of these proteins has been assigned an unambiguous biological role. NS1 has been detected in at least two different locations in infected cells. Some of the NS1 proteins synthesized in the cytoplasm migrate to the nucleus and accumulate in the nucleolus (Krug and Etkind, 1975). Their function in the nucleus is unknown. NS1 is also found in association with cytoplasmic ribosomes (Pons, 1972; Compans, 1973). Both ribosomal subunits bind significant amounts of NS1, but only in low-salt buffer, which raises doubts about the functional significance of the association (Krug and Etkind, 1975).

NS1 has almost the same electrophoretic mobility on polyacrylamide gels as the M protein, and several groups have compared the tryptic peptide patterns of these two proteins in order to assess the relationship between them. The results have been contradictory. In one study (Gregoriades, 1973) one-dimensional tryptic peptide analyses revealed considerable similarity between the fingerprints of NS1 and M, while in other studies (Lazarowitz *et al.*, 1971; Inglis *et al.*, 1976) distinctly different tryptic peptide maps of the two proteins were obtained. The recent finding (Krug, personal communication) that the smallest and next-smallest classes of complementary RNA isolated from infected cells contain the mRNAs for NS1 and M, respectively, supports the notion that each of these proteins is a unique viral gene product.

A small nonstructural protein NS2 having a molecular weight of 10,000–15,000 has been detected in fowl plague virus-infected cells (Skehel, 1972) and also in the nucleus of MDBK cells infected with the WSN strain (Krug and Etkind, 1975). Except for a small genome RNA segment recently detected by Palese and Schulman (1976), genome segments possessing the appropriate coding capacity for NS2 have not been routinely detected, and it is not known whether this polypeptide is a degradation product or a primary gene product.

2.2.2. Viral mRNA

Several recent studies have shown that viral mRNA, which is free from contamination by double-stranded RNA and viral genome RNA, can be isolated from influenza virus-infected cells, and that this mRNA contains sequences complementary to at least 80% of the viral genome

(Glass *et al.,* 1975; Etkind and Krug, 1975). These studies should pave the way for the separation and recovery of the viral mRNAs by a suitable technique such as formamide gel electrophoresis and the subsequent correlation of individual genome segments with each size class of mRNA by RNA-RNA hybridization. The isolated species of mRNA can also be assayed in cell-free protein-synthesizing systems to determine protein products. Krug and associates (personal communication) have recently made progress in this direction. They have separated cRNA extracted from infected cells on polyacrylamide gels and recovered three cRNA bands corresponding in size to genome segments 5, 7, and 8. Wheat germ extracts programmed with each of these cRNAs synthesized proteins which corresponded in electrophoretic mobility to NP, M, and NS1, respectively. At present, the correlation between the remaining genome segments and the polypeptide(s) encoded by each rests upon the analyses of recombinant viruses (Ritchey *et al.,* 1976b) and on the similarities in number and molecular weight (coding capacity) of the segments and the known viral proteins (Table 1). These studies are in agreement and do suggest that each virion RNA segment represents one gene coding for a single polypeptide.

Etkind and Krug (1975) have provided the strongest evidence that most of the proteins isolated from virions and as major species from infected cells are in fact virus coded. They prepared viral mRNA from MDCK (canine kidney) cells infected with WSN. Cordycepin was used to block the appearance of newly synthesized cellular mRNA in the cytoplasm, and cycloheximide was added to increase the ratio of single-stranded to double-stranded viral RNA. The addition of cordycepin rules out the presence of most newly synthesized cellular mRNA but not preexisting cellular mRNA which may have been activated by infection. Using these procedures, they were able to isolate RNA from the cytoplasm which was almost 100% single stranded, rendered almost 100% RNase resistant by annealing with genome RNA, and representing 84–90% of the genome. The viral mRNA was translated in wheat germ cell-free extracts. Four proteins were synthesized which comigrated on polyacrylamide gels with authentic P, NP, M, and NS. Three of these, NP, M, and NS, were further identified as authentic viral proteins by immunoprecipitation with specific antisera. Two candidates for nonglycosylated HA and NA were also detected among the products of cell-free synthesis. The cell-free synthesis of NP and M in wheat germ extracts programmed with poly(A)-containing RNA from fowl plague virus-infected cells has been confirmed by Content (1976). The products of cell-free translation were authenticated by tryptic peptide analyses.

The most rigorous test for virus-coded proteins—synthesis of viral mRNA by the detergent-activated virion-associated transcriptase followed by translation of the mRNA in cell-free protein synthesizing systems—has been hampered by technical difficulties with the *in vitro* polymerase reaction. Some of the major problems—low activity, small product size, and lack of poly(A)addition to the cRNA—have recently been overcome by the use of dinucleoside monophosphates to stimulate the polymerase reaction. McGeoch and Kitron (1975) found that GpG and GpC were effective in stimulating the virion-associated transcriptase. Krug *et al.* (personal communication) confirmed the effect of these dinucleoside monophosphates and also of ApG, which gave the largest stimulation (110-fold) in their studies. The product synthesized in the presence of ApG and GpG was similar to cRNA from infected cells in size, polarity, and in the possession of poly(A).

2.3. Replication and Assembly

Detailed accounts of the replication and assembly of influenza viruses have been presented in the chapter by Compans and Choppin in Volume 4 of this series, in *Influenza Viruses and Influenza* (1975), and also in the two-volume compendium *Negative-Strand Viruses* (1975). Less recent but still quite pertinent reviews are available by Kingsbury (1970) and Pons (1970) and in the collection of influenza virus papers in *The Biology of Large RNA Viruses* (1970). Therefore, we will only briefly consider two aspects of central importance in genetic studies, the mode of assembly of the genome into virions and the physical state of the replicative complexes.

2.3.1. Assembly

The mechanism of packaging of the genome into virions is thought to involve either a coordinate mechanism or the packaging of individual segments by a process of random envelopment. Compans *et al.* (1970) have pointed out that production of complete virions would be very inefficient if only the same number of segments as required for a complete genome were randomly assembled. For example, the probability of assembling a particle with an entire genome would be 0.04 if the complete genome contained five segments and only five are taken at random. However, packaging additional segments substantially increases the probability of obtaining a full genome complement, 0.12 if six segments are taken and 0.22 if seven are taken at random. Such a packaging mechanism should result in the production of partial diploids or heterozygous particles with rather high frequency. However, as suggested in Section 3.5, the occurrence of heterozygotes (or mixed aggregates) is infrequent.

Laver and Downie (1976) have recently presented results of a recombinant virus analysis which are more consistent with the existence of a coordinate packaging mechanism rather than a random one. Virus yields from cells mixedly infected by several different strains of influenza type A (BEL, Port Chalmers, Shearwater) were analyzed. The progeny were cloned at limiting dilution (eliminating phenotypically mixed particles) without antibody selection. Populations obtained in this manner were analyzed for markers which were distinguishable in the parental viruses—hemagglutinin and neuraminidase subunits were characterized antigenically and the M proteins were identified by one-dimensional peptide mapping. Analysis of recombinant viruses revealed two very interesting patterns. During recombination, segregation of the M protein was independent of either the hemagglutinin or neuraminidase proteins. Furthermore, none of the cloned virus populations possessed more than one parental type of hemagglutinin or neuraminidase subunit. This result strongly suggests that each plaque-forming particle contains only one active copy of each gene. If each gene indeed corresponds to a genome RNA segment, a coordinate packaging of the genome segments may occur during virus maturation. Alternatively, as Laver and Downie also suggested, the production of virus particles containing only a single copy of each segment may be favored by a selection process.

Several other lines of evidence lend support to the coordinate assembly hypothesis. In MDBK cells, the production of complete virus particles is very efficient (see Section 3.2.1), and it is difficult to reconcile this level of efficiency with a random envelopment process. Kingsbury (1970) has pointed out that populations of influenza virus and Newcastle disease virus, which has a continuous covalently linked genome, contain similar proportions of plaque-forming and non-plaque-forming particles, which might indicate a lack of gross differences in the efficiency of virus assembly. Clearly, the efficiency of production of complete influenza viruses varies dramatically with the particular host cell used (Section 3.2.1), and random assembly processes may predominate in some systems while a coordinate mechanism is favored in others, with a spectrum of possible combinations in between. In our opinion, the weight of evidence (albeit mostly circumstantial) has now shifted in favor of a coordinate assembly process by which genetically complete virions can be assembled with high efficiency. Presumably this coordinate process is perturbed in certain cell types (or perhaps under particular conditions of infection, such as serial undiluted passage) so that less than a complete complement of genomic segments is packaged. However, a perturbation involving the packaging of more than one copy of each gene per virion would be a rare event. We further assume that the capacity of coordinate assembly is an intrinsic property of the virus and not primarily the function of the particular host cell. Some evidence for this possibility is presented in the following section.

2.3.2. Replication

The crucial aspect of replication for understanding genetic interactions is the physical state of the parental and progeny genomes during infection. The overwhelming majority of genetic studies (see Section 2.1.3), especially those in which the genetic markers can be ascribed to a single gene such as HA, NA, and M, support the existence of independently replicating RNA segments, each containing a single gene. Only the study by Mackenzie (1970*b*) of temperature-sensitive mutants of influenza virus, in which additive recombination frequencies were reported, contradicts the random reassortment hypothesis (Section 4.1). However, even if we presume that the genome segments can reassort at near-random frequencies, we still do not know when this occurs during RNA replication, and whether or not the genome enjoys only a transient independence from a state in which the segments are associated in a specific order. Pons (1970) originally proposed the hypothesis that the genome RNA segments may be ordered on a "protein backbone" and that this complex is conserved during replication. He further suggested that newly synthesized positive strands may displace parental negative strands to create a replication template in which the original gene order is preserved. The RNA in such a ribonucleoprotein structure would have to be accessible to displacement, and, in fact, some evidence exists that the ribonucleoprotein complexes of influenza viruses are quite different from those of other negative-strand viruses such as Newcastle disease virus (NDV). In contrast to NDV, the RNA in influenza virus RNPs is sensitive to bovine pancreatic ribonuclease, while the nucleocapsid protein is protected from extensive proteolysis (Duesberg, 1969; Kingsbury and

Webster, 1969; Pons, 1970). Displacement of the RNA in the ribonucleoprotein complex can be accomplished by a polyanion, polyvinylsulfate, without significantly altering the morphology or sedimentation behavior of the complex, suggesting that the protein "backbone" provides the structural integrity for the RNP. Kingsbury (1970) has entertained the hypothesis that a consequence of a more open RNP structure may be to allow specific pairing among exposed bases on different RNA segments. Such base pairing could provide a mechanism for coordinating the assembly of the genome RNA segments. The extent of base pairing would have to be limited since influenza virion RNAs do not self-anneal to an appreciable extent (Duesberg and Robinson, 1967).

The question then becomes, is there any direct evidence for the existence of multisegmented complexes? Some evidence exists for noncovalent interactions between genome RNA segments. An aggregate of 3×10^6 daltons is obtained when RNA is extracted in the presence of divalent cations (Agrawal and Bruening, 1966; Pons, 1967a). After heating, this aggregate is converted to slower-sedimenting RNA species. Electron microscopic studies of RNA extracted by phenol/SDS from purified virions of three different strains of influenza virus have revealed molecules with average lengths of 2.4–2.7 μm, which correspond to 2.5–2.9 $\times 10^6$ daltons of RNA (Li and Seto, 1971). After a brief exposure at pH 3 or prolonged storage, only small RNA molecules were detected. Extraction of RNA, even by strong denaturants such as SDS and phenol, does not entirely rule out the existence of protein–nucleic acid interactions (Shatkin, 1971; Kubinski and Gibbs, 1970), and it is conceivable that a protein or small RNA "linker" is present in these RNA preparations. Also, Rochovansky and Hirst (1976) presented some evidence that the infectious ribonucleoprotein complexes which they isolated from virions readily form aggregates. Although these data suggest that interaction between segments may exist, evidence of specificity in these interactions is lacking. Furthermore, no multisegmented complexes have been successfully isolated from infected cells. Viral RNPs of both positive and negative polarity isolated from infected cells have sedimentation properties similar to those isolated from virions and characteristic of structures containing the different size classes of viral genome RNA (Duesberg, 1969; Krug, 1971, 1972; Pons, 1971, 1972; Compans and Caliguiri, 1973). Like other negative-strand viruses, RNPs of influenza virus with the expected properties of functionally active replicase complexes have not been routinely isolated from infected cells (for a possible exception, see Ruck *et al.,* 1969). However, RNase-resistant RNA which may represent base-paired replicative forms (Duesberg and Robinson, 1967; Nayak, 1970; Pons, 1967*b*) and partially base-paired RNA which may represent replicative intermediates (Nayak and Baluda, 1969; Nayak, 1970) have been isolated from infected cells. These "deproteinated" structures are of course compatible with a model of replication based on either independently replicating segments or segments ordered on a protein backbone or otherwise noncovalently linked.

3.   VIRUS POPULATION

3.1.   Plaque-Forming and Non-Plaque-Forming Particles

It is apparent from recent studies of influenza virus populations that the old descriptions of populations composed of "infectious" and "non-infectious" particles can be misleading. When the usual plaque assay techniques are used to quantify virus yields, populations may be more accurately described as containing plaque-forming (PF) and non-plaque-forming (NPF) particles (Hirst and Pons, 1973; Hirst, 1973).

Most influenza virus populations contain only 1–10% (Schulze, 1970) plaque-forming particles. The remainder of the population (NPF) may include particles which have been thermally inactivated or otherwise physically damaged, and randomly defective particles, subpopulations each missing different genomic segments. According to Hirst (1973), if two non-plaque-formers, each deficient in a different RNP segment, enter the same cell, complementation may occur, followed by mixing and random assembly of progeny RNP segments into virus particles, only a small proportion of which receive a full genomic complement of RNA.

The frequency with which non-plaque-forming particles enter a cell in close enough proximity to effectively complement one another can be significantly increased by particle aggregation. Such aggregation occurs naturally at low levels in stocks of influenza virus and can be enhanced for experimental studies by the use of polycations such as nucleohistone (Dahlberg and Simon, 1969; Hirst and Pons, 1973). The penetration of cells by such viral aggregates has been the subject of recent studies (Dales and Pons, 1976) which suggest that even virus particles clumped with an excess of inactive (UV-irradiated) virus are highly infectious.

Viral aggregation and the participation of non-plaque-forming particles in intracellular events may be important factors in genetic studies of the temperature-sensitive mutants of influenza virus. When chicken embryo cells were mixedly infected with *ts*12 and *ts*25, temperature-sensitive (*ts*) mutants of the WSN strain of influenza A (Simpson and Hirst, 1968), and incubated at the permissive temperature, about 6% of the progeny yield were scored as wild-type recombinants, virus capable of forming plaques similar to the wild-type strain at the nonpermissive temperature (Table 2). When the input multiplicity of infection was reduced tenfold, the frequency of recombinants in the progeny yield remained at 6%, despite a more than sixtyfold reduction in the theoretical fraction of mixedly infected cells. Subsequent studies showed that certain pairs of mutants formed mixed aggregates more readily than others and that recombinant-yielding cells were generated via a single-hit process by infection with these aggregates. Recombinant-yielding cells could also be generated by independent infection of the same cell by two different *ts* mutants, a two-hit process. Such recombinant-yielding cells were obtained using very low input multiplicities of infection, suggesting that non-plaque-forming particles were the principal source of recombinants. Recombinants could be obtained even when cells mixedly infected at low multiplicities by a pair of *ts* mutants were incubated only at the nonpermissive temperature. Hirst (1973) suggested that the initial events leading to recombinant formation must involve complementation, followed by synthesis and reassortment of progeny RNP segments. Recombinant viruses which packaged a full complement of unmutated genomic segments would produce wild-type plaques. In order to complement efficiently, the non-plaque-forming virus must have the capacity to enter cells and initiate macromolecular synthesis, at least messenger RNA

TABLE 2

WSN *ts* Mutants Grown in CEF Cells at Permissive Temperature[a]

Input MOI *ts*12	PFU/cell *ts*25	Calculated fraction of mixedly infected cells[b]	Wild-type recombinants percentage of 34°C yield[c]
0.65	0	0	0.001
0	0.51	0	0.0007
0.65	0.51	19%	6
0.065	0.051	0.3%	6.7

[a] Adapted from Table 2, Simpson and Hirst (1968).
[b] Formula: $(1 - e^{-M_A})(1 - e^{-M_B}) \times 100$, where M_A and M_B are input multiplicities of the infecting virus.
[c] Progeny virus capable of forming plaques at both permissive and nonpermissive temperatures.

and viral protein synthesis, although very low levels of synthesis may be adequate (see Section 4.2.2b).

3.2. Interference

3.2.1. von Magnus Virus

The original "von Magnus effect" was a progressive decrease in the ratio of plaque-forming particles to hemagglutinating particles (a measure of the number of physical particles) following serial undiluted passage in embryonated eggs (von Magnus, 1954). The defective particles produced under these conditions have been called "noninfectious hemagglutinating particles," "incomplete virus," or "von Magnus virus." In addition to reduced infectivity, populations of von Magnus virus possess aberrant virion morphologies (Almeida and Waterson, 1970), lower virion-associated transcriptase activity (Bean and Simpson, 1976), less total RNA (Ada and Perry, 1954), and altered proportions of genomic RNA segments (Duesberg, 1968; Pons and Hirst, 1969; Choppin and Pons, 1970). However, as recently demonstrated by Bean and Simpson (1976), the causal relationships between polymerase activity or RNA patterns and the loss of infectivity of von Magnus virus are ambiguous. For example, after the third undiluted passage in embryonated eggs, the specific infectivity of WSN decreased by a factor of 10^4, while virion-associated transcriptase activity was reduced only 2.7-fold. Hybridization studies revealed that all of the virion RNP segments were transcribed *in vitro*. Therefore, the loss of polymerase activity is not large enough to account for the loss of infectivity. Infectivity starts decreasing prior to any gross alterations in the relative proportions of the virion RNA segments. After the third passage, the amounts of large genomic RNA segments were reduced from 48% to 17% of the total virion RNA; however, none of the three largest segments was completely absent. In lieu of positive correlations among these phenomena, Bean and Simpson suggested that von Magnus virus may be composed of a large population of randomly defective particles similar to those postulated to exist in standard virus populations (Hirst, see Section 3.1). According to this hypothesis, the average defective particle would contain less than a genomic complement of RNA, which would be consistent with Ada and Perry's (1954) finding of less total RNA in von Magnus populations than in standard virus stocks. Instead of random defects, some observations on von Magnus virus seem more readily explicable by the existence of nonrandom defects. Specifically, von Magnus virus does not readily undergo multiplicity reactivation (Rott and Scholtissek, 1963), and recently it has been reported (Choppin *et al.,* 1975) that von Magnus virus has been placed in the same recombination–complementation group as Sugiura's group II (putative replicase defects) temperature-sensitive mutants.

Additional defects in populations of von Magnus virus have been reported. Morphological studies of von Magnus virus by electron microscopy show that the appearance of abnormal particles roughly parallels the reduction in the proportion of plaque-forming particles in the virus population (Almeida and Waterson, 1970). Several different aberrant particle morphologies were observed, the common feature being a defect in the assembly or composition of the viral envelope. Meier-Ewert and Dimmock (1970) have suggested another possibility for the formation of incomplete particles. The neuraminidase enzyme of the input inoculum may contribute to the production of von Magnus virus by concentrating around the nuclear membrane of infected cells and consequently altering the passage of viral products such as RNP between nucleus and cytoplasm.

It is apparent that populations of von Magnus virus possess a number of defects related to RNA replication and/or assembly, some of which may be random and others nonrandom. Furthermore, it is clear that various defects appear at different passage levels, and that the perturbation in virus reproduction responsible for the original von Magnus phenomenon (reduced PFU/particle ratio) is not yet understood.

The development (Choppin, 1969) of a virus–cell system in which the occurrence of the von Magnus phenomenon is minimal has proved useful for both genetic and molecular studies. Plaque-forming particles are produced efficiently in the MDBK line of bovine kidney cells. The populations contain relatively little incomplete virus capable of producing low yields when used as inoculum in other kinds of cells. Von Magnus virus can be produced in MDBK cells, but three or four serial, undiluted passages are required instead of one passage as in most cell types.

3.2.3. Unidirectional Interference

In addition to the von Magnus effect, which may be considered autointerference, a second type of interference, unidirectional and host dependent, has been reported (Noronha-Blob and Schulze, 1976). Two variants of influenza A_0/WSN have been isolated which have the same plaque morphology on chick cells and are indistinguishable in density, size, polypeptide composition, RNA-dependent RNA polymerase activity, hemagglutinating activity, neuraminidase activity, and infectivity. The variants can be distinguished by plaque morphology on MDBK cells, although after passage in these cells the variants are still similar in the other properties listed above. One variant, designated F, has a fuzzy plaque morphology, while the C variant forms clear plaques on MDBK cells. These variants exhibited nonreciprocal interference that resulted in the elimination of the F variant from the viral progeny of MDBK cells. The interference phenomenon did not occur when the variants were cocultivated in chick embryo cell cultures.

These observations may be very important for genetic studies. Cells which support unidirectional interference could be useful for selecting a desired recombinant from the progeny of mixedly infected cells. On the other hand, unidirectional interference could complicate the recovery or quantification of reciprocal recombinants. For example, there is some indication that the production of wild-type recombinants may be suppressed as a result of interference by one or both of the parental temperature-sensitive mutants (Sugiura, 1975) in some genetic crosses. The extent to which interference phenomena have affected recombination and complementation analyses of the temperature-sensitive mutants of influenza viruses is not known. A review of early studies of interference among influenza viruses and the significance of these phenomena for recombination studies has been presented by Kilbourne (1963).

3.3. Genetic Dimorphism

Kilbourne has proposed the term "genetic dimorphism" to describe the simultaneous, balanced maintenance in the influenza virus population of variants which possess distinct phenotypes. Such genetic heterogeneity would presumably confer a survival advantage on the population (Mowshowitz and Kilbourne, 1975). Particle morphology was one of the first dimorphic properties to be observed (Burnet and Lind, 1957; Kilbourne and Murphy, 1960; Kilbourne, 1963; Choppin, 1963). Virus populations of newly isolated strains often contain particles with both spherical and filamentous morphologies. Although the molecular basis for this alteration in virion structure is unknown, the production of filamentous particles has provided a useful marker in recombination experiments.

Another dimorphic property which has been recognized for a long time is receptor affinity (Choppin and Tamm, 1960a,b, 1964; Choppin et al., 1960). Influenza A_2 contains two populations of particles designated "plus" (+) and "minus" (−). The plus particles are very sensitive to neutralization by antibodies, serum inhibitors, and urinary mucoprotein, elute poorly from human erythrocytes, and agglutinate erythrocytes treated with neuraminidase. The minus particles have the opposite properties. Biochemical studies have not revealed significant differences in the protein compositions of either the morphological variants or the + variants (see Compans and Choppin, Vol. 4, this series).

Quantitative differences among subpopulations have been reported for variants of still another dimorphic characteristic, neuraminidase activity (Mowshowitz and Kilbourne, 1975; Palese and Schulman, 1974; Webster and Campbell, 1972; Kilbourne et al., 1967; Webster et al., 1968). In the most recent study of NA variants, Mowshowitz and Kilbourne (1975) showed that the variants designated NA^+ (high activity) and NA^- (low activity) were present in their standard virus stock of the Aichi H3N2 strain. These variants showed tenfold differences in the ratio of neuraminidase to hemagglutinin activities; polyacrylamide gel electrophoresis revealed a corresponding difference in the amounts of NA protein in the two variants. The NA^+ character was shown to be a genetically stable trait.

The F and C variants described by Noronha-Blob and Schulze (see Section 3.2.2) may also be an example of genetic dimorphism. When viral reproduction occurs in chick embryo cells, little selective pressure acts on the F/C property, and a balance which allows the survival of both variants is attained. In MDBK cells, the F variant is lost through an unknown selective mechanism which upsets the reproductive balance in the virus population. Mowshowitz and Kilbourne (1975) have suggested that the presence of incomplete particles in influenza virus populations may also be a form of genetic polymorphism, although the functional significance of this property is not clear. Dimorphic properties continue to provide useful genetic markers in the instances where variants can be separated and relatively homogeneous stocks prepared.

3.4. Phenotypic Mixing

Phenotypically mixed particles are readily produced in mixed infections of type A and B influenza viruses (Gottlieb and Hirst, 1954) and even of influenza viruses and paramyxoviruses (Granoff and Hirst, 1954). Given the ease with which phenotypic mixing occurs, a substantial portion of the progeny from mixed infections by influenza variants and strains undoubtedly consists of phenotypically mixed particles.

Phenotypic mixing is a potentially complicating factor in genetic analysis of temperature-sensitive mutants. Consider the following example. A mutant may possess lesions in two different structural genes. One lesion results in the synthesis of an M protein which is temperature sensitive but only in association with an altered NP protein which is not temperature sensitive and retains near-normal function. If such a mutant is crossed in a complementation test with another mutant possessing a ts defect in the M protein but having a normal gene for NP protein, the cross will give apparent complementation even though both mutants possess lesions in the same gene. Here, the mutant phenotype is only expressed in the presence of another mutation. The possible existence of such "sensitizing" mutations has been discussed in the context of phage genetics by Hartman and Roth (1973). The kind of pseudocomplementation described above could result in the assignment of mutants with the same phenotype to different complementation–recombination groups. Curiously, a number of investigators (see Section 4.2.2c) have obtained a mixture of phenotypes within a single recombination group of influenza temperature-sensitive mutants.

3.5. Genotypic Mixing

The existence of heterozygotes in influenza virus populations derived from mixed infection has been postulated for many years. However, none of the studies to date allows a clear distinction between heterozygotes and the occurrence of genotypically mixed aggregates of virus particles. The frequency of occurrence of heterozygotes and thus their significance in the genetic interactions of influenza virus were ambiguous even in early studies. For example, Hirst and Gottlieb (1955) found that 77 out of 220 clones from the progeny of a mixed infection behaved as heterozygotes; that is, these clones produced a virus population with both parental phenotypes on subsequent passages. In contrast, Lind and Burnet (1957) isolated only three clones out of 24 which behaved as heterozygotes in segregation analyses. Hirst (1962) used the frequent occurrence of heterozygotes as evidence in support of the hypothesis that the RNA content within individual virus particles was variable, presumably as a result of an imprecise virion assembly process.

Recent studies of mixed infection between different strains of influenza virus and between *ts* mutants do not support the contention that the formation of heterozygotes is a frequent event. Tobita (1971) isolated three clones out of 42 from the progeny of mixed infection by two different type A strains which segregated out parental markers on subsequent cultivation. Suguira *et al.* (1975) tested 12 clones which had been scored as presumptive wild-type recombinants from the progeny of a cross between two temperature-sensitive mutants. All 12 clones continued to behave as wild-type virus on subsequent passage.

It is important to rule out the possibility of frequent occurrence of heterozygotes since the presence of complementing heterozygotes can lead to an overestimation of recombination frequencies. The existence of mixed aggregates of virus particles which are infectious and capable of participating in genetic interactions (see Section 3.1) further complicates the interpretation of segregation analyses. The experimenter is left with the frustrating task of attempting to distinguish between virions possessing different genotypes, tenaciously bound together in a clump, and individual virus particles containing allelic copies of one or more genes. Either possibility would appear to be an equally plausible explanation for the studies in which parental markers segregated out.

It is instructive to consider the various theories of genome packaging from the viewpoint of heterozygote formation. If packaging occurs by a random, indiscriminate incorporation of genome segments, heterozygotes and their counterparts in single infections, homozygotes or partial diploids, should be formed rather frequently. On the other hand, a mechanism which assures that each infectious particle contains only one copy of each segment could relegate heterozygote formation to an improbable event. As we discussed in Section 2.3, this latter possibility seems to fit current data on the low frequency of occurrence of heterozygotes (or mixed aggregates) better.

4. TEMPERATURE-SENSITIVE MUTANTS

4.1. Genetic Interactions

4.1.1. Recombination

Simpson and Hirst (1968) provided the first evidence of genetic recombination among the temperature-sensitive mutants of influenza virus, and we have presented some of their experimental findings which support the occurrence of high-frequency recombination in Section 3.1 and in Table 2. There is among most of the studies of *ts* mutants (summarized in Table 3) remarkable agreement on the characteristics of recombination. We have already described one of these characteristics—the failure of recombination frequencies to decrease with decreasing input multiplicities of infection—and the attendant hypothesis that non-plaque-forming particles may be responsible for this phenomenon (Section 3.1). Sugiura *et al.* (1972) have suggested an alternative explanation. They speculated that virus replication might proceed at a faster rate in multiply infected cells than in singly infected cells, and as a result the progeny virus from mixedly infected cells would be overrepresented in the final yield.

Another characteristic which has been repeatedly corroborated is the all-or-none nature of recombination between pairs of *ts* mutants. For example, Simpson and Hirst (1968) found that cells mixedly infected with different pairs of mutants either yielded wild-type recombinants with a frequency of 5–20% or gave undetectable levels of recombination. The recombination frequencies reported by Sugiura *et al.* (1972) ranged from 0.43% to 16.8% between groups to less than 0.01% within a group. Seven to eight recombination groups have been identified in the studies involving the largest numbers of mutants (Simpson and Hirst, 1968; Hirst, 1973; Sugiura *et al.*, 1972, 1975) and it is tempting to equate each recombination group with an individual gene.

In several studies, the progeny derived from plaque isolates which would be scored as recombinants were analyzed further. Recombinant plaques generally yielded wild-type virus on further cultivation. Neither Simpson and Hirst (1968) nor Sugiura *et al.* (1975) found any clones which were temperature sensitive in plaque-forming ability. Therefore, it is not likely that either mixed aggregates or complementing heterozygotes contributed significantly to the observed recombination frequencies. Markushin and Ghendon (1973) made a similar observation for fowl plague virus mutants. Over 80% of the plaques which had been scored as recombinants exhibited the wild-type plaquing characteristics and probably represented truly recombinant viruses.

Variability has been a common problem in the studies of genetic recombination among the *ts* mutants. There is considerable variation (up to thirtyfold) in recombination frequencies obtained for the same pair of mutants in different experiments and also for replicate crosses within the same experiment. Although recombination frequencies for

TABLE 3
Temperature-Sensitive Mutants of Influenza Viruses

Wild type	Number[a] of mutants	Frequency of isolation (%)	Mutagen[b] (number of mutants)	Cells[c] virus stock (prep./expts.)	Temperature NPT/PT (°C)	EOP NPT/PT	Yield reduction (one-step growth) NPT/PT	Reference
WSN A(H0N1)	35 ind 6 sp	1.5–2.0	5-FU (23) NTG (9) HNO$_2$ (3)	CEC/CEC	39.5/34	10^{-4}	—	Simpson and Hirst (1968)
WSN A(H0N1)	15 sp	0.5	—	CEC/CEC	39.8/36	10^{-4}	10^{-2}–10^{-3}	Hirst (1973)
WSN A(H0N1)	16 ind	0.47 0.35	5-FU (11) HA (5)	Chick embryo/ AOS	39/33	10^{-3}	—	Mackenzie (1970a)
WSN A(H0N1)	15 ind	0.31	5-FU	MDBK/MDBK	39.5/33	10^{-3}	10^{-3}–10^{-6}	Sugiura et al. (1972)
WSN A(H0N1)	19 ind	4.6 0.17	5-FU (16) HA (3)	MDBK/MDBK	39.5/34	10^{-3}	—	Sugiura et al. (1975)
A(H2N2) 0389/1965	2 ind	—	5-FU	BK/BK	38/32	10^{-5}–10^{-6}	10^{-4}–10^{-5}	Mills and Chanock (1971)
A(H3N2)	9 ind 6 recomb	3.6	5-FU	Chick embryo/ BK/RMK	39/33	—	10^{-3}–10^{-6}	Spring et al. (1975b)
X-3311	6 ind	—	5-FU	1-5C-4/1-5C-4	38/31	10^{-4}	10^{-2}–10^{-3}	Ueda (1972)
FPV (Weibridge)	14 ind	0.005–0.01	HA (8) 5-FU (4) HNO$_2$ (1) NMU (1)	CEC/CEC	42/36	10^{-3}–10^{-5}	10^{-2}–10^{-3}	Markushin and Ghendon (1973)
FPV (Rostock)	4 ind	0.4	5-FU	Chick embryo/ CEC	40/33	10^{-4}–10^{-5}	10^{-4}	Scholtissek et al., (1974)
	25 ind	0.4	5-FU	Chick embryo/ CEC	40/33	10^{-5}–10^{-7}	—	Scholtissek and Bowles (1975)

[a] Abbreviations: ind, mutants induced by mutagens; sp, spontaneously occurring mutants; recomb, recombinant viruses.

[b] Abbreviations: 5-FU, 5-fluorouracil; NTG, nitrosoguanidine; HA, hydroxylamine; NMU, nitrosomethylurea.

[c] Abbreviations: CEC, chick embryo cells; AOS, allantois on shell; MDBK, bovine kidney; BK, calf kidney; RMK, rhesus monkey kidney; 1-5C-4, human conjunctival cell line.

different pairs cover a rather broad range, the frequencies are generally not additive and the groups usually cannot be arranged on a genetic linkage map. In contrast to the prevalent observations, Mackenzie obtained significant improvements in reproducibility when receptor-destroying enzyme (RDE), a crude neuraminidase preparation, was added immediately after virus adsorption and again to the culture medium during the viral reproductive cycle. RDE was postulated to act by stripping off cellular receptor sites and thus preventing subsequent infection by unadsorbed virus which might interfere with early replication events. The subsequent presence of RDE might aid the release of progeny virus from cells and prevent clumping. However, the effect of RDE was not mimicked by hyperimmune antiserum prepared against wild-type virus, and the actual mode of action of the RDE preparation is not known. Simpson and Hirst (1968) were not successful in applying RDE to control variability in their system. In Mackenzie's hands, the use of RDE resulted in a general lowering of recombination frequencies and a large improvement in reproducibility. Mutants could still be arranged in distinct clusters with frequencies greater than 1% between clusters and less than 1% within a group. In addition to RDE, variations in recombination frequencies were minimized by including a standard cross in each experiment to normalize day-to-day variations. Under these conditions, recombination frequencies among some mutants were additive and these mutants were ordered on a linear map. The map distances between terminal mutant loci were shorter than expected and the possibility was raised that the map might be circular. Mackenzie emphasized the preliminary nature of the map, particularly the need to analyze a larger number of mutants and the desirability of using three-factor crosses to confirm the map.

Fields (1971) has demonstrated the inadequacies of two-factor crosses for genetic mapping of reovirus *ts* mutants. A statistical analysis was used to determine whether or not apparent differences in the recombination frequencies between mutant pairs were attributable to drawing random samples from a normal population. Most *ts* crosses did not have significantly different recombination frequencies, even though the frequencies ranged from 3% to 8% for different pairs of mutants.

In some studies (Mackenzie, 1970*b*), no increases in recombination frequencies were observed between 4 and 24 h postinfection; consequently, recombination was postulated to be an early event involving a single round of mating. However, Sugiura *et al.* (1972) found a steady increase in the kinetics of recombination from 1% to 19% between 5 and 19 h after infection. Two possible mechanisms were suggested. Either multiple rounds of mating occur during replication, or the increase in recombination frequencies may be the result of a gradual overlapping of several replication matrices within the cell. These observations may not be contradictory, since the kinetics of recombination may be dependent on the location and nature of the sites of replication, factors which could vary with the particular host cell used.

4.1.2. Complementation

When cells mixedly infected with the pair of *ts* mutants described in Table 2 were incubated at the nonpermissive temperature, 78% of the progeny viruses showed a temperature-sensitive phenotype (Simpson and Hirst, 1968). This was the first evidence of complementation among the *ts* mutants of influenza virus. In addition to *ts* progeny, the mixed infection at the restrictive temperature yielded viruses with the plaquing properties of wild-type virus (18.5% of the yield). Apparently, complementation between the parental *ts* viruses is followed by genetic reassortment of the parental *ts* markers, giving rise to wild-type recombinants. Interestingly enough, the recombination frequency at the restrictive temperature was three times higher than the frequency at the permissive temperature for this particular pair of mutants (Table 2). Simpson and Hirst suggested that production of recombinant virus may be favored by a selective mechanism operating at the higher temperature. Markushin and Ghendon (1973) observed a similar effect of temperature on recombination frequencies among fowl plague virus mutants, and Sugiura *et al.* (1972) confirmed the observation for WSN mutants. Because of the frequent occurrence of recombination at the restrictive temperature, some investigators refer to their mutant groupings as "complementation–recombination" groups.

Sugiura *et al.* (1975) found a one-to-one correspondence between recombination groups and complementation–recombination groups. In "complementation" experiments, indices ranged from 21 to 17,900 for mutant pairs representing different recombination groups and less than 2 for mutants within the same group. In contrast, Simpson and Hirst (1968), Mackenzie (1970*b*), and Markushin and Ghendon (1973) observed instances of complementation in the absence of recombination. That is, some mutants within the same recombination group were able to complement one another at the restrictive temperature. If a recombination group corresponds to a single gene, this result would suggest the occurrence of intragenic complementation. It is also possible that some recombination groups are multigenic. Two possible physical arrangements of genes can be envisaged. Two genes may lie in the same RNA segment or two different RNA segments may be tightly linked, perhaps by base pairing, and consequently reassort as a unit.

In addition to falling into two complementation groups, mutants of Markushin and Ghendon's (1973) group I are unusual in another respect. All eight of the *ts* mutants isolated from stocks mutagenized by hydroxylamine belong to group I. Such a localization of mutants, apparently reflecting the action of the mutagen, is unusual among the influenza mutant studies and may be peculiar to fowl plague virus (Table 3). The target base for hydroxylamine is cytosine and the mutagen induces G-C to A-U transitions. It is possible that the localization of mutants in group I reflects a C-rich region and/or a hypermutable region in the genome RNA.

4.2. Isolation and Characterization

4.2.1. Determination of Mutant Phenotypes

4.2.1a. RNA Phenotypes

Our current knowledge of the processes of viral transcription and replication in influenza virus-infected cells is meager. Part of the problem has been the difficulties encountered in quantifying virus-specific RNA synthesis. Unlike other negative-strand viruses, influenza viral RNA synthesis is sensitive to actinomycin D. Therefore, this drug cannot be used to selectively inhibit cellular RNA synthesis, at least not early in infection. These same problems recur when attempts are made to determine the RNA phenotypes of temperature-sensitive mutants. The approaches taken by individual laboratories to overcome these problems are varied and are perhaps most conveniently divided into those approaches involving the use of actinomycin D and those relying on nucleic acid hybridization analyses.

If actinomycin D is added to infected cells between 0 and 2–3 h postinfection, viral RNA synthesis is almost completely inhibited. According to our present understanding of the genome strategy, the bulk of influenza cRNA is synthesized during this actinomycin D-sensitive period. After the first 4 h of infection, mainly vRNA is synthesized. Its synthesis is more resistant to actinomycin D than that of cRNA. For example, if the drug is added 3–4 h after infection, cRNA synthesis is inhibited by 90–95%, while vRNA synthesis is reduced by 50–60%. A number of investigators (Sugiura *et al.,* 1975; Ghendon *et al.,* 1973; Mackenzie and Dimmock, 1973) have assayed mutant phenotypes by adding actinomycin D at 3–4 h postinfection and measuring total radioactive uridine incorporation. If a mutant is unable to induce drug-resistant RNA synthesis at the nonpermissive temperature, it is considered to be defective in some aspect of viral RNA synthesis. As the following sections on the characterization of the *ts* mutants will show, some of the most ambiguous experiments are those involving the use of actinomycin D. The sources of the ambiguity may be hidden in the unknown nature of the drug-sensitive step or steps in viral RNA synthesis and in the indirect method of measuring viral RNA synthesis by radioactive uridine incorporation.

More direct methods of measuring viral RNA synthesis involve the use of nucleic acid hybridization techniques. In the assay developed by Scholtissek and Rott (1970), radioactively labeled RNA is extracted from infected cells and hybridized with an excess of either unlabeled virion RNA or a preparation of unlabeled complementary RNA. RNase-resistant radioactivity is measured and a background correction factor of 1.1 times the RNase resistance of uninfected cellular RNA is subtracted. The corrected radioactivity is taken as a measure of either vRNA or cRNA. Krug *et al.* (1975) employed a more direct assay to measure the amount of cRNA in infected cells. Unlabeled RNA extracted from infected cells was hybridized with an excess of radioactively labeled virion RNA of known specific activity. RNase-resistant radioactivity was taken as a measure of the quantity of cRNA. Krug and Taylor (personal communication) have recently measured the concentrations of both cRNA and vRNA in infected cells by Crt analysis using ^{125}I-labeled vRNA and ^{32}P-labeled cDNA (synthesized by reverse transcriptase) as hybridization probes.

Polymerase activity, either virion associated or in extracts of infected cells, is sometimes used as an indication of RNA-synthesizing capacity. However, unless the virion-associated transcriptase of a *ts* mutant exhibits approximately normal activity at 32°C *in vitro* and loss of activity at higher temperatures, it is difficult to relate the *in vitro* activity directly to the *ts* lesion. The polymerase activity of extracts from infected cells has the characteristics of a transcriptase activity when measured *in vitro.* It is not clear whether the replicase is inactive under these assay conditions or whether it is contributing to the apparent transcriptase activity. Therefore, the use of this assay as an indicator of mutant RNA phenotype is also of limited value.

Virus-specific RNA synthesis can also be monitored by isolating and quantifying the amounts of viral RNPs which accumulate in infected cells. Radioactively labeled RNPs have been isolated by several different procedures. Gregoriades and Hirst (1976) used Pon's (1971) method of selectively precipitating viral RNPs from detergent-treated cellular extracts by sodium acetate at pH 4.7. Viral RNPs can also be isolated from cellular extracts by CsCl equilibrium density gradient centrifugation (Choppin, 1969). After glutaraldehyde fixation, viral RNPs band at a density of 1.34 g/ml.

4.2.1b. Phenotypes of RNA⁺ Mutants

The three proteins and/or associated biological activities which are routinely measured for the characterization of influenza virus mutants are HA, NA, and NP. In most protocols, infected cells are scraped from tissue culture plates and subjected to several cycles of freezing and thawing, sometimes followed by dounce homogenization, and a low-speed centrifugation. The supernatant fraction is then assayed for infectious virus, hemagglutinin activity, neuraminidase activity, and nucleocapsid protein antigen. Hemagglutinating activity is usually measured by standard hemagglutination assays or by hemadsorption on the intact cell layers. Neuraminidase activity is monitored by spectrophotometric assays for N-acetylneuraminic acid using neuraminlactose or fetuin as substrates (Aminoff, 1961). The rate of elution of adsorbed erythrocytes is sometimes used as an indirect measure of neuraminidase activity (Mackenzie, 1970a), although this method does not always bear an unambiguous relationship to NA (Laver and Kilbourne, 1966). The presence of HA or NA antigen can also be detected (Mackenzie, 1970a) using recombinant viruses to prepare monospecific antisera directed against either the HA or NA antigen (Kilbourne et al., 1967). The nucleocapsid antigen is measured by standard complement fixation tests. Synthesis of the internal membrane protein M has not been routinely monitored in mutant analyses except in recent studies by Gregoriades and Hirst (1976) and Scholtissek and Bowles (1975) in which the accumulation of a protein with the electrophoretic mobility of M was followed by polyacrylamide gel electrophoresis. And recently the one-dimensional tryptic peptide maps of three different type A influenza viruses were shown to be sufficiently different to allow distinct peptides to serve as markers for M in the analysis of recombinant viruses (Laver and Downie, 1976).

4.2.2. WSN-Sugiura *et al.*

4.2.2a. Isolation

Sugiura *et al.* (1972, 1975) have isolated two sets of mutants derived from mutagenized stocks of WSN. The study is distinctive in that MDBK cells were used for both virus stock preparation and genetic studies, thereby minimizing the contribution of von Magnus virus. Initially, 15 *ts* mutants were arranged into five recombination groups. Later, 19 more were isolated and the number of recombination groups was extended to seven. Mutants were isolated by both the plaque-enlargement method and by testing individual clones at the two temperatures. Isolation was estimated to be about tenfold more efficient by the latter procedure.

4.2.2b. RNA⁻ Mutants

Representatives of the four RNA⁻ groups were studied further using temperature-shift experiments (Sugiura *et al.*, 1975). Mutant-infected cells were allowed to undergo transcription and replication at the permissive temperature for 4 h. Then actinomycin D was added and the cells were shifted to the nonpermissive temperature. Uridine incorporation ceased in cells infected by mutants from all four RNA⁻ groups. Replication is the main activity measured under these conditions, since actinomycin D inhibits transcription by 90–95% and replication by a smaller amount, 50–60%. Therefore, these results suggest that all RNA⁻ mutants are defective in negative-strand RNA synthesis.

The results of physiological tests to determine the phenotypic characteristics of mutants in various complementation–recombination groups are shown in Table 4. The RNA phenotype of the mutants was determined by their ability to incorporate radioactive uridine into acid-precipitable material in the presence of actinomycin D. Mutants in groups I, II, III, and V did not incorporate uridine above control levels. All mutants in groups IV, VI, and VII incorporated uridine over a 16–94% range relative to wild type. Some mutants scored as RNA⁻ by this

TABLE 4

Summary of Phenotypic Characterization of *ts*-Mutants of WSN[a]

Recom-bination group	RNA phenotype	RNP antigen (complement fixation)	HA[b] (hemagglu-tination)	NA[b] (enzyme activity)	Comments
I	cRNA⁻ vRNA⁻	−	−	−	1. Mixed group (RNP antigen, HA, NA, detected in several mutants) 2. Synthesize little or no (+) RNA at NPT 3. Over half the mutants were in I and II, I has a probable defect in transcriptase complex (Krug *et al.*, 1975)
II	cRNA⁺ vRNA⁻	+	+	+	1. Synthesis of (−)RNA deficient—possible defect in replicase function
III	cRNA⁻ vRNA⁻	−	−	±	1. Little or no (+)RNA at NPT—probable defect in transcriptase complex (Krug, *et al.*, 1975)
IV	cRNA⁺ vRNA⁺	+	−	−	1. Undetectable NA—only one this low 2. Lowest HA also 3. Altered NA which masks HA activity (Palese *et al.*, 1974)
V	cRNA⁺ vRNA⁻	−	±	+	1. Synthesis of (−)RNA deficient—possible defect in replicase function
VI	cRNA⁺ vRNA⁺	+	±	±	1. Altered HA (Ueda, unpublished) 2. Represented by one mutant
VII	cRNA⁺ vRNA⁺	+	±	+	

[a] Data from Sugiura *et al.* (1972, 1975), Palese *et al.* (1974), and Krug *et al.* (1975).
[b] +, 10–100% wild type; ±, 1–10% wild type; −, less than 1% of wild-type activity.

criterion were capable of synthesizing appreciable amounts of protein products including RNP antigen at the nonpermissive temperature. This result is similar to the anomalous behavior of Simpson and Hirst's *ts* mutants when assayed in the presence of actinomycin D (Gregoriades and Hirst, 1976). Temperature-sensitive mutants of fowl plague virus (Ghendon *et al.*, 1973) behaved in a similar manner. It is not clear whether these data reflect only partially defective mutant functions or problems in the assessment of RNA phenotype in the presence of actinomycin D.

Analysis of the RNA⁻ groups has been extended by Krug *et al.* (1975). In this study, viral RNA synthesis was monitored without the use of actinomycin D. The accumulation of viral plus-strand RNA was quantified by hybridization to radioactively labeled negative-strand RNA of known specific activity. Mutant-infected cells were incubated at the permissive temperature for 4–5 h and then shifted up to the restrictive temperature. Mutants in groups I and III produced little or no detectable plus-strand RNA after shiftup. It is likely that mutants from these groups contain a defect in the enzyme or template used for transcription. In contrast, mutants from groups II and V continued to synthesize plus-strand RNA after a shiftup. The *ts* defect in these mutants does not appear to reside in the transcriptase complex, and another aspect of RNA synthesis such as replication is likely to be the defective function.

Most mutants in groups I and III exhibited barely detectable levels of transcription at the restrictive temperature and directed the synthesis of almost no viral proteins detectable by immunological, enzymatic, and polyacrylamide gel analyses. Since groups I and III complement one another efficiently, these low levels of synthesis appear to be sufficient to effect this interaction.

4.2.2c. RNA$^+$ Mutants

Three groups of mutants (IV, VI, VII) had RNA$^+$ phenotypes. Mutants from all of these groups caused significant cytopathic effects (CPE) in cells incubated at the restrictive temperature. In contrast, none of the RNA$^-$ mutants caused detectable CPE despite the fact that detectable RNP antigen was present in some cases (perhaps due to leakiness or revertants in the mutant stocks). This observation was interpreted to indicate that entry of the virus particles *per se* and synthesis of RNP were not sufficient to cause CPE.

Two of the group IV mutants which exhibited low neuraminidase and hemagglutinin activities have been studied in greater detail (Palese *et al.*, 1974). These mutants had 10^3- to 10^4-fold lower infectivity titers than wild-type virus. However, electron microscopic studies revealed that morphologically intact virus particles were formed at the restrictive temperature. In contrast to infection at the permissive temperature, these particles accumulated in large aggregates at the cell surface. The aggregated particles contained neuraminic acid, and it was suggested that neuraminic acid-containing proteins on some virions serve as receptors for the hemagglutinin of other virus particles in the aggregate. Hemagglutinating activity, but not infectivity or neuraminidase activity, was restored by treatment of the aggregates with neuraminidase from *Vibrio cholerae*. These results suggest that the defect in group IV mutants is in the neuraminidase protein, and that this defect masks hemagglutinating activity. It was proposed that neuraminidase is essential for the dissemination of influenza virus particles (but not for formation of intact particles by budding) and is required to remove neuraminic acid containing receptors from the viral envelope, thus avoiding viral aggregation. On the other hand, genetically defective virus particles containing some neuraminic acid could presumably participate more readily in aggregation. According to Hirst's hypothesis, this could be advantageous in acquiring a full genome complement in an infected cell. It has been shown that viral aggregates are readily taken up by cells (Dales and Pons, 1976).

While Table 4 provides a useful summary, it tends to give an idealized view of the relationship between phenotypes and recombination group. As in virtually all of the mutant studies, there were two main difficulties in making this correlation. Mutants within a group (especially groups I, II, III) exhibited mixed phenotypes, perhaps simply reflecting different rates of reversion or degrees of leakiness. On the other hand, some mutants from different recombination groups had similar phenotypes, suggesting the possibility that mutants with different primary defects may share a common phenotype. Sugiura suggested that influenza virus mutants may exhibit asymmetric covariation of phenotypes. A similar phenomenon was described by Cooper (1969) for poliovirus mutants.

4.2.3. WSN–Mackenzie

Mackenzie (1970a) isolated a set of 16 temperature-sensitive mutants derived from mutagenized stocks of strain WSN. The original WSN stock was recloned twice at 38.8°C to minimize the probability of isolating multiple mutants derived from mutagenesis of preexisting ts mutants. The resulting stock was designated WSN_p. The mutants were grouped into five distinct clusters on the basis of recombination frequencies.

A summary of physiological studies of these mutants is presented in Table 5. None of the mutants differed significantly from WSN_p in its growth capacity during a single cycle at the permissive temperature. In this respect, the mutants appear to be different than most of Simpson and Hirst's mutants, which did not reproduce well at the permissive temperature. RNA phenotypes were determined by measuring radioactive uridine incorporation in the presence of actinomycin D. Only mutants from group II showed a large decrease in uridine incorporation. However, some RNP and neuraminidase antigens (but not hemadsorbing activity) were detected under restrictive conditions. This phenotype may be indicative of a rather leaky mutation in replicase function, allowing limited gene amplification and transcription. Most

TABLE 5

Summary of Physiological Experiments on Representatives of the Recombination Groups of WSN_p [a]

Recombination group	Uridine Incorporation[b]	Ribonucleoprotein (fluorescent antibody)	Hemadsorption	Neuraminidase activity (elution after hemadsorption)	Comments
I	(+)	+	+	+	1. One mutant has a block in exit of RNP from nucleus
II	±	+	−	ND[c]	1. Detectable neuraminidase antigen present
III	+	+	−	ND	1. Intracellular HA and fluorescent antibody staining for HA detected in some mutants 2. Detectable neuraminidase antigen present
IV	+	+	+	−	1. Enzymatically active neuraminidase present
V	(+)	+	+	+	

[a] Adapted from Mackenzie (1970b) and Mackenzie and Dimmock (1973).
[b] [³H]Uridine incorporation measured after delayed addition of actinomycin D. +, 75% wild type; +, 31–75% wild type; ±, 20–23% wild type.
[c] Not determinable.

group I mutants were not significantly different from wild type in the properties measured. They did exhibit slightly lower levels of uridine incorporation, and, in one mutant, RNP antigen remained localized in the nucleus. This phenotype might result from an altered nucleocapsid protein which, upon assembly into RNPs, changes their template and/ or transport properties. Cells infected by group III mutants were defective in hemadsorption, and in at least one mutant the HA protein was not assembled into plasma membranes in an active form. Erythrocytes adsorbed to the surface of cells infected by group IV mutants did not elute, and these mutants are presumed to have a neuraminidase defect. Cells infected by some of these mutants contained an active neuraminidase in the cytoplasm but were unable to incorporate the NA protein into plasma membranes in a functional form. Group V mutants gave normal responses except for slightly depressed levels of uridine incorporation.

The virulence of the mutants was tested by intranasal inoculation of mice. The presence of *ts* lesions was associated with a decrease in virulence and mutants fell into one of two patterns: either the mutants were avirulent, or deaths occurred over a longer period than after wild-type infection. No obvious correlation of virulence with other characters of the mutants was claimed, although other investigators found a correlation between the shutoff temperature (temperature at which a tenfold decrease in plating efficiency occurs) and virulence (Mills *et al.*, 1969*a*).

4.2.4. WSN—Simpson and Hirst

Two sets of temperature-sensitive (*ts*) mutants of the WSN strain of influenza type A have been isolated by Hirst and co-workers. The original set was isolated from mutagenized virus stocks (Simpson and Hirst, 1968) and the second set was composed of spontaneously occurring mutants (Hirst, 1973). The latter set is of current interest because these mutants have been further characterized biochemically (Gregoriades and Hirst, 1976), while the former set was used in the first recombination and complementation analyses (discussed in Section 4.1) of *ts* mutants which provided many of the seminal observations of this new phase of influenza virus genetics.

The spontaneously occurring *ts* mutants were originally isolated with the hope that these mutants would be less likely to contain multiple lesions than those obtained from mutagenized stocks. The mutants were arranged into eight complementation–recombination groups and prototype strains were selected for each group. These prototype strains included seven spontaneous mutants (*ts* 40, 41, 42, 43, 44, 50, 59) and one mutant (*ts*24) derived from nitrosoguanidine-treated stocks. Several problems were encountered in preparing stocks of the mutants, problems which continue to plague investigators. None of the mutants was sufficiently stable to be propagated serially without frequent recloning. The properties of certain *ts* mutants were shown to change after successive recloning; the risks of additional mutations and changing phenotypes with the preparation of new stocks were not imaginary. Occassionally a strain failed to yield recombinants during mixed infections with representatives from more than one recombination group, suggesting that multiple lesions were present in a significant portion of the spontaneously occurring mutants.

In order to characterize the mutants, two general types of studies were carried out: (1) analyses of purified virions grown at the permissive temperature and (2) analyses of viral proteins in infected cells at the permissive and nonpermissive temperatures. Virions were assayed for particle-associated neuraminidase activity (NA), hemagglutinating activity (HA), plaque-forming capacity (PFU), and protein content. The HA per milligram of protein was roughly comparable to that of wild-type virions for all except one mutant. However, the PFU per milligram of protein was low for all mutants tested relative to that of wild type. Three of the mutants (ts40, 41, 50) had less than 10% NA/ mg protein compared to wild-type virions. Cells infected by these three mutants were also low in NA even at the permissive temperature. The possibility must be considered that many of these mutants contain multiple mutations, some of which may not be temperature sensitive. No heat-labile virion-associated activities were found, although this class of mutants may have been selected against by the plaque enlargement technique used in the isolation of these mutants.

The RNA phenotype of prototype mutants was analyzed by measuring acid-precipitable radioactive uridine incorporation in mutant-infected cells. The results were somewhat equivocal. In the absence of actinomycin D, all mutant-infected cells incorporated uridine in excess of uninfected control levels. However, if actinomycin D was added after the actinomycin-sensitive stage, all of the mutant strains were RNA negative. The results obtained using actinomycin D contradict the finding that all but one mutant synthesized viral RNP as detected by precipitation of viral RNPs from cell extracts at pH 4.7 by the method of Pons (1971). Ts25, which failed to synthesize acid-precipitable viral RNP at nonpermissive temperature, is considered to be a likely candidate for a defect in either RNA synthesis or RNP assembly.

Mutant-infected cells were also assayed for cytoplasmic and plasma membrane-associated hemagglutinin and neuraminidase activity. Some mutants produced low levels of hemagglutinin activity; the residual HA tended to concentrate in plasma membranes. No mutants were completely deficient in NA, and the mutants having the lowest levels of activity showed the deficiency at both restrictive and permissive temperatures. Neither the HA phenotype nor the NA phenotype was clearly localized in one recombination group.

The most unusual observations involved the internal membrane protein, M. No detectable M protein could be extracted with acidified chloroform–methanol from cells infected by any of the prototype mutants. No proteins with the expected size of either M or NS accumulated in mutant-infected cells, as analyzed by polyacrylamide gel electrophoresis. And in contrast to plasma membranes derived from cells infected by wild-type virus, membranes isolated from mutant-infected cells by several different techniques lacked the M polypeptide. Gregoriades and Hirst (1976) suggested that all of the recombination groups share a common phenotype, a defect in M synthesis. In our opinion, the data can be interpreted to mean that the mutants all have a defect in the accumulation of NS as well. Also, the possibility that both M and NS are still synthesized but rapidly degraded has not been rigorously excluded. Surprisingly, cells coinfected by two of the mutants (*ts*24 and *ts*40) which exhibit high recombination frequencies supported the accumulation of a 25,000 dalton polypeptide at the restrictive temperature. If these groups share a common phenotype, they are nevertheless capable of undergoing complementation. These observations are difficult to reconcile. It is possible that the failure of mutant-infected cells to accumulate M and NS is a secondary consequence of a number of different primary defects.

Bean and Simpson (1976) measured the virion-associated transcriptase activity of mutants representing each of Hirst's seven recombination–complementation groups (*ts*11, 24, 40, 41, 42, 44, 50). All of the mutants tested had diminished transcriptase activity relative to the wild type. None of the mutants possessed a heat-labile virion-associated polymerase; heat-sensitive polymerases have been detected among fowl plague virus mutants (Ghendon *et al.*, 1973; Scholtissek *et al.*, 1974).

The mutant *ts*24, which did not have any detectable polymerase activity at 37°C and less than 5% of the wild-type activity at 32°C, was studied in detail. The virion-associated polymerase activity of this mutant could not be stimulated by changing the temperature or detergent and divalent cation concentrations in the *in vitro* reaction. Using this mutant, Bean and Simpson (1976) detected only low levels of polymerase activity from extracts of infected cells incubated at the permissive temperature, while Gregoriades and Hirst (1976) obtained roughly 25% of the wild-type levels of vRNP from *ts*24-infected cells, again incubated at permissive temperature. Both of these observations suggest that the mutant-induced infection does not progress normally even at the permissive temperatures (although the yields of infectious virus obtained in a one-step growth experiment were comparable to those of the other representative mutants, Gregoriades and Hirst, 1976).

It is not clear how the transcriptase defect as measured *in vitro* is related to the activity of the polymerase in cells. Also, the relationship between decreased *in vitro* transcriptase activity (which all of the representative mutants appear to share) and the *ts* character of the mutants is not straightforward.

Rochovansky and Hirst (1976) have recently obtained evidence that at least some of the lesions in the *ts* mutants isolated by Hirst are in different viral RNA segments. These workers have succeeded in preparing infectious ribonucleoprotein complexes from purified virions containing only viral RNA, nucleocapsid protein, and two P proteins. Successful infections required the cooperation of at least seven RNP segments, and the infectivity of the complexes was sensitive to RNase, pronase, and conditions which removed the P proteins from the ribonucleoprotein. The infectious ribonucleoprotein complexes were used to rescue temperature-sensitive mutants representing different complememtation–recombination groups. The complexes were first separated into three major size classes by sedimentation on linear glycerol gradients. The large, medium, and small size classes of infectious RNP were enriched for the three large RNA segments, the three medium-sized segments, and the two small segments, respectively. Each class of infectious RNP was tested for its ability to rescue a particular *ts* mutant after coinfection of chicken embryo cell cultures at the nonpermissive temperature. *Ts*40 and *ts*44 were rescued most efficiently by the large RNP segments, while *ts*42 was rescued using the small RNP segments. *Ts*24 could be rescued by all classes, but most efficiently by the medium size class. An analysis of the efficiency of rescue as a function of the concentration of the infectious RNP complexes suggested that one genomic segment was required to rescue *ts*40 while two different segments were needed to rescue *ts*42. The successes of these initial rescue experiments by Rochovansky and Hirst raise hopes that infectious RNP complexes will provide a significant new tool for mapping the lesions of the *ts* mutants of influenza viruses. Technological improvements in the methods available for fractionating the infectious complexes should allow investigators to identify the individual genomic segment on which a mutation is located.

4.2.5. Fowl Plague Virus—Markushin and Ghendon

4.2.5a. Isolation

Fourteen temperature-sensitive mutants have been isolated from mutagenized stocks of fowl plague virus (FPV Weibridge). The mutants could be arranged into five complementation–recombination groups (A–E). Preliminary tests showed that the thermostability of both infectivity and hemagglutinin activity was similar for the mutants and the wild-type virus. A summary of the biochemical characterization of representative mutants from each complementation–recombination group is presented in Table 6.

4.2.5b. RNA⁻ Mutants

Information on the capacity of the mutants to synthesize RNA was obtained from a variety of experiments. Detergent-activated virion-associated transcriptase activity was measured at the permissive and nonpermissive temperatures. The wild-type virus and most of the mutants exhibited a 16% or less reduction in activity at the restrictive temperature relative to the permissive temperature. The group D mutant, however, showed a 67–88% reduction in activity. *In vivo* RNA synthesis was measured by incubating infected cells for 3 h at either the restrictive or permissive temperature, then treating the cultures with actinomycin D for ¾ h, followed by a 3-h incubation in the presence of radioactive uridine. Cells infected by mutants in groups A–D incorporated 5–8% as much radioactivity at the restrictive temperature relative to the permissive, and these mutants were considered to have RNA⁻ phenotypes. Cells infected by the group E mutant showed only a 30% reduction in radioactive uridine incorporation, and this mutant was considered to have an RNA⁺ phenotype. Mutant-infected cells were also assayed for the presence of viral RNPs, again by radioactively labeling infected cultures at the restrictive temperature in the presence of actinomycin D. Any material containing both radioactive uridine and amino acids and which migrated as a 60–70 S component by sedimentation velocity in a sucrose linear gradient was considered viral RNP. By this criterion, only cells infected by the group E mutant synthesized detectable levels of viral RNP.

The RNA-synthesizing capacity of the *ts* mutants was analyzed in greater detail in a subsequent study (Ghendon *et al.*, 1975). The synthesis of complementary RNA was measured by annealing the radioactive RNA isolated from mutant-infected cells to negative-strand RNA (vRNA) isolated from virions. Positive-strand RNA (cRNA) was then measured as RNase-resistant radioactivity. Negative-strand RNA synthesis was measured indirectly as actinomycin D-resistant radioactive uridine incorporation late in infection. Two mutants representing groups C and D failed to synthesize detectable amounts of positive-

TABLE 6
Characterization of the *ts* Mutants of Fowl Plague Virus[a]

Complementation recombination group	Recombination group representative mutant	RNA phenotype[b] (1975 study)	RNA phenotype 1973 study (uridine incorporation + actinomycin D)	Viral RNP (uridine incorporation + actinomycin D)	HA activity	NA activity	Viral protein synthesis at NPT	In vitro transcriptase activity at NPT
A	I ts43	cRNA+ vRNA-	-	-	-	-	+	+
B	I ts166	cRNA+ vRNA-	-	-	-	-	+	+
C	II ts29	cRNA- vRNA-	-	-	-	-	+	+
D	III ts131	cRNA- vRNA-	-	-	-	-	-	-
E	IV ts5	cRNA+ vRNA+	+	+	+	+	+	+

[a] Taken from Markushin and Ghendon (1973) and Ghendon *et al.* (1973, 1975).
[b] cRNA, complementary to genome strand; vRNA, negative genome strand.

strand RNA by this criterion, while only the group E mutant synthesized negative-strand viral RNA. Experiments in which infected cultures were incubated for varying lengths of time at permissive temperature and then placed at the nonpermissive temperature (shift up) indicated that all of the mutants possessed defects which were manifested at later times in the infectious cycle. When mutants from groups A, B, and E were incubated first at the nonpermissive temperature for 5 h and then shifted down to permissive temperature, substantial amounts of infectious virus were produced, suggesting that these mutants are defective in "late" functions. Mutants from groups C and D, on the other hand, produced little virus after a shiftdown, suggesting the defect is in a function required both early and late in infection. The authors defined late functions as those occurring after 4.5 h of the infectious cycle (8–9 h long). We assume that this point in the cycle roughly corresponds to the end of the actinomycin D-sensitive phase.

Groups C and D both have the same RNA phenotype (cRNA⁻vRNA⁻). The Group D mutant manifests a temperature-sensitive virion-associated transcriptase *in vitro*. It was hypothesized that the group C mutant also has a defect in the transcriptase complex, but that once synthesized and assembled at the permissive temperature this complex can function at the nonpermissive temperature. The existence of two different complementation–recombination groups defective in positive-strand RNA synthesis suggests that at least two viral proteins participate in the transcriptase complex, perhaps NP and P. Krug *et al.*, (1975) also found two groups of mutants (Sugiura's groups I and III mutants, Table 4) with RNA phenotypes similar to those of Ghendon's group C and D mutants. In addition to the two putative transcriptase-defective groups, both laboratories found two additional RNA⁻ groups (Ghendon's groups A and B and Sugiura's groups II and V) which may be involved in replicase function.

The absence of actinomycin D-resistant radioactive uridine incorporation after a shift up in cells infected with group C and D mutants, the putative transcriptase defectives, may indicate that negative-strand RNA synthesis is blocked as well. Several investigators, including Scholtissek *et al.* (1974), Ghendon *et al.* (1975), and Krug *et al.* (1975), have interpreted this behavior as an indication that the replicase and transcriptase complexes of influenza virus may share a common subunit. A similar hypothesis has been advanced for RNA⁻ temperature-sensitive mutants of vesicular stomatitis virus (see Pringle, this volume).

4.2.5c. RNA⁺ Mutants

The proteins synthesized in mutant-infected cells at the permissive and nonpermissive temperatures were analyzed on polyacrylamide gels. Protein patterns similar to wild-type infection were obtained for all of the mutants except group D, which synthesized primarily low molecular weight polypeptides at the restrictive temperature. We are left with the apparent paradox that groups A–C have an RNA⁻ phenotype, and yet substantial amounts of viral proteins are synthesized at the restrictive temperature (see Section 4.2.2b). Ghendon *et al.* (1973) point out that the RNA phenotype refers only to later stages of infection when primarily negative-strand synthesis is occurring. They suggest that the high-input multiplicity of infection used in these experiments (300–500 PFU/cell) might allow for the synthesis of detectable levels of viral proteins as a result of primary transcription of input genomes.

Only the group E mutant directed the synthesis of either hemagglutinin or neuraminidase activity. However, none of the mutants, including the group E mutant, formed particles at the restrictive temperature with the characteristic sedimentation properties of virions. The defect in group E mutants was not obvious. The temperature-shift experiments favor a late function; perhaps a defect in the M protein affecting maturation of virus particles is a possibility.

4.2.6. Fowl Plague Virus—Scholtissek *et al.*

4.2.6a. Isolation

Scholtissek and Bowles (1975) isolated 25 mutants from mutagenized stocks of the Rostock strain of fowl plague virus. Twenty-three of the mutants were arranged into six recombination groups having less than a 0.1% frequency of recombination between members of the same group. Scholtissek and Bowles considered the recombination data to be inconclusive for two mutants, *ts*18 (RNA⁺) and *ts*236 (RNA⁻). They either belong to group III or comprise two additional recombination groups. The characterization of these mutants is summarized in Table 7.

4.2.6b. RNA⁻ Mutants

The RNA phenotype of these mutants was analyzed in two ways. The viral RNA polymerase in extracts of infected cells incubated at

TABLE 7

Characterization of the *ts* Mutants of Fowl Plague Virus[a]

Recombination group Representative mutant	RNA phenotype	*In vitro* transcriptase activity at NPT	HA (hemagglutination)	NA (enzyme activity)	Transport of RNP complex from nucleus at PT
I	cRNA⁻ vRNA⁻	−	−	−	+
*ts*3					
II	cRNA⁻ vRNA⁻	−	−	−	+
*ts*263					
III	cRNA⁺ vRNA⁺	+	−	±	−
*ts*90					
IV	cRNA⁺ vRNA⁺	±	+	−	+
*ts*113					
V	cRNA⁺ vRNA⁺	+	−	+	+
*ts*227					
VI					
*ts*19	cRNA⁺ vRNA⁺	+	+	+	+
*ts*81	cRNA⁻ vRNA⁻	−	−	−	+

[a] Adapted from Scholtissek and Bowles (1975) and Scholtissek *et al.* (1974).

either permissive or nonpermissive temperature was assayed *in vitro* at 32°C. Virus-specific RNA synthesis *in vivo* was measured by labeling cells with radioactive uridine, followed by hybridization of the isolated radioactive RNA with an excess of either unlabeled vRNA or cRNA.

Mutants having an RNA-negative phenotype were found in three recombination groups and possibly a fourth one. Groups I and II contain only RNA⁻ mutants, group VI contains an RNA⁻ mutant (*ts*81) but also RNA⁺ mutants (*ts*19), and another RNA⁻ mutant *ts*236 either belongs to group III or represents a new group. Cells infected by most of the mutants in groups I and II possessed less than 5% of the viral RNA polymerase activity at the nonpermissive temperature as compared with the permissive temperature. The heat stability of the polymerase synthesized in cells infected by each of three mutants from groups I and II was as heat stable as the wild-type enzyme. Once synthesized at the permissive temperature, the viral polymerase activity of cells infected by group I and II mutants is stable after a shift to the nonpermissive temperature. Viral RNA synthesis, as measured by hybridization, is inhibited either after incubation at the nonpermissive temperature or after a shiftup in cells infected by mutants from groups I and II and also by *ts*236. Essentially no differences in phenotype were found between the mutants of groups I and II. Both groups are deficient in the synthesis of both cRNA and vRNA, and are likely candidates for defects in transcriptase function.

When the polymerase activity in extracts of cells infected by the two group III mutants was assayed, no activity was detected in the cytoplasm at either permissive or nonpermissive temperature. However, polymerase activity was recovered in the nuclear fraction from infected cells, suggesting the possibility that these mutants possess either an altered RNP complex or a defect in a protein needed for transport of RNP complexes from the nucleus (see Mackenzie, Section 4.2.3 for a similar mutant). On continuous incubation at the nonpermissive temperature, cells infected by group III mutants synthesize wild-type levels of RNA, but if RNA synthesis was measured after a shiftup, it was markedly reduced. The basis for this phenomenon is not understood.

Cells infected by mutants from groups IV, V, VI, and *ts* 18 synthesize wild-type levels of viral RNA after incubation at the nonpermissive temperature and are considered to have an RNA$^+$ phenotype. The mutant *ts*81 does not direct the synthesis of significant amounts of viral RNA under these same conditions, even though it belongs to a recombination group containing mutants with RNA$^+$ phenotypes.

4.2.6c. RNA$^+$ Mutants

Most of the RNA$^-$ mutants of groups I and II do not direct the synthesis of detectable amounts of hemagglutinin or neuraminidase activity in infected cells. A few of the mutants in these groups, which are considered to be leaky mutants by other criteria (e.g., polymerase activity, PFU titer), produce almost wild-type amounts of HA and NA. The behavior of these mutants is consistent with the hypothesis that they have an altered transcriptase which retains some activity. Even a low level of transcriptase activity could lead to genome amplification, and, consequently, the production of significant amounts of viral protein.

The mutants in group IV are defective in the production of neuraminidase activity. The characteristics of these mutants are considerably different than the WSN mutants isolated by Sugiura and analyzed by Palese and colleagues (Section 4.2.2c). Sugiura's mutants directed the synthesis of a heat-labile enzyme, and these mutants were also deficient in hemagglutinin activity. The neuraminidase enzyme synthesized by Scholtissek's mutants is heat stable, and cells infected by the mutants possess at least some hemagglutinin activity. Whereas neuraminidase treatment resulted in a restoration of hemagglutinin activity to Sugiura's mutants, external addition of the enzyme to Scholtissek's mutants did not affect their hemagglutinin activity.

Scholtissek's group IV mutants possessed several additional interesting properties. Although they produced wild-type levels of infectious virus at the permissive temperature, cell-associated neuraminidase activities were only 1–10% of wild type. Also, virus release proceeded at the nonpermissive temperature in the absence of detectable NA, and the released virus formed plaques at permissive temperature. These results suggest that budding and virus release may occur in the absence of NA, but it is required for subsequent infection (or at least plaque formation).

Mutants of group V have a defect in the production of hemagglutinin activity as measured in cell homogenates. Analysis by polyacrylamide gel electrophoresis of the viral proteins synthesized in mutant-infected cells at the nonpermissive temperature revealed that uncleaved HA protein accumulated in relatively large amounts. This finding supports the hypothesis that group V mutants have a primary lesion in the gene coding for hemagglutinin protein. Group III mutants are also negative for hemagglutinin activity. However, Scholtissek and Bowles (1975) consider the primary defect of this group to be in the structure or functions of viral RNP; the effects on HA and NA activity may be secondary.

Except for $ts81$, which has an RNA$^-$ phenotype, the defect(s) in the group VI mutants has not been identified. Analysis by polyacrylamide gel electrophoresis of the proteins synthesized in cells infected by the group VI mutant $ts19$ at the nonpermissive temperature showed reduced accumulation of either M or NS or both (these proteins were not separated). The gel electropherogram of $ts19$ is similar in this respect to the patterns obtained by Gregoriades and Hirst (Section 4.2.4) for Hirst's mutants; $ts19$ is considered a possible candidate for a defect in virus maturation.

4.2.7.   X-3311—Ueda *et al.*

Six temperature-sensitive mutants of influenza A (clone X-3311, obtained from a mixed infection of active A_1/CAM and inactivated A_0/NWS) have been isolated by Ueda (1972). These mutants were obtained after a rather long exposure of infected cells to 5-fluorouracil (4 days at 31°C). Mutant-infected cells were analyzed for the production of plaque-forming units, hemagglutinin activity, cytopathic effects, and ribonucleoprotein antigen. Five of the mutants had similar phenotypes. They all directed the synthesis of hemagglutinin and caused cytopathic effects, while at the same time producing significantly less RNP antigen than the wild-type infection at the nonpermissive temperature. One mutant, $ts7$, exhibited a large decrease in RNP antigen accumulation at the restrictive temperature (3 $\log_2$), and yet the amount of hemagglutinating activity was approximately the same at either temperature. The phenotype of $ts5$ differed from that of the other five mutants. This mutant failed to induce the synthesis of hemagglutinating activity or produce cytopathic effects at the nonpermissive temperature. Like the other mutants, $ts5$ produced low levels of RNP antigen at the restrictive temperature. RNA phenotypes were not determined for the mutants, and the results of complementation–recombination analysis were reported for only one pair of mutants; $ts5$ and $ts9$ complemented one another.

4.3. Variants

Viruses with temperature-sensitive (ts) properties are under evaluation as live, attenuated vaccine strains for human use. Although a detailed analysis of these studies is outside the limits of this chapter, the application of ts viruses to vaccine production is an area of both scientific and public concern; therefore, we have provided a very brief introduction to current research.

The problem of isolating ts mutants with the desired characteristics for vaccine use has been approached in two different ways. Viruses have been attenuated in virulence for both laboratory animals and humans by adaptation to reproduction at suboptimal temperatures. In addition, ts mutants have been isolated from mutagenized stocks and used in mixed infections with wild-type strains to produce ts recombinants which are both genetically stable and attenuated in virulence. The goal of the mutant-isolation studies described in Sections 4.1–4.2 was to isolate and characterize ts mutants possessing single lesions. The vaccine studies are different (at least by intention if not always in practice) in that the primary goal is to isolate stable ts mutants with a particular set of properties. In fact, the mutants which are selected are likely to contain multiple lesions, and we refer to them as "ts variants."

4.3.1. Cold-Adapted Variants

Aleksandrova and Kugel (1961) made the original observation that influenza viruses cultivated at suboptimal temperatures (25–26°C) are attenuated in virulence and may be suitable for use as human vaccine strains. The most comprehensive investigation of "cold variants" has been conducted by Maassab and co-workers; the reader is referred to Maassab (1975) and the previous publications by this group which are also listed in the references section for a more detailed summary and for references to other workers.

In the initial studies, viruses were cold-adapted by gradually lowering the incubation temperature during multiple cycles of reproduction. Four to eight months were required to produce attenuated variants which were still immunogenic in animals and humans. The variants, which had acquired the ability to reproduce at 25°C, were no longer able to reproduce efficiently at optimal temperatures (35–40°C). Several of the newly acquired properties of the cold variants—growth capacity at 25°C, temperature sensitivity, attenuation, and *in vivo* growth—were shown to be relatively stable markers which could be transferred to other strains by recombination at 25°C. Based on the ability of the cold variants to participate in genetic reassortment at 25°C, the following strategy for constructing a vaccine strain was devised: Cells are first mixedly infected at 25°C with the cold variant of an influenza A virus and the current epidemic strain. The progeny virus from the mixed infection are then passaged in the presence of antisera against the parental attenuated cold variant to facilitate the selection of a "cold hybrid," a recombinant virus containing surface antigens of the epidemic strain and the attenuation and growth properties of the cold variant. Cold hybrids of influenza A viruses from both human and animal sources have been produced in approximately 4 weeks by recombination selection at 25°C.

Extensive biochemical characterization of cold variants has not been reported. However, Kendal *et al.* (1973) have compared the polypeptides of virions and cells infected at optimal and suboptimal temperatures with either a wild-type virus or its cold variant by polyacrylamide gel electrophoresis. No glycopolypeptide with the expected electrophoretic mobility of HA was detected in variant-infected cells at 40°C. Serological studies indicated that the hemagglutinin of the cold variant lacked some of the antigenic sites present on the wild-type virus. Therefore, it is likely that the variant possesses lesions in the gene coding for hemagglutinin glycopolypeptide. Additional lesions may also exist.

4.3.2. Temperature-Sensitive Recombinants

The second major approach to the development of a live vaccine strain stemmed from the observations that many of the *ts* mutants of influenza virus were attenuated in virulence for laboratory animals. Furthermore, the extent of attenuation in animals seemed to be closely correlated with the shutoff temperature of the *ts* mutants (see Section 4.2.3) in cell culture. Shutoff temperature has proved to be a useful marker for screening *ts* mutants for attenuated virulence. Chanock and co-workers have undertaken the most extensive studies in this area, and the reader is referred to Richman *et al.* (1975) and the earlier papers also listed in the references section for a more detailed summary and references to related investigations.

The overall goal of the second approach is very similar to the previous studies using cold variants: to produce a genetically well-characterized, attenuated *ts* donor virus. However, the methods employed to construct the donor virus were quite different. Mills and Chanock (1971) first isolated several *ts* mutants from stocks [A/Great Lakes/1965(H2N2)] mutagenized by prolonged growth in the presence of 5-flurouracil followed by passage in cell culture to facilitate the selection of stable mutants. One of these mutants, *ts*1, has been the object of much of the subsequent research. This mutant had the desirable properties of failing to produce plaques above 37°C (and consequently failing to grow and produce symptoms in the lower respiratory tract) while retaining the ability to grow at 34°C (and presumably also in the passages of the upper respiratory tract where its reproduction would stimulate an immune response).

The mutant *ts*1 was used as the parental *ts* donor in a mixed infection with another influenza A virus [Hong Kong/1968 (H3N2)] to produce the *ts* recombinant *ts*1 [E] (H3N2). This recombinant possessed the necessary balance between attenuated virulence and ability to stimulate the host immune system needed for a vaccine strain. Furthermore, *ts*1 [E] was genetically stable in humans and was not readily communicable. Subsequent characterization of *ts*1 [E] revealed that it contains two distinct genetic lesions (Murphy *et al.*, 1973*b*) and that both *ts* lesions segregate independently of the HA and NA genes.

These *ts* lesions can be transferred along with the characteristic level of attenuation of the *ts* donor to an influenza virus with different HA and/ or NA surface antigens.

Additional *ts* mutants of influenza A (H3N2) have been isolated in order to analyze the relationships among attenuation, sites of genetic lesions, and levels of temperature sensitivity in detail (Spring *et al.*, 1975*b*). Fifteen *ts* mutants, including nine isolated from mutagenized stocks and six recombinant viruses, were assigned to seven complementation–recombination groups. Biological and biochemical characterization of these mutants is under way, and they should provide useful tools for further characterization of potential *ts* recombinant vaccine strains.

5. CONCLUSION

The concept of one gene corresponding to one RNA segment corresponding to one recombination group remains a valuable hypothesis, and the assumptions that the genome RNA segments are unique and that each segment is transcribed and translated into a unique virus-specific protein in infected cells have received firm experimental support (McGeoch *et al.*, 1976; and Ritchey *et al.*, 1976*b*, respectively). At this juncture, the magic number appears to be eight genes, assuming that NS2 is not a primary gene product.

Attempts to establish unambiguous phenotypes for the temperature-sensitive mutants in each recombination group have often been disappointing. The masking of hemagglutinin activity in *ts* mutants defective in neuraminidase function dramatizes the complication which the occurrence of pleiotropism creates for phenotypic analyses. Pleiotropic effects may be largely responsible for the lack of localization of specific phenotypes within each recombination group. The molecular organization of influenza viruses—the close proximity of the hemagglutinin and neuraminidase spikes, the apparent need for proteins such as M with multiple recognition sites, protein–membrane interactions, and protein–protein and protein–RNA interactions in ribonucleoprotein complexes—readily lends itself to pleiotropic phenomena. It is also important to use the most direct and unambiguous methodology available to characterize the mutants phenotypically so that primary defects can be detected with greater certainty. The neglect of this principle can result in substantial confusion, as illustrated by some of the studies of RNA phenotype.

TABLE 8

Summary of Defects in *ts* Mutants of Influenza Virus

	Defective function				
Possible defective protein(s)	cRNA synthesis (P1–3, NP)	vRNA synthesis (P1–3, NP)	Hemagglutination/ hemadsorption (HA)	Neuraminidase activity (NA)	Unknown (?)
WSN (Sugiura *et al.*)	I(A),[a] III(C)	II(B), V(E)	VI(F)	IV(D)	VII(G)
FPV (Ghendon *et al.*)	II(C), III(D)	I(A), I(B)	—	—	IV(E)
FPV (Scholtissek *et al.*)	I, II	—	V	IV	III, VI

[a] Roman numerals denote recombination groups, letters denote complementation–recombination groups.

The extent of the initial difficulties encountered in working with the *ts* mutants indicates that easy answers to the molecular questions about influenza virus reproduction and genetics are not in the offing. In fact, mutant analysis has shown as much facility in uncovering new genetic mysteries as in providing solutions to venerable enigmas. Additional clues to both the old and new genetic mysteries will have to be provided by continued technological advances in the molecular studies of RNA replication and genome assembly and in the biological and physical characterization of influenza virus populations.

In Table 8 we have tentatively arranged the recombination groups from the most extensively characterized sets of mutants according to their putative phenotypes. These classifications include candidates for lesions in the genes coding for P1–3, NP, HA, and NA. The groups listed in the column designated "unknown" may include mutants having maturation defects, perhaps due to alterations in M or NS.

One takes heart in these recent demonstrations that at least some of the mutants are amenable to incisive characterization. These developments presage the potential usefulness of the *ts* mutants in studies at the molecular level; however, we hope that the timidity on the part of the present reviewers in remaining paramyxovirologists will be pardoned.

ACKNOWLEDGMENTS

We are grateful to Pat Klitzke for her excellent assistance in preparing the manuscript; to Richard W. Compans, Robert M. Krug, and

Irene T. Schulze for critical readings and helpful comments; to numerous investigators in the field who provided us with preprints; to our colleagues Charles H. Madansky, C. Worth Clinkscales, L. Andrew Ball, Robert C. Warrington, and Robert T. Vinopal for many discussions and suggestions; and to the National Science Foundation (BMS 75-05024) and the National Institutes of Allergy and Infectious Diseases (AI-12467) for support to M. A. B., and the University of Connecticut Research Foundation, the National Cancer Institute (CA-14733), and the National Heart and Lung Institute (HL-19490) for support to L. E. H.

6. REFERENCES

Ada, G. L., and Perry, B. T., 1954, The nucleic acid content of influenza virus, *Aust. J. Exp. Biol. Med. Sci.* **32**:453.

Agrawal, H. O., and Bruening, G., 1966, Isolation of high molecular weight P^{32}-labeled influenza virus ribonucleic acid, *Proc. Natl. Acad. Sci. USA* **55**:3818.

Aleksandrova, G. I., and Kugel, S. M., 1961, Materials on the preparation of an areactogenic live anti-influenza vaccine for immunization of infants (in Russian), in: *Problema Grippa,* p. 29, Leningrad.

Almeida, J. D., and Waterson, A. P., 1970, Two morphological aspects of influenza virus, in: *The Biology of Large RNA Viruses* (R. D. Barry and B. W. J. Mahy, eds.), pp. 27–52, Academic Press, New York.

Aminoff, D., 1961, Methods for the quantitative estimation of *N*-acetylneuraminic acid and their application to hydrolysates of sialomucoids, *Biochem. J.* **81**:384.

Andrewes, C. H., Bang, F. B., and Burnet, F. M., 1955, A short description of the myxovirus group (influenza and related viruses), *Virology* **1**:176.

Apostolov, K., and Flewett, T. H., 1969, Further observations on the structure of influenza viruses A and C, *J. Gen. Virol.* **4**:365.

Apostolov, K., Flewett, T. H., and Kendall A. P., 1970, Morphology of influenza A. B. C. and infectious bronchitis virus (IBV) virions and their replication, in: *The Biology of Large RNA Viruses* (R. D. Barry and B. W. J. Mahy, eds.), pp. 3–26, Academic Press, New York.

Armstrong, S. J., and Barry R. D., 1975, The detection of virus-induced RNA synthesis in the nuclei of cells infected with influenza viruses, in: *Negative Strand Viruses,* Vol. 1 (B. W. J. Mahy and R. D. Barry, eds.), pp. 491–499, Academic Press, New York.

Bachi, T., Gerhard, W., Lindenmann, J., and Muhlethaler, K., 1969, Morphogenesis of influenza A virus in Ehrlich ascites tumor cells as revealed by thin-sectioning and freeze-etching, *J. Virol.* **4**:769.

Baron, S., and Jensen, K. E., 1955, Evidence for genetic interaction between non-infectious and infectious A viruses, *J. Exp. Med.* **102**:677.

Barry, R. D., 1961, The multiplication of influenza virus. II. Multiplicity reactivation of ultraviolet-irradiated virus, *Virology* **14**:398.

Barry, R. D., and Mahy, B. W. J., eds., 1970, *The Biology of Large RNA Viruses,* Academic Press, New York.

Barry, R. D., Ives, D. R., and Cruickshank, J. G., 1962, Participation of deoxyribonucleic acid in the multiplication of influenza virus, *Nature (London)* **194**:1139.

Bean, W. J., Jr., and Simpson, R. W., 1976, Transcriptase activity and genome composition of defective influenza virus, *J. Virol.* **18**:365.

Bishop, D. H. L., Obijeski, J. F., and Simpson, R. W., 1971, Transcription of the influenza ribonucleic acid genome by a virion polymerase. II. Nature of the *in vitro* polymerase product, *J. Virol.* **8**:74.

Bishop, D. H. L., Roy, P., Bean, W. J., Jr., and Simpson, R. W., 1972, Transcription of the influenza ribonucleic acid genome by a virion polymerase. III. Completeness of the transcription process, *J. Virol.* **10**:689.

Blair, C. D., and Duesberg, P. H., 1970, Myxovirus ribonucleic acids, *Annu. Rev. Microbiol.* **24**:539.

Bromley, P. A., and Barry, R. D., 1973, *Arch Ges Virusforsch.* **42**:182.

Burnet, F. M., 1956, Structure of influenza virus, *Science* **123**:1101.

Burnet, F. M., and Lind, P. E., 1949, Recombination of characters between two influenza virus strains, *Aust. J. Sci.* **12**:109.

Burnet, F. M., and Lind, P. E., 1951, A genetic approach to variation in influenza viruses. 4. Recombination of characters between the influenza virus A strain NWS and strains of different serological subtypes, *J. Gen. Microbiol.* **5**:67.

Burnet, F. M., and Lind, P. E., 1952, Studies on recombination with influenza viruses in the chick embryo. III. Reciprocal genetic interaction between two influenza virus strains. *Aust. J. Exp. Biol. Med. Sci.* **30**:469.

Burnet, F. M., and Lind, P. E., 1954, Reactivation of heat inactivated influenza virus by recombination, *Aust. J. Exp. Biol. Med. Sci.* **32**:133.

Burnet, F. M., and Lind, P. E., 1957, Studies on filamentary forms of influenza virus with special reference to the use of dark-ground microscopy, *Arch. Ges. Virusforsch.* **7**:413.

Caliguiri, L. A., and Compans, R. W., 1974, Analysis of the *in vitro* product of an RNA-dependent RNA polymerase isolated from influenza virus-infected cells, *J. Virol.* **14**:191.

Choppin, P. W., 1963, Multiplication of two kinds of influenza A_2 virus particles in monkey kidney cells, *Virology* **21**:342.

Choppin, P. W., 1969, Replication of influenza virus in a continuous cell line: High yield of infective virus from cells inoculated at high multiplicity, *Virology* **38**:130.

Choppin, P. W., and Pons, M. W., 1970, The RNA's of infective and incomplete influenza virions grown in MDBK and HeLa cells, *Virology* **42**:603.

Choppin, P. W., and Tamm, I., 1960a, Studies of two kinds of virus particles which comprise influenza A_2 virus strains. I. Characterization of stable homogeneous substrains in reactions with specific antibody, mucoprotein inhibitors, and erythrocytes, *J. Exp. Med.* **112**:895.

Choppin, P. W., and Tamm, I., 1960b, Studies of two kinds of virus particles which comprise influenza A_2 virus strains. II. Reactivity with virus inhibitors in normal sera, *J. Exp. Med.* **112**:921.

Choppin, P. W., and Tamm, I., 1964, Genetic variants of influenza virus which differ in reactivity with receptors and antibodies, in: *Ciba Foundation Symposium: Cellular Biology of Myxovirus Infections,* Little, Brown, Boston.

Choppin, P. W., Murphy, J. S., and Tamm, I., 1960, Studies of two kinds of virus particles which comprise influenza A₂ virus strains. III. Morphological characteristics: Independence of morphological and functional traits, *J. Exp. Med.* **112**:945.

Choppin, P. W., Kilbourne, E. D., Dowdle, W., Hirst, G. K., Joklik, W. K., Simpson, R. W., and White, D. O., 1975, Genetics, replication, and inhibition of replication of influenza virus—Summary of influenza workshop VII, *J. Infect. Dis.* **132**:713.

Compans, R. W., 1973, Influenza virus proteins. II. Association with components of the cytoplasm, *Virology* **51**:56.

Compans, R. W., and Caliguiri, L. A., 1973, Isolation and properties of an RNA polymerase from influenza virus-infected cells, *J. Virol.* **11**:441.

Compans, R. W., and Choppin, P. W., 1975, Reproduction of myxoviruses, in: *Comprehensive Virology,* Vol. 4 (H. Fraenkel-Conrat and R. R. Wagner, eds.), pp. 179–252, Plenum Press, New York.

Compans, R. W., and Dimmock, N. J., 1969, An electron microscopic study of single-cycle infection of chick embryo fibroblasts by influenza virus, *Virology* **39**:499.

Compans, R. W., Dimmock, N. J., and Meier-Ewert, H., 1969, Effect of antibody to neuraminidase on the maturation and hemagglutinating activity of an influenza virus A₂, *J. Virol.* **4**:528.

Compans, R. W., Dimmock, N. J., and Meier-Ewert, H., 1970, An electron microscopic study of the influenza virus-infected cell, in: *The Biology of Large RNA Viruses* (R. D. Barry and B. W. J. Mahy, eds.), pp. 87–108, Academic Press, New York.

Compans, R. W., Content, J., and Duesberg, P. H., 1972, Structure of the ribonucleoprotein of influenza virus, *J. Virol.* **10**:795.

Content, J., 1976, Cell-free translation of influenza virus mRNA, *J. Virol.* **18**:604.

Content, J., and Duesberg, P. H., 1971, Base sequence differences among the ribonucleic acids of influenza virus, *J. Mol. Biol.* **62**:273.

Cooper, P. D., 1969, The genetic analysis of poliovirus, in: *The Biochemistry of Viruses* (H. B. Levy, ed.), pp. 177–218, Dekker, New York.

Dahlberg, J. E., and Simon, E. H., 1969, Recombination in Newcastle disease virus (NDV): The problem of complementing heterozygotes, *Virology* **38**:490.

Dales, S., and Pons, M. W., 1976, Penetration of influenza examined by means of virus aggregates, *Virology* **69**:278.

Duesberg, P. H., 1968, The RNA's of influenza virus, *Proc. Natl. Acad. Sci. USA* **59**:930.

Duesberg, P. H., 1969, Distinct subunits of the ribonucleoprotein of influenza virus, *J. Mol. Biol.* **42**:485.

Duesberg, P. H., and Robinson, W. S., 1967, On the structure and replication of influenza virus, *J. Mol. Biol.* **25**:383.

Emerson, S. U., and Wagner, R. R., 1973, L protein requirement for *in vitro* RNA synthesis by vesicular stomatitis virus, *J. Virol.* **12**:1325.

Etkind, P. R., and Krug, R. M., 1975, Purification of influenza viral complementary RNA: Its genetic content and activity in wheat germ cell-free extracts, *J. Virol.* **16**:1464.

Fazekas de St. Groth, S., 1970, Evolution and hierarchy of influenza viruses, *Arch. Environ. Health* **21**:292.

Fenner, F., 1969, Conditional lethal mutants of animal viruses, *Curr. Top. Microbiol.* **48**:1.

Fenner, F., 1970, The genetics of animal viruses, *Annu. Rev. Microbiol.* **24:**297.

Fields, B. N., 1971, Temperature-sensitive mutants of reovirus type 3: Features of genetic recombination, *Virology* **46:**142.

Floyd, R. W., Stone, M. P., and Joklik, W. K., 1974, Separation of single-stranded ribonucleic acids by acrylamide–agarose–urea gel electrophoresis, *Anal. Biochem.* **59:**599.

Frisch-Niggemeyer, W., and Hoyle, L., 1956, The nucleic acid and carbohydrate content of influenza virus A and of virus fractions produced by ether disintegration, *J. Hyg.* **54:**201.

Furuichi, Y., Muthukrishnan, S., and Shatkin, A. J., 1975, 5′-Terminal M⁷G(5′) ppp (5′) G p *In vivo*: Identification in reovirus genomic RNA, *Proc. Natl. Acad. Sci. USA* **72:**742.

Ghendon, Y. Z., 1972, Conditional lethal mutants of animal viruses, *Prog. Med. Virol.* **14:**68.

Ghendon, Y. Z., Markushin, S. G., Marchenko, A. T., Sitnikov, B. S., and Ginzburg, V. P., 1973, Biochemical characteristics of fowl plaque virus TS mutants, *Virology* **55:**305.

Ghendon, Y. Z., Markushin, S. G., Blagovczhenskaya, O. V., and Genkina, D. B., 1975, Study of fowl plague virus RNA synthesis in *ts* mutants, *Virology* **66:**454.

Glass, S. E., McGeoch, D., and Barry, R. D., 1975, Characterization of the mRNA of influenza virus, *J. Virol.* **16:**1435.

Gottlieb, T., and Hirst, G. K., 1954, The experimental production of combination forms of virus. III. The formation of doubly antigenic particles from influenza A and B virus and a study of the ability of individual particles of X virus to yield separate strains, *J. Exp. Med.* **99:**307.

Granoff, A., and Hirst, G. K., 1954, The experimental production of combination forms of virus. IV. Mixed influenza A Newcastle disease virus infections, *Proc. Soc. Exp. Biol.* **86:**84.

Granoff, A., and Kingsburg, D. W., 1964, Effect of actinomycin D on the replication of Newcastle disease and influenza virus, in: *Cell Biology of Myxovirus Infection* (G. E. W. Wolstenholme and J. Knight, eds.), pp. 99–119, Little, Brown, Boston.

Gregoriades, A., 1970, Actinomycin D and influenza virus multiplication in the chick embryo fibroblast, *Virology* **42:**905.

Gregoriades, A., 1973, The membrane protein of influenza virus: Extraction from virus and infected cell with acidic chloroform–methanol, *Virology* **54:**369.

Gregoriades, A., and Hirst, G. K., 1976, Mechanism of influenza recombination. III. Biochemical studies of temperature-sensitive mutants belonging to different recombination groups, *Virology* **69:**81.

Griffith, I. P., 1975, The fine structure of influenza virus, in: *Negative Strand Viruses,* Vol. 1 (B. W. J. Mahy and R. D. Barry, eds.), p. 121, Academic Press, New York.

Hartman, P. E., and Roth, J. R., 1973, Mechanisms of suppression, *Adv. Genet.* **17:**1.

Hastie, N. D., and Mahy, B. W. J., 1973, RNA-dependent RNA polymerase in nuclei of cells infected with influenza virus, *J. Virol* **12:**951.

Hay, A. J., and J. J. Skehel, 1975, Studies on the synthesis of influenza virus, in: *Negative Strand Viruses,* Vol. 2 (B. W. J. Mahy and R. D. Barry, eds.), pp. 635–655, Academic Press, New York.

Hefti, E., Roy, P., and Bishop, D. H. L., 1975, The initiation of transcription by influenza virion transcriptase, in: *Negative Strand Viruses,* Vol. 1 (R. D. Barry and B. W. J. Mahy, eds.), pp. 307–326, Academic Press, New York.

Henle, G., Girardi, A., and Henle, W., 1955, A non-transmissable cytopathogenic effect of influenza virus in tissue culture accompanied by formation of non-infectious hemagglutinins, *J. Exp. Med.* **101**:25.

Henle, W., and Liu, O. C., 1951, Studies on host–virus interactions in the chick embryo–influenza virus system. VI. Evidence for multiplicity reactivation of inactivated virus, *J. Exp. Med.* **94**:305.

Hillis, W. D., Moffat, M. A. J., and Holtermann, O. A., 1960, The development of soluble (s) and viral (v) antigens of influenza A virus in tissue culture as studied by the flourescent antibody technique. 3. Studies on the abortive cycle of replication in HeLa cells, *Acta Pathol. Microbiol. Scand.* **50**:419.

Hirst, G. K., 1962, Genetic recombination with Newcastle disease virus, poliovirus and influenza, *Cold Spring Harbor Symp. Quant. Biol.* **27**:303.

Hirst, G. K., 1973, Mechanism of influenza recombination. I. Factors influencing recombination rates between temperature-sensitive mutants of strain WSN and the classficiation of mutants into complementation–recombination groups, *Virology* **55**:81.

Hirst, G. K., and Gottlieb, T., 1955, The experimental production of combination forms of virus. V. Alterations in the virulence of neurotropic influenza virus as a result of mixed infection, *Virology* **1**:221.

Hirst, G. K., and Pons, M., 1972, Biological activity in ribonucleoprotein fractions of influenza virus, *Virology* **47**:546.

Hirst, G. K., and Pons, M. W., 1973, Mechanism of influenza virus recombination. II. Virus aggregation and its effect on plaque formation by socalled noninfectious virus, *Virology* **56**:620.

Horne, R. W., Waterson, A. P., Wildy, P., and Farnham, A. E., 1960, The structure and composition of the myxoviruses. I. Electron microscope studies of the structure of the myxovirus particles by negative staining techniques, *Virology* **11**:79.

Horst, J., Content, J., Mandeles, S., Fraenkel-Conrat, H., and Duesberg, P., 1972, Distinct oligonucleotide patterns of distinct influenza virus RNA's, *J. Mol. Biol.* **69**:209.

Hoyle, L., 1968, The influenza viruses, *Monogr. Virol.* **4**:1.

Hoyle, L., Horne, R. W., and Waterson, A. P., 1961, The structure and composition of the myxoviruses. II. Components released from the influenza virus particle by ether, *Virology* **13**:448.

Inglis, S. C., Carroll, A. R., Lamb, R. A., and Mahy, B. W. J., 1976, Polypeptides specified by the influenza virus genome. I. Evidence for eight distinct gene products specified by fowl plague virus, *Virology* **74**:489–503.

Isaacs, A., and Donald, H. B., 1955, Particle counts of hemagglutinating viruses, *J. Gen. Microbiol.* **12**:241.

Joss, A., Gandhi, S. S., Hay, A. J., and Burke, D. C., 1969, Ribonucleic acid and protein synthesis in chick embryo cells infected with fowl plague virus, *J. Virol.* **4**:816.

Kendal, A. P., Kiley, M. P., and Maassab, H. F., 1973, Comparative studies of wildtype and "cold-mutant" (temperature-sensitive) influenza viruses: Polypeptide synthesis by an Asian (H2N2) strain and its cold-adapted variant, *J. Virol.* **12**:1503.

Kilbourne, E. D., 1955, Reactivation of non-infective virus in a cortisone-infected host, *J. Exp. Med.* **101**:437.

Kilbourne, E. D., 1963, Influenza virus genetics, *Prog. Med. Virol.* **5**:79.

Kilbourne, E. D., 1969, Future influenza vaccines and the use of genetic recombinants, *Bull. WHO* **41**:643.

Kilbourne, E. D., 1973, The molecular epidemiology of influenza, *J. Infect. Dis.* **127**:478.

Kilbourne, E. D., ed., 1975, *The Influenza Viruses and Influenza,* Academic Press, New York.

Kilbourne, E. D., and Murphy, J. S., 1960, Genetic studies of influenza virus. I. Viral morphology and growth capacity as exchangeable genetic traits: Rapid *in ovo* adaptation of early passage Asian strain isolated by combination with PR8, *J. Exp. Med.* **111**:387.

Kilbourne, Edwin D., Lief, F. S., Schulman, J. L., Jahiel, R. I., and Laver, W. G., 1967, Antigenic hybrids of influenza viruses and their implications, *Perspect. Virol.* **5**:87.

Kilbourne, E. D., Laver, W. G., Schulman, J. L., and Webster, R. G., 1968, Antiviral activity of antiserum specific for an influenza virus neuraminidase, *J. Virol.* **2**:281.

Kilbourne, E. D., Choppin, P. W., Schulze, I. T., Scholtissek, C., and Bucher, D. L., 1972, Influenza virus polypeptides and antigens—Summary of influenza workshop I, *J. Infect. Dis.* **125**:447.

Kingsbury, D. W., 1970, Replication and functions of myxovirus ribonucleic acids, *Prog. Med. Virol.* **12**:49.

Kingsbury, D. W., and Webster, R. G., 1969, Some properties of influenza virus nucleocapsids, *J. Virol.* **4**:219.

Klenk, H. D., Scholtissek, C., and Rott, R., 1972, Inhibition of glycoprotein biosynthesis of influenza virus by D-glucosamine and 2-deoxy-D-glucose, *Virology* **49**:723.

Krug, R. M., 1971, Influenza viral RNP's newly synthesized during the latent period of growth in MDCK cells, *Virology* **44**:125.

Krug, R. M., 1972, Cytoplasmic and nucleoplasmic viral RNPs in influenza virus-infected MDCK cells, *Virology* **50**:103.

Krug, R. M., and Etkind, P. R., 1975, Influenza virus-specific products in the nucleus and cytoplasm of infected cells, in: *Negative Strand Viruses,* Vol. 2 (B. W. J. Mahy and R. D. Barry, eds.), pp. 555–572, Academic Press, New York.

Krug, R. M., Ueda, M., and Palesa, P., 1975, Temperature-sensitive mutants of influenza WSN virus defective in Virus-specific RNA synthesis, *J. Virol.* **16**:790.

Kubinski, H., and Gibbs, P., 1970, Tenacious binding of nucleic acids to basic proteins *in vitro*: Influence of antibiotics, *Fed. Proc.* **29**:877A.

Lamb, R. A., and Choppin, P. W., 1976, Synthesis of influenza virus proteins in infected cells: Translation of viral polypeptides, including three P polypeptides, from RNA produced by primary transcription, *Virology* **74**:504–519.

Laver, W. G., 1973, The polypeptides of influenza viruses, *Adv. Virus Res.* **18**:57.

Laver, W. G., and Downie, J. C., 1976, Influenza virus recombination. I. Matrix protein markers and segregation during mixed infections, *Virology* **70**:105.

Laver, W. G., and Kilbourne, E. D., 1966, Identification in recombinant influenza virus of structural proteins derived from both parents, *Virology* **30**:493.

Lazarowitz, S. G., Compans, R. W., and Choppin, P. W., 1971, Influenza virus structural and non-structural proteins in infected cells and their plasma membranes, *Virology* **46**:830.

Lewandowski, L. J., Content, J., and Leppla, S. H., 1971, Characterization of the subunit structure of the ribonucleic acid genome of influenza virus, *J. Virol.* **8**:701.

Li, K. K., and Seto, J. T., 1971, Electron microscope study of ribonucleic acid of myxoviruses, *J. Virol.* **7**:524.

Lind, P. E., and Burnet, F. M., 1957, Recombination between virulent and non-virulent strains of influenza virus. I. The significance of heterozygosis, *Aust. J. Exp. Biol. Med. Sci.* **35**:57.

Maassab, H. F., 1967, Adaptation and growth characteristics of influenza virus at 25°C, *Nature (London)* **213**:612.

Maassab, H. F., 1968, Plaque formation of influenza virus at 25°C, *Nature (London)* **219**:645.

Maassab, H. F., 1969, Biologic and immunologic characteristics of cold-adapted influenza virus, *J. Immunol.* **102**:728.

Maassab, H. F., 1970, Development of variants of influenza virus, pp. 542–566. in: *The Biology of Large RNA Viruses* (R. D. Barry and B. W. J. Mahy, eds.), pp. 542–566, Academic Press, New York.

Maassab, H. F., 1975, Properties of influenza virus "cold" recombinants, in: *Negative Strand Viruses,* Vol. 2 (B. W. J. Mahy and R. D. Barry, eds.), pp. 755–765, Academic Press, New York.

Mackenzie, J. S., 1969, Virulence of temperature-sensitive mutants of influenza virus, *Br. Med. J.* **3**:757.

Mackenzie, J. S., 1970a, Isolation of temperature-sensitive mutants and the construction of a preliminary genetic map for influenza virus, *J. Gen. Virol.* **6**:63.

Mackenzie, J. S., 1970b, Studies with temperature-sensitive mutants of influenza virus, in: *The Biology of Large RNA Viruses,* (R. D. Barry and B. W. J. Mahy, eds.), pp. 507–534, Academic Press, London.

Mackenzie, J. S., 1971, The use of temperature-sensitive mutants in live virus vaccines, *Proc. Symp. Live Influenza Vaccine,* p. 35.

Mackenzie, J. S., and Dimmock, N. J., 1973, A preliminary study of physiological characteristics of temperature-sensitive mutants of influenza virus, *J. Gen. Virol.* **19**:51.

Mahy, B. W. J., and Barry, R. D., eds., 1975, *Negative Strand Viruses,* Vols. 1 and 2, Academic Press, New York.

Mahy, B. W. J., and Bromley, P. A., 1970, *In vitro* product of a ribonucleic acid polymerase induced by influenza virus, *J. Virol.* **6**:259.

Markushin, S. G., and Ghendon, Y. Z., 1973, Genetic classification and biological properties of temperature-sensitive mutants of fowl plague virus, *Acta Virol.* **17**:369.

McCahon, D., Hay, A. J., and Skehel, J. J., 1975, Genetic analysis of influenza virus by marker rescue, in: *Negative Strand Viruses,* Vol. 2 (B. W. J. Mahy and R. D. Barry, eds.), pp. 725–740, Academic Press, New York.

McGeoch, D., and Kitron, N. 1975, Influenza virion RNA-dependent RNA Polymerase: stimulation by guanosine and related compounds, *J. Virol.* **15**:686.

McGeoch, D., Fellner, P., and Newton, C., 1976, The influenza virus genome consists of eight distinct RNA species, *Proc. Natl. Acad. Sci. USA* (in press).

McSharry, J. J., Compans, R. W., and Choppin, P. W., 1971, Proteins of vesicular stomatitis virus (VSV) and of phenotypically-mixed VSV-SV5 virions, *J. Virol.* **8**:722.

Medvedeva, T. E., Aleksandrova, G. I., and Smorodintsev, A. A., 1969, Pathogenicity of cryophilic and thermophilic strains of influenza type A2 virus for developing chick embryo and albino mice, *Acta Virol.* **13**:379.

Meier-Ewert, H., and Dimmock, N. J., 1970, The role of the neuraminidase of the infecting virus in the production of noninfectious (von Magnus) influenza virus, *Virology* **42**:794.

Meier-Ewert, H., Gibbs, A. J., and Dimmock, N. J., 1970, Studies on antigenic variations of swine influenza virus isolates, *J. Gen. Virol.* **6**:409.

Melnick, J. L., 1973, Classification and nomenclature of viruses, *Prog. Med. Virol.* **15**:380.

Mills, J. V., and Chanock, R. M., 1971, Temperature-sensitive mutants of influenza virus. I. Behavior in tissue culture and in experimental animals, *J. Infect. Dis.* **123**:145.

Mills, J., Chanock, R. M., and Alling, D. W., 1969a, Mutants of influenza virus, *Br. Med. J.* Dec. 13, 690.

Mills, J., van Kirk, J., Hill, D. A., and Chanock, R. M., 1969b, Evaluation of influenza virus mutants for possible use in a live virus vaccine, *Bull. WHO* **41**:599.

Mowshowitz, S., and Kilbourne, E. D., 1975, Genetic dimorphism of the neuraminidase in recombinants of H3N2 influenza virus, in: *Negative Strand Viruses,* Vol. 2 (B. W. J. Mahy and R. D. Barry eds.), pp. 765–775. Academic Press, London.

Murphy, B. R., Chalhub, E. G., Nusinoff, S. R., and Chanock, R. M., 1972, Temperature-sensitive mutants of influenza virus. II. Attenuation of ts recombinants for man, *J. Infect. Dis.* **126**:170.

Murphy, B. R., Baron, S., Chalhub, E. G., Uhlendorf, C. P., and Chanock, R. M., 1973a, Temperature-sensitive mutants of influenza virus. IV. Induction of interferon in the nasopharynx by wild-type and a temperature-sensitive recombinant virus, *J. Infect. Dis.* **128**:488.

Murphy, B. R., Chalhub, E. G., Nusinoff, S. R., Kasel, J., and Chanock, R. M., 1973b, Temperature-sensitive mutants of influenza virus. III. Further characterization of the ts-1 [E] influenza A recombinant (H_3N_2) virus in man, *J. Infect. Dis.* **128**:479.

Murphy, B. R., Hodes, D. S., Nusinoff, S. R., Spring-Stewart, S., Tierney, E. L., and Chanock, R. M., 1974, Temperature-sensitive mutants of influenza virus. V. Evaluation in man of an additional *ts* recombinant virus with a 39°C shutoff temperature, *J. Infect. Dis.* **130**:144.

Nayak, D. P., 1969, Influenza virus: Structure, replication and defectiveness, *Fed. Proc.* **28**:1858.

Nayak, D. P., 1970, The replication of influenza virus RNA, in: *The Biology of Large RNA Viruses* (R. D. Barry and B. W. J. Mahy, eds.), pp. 371–391, Academic Press, New York.

Nayak, D. P., 1972, Defective virus RNA synthesis and production of incomplete influenza virus in chick embryo cells, *J. Gen. Virol.* **14**:63.

Nayak, D. P., and Baluda, M. A., 1969, Characterization of influenza virus ribonucleic acid duplex produced by annealing *in vitro, J. Virol.* **3**:318.

Nordling, S., and Mayhew, E., 1966, *Exp. Cell. Res.* **44**:552.

Noronha-Blob, L., and Schulze, I. T., 1976, Viral interference-mediated selection of a plaque-type variant of influenza virus, *Virology* **69**:314.

Palese, P., and Schulman, J. L., 1974, Isolation and characterization of influenza virus recombinants with high and low neuraminidase activity, *Virology* **57**:227.

Palese, P., and Schulman, J. L., 1976, Differences in RNA patterns of influenza A virus, *J. Virol.* **17**:876.

Palese, P., Tobita, K., Ueda, M., and Compans, R. W., 1974, Characterization of temperature-sensitive influenza virus mutants defective in neuraminidase, *Virology* **61**:397.

Pons, M. W., 1967*a*, Studies on influenza virus ribonucleic acid, *Virology* **31**:523.

Pons, M. W., 1967*b*, Some characteristics of double-stranded influenza virus ribonucleic acid, *Arch. Ges. Virusforsch.* **22**:203.

Pons, M. W., 1970, On the nature of the influenza virus genome, *Curr. Top. Microbiol. Immunol.* **52**:142.

Pons, M. W., 1971, Isolation of influenza virus ribonucleoprotein from infected cells: Demonstration of the presence of negative-stranded RNA in viral RNP, *Virology* **46**:149.

Pons, M. W., 1972, Studies on the replication of influenza virus RNA, *Virology* **47**:823.

Pons, M. W., 1973, The inhibition of influenza virus RNA synthesis by actinomycin D and cycloheximide, *Virology* **51**:120.

Pons, M. W., 1976, A reexamination of influenza single- and double-stranded RNAs by gel electrophoresis, *Virology* **69**:789.

Pons, M. W., and Hirst, G. K., 1968, Polyacrylamide gel electrophoresis of the replicative form of influenza virus RNA, *Virology* **35**:182.

Pons, M. W., and Hirst, G. K., 1969, The single- and double-stranded RNA's and the proteins of incomplete influenza virus, *Virology* **38**:68.

Richman, D. D., Murphy, B. R., Spring, S. B., Coleman, M. T., and Chanock, R. M., 1975, Temperature-sensitive mutants of influenza virus. IX. Genetic and biological characterization of TS-1 [E] lesions when transferred to a 1972 (H3N2) influenza A virus, *Virology* **66**:551.

Ritchey, M. B., Palese, P., and Kilbourne, E. D., 1976*a*, RNAs of influenza A, B, and C viruses, *J. Virol.* **18**:738.

Ritchey, M. B., Palese, P., and, Schulman, J. L., 1976*b*, Mapping of the influenza virus genome. III. Identification of genes coding for nucleoprotein, membrane protein, and nonstructural protein, *J. Virol.* **20**:307–313.

Rochovansky, O. M., and Hirst, G. K., 1976, Infectivity and marker rescue activity of influenza virus ribonucleoprotein–polymerase complexes, *Virology* **73**:339–349.

Rott, R., and Scholtissek, C., 1963, Investigations about the formation of incomplete forms of fowl plague virus, *J. Gen. Microbiol.* **33**:303.

Ruck, B. J., Brammer, K. W., Page, M. G., and Coombes, J. D., 1969, The detection and characterization of an induced RNA polymerase in the chorioallantoic membranes of embryonated eggs infected with influenza A_2 viruses, *Virology* **39**:31.

Scholtissek, C., and Bowles, A., 1975, Isolation and characterization of temperature-sensitive mutants of fowl plague virus, *Virology* **67**:576.

Scholtissek, C., and Rott, R., 1964, Behavior of virus-specific activities in tissue cultures infected with myxoviruses after chemical changes of the viral ribonucleic acid, *Virology* **22**:169.

Scholtissek, C., and Rott, R., 1969, Ribonucleic acid nucleotidyl transferase induced in chick fibroblasts after infection with an influenza virus, *J. Gen. Virol.* **4**:125.

Scholtissek, C., and Rott, R., 1970, Synthesis *in vivo* of influenza virus plus and minus strand RNA and its preferential inhibition by antibiotics, *Virology* **40**:989.

Scholtissek, C., Kruczinna, R., Rott, R., and Klenk, H. D., 1974, Characteristics of an influenza mutant temperature-sensitive for viral RNA synthesis, *Virology* **58**:317.

Schulze, I. T., 1970, The structure of influenza virus. I. The polypeptides of the virion, *Virology* **42**:890.

Schulze, I. T., 1973, Structure of the influenza virion, *Adv. Virus Res.* **18**:1.

Shatkin, A. J., 1971, Viruses with segmented ribonucleic acid genomes: Multiplication of influenza versus reovirus, *Bacteriol. Rev.* **35**:250.

Simpson, R. W., and Hirst, G. K., 1961, Genetic recombination among influenza viruses. I. Cross reactivation of plaque forming capacity as a method for selecting recomginants from the progeny of crosses between influenza A strains, *Virology* **15**:436.

Simpson, R. W., and Hirst, G. K., 1968, Temperature-sensitive mutants of influenza A virus: Isolation of mutants and preliminary observations on genetic recombination and complementation, *Virology* **35**:41.

Skehel, J. J., 1971*a,* Estimations of the molecular weight of the influenza virus genome, *J. Gen. Virol.* **11**:103.

Skehel, J. J., 1971*b,* The characterization of subviral particles derived from influenza virus, *Virology* **44**:409.

Skehel, J. J., 1972, Polypeptide synthesis in influenza virus-infected cells, *Virology* **49**:23.

Spring, S. B., Nusinoff, S. R., Mills, J., Richman, D. D., Tierney, E. L., Murphy, B. R., and Chanock, R. M., 1975*a,* Temperature-sensitive mutants of influenza virus. VI. Transfer of *ts* lesions from the Asian subtype of influenza A virus (H2N2) to the Hong Kong subtype (H3N2), *Virology* **66**:522.

Spring, S. B., Nusinoff, S. R., Tierney, E. L., Richman, D. D., Murphy, B. R., and R. M., Chanock, 1975*b,* Temperature-sensitive mutants of influenza. VIII. Genetic and biological characterization of TS mutants of influenza virus A (H3N2) and their assignment to complementation groups, *Virology* **66**:542.

Sugiura, A., 1975, Influenza virus genetics, in: *The Influenza Viruses and Influenza* (E. D. Kilbourne, ed.), Academic Press, New York.

Sugiura, A., and Kilbourne, E. D., 1965, Genetic studies of influenza viruses. II. Plaque formation by influenza viruses in a clone of a variant human heteroploid cell line, *Virology* **26**:478.

Sugiura A., and Kilbourne, E. D., 1966, Genetic studies of influenza viruses. III. Production of plaque type recombinants with A0 and A1 strains, *Virology* **29**:84.

Sugiura, A., and Ueda, M., 1971, Marker rescue with ultraviolet inactivated influenza virus, *J. Virol.* **7**:499.

Sugiura, A., Tobita, K., and Kilbourne, E. D., 1972, Isolation and preliminary characterization of temperature-sensitive mutants of influenza virus, *J. Virol.* **10**:639.

Sugiura, A., Ueda, M., Tobita, K., and Enomoto, C., 1975, Further isolation and characterization of temperature-sensitive mutants of influenza virus, *Virology* **65**:363.

Tobita, K., 1971, Genetic recombination between influenza viruses A0/NWS and A2/Hong Kong, *Arch. Ges. Virusforsch.* **34**:119.

Tobita, K., 1972, Kinetics of genetic recomtination between influenza viruses A0/NWS and A2/Hong Kong, *Arch. Ges. Virusforsch.* **38**:100.

Tobita, K., and Kilbourne, E. D., 1974, Genetic recombination for antigenic markers of antigenically different strains of influenza B virus, *J. Virol.* **13**:347.

Tumova, B., and Pereira, H. G., 1965, Genetic interaction between influenza A viruses of human and animal origin, *Virology* **27**:253.

Ueda, M., 1972, Temperature-sensitive mutants of influenza virus, *Arch. Ges. Virusforsch.* **39**:360.

von Magnus, P., 1954, Incomplete forms of influenza virus, *Adv. Virus Res.* **2**:59.

Wagner, R. R., 1975, Reproduction of rhabdoviruses, in: *Comprehensive Virology*, Vol. 4 (H. Fraenkel-Conrat and R. R. Wagner, eds.), pp. 1–93, Plenum Press, New York.

Webster, R. G., 1972, On the origin of pandemic influenza viruses, *Curr. Top. Microbiol. Immunol.* **59**:75.

Webster, R. G., and Campbell, C. H., 1972, The *in vivo* production of "new" influenza viruses. II. *In vivo* isolation of "new" viruses, *Virology* **48**:528.

Webster, R. G., and Granoff, A., 1974, Evolution of orthomyxoviruses, in: *Viruses, Evolution, and Cancer* (E. Kurstak, and K. Maramorosch, eds.), pp. 625–649, Academic Press, New York.

Webster, R. G., and Laver, W. G., 1971, Antigenic variation in influenza virus biology and chemistry, *Prog. Med. Virol.* **13**:271.

Webster, R. G., Laver, W. G., and Kilbourne, E. D., 1968, Reactions of antibodies with surface antigens of influenza virus, *J. Gen. Virol.* **3**:315.

White, D. O., 1974, Influenza viral proteins: Identification and synthesis, *Curr. Top. Microbiol. Immunol.* **63**:1.

White, D. O., and Cheyne, I. M., 1965, Stimulation of Sendai virus multiplication by puromycin and actinomycin D, *Nature (London)* **208**:813.

Young, R. J., and Content, J., 1971, 5′-Terminus of influenza virus RNA, *Nature (London) New Biol.* **230**:140.

Zhdanov, V. M., 1965, A suggested genetic map of influenza virus, *Lancet,* April 3, p. 738.

Index

Actinomycin D, 223, 507, 564, 565, 567, 568, 570, 573, 576, 578
Adenosine monophosphate, cyclic (AMP), 396
Adenosine triphosphatase, viral, 469
Adenovirus, 27-88, 150
  antibodies, 30
  antigen, soluble, 28, 40
  architecture, 29-30
  assembly, 40-41, 50
  biosynthesis, 34-41
  capsid, 28
    empty, 40
  capsomere, 30
  complementation, 67-68
    group, 49
    index, 49
  discovery, 27
  DNA, viral, 37-38, 65, 67-68
  fiber, 30, 32, 50, 64
  genes, 62-63
  genetics, 27-88
    analysis, 47
    system 47-62
  genome, 27
  helper, 73-74
  hexon, 30, 39, 50, 63, 69-70
  hybrid with SV40, 14-15
  inclusion body, intranuclear, 40
  mapping, 54-62, 76-78
  molecular weight, 31
  mutagens, listed, 29, 42-44
  mutants, 41-47
    assembly, 64-65
    DNA minus, 71, 73, 75
    fiber, 64
    frequency, 43
    genetic constitution, 46-47

Adenovirus (*cont'd*)
  mutants (*cont'd*)
    growth cycle, prior, 43
    hexon, 63
      protein transport, 69-70
    host range, 66-67
    isolation, 29, 44-46
    late, 77
    plaque morphology, 66-67
    temperature-sensitive, 62-65, 72
    types, 41-42
  particle, 31
  penton, 30, 32, 50
  phenotype, 62-67
  protein, 30-32, 69-70
    synthesis, 39-40
  recombination, 54-57, 62, 74-76
  replication, 34-36
  reviews, 28
  subgroups A, B, and C, 33
  transcription, 36-37, 68-69
  transformation, 70-73
Alkylating agents, 215
Alphavirus, 209
α-Amanitin, 36, 344
AMP, *see* Adenosine monophosphate
Antigen
  soluble, 28, 40
  tumor-specific, surface (TSSA), 395
Aphthovirus, 134, 136, 137, 142
  genetic map of, 157-158
Assay, infectious center-, 305
Assembly, 40, 41, 50, 194, 318-322
  coordinate, 549
  viral, 548-550
ATPase, *see* Adenosine triphosphatase
Autointerference, 555

Avian erythroblastosis virus, 360
Avian leukosis virus, 269, 342, 382, 415
  and chicken fibroblast, 374
  host range variant, 372-376
  plaques, 397
Avian myeloblastosis virus, 360, 423
  replication defective, 361
Avian sarcoma virus, 342, 372, 379, 382,
      384, 388
  and chicken fibroblast, 374
  focus formation, 375
  host range variant, 372-376
  mutants
    C (coordinate), 390-398, 401-406, 408
    early, 391-392
    late, 391-392
    R, 390-398, 401-402, 405-407
    T (41°C), 390-398
    temperature-sensitive, 390-392
  replication defective, 354-360
  transformation defective, 362-365
  see Rous sarcoma virus
5-Azacytidine, 215, 246, 285

Baboon, type C virus in, 414
Back mutation rate, 215
Bacteriophage T4, 215
Bromodeoxyuridine, 42, 95, 100, 102

C protein, 226-228, 231
Calicivirus, 136, 137
Cardiovirus, 134, 136, 137
Cat virus RD 114, 351
Cell transformation, see Transformation
Chandipura virus, 239, 240, 242, 245, 253,
      255, 271
Cistron, 135, 146
Cleavage enzyme, 181-182
Cold-adapted variants of influenza virus, 584-585
Complementation, genetic, 47-54, 103-106,
      120-122, 145-147, 218-221, 250-254,
      304-306, 380-383, 411, 503, 504
      509, 515, 563-564
  analysis, 48, 52, 103, 104
  between enteroviruses, 146
  defined, 380
  efficiency, 250
  first evidence, 563
  groups, 49-52, 106, 252-260
  index, 49, 250, 304
  interstrain, 253-254
  intertypic, 120-122
  intracistronic, 8, 218
  method for, 305
  one-sided, 149
  reaction, 103

Complementation, genetic (cont'd)
  symmetrical, 251
  tests, 47, 52-54, 104-106
    filter paper disk, 105
    infectious center formation, 104-105
    mixed morphology plaques, 105
    yield complementation, 104
  without recombination, 563
Coordinate mutant, see Avian sarcoma virus,
      C mutant
Cordycepin, 547
Covariation, 486
Coxsackie virus, 182, 183
  strain A9, 167
Crossing-over, viral, 385-388
  high frequency of, 387
Cytolysis, 468
Cytosine arabinoside, 95

Defective virus, 354-372, see also Particle,
      defective
Deoxycytidine kinase, 95-96
  viral, 119-120
Deoxyribonucleic acid, see DNA
Dextran sulfate, 182
Dimethylsulfate, 485
Dimorphism, genetic
  C variant, 557
  F variant, 557
  and neuraminidase activity, 557
  and particle morphology, 556
  and receptor affinity, 557
DI particle, see Particle, defective-interfering
DNA
  -binding protein, 38, 39
  cellular, 65
    repressed by poliovirus, 164-165
  closed circular, viral, 428
  dimeric circle model, 425
  G + C content, 107
  infectious, 118-119
    size of, 348
  mitochondrial, 397
  phenotype, 107
  probe, (cDNA$_{sarc}$), 417
  provirus, 344
  replication, viral, 37-39, 67-68
  restriction enzyme, 418, 429
  -RNA hybridization, 37, 348, 349
  supercoiled, 428
  synthesis shut-off by host cell, 109
  viral, 32-34, 65, 107-108
DNA polymerase
  -RNA dependent, 343, 345, 353, 404, 469,
      520
  viral, 108, 109, 402-405, 410

Drosophila, 243, 278-280
  virus of, 239, *see also* Sigma virus

Eastern equine encephalitis virus, 214, 217,
      226, 233
EMC virus, 173, 175
Encephalitis due to reovirus, 334-335
Encephalomyocarditis virus (EMC virus),
      173, 175
Enterovirus, 136, 137
  strain GDVII (murine poliovirus), 167
Equestron concept, 162, 185-188, 190-193
Escherichia coli
  endonuclease, 33
  phage T4, 142
  restriction enzyme, 3
Esterase, viral, 469
Ethidium bromide, 343
Ethylethane sulfonate, 485
Ethylmethane sulfonate, 246

Factory, viral, 313, 318, 332
Feline sarcoma virus, 365, 367, 372
Fibroblast, avian, 375
Fingerprint pattern of oligonucleotides,
      418-419, 421, 422
5-Fluorouracil, 139, 153, 172, 215, 246, 294,
      485, 506, 508, 512, 561
Focus assay for transformation, 360, 370
Foot-and-mouth disease virus, 134, 249
Fowl plague virus
  strain Markushin and Ghendon, 575-579
    isolation, 575-576
    RNA minus mutant, 576-578
    RNA plus mutant, 579
    temperature-sensitive mutant, 577
  strain Scholtissek, 579-586
    isolation, 579
    RNA minus mutant, 579-581
    RNA plus mutant, 581-582
    temperature-sensitive mutant, 580
Fragment rescue technique, 10
Friend leukemia virus, 370, 371
Fusion, 467-468

Genome, *see* separate viruses
Genotypic mixing, 558-559
Glycoprotein, 353, 373-376, 494, 508
  entry, 343
  F, 479
  HA, 544
  HN, 467
  mutant, 262-263
  NA, 545
  of viral envelope, 374

Growth inhibitors against virus, 182-184
  dextran sulfate, 182
  S-7-(ethyl-2-methylthio-4-methyl-5-
      pyrimidine carboxylate), 184
  guanidine hydrochloride, 182
  hydantoin, 184
  2-(α-hydroxylbenzyl)benzimidazole, 184
  oxadiazole, 184
Guanidine hydrochloride, 182

Haemophilus aegyptius, 3
H. influenzae, 3
H. parainfluenzae, 3, 34
  endonuclease, 34
Helper virus, 15-18, 73-74, 355, 365, 370-
      371, 389
Hemadsorption, viral, 229-231, 467, 571,
      587
Hemagglutination, viral, 229, 467, 475-476,
      544, 566, 568, 577, 580, 582, 587
Hemolysis, 468
Herpesvirus, 89-131, 150, 269
  "chromosomes" of, 92
  complementation, 103-105
    groups, 106
    intertypic, 120-122
    test, 106
  DNA
    arrangement of molecules, 90-92
    infectious, 118-119
    synthesis, cellular, 109
      viral, 107-108
  dog kidney cells, 94
  enzyme, virus-specified, 108-109
  genes of, 117
  genetics, 89-131
  genome, 89
    effective, 115-116
  latency, 124-125
  linkage map, 114-115
  marker rescue, 118-119
  mutagenization, 100
  mutants, 97-113
    conditional lethal, 96-97
    host range, 94
    leakiness, 98-99
    plaque morphology, 94, 117-122
    resistant to
      bromodeoxyuridine, 95-96
      cytosine arabinoside, 95-96
      phosphonoacetic acid, 95
      toxic compounds, 95
    reversion, 99-100
    specialized, 93-96
      defined, 93
    temperature-sensitive, 97-105

Herpesvirus (*cont'd*)
  mutation, multiple, 100-101
  particles, 112
  phenotypes, 112-113
  plaques of mixed morphology, 117-122
  polypeptides, 109-112
  proteins, 109-112
  recombination, 113-115, 120-122
    analysis, 114, 116-117
  temperature shift experiment, 112
  thymidine kinase, 119-120
  transformation, 122-124
Heterozygote, 425-426, 494-497
  defined, 494
  genomes of, 496
  in influenza virus populations, 558-559
Host-induced modification, 478-480
Host range mutants, 66-69, 94, 211-212,
    372-378
Hydantoin, 184
2-(α-Hydroxybenzyl)benzimidazole, 184
Hydroxylamine, 8, 42, 100, 139, 215, 295,
    485, 561

Infection
  abortive, 2
  carrier state, 471
  lytic, 2
  persistent, 470-471, 515-522
    and interferon, 516
    variants, 516-517
Influenza virus, *see* Orthomyxovirus
Interference
  among poliovirus, 147-150
    with multiplication, 147-148
    without multiplication, 149-150
  defined, 222
  heterologous, 150
  homologous, 147-148, 222
  intrinsic, 470
  and mixed infection, 222
  surface, 470
  see Autointerference
Interferon, 151, 232, 333-334, 516
Iododeoxyuridine, 18

Kirsten murine sarcoma virus, *see* Murine
    sarcoma virus, Kirsten strain

Lactic dehydrogenase virus, 216
Lagos bat virus, 246
Latency, viral, 124-125
Leakiness, 8, 98-99, 216, 487
Lettuce necrotic yellows virus, 239, 240
Leucine aminopeptidase, viral, 469

Leukosis virus, *see* Avian leukosis virus
Leukovirus, *see* Avian leukovirus, Murine
    leukovirus
Lipid metabolism, 165-166
Lymphoid leukemia virus, 370

M-band technique, 38
M protein of influenza virus, 545
Macrophage of chicken, 361
  von Magnus
    effect, 554
      autointerference, 555
    virus, 554-555
Mammalian sarcoma virus, 365-370
  coordinately defective, 365-370
  replication defective, 365-370
  rescued, 368
Mapping of genome, 3, 54-62, 76-78,
    114-115, 152-168, 173, 266-268,
    418-423, 429
  biochemical, 59
  correlations, 60-62
  genetic, 54-58, 418, 421, 423
  physical, 58-60, 266-268
  recombinant, 420-421
Marker rescue technique, 118-119, 139, 543
Masking, genomic, *see* Transcapsidation
Measles virus, 493, 499, 519
  hydrocephalus due to, 522
  mutants, 510
  noninfectious particle, 517
  RNA group, 514
  temperature-sensitive mutant, 508-513
Membrane, 165-166
  protein M, 573
Meningovirus, 167, 173, 175, 182
N-Methyl-N'-nitro-N-nitrosoguanidine, 246
Microtubule, cellular, 322-333
Missense substitution, 97
Mitomycin C, 372
Mixing
  genetic, *see* Genotypic mixing
  phenotypic, *see* Phenotypic mixing
Modification
  host-controlled, 166-168, 271-272
  host-induced, 478-480
Mokola virus, 240, 246
Moloney murine leukemia virus (MuLV),
    see Murine sarcoma virus
Monkey kidney cell, 538
Mouse
  Fv-1 locus, 376-378
  Fv-1 restriction, 377, 378
  see Murine
MSV, *see* Murine sarcoma virus

Multiple sclerosis, 470
Multiplicity reactivation, 307-308, 497-499, 542
  defined, 498
Multiploid particle, 494-497
MuLV, *see* Murine sarcoma virus, Moloney strain
Mumps virus, 499
Murine leukemia virus (MLV), 342, 385
  Abelson strain, 371
  complementation, 411
  focal transformation, 371
  helper-dependent, 370-371
  host range
    amphotropic, 378
    N-tropic, 378
    xenotropic, 378, 380
  mutant
    early, 408-409
    late, 408-409
  postpenetration, early, 376-378
  recombination, 411
  replication defective, 370-371
  transformation, 411
    focal, 371
Murine leukovirus, 269
Murine poliovirus, 167
Murine sarcoma virus, 377
  mutant
    cold-sensitive, 412-413
    temperature-defective, 372
  strain
    Harvey, 365
    Kirsten, 347, 365, 412
    Moloney, 346, 347, 365, 370
Murine type C virus, ectotropic, 372-373
Mutagen, 8, 484-486
  base analogue, incorporated, 484
  changing nucleotide base, 484
  listed, 246, 485, 561
Mutagenization, 100
Mutants
  defective, 13
  definition, 482
  deletion, 13
  enrichment technique, 44
  insertion, 14
  temperature-sensitive, 11-12
  see separate viruses
Mutation
  conditional, 407-408
  multiple, 405, 406, 487
  single point, 486
  see separate viruses
Myotube, degeneration of, 397

Myxovirus, 535, *see also* Orthomyxovirus

Neuraminidase, viral, 467, 475, 487, 545, 557, 562, 566, 568, 571, 577, 580, 581, 587
  bacterial, 569
Neurotropism, viral, 274-277
Newcastle disease virus, 150, 306, 480
  budding through the plasma membrane, 477
  in cell culture, 477, 478
  cloning, 473
  complementation groups, 515
  DNA polymerase, RNA-dependent, 520
  hemagglutinin, 475-476
  Herts strain, 477, 478, 518
  mutants, 505
  noninfectious particle, 501
  particle size, 475-478
  polypeptide, 466
  repository at the University of Wisconsin, 472
  RNA
    defective, 519
    -dependent DNA polymerase, 520
    groups, 514
    temperature-sensitive mutant, 503-506
    ultraviolet, inactivation by, 495, 497-499
  virulence, 472
Nitrosoguanidine, 8, 42, 100, 102, 139, 153, 485, 506, 508, 561
Nitrosomethylurea, 561
Nitrous acid, 8, 42, 100, 102, 139, 153, 246, 294, 296, 485, 505-506
Nonsense codon mutation, 96
Nucleic acid
  homology, 414
  see DNA, RNA
Nucleocapsid protein of influenza virus, 545
Nucleoprotein mutant, 263

Oligonucleotide, 322-324
  fingerprinting, 348
Oligopolymerase, 323
Oncoviridae, 342
Oncornavirus, 270-271
Orthomyxovirus
  assembly, 548-550
  clone X-3311 – Ueda *et al.*, 582-583
  complementation, 563-564
  dimorphism, genetic, 556-557
  gene product, 543-548
  genetics, 535-598
  genome, 540-543
    chemical nature of, 540-541

Orthomyxovirus (*cont'd*)
 genome (*cont'd*)
  molecular biology of, 540-552
  segmented, 541-543
  size, 540-541
 genotypic mixing, 558-559
 history, 537-539
 influenza virus, 306, 385, *see also* Orthomyxovirus in general
 interaction, genetic, 559-564
 interference, 554-556
  unidirectional, 555-556
 mixing, genotypic, 558-559
 mixing, phenotypic, 557-558
 mutant phenotype, 564-567
 plaque-forming particles, 552-554
 phenotypic mixing, 557-558
 polypeptide, 543-546
 population, 552-559
 protein product, 543-546
 recombinant, temperature-sensitive, 585-
  587
 recombination, 559-563
 and reovirus, 536
 replication, 550-552
 research, milestones of, 537-539
 reviews on, 536, 539
 RNA, 540-552
  messenger, 546-548
  phenotype, 564-566
  plus mutant, 566-567, 569-570
 strain
  Mackenzie, 570-572
  Simpson and Hirst, 572-575
  Sugiura, 567-570
   isolation, 567
   RNA minus mutant, 567-569
   temperature-sensitive mutant, 568
 temperature-sensitive mutant, 559-586
  discovered, 539
  listed, 561
 variant, cold-adapted, 584-585
Oxadiazole, 184

Pactamycin, 172, 173
 maps of gene product, 173
Panencephalitis, subacute sclerosing, 470
Paramyxovirus
 attachment, 460
 cell-associated (CAV), 477-478
  a valuable tool in evaluating infection,
   478
 cytolysis, 468
 defectiveness, 470
  in mutant, 483
  in virus, 499-501

Paramyxovirus (*cont'd*)
 description of virion, 460
 enzymes, viral, 469-470
 fusion, 467-468
 genetics, 457-533
  analysis, 459-472
 hemadsorption, 467
 hemagglutination, 467
 hemagglutinin, 475-476, 509
 hemolysis, 468
 heterozygote, 494-497
 and host cell, 461
 incomplete virus, 499-501
 infection, 460-461
 infectivity, 476-477
 interference, 470
 multiplicity reactivation, 497-499
 multiploid particle, 497-499
 mutants, 482-492
  defective, 483
  induced, 483-484
  plaque size, 489-490
  plaque type, 489
  red plaque, 490-491
  spontaneous, 483-484
  turbid plaque, 491-492
 neuraminidase, viral, 467
 particle, noninfectious, 476-477
 penetration, 460
 persistent infection, 515-522
 phenotypic mixing, 493-494
 plaque-forming ability, 476-477, *see also*
  mutants above
 poly(A)-adding activity, 468
 population, 472-483
  adaptation, 473-474
  selection, 473-474
  stocks in eggs, 474-475
 production of virion, 460-461
 protein, viral, 461-462
 recombination, 492-493
 RNA, 480
  intracellular, 463-464
  synthesis, 468-469
  viral, 462-465
 serotype, 480-481
 strains, 481-482
  definition, 481
  temperature-sensitive mutant, 501-515
  complementation groups, 503, 504,
   509
  complementation index, 509
  input virus, 502
  multiplicity of infection, 501
  temperature, 502
 transcriptase, 464, 468

Paramyxovirus (*cont'd*)
  transcription, 464-465
    primary, 465
    secondary, 465
  vaccine, 522
  variant, 482
  virion
    description, 460
    production, 460-461
    structure, 460-461
  virulence, 471-472, *see also* Measles virus,
      Mumps virus, Newcastle disease virus,
      Parainfluenza virus, Rinderpest
Particle
  aggregation, 552
  defective, 538, 554
    interfering(DI), 148-149
  morphology, 556
  noninfectious hemagglutinating, 554
  nonplaque-forming, 552-554
  plaque-forming, 552-554
Persistent infection, 272-278
Phagocytosis, 35
Phenotypic mixing, 147, 216-217, 268-271,
      380-383, 493-494, 557-558,
  among unrelated virions, 382-383
  classical case, 381
  discovered, 493
Phosphonoacetic acid, 95
Picornaviridae, 134
Picornavirus
  assembly, 194
  classification, 136-138
    genera, 137
  cleavage
    enzymes, 181-182
    pathways, 173-175
  complementation, genetic, 145-147
  definition, 134
  gene
    function, 151, 168
    product, 169-182
  genetic maps, 152-168
    of aphthovirus, 157
    of poliovirus, 152-155
  genetic methods, 138-140
    covariant reversion, 139-140
    marker, 139
    mutant isolation, 139
    temperature shift experiment, 140
  genetics, 133-207
  genome, 141-152
    expression, 188-190
    interactions, 141-152
    strategy, 184-195
  growth inhibitor, 182-184

Picornavirus (*cont'd*)
  growth process, 190-192
  infection, establishment of, 192-193
  interference
    heterologous, 150
    with multiplication, 147-148
    without multiplication, 149-150
  interferon, 151
  late effects, 194-195
  map, genetic, 152-168
  method, genetic, 138-140
  multiplication, interference with, 147-
      148
  5'-3'-orientation, 172-173
  particle, defective interfering, 148-149
  phenotypic mixing, 147
  polysome, predominance of, 193
  properties, 134
    capsid, 134
    capsomere, 134
    RNA, 134
  protein, structural, 169-170
  reactivation, genetic, 147
  recombination
    genetic, 141-145
    map, 152-157
      of poliovirus, 152-155
  regulation
    mechanism, 184-188
    start of, 193
  RNA
    cistron concept, 176-181
    strand completion, 193-194
    translation unit, 176-181
  schizon, 135
  temperature-sensitive mutant, 156-157
  translation, *in vitro*, 175-176
Pig, type C virus, 414
Piry virus, 242
Plaque
  assay, 537
  -forming particles, 552-554
  morphology
    mixed, 117-122
    mutant, 66-67, 94, 117-122, 211, 397,
        489-492
  mutant, 489
  red, 490-491
  screening, 44-45
  size, 489-490
  turbid, 491-492
Plasma membrane, 395
Point mutation, 483
Poliovirus, 134, 249
  cytology changes, late, 163-164
  DNA synthesis, repression of, 164-165

Poliovirus (*cont'd*)
  gene function
    primary, 157-161
    secondary, 161-162
  genome
    RNA, 189, 192
    strategy, 136
  growth, 190-192
  map, 152-153
    properties of, 153-154
      asymmetrical covariation, 153
      linear, 153
      three genes, 154
  maturation factor, 165
  membrane and lipid metabolism, 165-166
  modification, host-controlled, 166-168
  mutant, temperature-sensitive, 152, 154,
      156-157, 160
  protein, structural, 156
  replicase, half-life, 148
  repression
    early metabolic, 162-163
    of host DNA, 163-165
    of host protein synthesis, 162-163
    of host RNA, 163
  RNA
    c, 193-194
    double-stranded is cytotoxic, 164
    molecular weight, 155
    temperature-sensitive mutant, 152, 154,
      156-157, 160
  translation, 172-173
  virulence, 166
Polymerase mutant, 257-262
Polyoma virus
  defective mutant, 13-14
  DNA
    cellular, 15-16
    replication, 4-5
  fragment rescue technique, 10
  genetics, 1-26
  genome
    early region, 15-18
    map, 3
  host range mutant, 12-13
  lytic growth cycle, 4-8
  mutants, 2, 8-15
  proteins, 6-8
  T antigen, 17
  temperature-sensitive mutant, 11-12
  transcription, 5-6
Polypeptide, viral, 109-112, 546
Polysome, predominance, 193
Potato yellow dwarf virus, 240, 241
  RNA, molecular weight, 242

Precipitation, immunological technique, 314,
    315
Proflavine, 246, 296, 485
Protease
  activation mutant, 488
  excretion, 395
Protein
  G, 262
  large external transformation specific
      (LETS), 396
  M, 263, 545
  N, 263
  P, 545
  of plasma membrane, 395
Protein kinase, viral, 469
Provirus, 344, 349
Pseudorabies virus, 102
Pseudotype, 268-271, 368, 381, 383, 409,
    493

Rabies virus, 239, 245
  pathogenesis in the mouse, 277-278
  RNA, molecular weight, 242
Random reassortment hypothesis, 550
Rat, type C virus, 416
RDE, *see* Receptor-destroying enzyme
Reactivation, genetic, 147
Reassortment, genetic, 298, 299, 301, *see
    also* Recombination
Receptor
  affinity, 557
  -destroying enzyme(RDE), 562
Recombinant, 303-304
  formula, 296
  frequency, 297
Recombination, 54-57, 62, 74-76, 113-117,
      120-122, 141-145, 383-389, 400-
      401, 411, 423-426, 492-493, 559-563
  analysis of herpesvirus, 114
    validity of, 116-117
  artifacts, 143-144
  assumptions of, 116
  between RNA tumor viruses, 383-389
  circular, 424
  crossing-over, viral, 385-388
  defective, 388-389
  discovered, 113, 537
  endonuclease technique, 77
  frequency, 57, 297, 307, 537, 538
  genetic, 54, 93, 120-122, 141, 217, 249-
      250, 296-301, 369, 492-493, 559-
      563
  heterotypic, 61
  linear, 424
  mechanism, 144-145

Recombination (*cont'd*)
  model for, 423
  occurrence, 141-142
  properties, 141
  reciprocity, 142
  test, 55
  for vaccine, 538
  variability, 560
Reovirus, 385
  as the most novel animal viral genetic sys-
      tem, 294
  assembly, 318-322
  capsid, 322
    double-shelled, 291, 319
    empty, 321
  complementation, 304-306
  crosses
    three-factor, 301-304, 330-331
    two-factor, 295-301
  cytopathic effect, 331-332
  Dearing strain, 295
  defective particle, 308-309
  deletion mutant, 308-309, 329-330
  and disease, 334-336
    encephalitis, lethal in rat, 334-335
  gene
    function, 309-331
    lesion, 324
  genetics, 291-340
  genome, 291
  host, effect on, 331-336
  interaction, genetic, 294-309
  interferon, 333-334
  microtubule, 332-333
  multiplication cycle, 293
  multiplicity reactivation, 307-308
  mutant
    conditional lethal, 294-295
    temperature-sensitive, 294-296
  oligonucleotide, 322-324
  particle
    aberrant, 329
    defective, 308-309
  phenotype, 309-310
  plaques, 306
  polypeptide, viral, 325-329
    synthesis, 314, 315, 318
  recombinant formula, 296
  replication, 291-294, 312-313
  RNA
    double-stranded, 292
    early, 312
    hybrid, 324-325
    late, 312
    synthesis, 312-313, 316-317

Reovirus (*cont'd*)
  structure, 291-294
  transcription, 310-312
  translation, 314-318
  temperature-sensitive mutant, 309, 310
Replica plating, 139
Replicase, 159, 162, 165, 168, 170-172, 190,
      240, 309
  polypeptides of, 170-172
  proteins, 170-172
  see also RNA polymerase, RNA-dependent
Replication, viral, 34-39, 67-68, 209-211,
      291-294, 312-313, 550-552
  defective, 354-372
Restriction endonuclease
  bacterial, 33, 34
  for recombinant analysis, 62
Restriction enzyme
  bacterial, 3
  and genome map, 3
  mapping, 429
Reticuloendothelial virus, 382, 415
Retroviridae, 342
Reversion, 99-100
  covariant, 139-140
  defined, 99
Rhabdovirus
  biosynthesis, 261
  cell-killing, 278
  complementation, 250-254
    group, 254-260
    interstrain, 253-254
    temperature-sensitive, 252-253
  defectiveness, 265-268
    in particles, 517
  features, biological, 239-241
  genetics, 239-289
  genome, 517
    coding capacity, 241-242
    mapping, physical, 266-268
  glycoprotein mutant, 263
  host, 239
    -controlled modification, 271-272
  infection, persistent, 272-278
  matrix protein, mutant, 263
  modification, host-controlled, 271-272
  mutants
    glycoprotein, 262-263
    induced, 246-247
    isolation technique for, 247-248
    listed, 244-245
    matrix protein, 263
    nucleoprotein, 263
    phenotype, 242-243
    polymerase, 257-262

Rhabdovirus (*cont'd*)
  mutants (*cont'd*)
    RNA minus, 254, 255
    RNA plus, 254, 255
    spontaneous, 243-246
    temperature-sensitive, 243-248, 252-264, 274-278
    thermolabile, 248-249
  neurotropism, 274-277
  nucleoprotein mutant, 263
  particle
    defective, 517
    T, 264-266, 272-274
  phenotype, 254-257
    mutant, 242-243
  phenotypic mixing, 268-271
  polymerase mutant, 257-262
  pseudotype, 268-271
  recombination is absent, 249-250
  RNA
    molecular weight, 241
    mutants, 254-255
  T particle, 264-266, 272-274
  temperature-sensitive mutant, 243-246
  thermolabile mutant, 248-249
  transcription, 260
  virulence, 277-278
Rhinovirus, 134, 136, 137, 173
Ribonucleic acid, *see* RNA
Ribonucleoprotein complex of
  fowl plague virus, 577, 580
  influenza virus, 575
Rifampin, 243
RNA
  cellular, 345-346
  -DNA hybridization, 37, 348, 349
  factories, 171
  fingerprint pattern, 418
  messenger, 546-548
  molecular weight, 346, 350
  mutants, minus, 567-569, 576-581
    plus, 566-567, 569-570, 579, 581-582
  phenotype, 564-566
  polymerase, *see* RNA polymerase
  -RNA hybridization, 547
  sarcoma virus, 344
  spreading technique for, 350
  synthesis, virus-specific, 565-566
  viral, 345-346, *see also* RNA tumor viruses
RNA polymerase, 171, 225, 565, 574
  II, 36, 344, 360
  RNA dependent, *see* Replicase
RNA tumor viruses, 306
  complementation, 380-383
  crossing-over, 385-388

RNA tumor viruses (*cont'd*)
  defective, 354-372
    in infectious progeny, 360-362
    pol defective, 358-360
    replication defective, 354-358, 365-371
    transformation defective, 362-365
  description, 342
  DNA polymerase, viral, 402-405
  DNA restriction enzyme, 429
  genetics, 341-455
    biochemical, 413-423
  genome
    diploid, 348-349
    model, 352
    properties, 345-353
  glycoprotein, 373-376
  host, 413-416
  infection by, 342-345
  interaction between, 380-389
    virus-cell genomes, 428-429
  map, genetic, 418-423
  markers for transformation, 353-380, 400-401
  mixing, phenotypic, 380-383
  mutants
    class C, 401-402, 405-406
    class R, 401-402, 405
    class T, 392-401
    conditional, 389-413
    deletion, 354-356, 381, 388-389
    host range, 372-378
    nonconditional, 353-380
    temperature-sensitive, 390-398, 406-413
  phenotypic mixing, 380, 383
  recombination, 383-389, 400-401, 423-426
  RNA, viral, 345-346
    35S, 346-350
    60-70S, 346, 350-352
    60-70S an inverted dimer, 350-352
    cellular in virus, 345-346
    molecular weight, 346
  species of virus, 413-416
  src
    product, 426-427
    region, 362-365, 416-418
  transformation
    gene, 411-413
    protein, 398-399
    markers, 353-380, 400-401
Rous sarcoma virus, 346
  envelope defective, 358-360
  polymerase defective, 358-360
  strains
    Bryan high titer, 354
    Schmidt-Ruppin, 354, 362

Salmonella typhimurium phage P*22,* 40
Sarcoma virus, *see* Avian, Feline, Mammalian,
     RNA, Rous, Simian
Sarkosyl technique, 38
Schizomer, 134, 169-170, 174, 181
Schizon, defined, 134
Sclerosis, multiple, *see* Multiple sclerosis
Semliki forest virus, 209, 210, 212, 214,
     224-227, 229, 231, 234
Sendai virus, 367, 470, 479, 480, 499, 500, 519
  hemagglutinin, 476
  polymerase polypeptide, 513
  polypeptide NP, 464
  protease activation, 488
    mutant, 522
  RNA
    18S, 463, 464
    22S, 463
    35S, 465
    50S, 463
    groups, 514
    temperature-sensitive, 506-508
    transcription, 469
Sigma virus, 239, 240, 245, 250, 278-280
  in *Drosophila,* 239
  and germinal transmission, 278-280
  Rho strains, 279
Simian virus *5,* 499
Simian virus *40*
  -adenovirus hybrid, 14-15
  defective mutant, 13-14
  DNA
    cellular, 15-16
    replication, 4-5
  fragment rescue technique, 10
  genetics, 1-26
  genome
    early region, 15-18
    mpa, 3
  helper function, 15-18
  lytic growth cycle, 4-8
  mutants, 2, 8-15
  proteins, 6-8
  T antigen, 17
  temperature-sensitive mutant, 11-12
  transcription, 5-6
Simian sarcoma virus, 365, 367, 368
  defective, 368
Sindbis virus, 212, 214, 217, 219-221,
    223, 225, 227, 230-233
Slow virus diseases, 275, 277
Spot test, 139
Spreading technique for RNA, 350
src gene of avian sarcoma virus, 416-418
  product, 426-427

Substitution, 97, 98
Syncytia, 94

T antigen, 4, 17
T mutants, 398-401
  of avian sarcoma viruses
    colony formation in agar, 394
    focus formation in fibroblast, 394
    high-density growth cell culture, 394
    protease excretion, 395
    tumor-specific surface antigen, 395
  recombination, 400-401
  transformation, cooperative, 400-401
T particle, 251, 254, 264-268
  and virulence, 272-274
Temperature-sensitive mutant, 11-12, 62-65,
    72, 97-105, 152-157, 160, 214-216,
    223-233, 243-248, 252-264, 274-
    278, 294-296, 309-310, 372, 390-
    398, 406-413, 501-515, 559-587
Temperature sensitivity, 518-520
Temperature shift experiment, 140
Thymidine kinase, 95-96
  viral, 119-120
Togavirus, 210
  back mutation rate, 215
  and cellular synthesis, 231-232
  complementation, 218-221
  envelope protein, defective, 229-231
  genetics, 209-238
  genome, 210
  interference, 222
  leakiness, 216
  mixing, phenotypic, 216-217
  mutants, 211-216
    defective-interfering, 213-214
    heat-resistant, 212
    host range, 211-212
    in mixed infections, 216-222
    morphology altered, 213
    plaque morphology, 211
    size altered, 213
    temperature-sensitive, 214-216, 223-233
    virulence reduced, 213
  nucleocapsid assembly defective, 226-229
  phenotypic mixing, 216-217
  recombination, 217
  replication, 209-211
  RNA, 210
    mutant, minus, 219, 220, 223, 224, 228
    plus, 219, 221, 223
    synthesis altered, 223-226
    structure, 209-211
    temperature-sensitive mutant
      physiological defect, 223-233

Togavirus (*cont'd*)
  temperature-sensitive mutant (*cont'd*)
    RNA synthesis defective, 223-226
    virulence, 232-233
  virion
    abnormal, 213
    defective, 213-214
    description, 209
  virulence of *ts* mutant, 232-233
Transcapsidation, 147
Transcription, 5-6, 36-37, 67-69, 310-312,
    574, 578, 580
  primary, 240
  viral, 257, 259, 464
Transfer RNA nucleotidyltransferase, 469
Transformation, 18-22, 70-73, 122-124, 353-
    380, 398-401, 411-413
  of cell, 1, 2
  cooperative, 400-401
  of defective virus, 362-365
  focus assay for, 360
  gene, 411-413
  of hamster embryo cell, 122-124
  marker, 378-380
  neoplastic, 18
  protein, 426-427
  viral, 18-22, 353
Translation, 175-181, 314-318
  two-cistron concept of, 176-181
Transmission, germinal
  and sigma virus, 278-280

TSSA, *see* Antigen
Type C virus, *see* RNA tumor viruses, Rat

Ultraviolet irradiation, 42, 102, 246
Uridine incorporation, 571, 577

Vaccine, viral, 277
Venezuelan equine encephalitis virus, 213,
    229
Vesicular stomatitis virus(VSV), 150, 239,
    240, 271, 306, 383
  glycoprotein, 272
  pseudotype, 377
  strains
    C, 242
    Cocal, 242, 244, 253-256
    Indiana, 244, 252-261
    M, 242
    New Jersey, 244, 253-256
  virulence, 276
Vibrio cholerae neuraminidase, 569
Virulence, 166, 232-233, 272-278, 471-472,
    517
Virus, *see* separate viruses
VSV, *see* Vesicular stomatitis virus

Western equine encephalitis virus, 214, 217,
    225, 232
WSN, *see* Orthomyxovirus under influenza
    virus strains